Bone Disease of Organ Transplantation

Bone Disease of Organ Transplantation

Edited by
Juliet Compston, M.D.
University of Cambridge School of Medicine

Elizabeth Shane, M.D.
Columbia University College of Physicians and Surgeons

ELSEVIER
ACADEMIC
PRESS

AMSTERDAM • BOSTON • HEIDELBERG • LONDON • NEW YORK
OXFORD PARIS • SAN DIEGO • SAN FRANCISCO
SINGAPORE • SYDNEY • TOKYO

Elsevier Academic Press
30 Corporate Drive, Suite 400, Burlington, MA 01803, USA
525 B Street, Suite 1900, San Diego, California 92101-4495, USA
84 Theobald's Road, London WC1X 8RR, UK

This book is printed on acid-free paper.

Library of Congress Cataloging-in-Publication Data

Bone disease of organ transplantation / edited by Juliet Compston and Elizabeth Shane.
p. ; cm.
Includes bibliographical references and index.
ISBN 0-12-183502-2 (alk. paper)
1. Bones–Diseases. 2. Osteoporosis. 3. Transplantation of organs, tissues, etc.–Complications.
[DNLM: 1. Bone Diseases–etiology. 2. Organ Transplantation–adverse effects. WE 225 B71258 2005] I. Compston, Juliet. II. Shane, Elizabeth, MD.
RC930.B663 2005
616.7′1–dc22 2004015214

British Library Cataloging in Publication Data
A catalogue record for this book is available from the British Library

For all information on all Elsevier Academic Press publications visit our Web site at www.books.elsevier.com

Printed in the United States of America

04 05 06 07 08 09 9 8 7 6 5 4 3 2 1

Contents

PART II

Pathogenesis of Transplantation-Related Bone Disease

PART III

Clinical Features of Transplantation Bone Disease

PART IV

Management

Preface

Bone disease, particularly osteoporosis, has emerged as a common and serious complication of solid organ transplantation. In recent years there have been real advances in our understanding of the pathogenesis and pathophysiology of bone loss but treatment studies have been relatively sparse and successful strategies to reduce skeletal morbidity after transplantation remain to be clearly established. This partly reflects the difficulties associated with studies of these patients, who are highly heterogeneous in terms of their clinical profile, pre-existing bone disease, and the immunosuppressive regimens used. In addition, appropriate recognition of the significant morbidity attributable to post-transplantation bone disease has until recently been lacking, as witnessed by its absence from many textbooks on bone disease.

Bone Disease of Organ Transplantation offers for the first time a comprehensive review of scientific and clinical aspects of bone disease in transplant recipients. The role of glucocorticoids and other immunosuppressive drugs is discussed in detail and there is a chapter devoted to the neglected but important area of interactions between bone and the immune system. Bone biology and mineral metabolism are reviewed and our current state of knowledge about the pathogenesis and pathophysiology of this bone disease is covered in some detail. Different types of transplantation are discussed separately, since both pre-existing and postoperative bone disease may differ according to the organ transplanted. Not only are the more common transplants covered (kidney, liver, heart, and lung), but the reader will also find reviews of bone disease occurring after kidney–pancreas and pancreas transplantation and bone marrow transplantation. There is also a chapter on the effects of transplantation during childhood and adolescence, a topic that has previously received little coverage. Finally, the management of transplantation bone disease is discussed in detail, with respect both to optimization of skeletal health prior to and prevention and treatment of bone loss after transplantation.

Whatever the future holds, the management of transplantation bone disease currently provides a difficult challenge for physicians and surgeons. With increasing use of organ transplantation and improvements in life expectancy, the prevention of skeletal morbidity is an important priority. This book provides a unique resource for the many health professionals involved with transplantation bone disease, both in terms of its scientific background and in the management of the disease in clinical practice.

Juliet Compston, M.D.
Elizabeth Shane, M.D.

Contributors

Robert M. Aris, Associate Professor of Medicine, Division of Pulmonary and Critical Care Medicine, School of Medicine CB #7020, 4131 Bioinformatics, University of North Carolina, Chapel Hill, NC 27599-7524

Helen Baron, Department of Medicine, Columbia University College of Physicians and Surgeons, New York Presbyterian Hospital-Milstein Hospital Building, 177 Ft. Washington Avenue, 5th floor–Room 5-407, New York, NY 10032

John P. Bilezikian, Professor of Medicine and of Pharmacology, Chief, Division of Endocrinology, Department of Medicine, Columbia University College of Physicians and Surgeons, 630 West 168th Street (PH 8W–Rm. 864), New York, NY 10032

Ernesto Canalis, Director, Department of Research, Saint Francis Hospital and Medical Center, 114 Woodland Street, Hartford, Connecticut 06105-1299, Professor, Department of Medicine, The University of Connecticut School of Medicine, Farmington, CT 06030

Bart L. Clarke, Assistant Professor of Medicine, Chair, Division of Metabolic Bone Disease, Division of Endocrinology, Metabolism, Diabetes, and Nutrition, Mayo Clinic W18-A, 200 1st Street S.W., Rochester, MN 55905

Adi Cohen, Department of Medicine, Duke University and Durham Veterans Affairs Medical Center, Durham, NC

Juliet Compston, Box 157, Department of Medicine, Addenbrooke's Hospital, Cambridge, CB2 2QQ UK

Annie M. Cooper, Metabolic Bone Centre, Northern General Hospital, Herries Road, Sheffield, South Yorkshire, S5 7AU UK

John Cunningham, Professor of Nephrology, University College London and University College London Hospitals, The Middlesex Hospital, Mortimer Street, London, W1T 3AA UK

Mario C. Deng, ISHLT MCSD Database Medical Director, Director of Cardiac Transplantation Research, Columbia University, Department of Medicine, Division of Cardiology, 622 West 168th Street, PH 12 Room 1291, New York, NY 10032

Richard Eastell, Professor of Bone Metabolism, Research Dean for the Medical School, R&D Director for the Sheffield Teaching Hospital Trust, University of Sheffield Clinical Sciences Centre, Northern General Hospital, Herries Road, Sheffield, South Yorkshire, S5 7AU UK

Peter R. Ebeling, Departments of Diabetes and Endocrinology and Medicine, The Royal Melbourne Hospital, Parkville, Victoria 3050, Australia

Solomon Epstein, Professor of Medicine and Geriatrics, Mount Sinai Bone Program, Department of Medicine, Division of Endocrinology (1055), Mount Sinai School of Medicine, Bronx VA Medical Center, One Gustave L. Levy Place, New York NY 10029

S.L.-S. Fan, Department of Nephrology and Transplantation, The Royal London Hospital, Whitechapel, London, E1 1BB UK

Nuria Guañabens, Metabolic Bone Diseases Unit, Department of Rheumatology, Hospital Clínic, Villarroel 170, 08036 Barcelona, Spain

Neveen A.T. Hamdy, Department of Endocrinology and Metabolic Diseases, Leiden University Medical Center, Albinusdreef 2 2333 ZA Leiden, The Netherlands

Angela M. Inzerillo, Mount Sinai Bone Program, Department of Medicine, Division of Endocrinology (1055), Mount Sinai School of Medicine, Bronx VA Medical Center, One Gustave L. Levy Place, New York NY 10029

Silviu Itescu, Departments of Medicine, Surgery, and Pathology, Columbia University College of Physicians and Surgeons, New York Presbyterian Hospital–Milstein Hospital Building, 177 Ft. Washinton Avenue, 5th floor–Room 5-407, New York, NY 10032

Ranjit John, Department of Surgery, University of Minnesota, Minneapolis, MN 55455

Craig B. Langman, Isaac A. Abt, MD Professor of Kidney Diseases, Feinberg School of Medicine, Northwestern University, Head, Division of Kidney Diseases, Children's Memorial Medical Center, 2300 Childrens Plaza, MD #37, Chicago IL 60614

Gudrun Leidig-Bruckner, Department of Nuclear Medicine, Klinikum Ludwigshafen, Bremserstr. 79, 67063 Ludwigshafen, Germany

Mary B. Leonard, Assistant Professor of Pediatrics and Epidemiology, Department of Pediatrics, Children's Hospital of Philadelphia, Department of Biostatistics and Epidemiology, University of Pennsylvania, CHOP North Room 1564, 34th Street and Civic Center Blvd., Philadelphia, PA 19104

Hartmut H. Malluche, University of Kentucky Medical Center, Division of Nephrology, 800 Rose Street, Rm MN564, Lexington, KY 40536-0298

Ana Monegal, Metabolic Bone Diseases Unit, Department of Rheumatology, Hospital Clínic, Villarroel 170, 08036 Barcelona, Spain

Marie-Claude Monier-Faugere, University of Kentucky Medical Center, Division of Nephrology, 800 Rose Street, Room MN564, Lexington, KY 40536-0298

Kim E. Naylor, Bone Metabolism Group, Division of Clinical Sciences (North), University of Sheffield, University of Sheffield Clinical Sciences Centre, Northern General Hospital, Herries Road, Sheffield, South Yorkshire, S5 7AU UK

David A. Ontjes, Professor of Medicine and Pharmacology, Division of Endocrinology, 257 MacNider, CB #7527, University of North Carolina School of Medicine, Chapel Hill, NC 27599-7527

Susan M. Ott, Associate Professor, Medicine, Division of Metabolism, 1959 NE Pacific Street, Room BB545, University of Washington, Box 356426, Seattle, WA 98195-6426

Roberto Pacifici, Herndon Professor of Medicine, Director, Division of Endocrinology, Metabolism and Lipids, Emory University School of Medicine, 101 Woodruff Circle, WMRB, Room 1301, Atlanta, GA 30322

Lawrence G. Raisz, Board of Trustees Distinguished Professor of Medicine, Director, UConn Center for Osteoporosis, University of Connecticut Health Center, 263 Farmington Ave., MC-3805, Farmington, CT 06030

Ian R. Reid, Department of Medicine, University of Auckland, Private Bag 92019, Auckland, New Zealand

Mishaela R. Rubin, Instructor in Clinical Medicine, Columbia University College of Physicians and Surgeons, 630 West 168th Street (PH 8W – Rm. 864), New York, NY 10032

Philip Sambrook, Professor of Rheumatology, University of Sydney, Institute of Bone and Joint Research, Level 4, Block 4, Royal North Shore Hospital, St Leonards, Sydney 2065, Australia

Adina E. Schneider, Mount Sinai Bone Program, Department of Medicine, Division of Endocrinology (1055), Mount Sinai School of Medicine, Bronx VA Medical Center, One Gustave L. Levy Place, New York NY 10029

Elizabeth Shane, Professor of Clinical Medicine, Columbia University College of Physicians and Surgeons, Department of Medicine, PH8-864, 630 West 168th Street, New York, NY 10032

Nicole Suciu-Foca, Departments of Medicine, Surgery, and Pathology, Columbia University College of Physicians and Surgeons, New York Presbyterian Hospital–Milstein Hospital Building, 177 Ft. Washinton Avenue, 5th floor–Room 5-407, New York, NY 10032

Stuart M. Sprague, Chief, Division of Nephrology and Hypertension, Professor of Medicine, Northwestern University Feinberg School of Medicine, Evanston Northwestern Healthcare, 2650 North Ridge Avenue, Evanston, IL 60201

Emily Stein, Columbia University College of Physicians and Surgeons, Department of Medicine, PH8-864, 630 West 168th Street, New York, NY 10032

Hans-Ulrich Stempfle, Department of Cardiology, Medizinische Poliklinik—Innenstadt, Ludwig–Maximilians–University Munich, Ziemssenstrasse 1, 80336 Munich, Germany

M. Neale Weitzmann, Division of Endocrinology, Metabolism and Lipids, Emory University School of Medicine, 101 Woodruff Circle, WMRB, Room 1301, Atlanta, GA 30322

Mone Zaidi, Professor of Medicine, Geriatrics and Physiology, Director, Mount Sinai Bone Program, Chief, Division of Endocrinology (VA), 1055, Endocrinology, Mount Sinai School of Medicine, One Gustave L. Levy Place, New York NY 10029

PART I

Basic Transplantation and Bone Biology

CHAPTER 1

Principles of Transplantation Immunology

Mario C. Deng, MD
Ranjit John, MD*
Helen Baron, MD
Silviu Itescu, MD
Nicole Suciu-Foca, PhD
Departments of Medicine, Surgery, and Pathology
Columbia University College of Physicians and Surgeons
New York, NY

*University of Minnesota, Minneapolis, MN

I. IMMUNOLOGICAL MECHANISMS

A. General Principles

Within the human genome, on chromosome 6, a group of genes called the major histocompatibility complex (MHC) codes for cell surface proteins that allow for identification of the cell as belonging to the individual. These proteins are termed human leukocyte antigen (HLA). Another group of genes codes for antigens of the AB0 blood types. If person A is exposed to cells or tissue of person B, the proteins on the surfaces of cells or tissue of person B (antigens) will be recognized as foreign by immune competent cells of person A (leukocytes). The reaction initiated by person A upon recognition of these foreign antigens is called the alloimmune response. The immune response leads to destruction of the foreign cells or tissue. It consists of the following steps, illustrated in Figure 1.

The foreign antigens are presented either by the foreign cells or tissue of person B or by leukocytes of person A. Upon presentation of foreign antigens, T-lymphocytes of person A develop to T-helper cells (CD4 T-cells) and cytotoxic T-cells (CD8 T-cells), and B-lymphocytes develop to plasma cells producing specific clones of antibodies. These immunocompetent cells destroy the foreign cells. In addition, an inflammatory response involving monocytes and macrophages participates in this alloimmune response. The

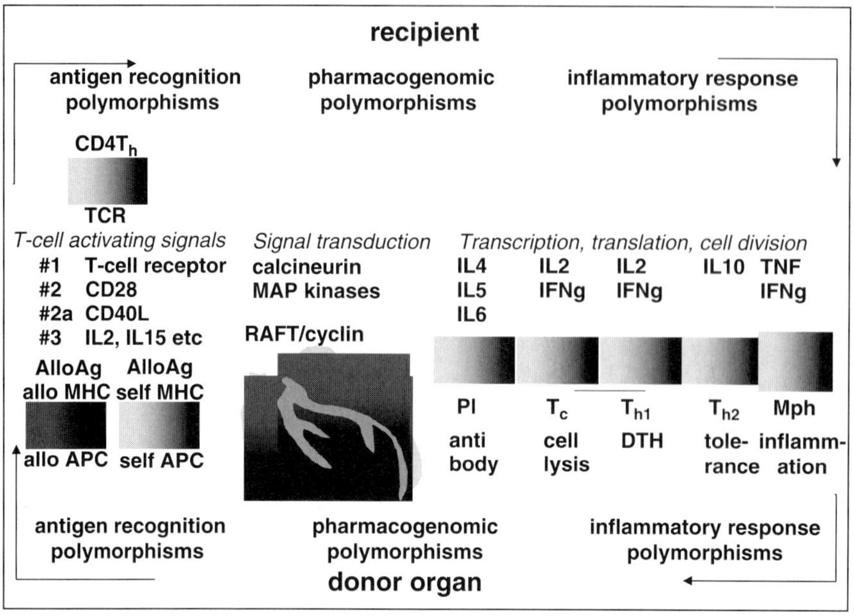

FIGURE 1 Steps in the alloimmune response

differentiation of this alloimmune response is orchestrated by a subtle regulation of soluble immune mediators, called cytokines.

Successful organ transplantation requires inhibition of this alloimmune response. First, matching the AB0 blood type is important. The recipient (person A) must be compatible with the donor organ within the AB0 system. Organs with blood type 0 can be used as universal donors; persons with blood type AB are considered universal recipients. Preoperative matching of the HLA formulae of recipient and donor is not yet feasible in cardiac transplantation due to short cold ischemic times of <4h. The exclusion of preformed HLA-specific antibodies in the recipient (person A), mediated by previous pregnancies, Mechanical Circulatory Support Devices (MCSD), or blood transfusions, against a panel of the population (persons B–Z) is another important step to allograft acceptance. In case of positivity of the panel-reactive antigens, a donor-specific crossmatch must be completed prior to transplantation. To prevent allograft rejection, pharmacologic immune prophylaxis, continuous immune and allograft function monitoring, and, if nessessary, augmentation of immunosuppression must be conducted.

B. Antigen Presentation

It is generally accepted that two pathways of allorecognition, direct and indirect, contribute to allograft rejection. It has been suggested that the direct pathway predominates during acute rejection while the indirect pathway provides a continuous supply of alloantigen responsible for chronic rejection [1, 2]. The true relative contribution of each pathway to the overall rejection process is still not entirely known. It is clear, however, that any strategies designed to achieve the ultimate goal in transplantation, the induction of tolerance, will need to take into account both pathways [3].

C. T-Cell Mediation of Acute Allograft Rejection

In the acute cellular rejection process, T-cells play a major role. CD4+ T-cells are absolutely required to initiate allograft rejection, but CD8+ T-cells are not [4]. Long-term graft acceptance appears to be associated with reduced direct recognition of donor alloantigens by recipient CD4 T-cells [5, 6]. Regulatory T-cells play an important role [7, 8, 9, 10].

D. B-Cell Mediation of Acute Allograft Rejection

Although T-cell-mediated rejection is the most common form of acute rejection, humoral rejection seems to account for a substantial fraction of rejection in patients with heart allografts, and it probably causes the majority of acute graft losses. The clinico-pathological entity of acute humoral rejection, although controversial over the last decade [11], is increasingly accepted in heart transplantation. Detection of circulating anti-donor reactive antibody (usually reactive to donor HLA antigens) confirms the diagnosis. The capillary endothelium, expressing HLA class II antigens constitutively and class I and II antigens inducibly upon stimulation with proinflammatory cytokines such as interferon-gamma (IFNγ), appears to be a major target of circulating HLA antibodies [12]. The complement system may play an important role in initiating humoral rejection. Complement activation may promote tissue injury and provide a potential target for future treatment. Staining for the complement protein C4d in tissues is more sensitive than histological features. However, ischemic changes after heart transplantation are also associated with complement activation [13, 14].

E. T-Cell/B-Cell/Monocyte–Macrophage Relationship

The relationship between T-cell-mediated and B-cell-mediated rejection is not well understood. T-cell mediation may be required for all phases of the alloimmune response, while B-cell-mediated antibodies may have a role in the complex choreography of the progressing alloimmune response [15]. It may also reflect a complementary interaction between the innate and adaptive immune systems [12, 14]. Primary rejections appear always to be accompanied by recipient T-cell recognition of a dominant HLA-DR allopeptide presented by self-antigen-presenting cells, whereas recurrent rejections, as well as the onset of transplantation vasculopathy, appear to be accompanied by inter-molecular and intra-molecular spreading and T-cell recognition of multiple donor HLA-DR alloantigenic determinants [6, 16].

F. $T_{helper1/2}$-Paradigm

The functions of proinflammatory cytokines such as IL6 in the regulation of T-cell and B-cell function can be interpreted within the context of the $T_{helper1/helper2}$ paradigm. Within this paradigm, naive T-cells ($T_{helper0}$ cells) polarize their cytokine production profile towards a $T_{helper1}$ pattern (IFNγ, TNFα, IL2) or $T_{helper\ 2}$ pattern (IL4, IL5, IL10) upon stimulation with a "master switch" cytokine, IL12 [17]. The $T_{helper\ 1}$ pattern is potentially associated with acute cellular rejection, while the $T_{helper\ 2}$ pattern has been associated with both antibody-mediated rejection and graft tolerance. Immunomodulatory cytokines have been inconsistently implicated as part of the $T_{helper\ 2}$ pattern.

G. Chronic Rejection

Chronic cardiac allograft rejection, also termed transplant vasculopathy, constitutes the dominant cause of death after the second year of cardiac transplantation [18]. As opposed to native atherosclerosis, transplant vasculopathy is characterized by concentric, diffuse luminal narrowing, involving proximal as well as distal segments of the coronary arterial tree. Pathophysiologically, transplant vasculopathy must be viewed within the context of an encounter of the recipient and donor immune system [19, 20]. The presentation of alloantigens by antigen-presenting donor cells as well as by recipient cells leads to a concerted response pattern. This pattern includes antigen-specific T-cell proliferation, CD4 T-cell proliferation with a differentiation into a $T\text{-}_{helper1}$ and a $T\text{-}_{helper2}$ profile, and non-antigen-specific proliferation of inflammatory cell responses. The donor coronary endothelium is invaded by recipient inflammatory cells. Upon diapedesis, these cells liberate specific cytokines, which in turn cause migration of medial smooth muscle cells into the intimal layer. During this process, these smooth muscle cells change from a contractile to a synthetic phenotype and initiate the intimal hyperplasia process characteristic of transplant vasculopathy. Diagnostically, the advent of intracoronary ultrasound has quickly set the gold standard for assessing this disease. Since this technique was established at Stanford University, the Stanford classification is most widely used [20].

H. Complex Networking of Allograft Rejection

Transplantation of foreign tissue initiates complex inflammatory responses that are mediated by cytokines and that, in the absence of immunosuppression, usually result in acute graft rejection and graft destruction. Thus, the study of cytokines in transplantation research has been pursued with great interest. Early cytokine biology focused on the identification and cataloguing of newly discovered cytokines. Now the field addresses the complexity of cytokine interactions with other cytokines and biologic mediators and with the extracellular matrix, as well as the diversity of cytokine effects upon both lymphoid and nonlymphoid cell types [21]. An understanding of acute allograft rejection has eluded investigators for many years, despite major research efforts in this area. This understanding may not be achievable, given the current philosophic approach to the study of immune processes. An alternative approach, as outlined in this chapter, would require investigators to develop an appreciation of the strengths and limitations of complex, adaptive networks like the interdigitated inflammatory, immune, and physiologic processes that are at work in transplanted allografts [22].

I. Transplantation Tolerance

Despite the dramatic improvement in early graft survival after the introduction of cyclosporine, late graft loss due to transplant coronary artery disease and the major consequences of long-term immunosuppression, such as infection and malignancy, remain an obstacle to longer allograft recipient survival. The development of tolerance to the allograft would eliminate these problems [23]. Tolerance is defined as the lack of detrimental immune reactivity to the donor antigen (allograft) with normal immune reactivity to other antigens occurring in the absence of ongoing immunosuppression [24]. Despite the discovery of the phenomenon of immunological tolerance by Billingham, Brent, and Medawar almost 50 years ago, true immunological tolerance remains the "Holy Grail" of transplantation [25].

Clinical and experimental evidence that transplantation tolerance is an achievable goal is mounting. The beneficial effect of blood transfusions on kidney allograft survival raised the possibility of inducing nonspecific hyporesponsiveness by infusing foreign cells [26]. Salvatierra et al. showed that donor-specific blood transfusions improve survival of kidney transplants coming from the same donor, suggesting that donor-derived cells could play a role in improving graft acceptance [27]. The observation that liver transplant recipients can maintain graft survival despite discontinuation of immunosuppression has been reported [28]. Further, long-term acceptance of allografts in nonhuman primates has been obtained using strategies with reduced toxicity, such as co-stimulation blockade or induction of mixed chimerism [23]. Chimerism is the condition in which cells of the donor engraft without further immunosuppressive therapy; microchimerism and macrochimerism are the two major types. Microchimerism exists when only a low percentage of cells are of donor origin (donor $<1\%$). This phenomenon has been well described by Starzl et al., who identified cells of donor origin in a variety of tissues in functionally tolerant liver transplant patients [29]. Macrochimerism exists when all cells are of donor origin (full chimerism) or when there is coexistence of cells of both donor and recipient origin (mixed chimerism, donor >1% but <100%). The transplantation of donor hematopoietic stem cells has been used successfully in numerous experimental settings to induce donor-specific tolerance. Other cells have also been used for the induction of tolerance, however. These include dendritic cells, regulatory T cells, and embryonic stem cells. Ideally, attempts to induce tolerance using cell therapy should precede transplantation. In the case of hematopoietic stem-cell transplantation for induction of mixed chimerism, it is suggested that the time interval between stem-cell and organ transplantation should be approximately 4–6 weeks to allow recovery of hematopoiesis between transplant surgeries [23, 30]. Several questions need to be answered before the initiation of clinical trials, however. These include the type of cells to be infused, the route and timing of infusion, and whether there is a need for a conditioning regimen or associated immunosuppressive therapy in addition to the infusion of donor-derived cells.

II. IMMUNOSUPPRESSANTS

A. General Principles

Only true "immunologic" tolerance can provide the outcome we pursue, namely, prolonged allograft function and otherwise normal immune function, without chronic immunosuppressive therapy and its risks. Until a successful tolerance-inducing protocol is developed, we must use the current and up-coming immunosuppressive agents and techniques [24].

Since the early 1980s, a three-drug regimen comprising cyclosporine, azathioprine, and usually glucocorticoids has been the mainstay of immunosuppression for patients undergoing cardiac and other forms of solid organ transplantation. This regimen, however, has a variety of inherent toxicities and is not associated with a lower incidence of graft coronary artery disease than earlier regimens. For these reasons, there has been a widely perceived need for the introduction of improved immunosuppressive agents. Two such agents have thus far been introduced: mycophenolate mofetil and tacrolimus. Mycophenolate mofetil (MMF) is used as a substitute for azathioprine and has been shown to result in significantly lower mortality rates and freedom from rejection in heart transplant recipients. Tacrolimus can be used as a substitute for cyclosporine but (at least in the short term) seems to offer no important advantage in terms of survival or rejection. The combination of these two new agents seems to have no short-term disadvantage; longer-term follow-up is pending [31].

The degree of selectivity of immunosuppressive methods determines their side effects. The following table summarizes current drugs:

Method	*Target*	*Selectivity*
Total body irradiation	Bone marrow	+
Glucocorticoids	Lymphocytes/RES	+
Thoracic duct drainage	Lymphocytes	++
Anti-lymphocyte globulin	Lymphocytes	++
Azathioprine	Lymphocytes	++
Plasmapheresis	Antibodies	++
Cyclophosphamide	B-lymphocytes	++
Anti-thymocyte globulin	T-lymphocytes	++
Monoclonal CD3 antibodies	CD3+ T-lymphocytes	+++
Monoclonal CD4 antibodies	CD4+ T-lymphocytes	+++
Mycophenolate	*De novo* purine synthesis in lymphocytes	++++
Cyclosporine	IL2 inhibition in T-lymphocytes	++++
Tacrolimus	IL2 inhibition in T-lymphocytes	++++
Daclizumab	IL2 receptor antibodies	++++

B. Cyclosporine A

The immunosuppressants cyclosporine A (CsA), FK506, and rapamycin suppress the immune response by inhibiting evolutionary conserved signal transduction pathways. CsA, FK506, and rapamycin bind to their intracellular receptors, immunophilins, creating composite surfaces that block the activity of specific targets. For CsA and FK506 the target is calcineurin. Because of the large surface area of interaction of the drug-immunophilin complex with calcineurin, FK506 and CsA have a specificity for their biologic targets that is equivalent to growth factor–receptor interactions. To date, all the therapeutic as well as toxic effects of these drugs have been shown to be due to inhibition of calcineurin. Inhibition of the action of calcineurin results in a complete block in the translocation of the cytosolic component of the nuclear factor of activated T cells (NF-AT), resulting in failure to activate the genes regulated by the NF-AT transcription factor. These genes include those required for B-cell help such as IL4 and CD40 ligand, as well as those necessary for T-cell proliferation, such as IL2 [32].

Cyclosporine has been the single most important factor associated with improved outcomes after cardiac and other solid organ transplantation over the past two decades. A review of the first decade of experience with heart transplantation revealed a total of 379 cardiac allograft recipients worldwide; actuarial survival rates in this cohort of patients at 1 year and 5 years were 56% and 31%, respectively, the main causes of death being acute rejection and the side effects of immunosuppression. With the introduction and widespread use of CsA over the next decade, survival rates dramatically improved to 85% and 75% at 1 and 5 years, respectively [33]. Sarris et al. reported on 496 patients who underwent cardiac transplantation since the introduction of

CsA (between 1980 and 1993) with 82%, 61%, and 41% survival at 1, 5, and 10 years, respectively [34]. Olivari et al. reported outstanding results on a group of patients receiving cardiac transplants between 1983 and 1988; 1- and 5-year survival rates were 92% and 78%, respectively [35]. CsA-based regimens were associated with significant prolongation in survival after cardiac transplantation [36, 37, 38].

CsA first binds to a cytosolic protein, cyclophilin (CyP), at the cellular level. The CsA–CyP complex then binds to calcineurin and subsequently blocks IL2 transcription. The binding of IL2 to the IL2 receptors on the surface of the T lymphocyte is a key stimulant in promoting lymphocyte proliferation and activation. The major adverse effects of CsA are nephrotoxicity, hypertension, neurotoxicity, and hyperlipidemia; less common side effects include hirsutism, gingival hyperplasia, and liver dysfunction. CsA nephrotoxicity can manifest as either acute or chronic renal dysfunction and may be potentiated by aminoglycosides, amphotericin B, and ketoconazole. Glucocorticoids also potentiate some of the side effects of CsA, such as hypertension, hyperlipidemia, and hirsutism [39]. To lessen these side effects, steroid weaning is practiced, as discussed later in this chapter.

The pharmacokinetics and pharmacodynamics of CsA are complex. Frequent monitoring of the serum level is essential to minimize adverse effects. One of the major limitations of the original oil-based CsA formulation (Sandimmune) is its variable and unpredictable bioavailability. In the mid-1990s, the introduction of Neoral, a new microemulsion formula of CsA, was a major advance; it has greater bioavailability and more predictable pharmacokinetics than Sandimmune [40, 41]. A study involving 380 recipients at 24 centers compared the safety and efficacy of these two CsA preparations in a double blind randomized trial. The results of this study showed fewer Neoral patients needing anti-lymphocyte therapy to treat rejection, fewer rejection episodes among female patients receiving Neoral, fewer infections in the Neoral group, and equivalent tolerability of the two formulations [42].

C. Azathioprine

Azathioprine has been available for more than 35 years and is still useful as an immunosuppressive agent. Following administration, azathioprine is converted into 6-mercaptopurine, with subsequent transformation to a series of intracellularly active metabolites. These inhibit both an early step in *de novo* purine synthesis and several steps in the purine salvage pathway. The net effect is depletion of cellular purine stores, thus inhibition of DNA and RNA synthesis, the impact of which is most marked on actively dividing lymphocytes responding to antigenic stimulation [39].

In currently used immunosuppressive protocols, azathioprine is used as part of a triple-therapy regimen along with CsA or tacrolimus and prednisone. As discussed later, the improved efficacy of mycophenolate mofetil has led many centers to replace azathioprine with MMF.

D. Prednisone

Since the inception of organ transplantation, glucocorticoids have been a mainstay in both induction and maintenance immunosuppression. Glucocorticoids are effective agents for reducing the incidence of allograft rejection. Their action is ubiquitous and begins at an early stage of the immunological cascade by influencing antigen presentation of the antigen-presenting cell and by inhibiting cytokine expression. The addition of glucocorticoids to the immunosuppressive regimen affects the quality of life of the successful transplant patient. The adverse effects of glucocorticoids on the cardiovascular system—the development of diabetes mellitus, arterial hypertension, prothrombotic state, and lipid metabolism dysregulation—are well documented, and they are responsible for osteo-articular and muscular problems, cataract formation, growth retardation, body disfiguration, and, last but not least, interference with the psychological well-being of the recipient. They may also play a role in the increased risk of infection and tumor formation in transplant patients, and there is evidence that they interfere with the tolerogenic pathway of organ acceptance [43].

E. Mycophenolic Acid

With the development of new immunosuppressive agents, the focus of anti-rejection therapy has shifted from prevention of acute allograft rejection to an emphasis on sufficient immunosuppression with minimal toxicity. Mycophenolate mofetil (MMF) is a recently developed immunosuppressive drug, which acts to inhibit T- and B-cell proliferation by blocking the production of guanosine nucleotides required for DNA synthesis. It also prevents the glycosylation of adhesion molecules, which are involved in attachment of lymphocytes to endothelium and potentially in leukocyte infiltration of an allograft during an immune response [44].

High-quality randomized clinical trials have demonstrated that MMF, when used with CsA and glucocorticoids, reduces the frequency and severity of acute rejection episodes in kidney and heart transplants, improves patient and graft survival in heart allograft recipients, and increases renal allograft survival at three years [45, 46, 47, 48, 49, 50, 51]. It has also been effective in reversing acute and resistant rejection episodes in heart, kidney, and liver recipients.

The ability of MMF to facilitate sparing of other immunosuppressive agents, particularly in CsA-related nephrotoxicity, is also promising. By permitting reduction in CsA doses, MMF may stabilize or improve renal graft function in patients with CsA-related nephrotoxicity or chronic allograft nephropathy.

Early results of phase I and II trials evaluating MMF therapy in liver and combined pancreas–kidney transplant recipients are encouraging. The main adverse effects associated with oral or intravenous MMF are gastrointestinal and hematologic in nature. Although the direct costs of using MMF versus azathioprine are higher, the decreased incidence and treatment of acute rejection in patients treated with MMF supports its use as a cost-effective option during the first year following transplantation. Ongoing issues to be resolved in clinical trials include the role of MMF in the absence of other potent agents, e.g., as monotherapy or with glucocorticoids but without calcineurin inhibitors; whether MMF will have an impact on chronic allograft dysfunction; and the cost effectiveness of treatment following the first year of transplantation [52].

F. Tacrolimus

Tacrolimus (FK506) is a macrolide antibiotic that inhibits T-cell activation and proliferation and inhibits production of other cytokines [53]. The product of *Streptomyces tsurubaensis* fermentation, FK 506 was discovered in 1984 and first used in clinical studies in 1988 [54]. Tacrolimus-based immunosuppression seems safe and effective in liver and kidney transplantation. The use of tacrolimus in heart transplantation began in the early 1990s, initially as "rescue therapy" and later as primary therapy [55]. Taylor et al. recently reviewed the guidelines for the use of tacrolimus in cardiac transplant recipients [53].

The initial trial comparing tacrolimus with CsA in clinical heart transplantation showed that patients receiving tacrolimus had a lower risk of hypertension and required a lower dose of steroids. Although the mean serum creatinine concentration at one year was higher in the tacrolimus group, this difference disappeared after two years. This study concluded that tacrolimus compares favorably with CsA as a primary immunosuppressant in cardiac transplant recipients [55]. An improved understanding of the efficacy and pharmacokinetics of tacrolimus came from the European and US multicenter trials [56, 57]. Patient survival and the probability of freedom from rejection were similar in the two treatment groups in both trials, and the overall rates of infection, impaired renal function, and glucose intolerance did not differ significantly between the tacrolimus and CsA groups. Tacrolimus-treated patients seemed to have a reduced requirement for antihypertensive therapy. Also, serum cholesterol and triglycerides were higher in patients treated with CsA. The conclusion drawn from these trials was that tacrolimus-based immunosuppression is effective for rejection prophylaxis after cardiac transplantation and may be associated with less hypertension and hyperlipidemia and comparable renal function and infection risk when compared to CsA.

It has been suggested, however, that some groups of patients may benefit from tacrolimus rather than CsA as primary immunosuppressive therapy after cardiac transplant [58]. Hirsutism and gingival hyperplasia occur infrequently with tacrolimus, which is not the case with CsA; thus, tacrolimus-based therapy may improve compliance and quality of life in female and pediatric transplant recipients. Alopecia has been documented with tacrolimus, but it is known to improve with dose reductions. The decreased incidence of hypertension and hyperlipidemia with tacrolimus makes it preferable to CsA in patients with difficult to treat hypertension or hyperlipidemia. Tacrolimus is also beneficial as a rescue immunosuppressant in cardiac transplant recipients on CsA with refractory rejection or intolerance to immunosuppression (severe side effects) [59]. In the experience of Baran et al. with tacrolimus monotherapy in cardiac transplant recipients, the use of tacrolimus alone after steroid weaning provides effective immunosuppression with a low incidence of rejection, infection, and transplant vasculopathy [60].

Since tacrolimus is metabolized using the same cytochrome P450 enzyme system as CsA, drug interactions are essentially the same. Drugs that induce this system therefore may increase the metabolism of tacrolimus, thereby decreasing its blood levels. Conversely, drugs that inhibit the P450 system decrease the metabolism of tacrolimus, thereby increasing its blood levels. It is important to note that some studies have indicated a higher incidence of nephrotoxicity with tacrolimus as compared to CsA. Tacrolimus-based immunosuppression seems safe and effective in liver and kidney transplantation.

G. Sirolimus

Sirolimus (rapamycin), a microbial product isolated from the actinomycete *Streptomyces hygroscopicus*, was discovered initially as an antifungal agent in the mid-1970s [61]. It is structurally related to tacrolimus, and retains a pharmacokinetic and drug interaction profile similar to that of the calcineurin inhibitors, cyclosporine and tacrolimus. The novel mechanism of action of sirolimus differs significantly from these agents, however, as does its adverse effect profile. The most significant adverse reaction is hyperlipidemia. Clinical experience with sirolimus has allowed transplant centers to expand its use into other areas of transplantation as well as certain autoimmune disorders [62].

In contrast to CsA or tacrolimus, sirolimus does not affect the activity of calcineurin or transcription of lymphokine genes. It selectively inhibits proteins associated with cell cycle phase G1 and ribosomal proteins that cause prolongation of cell cycle at G1/S interphase. In addition, sirolimus inhibits IL2-induced binding of transcription factors in the proliferating cell nuclear antigen promoter, thus inhibiting progression to DNA synthesis and S phase. The consequences of these actions make sirolimus a unique immunosuppressive agent. Although it is a less potent inhibitor of cytokine synthesis than CsA, sirolimus is able to inhibit immune functions such as B-cell Ig synthesis, antibody-dependent cellular cytotoxicity, and killer cell activity. Also important is its ability to exert an antiproliferative effect, thereby suggesting a potential benefit of sirolimus in chronic rejection and transplant vasculopathy. It has been shown that sirolimus can reverse established allograft vascular disease in a rat cardiac allograft model and a monkey aortic allograft model [63, 64].

The efficacy of sirolimus as an immunosuppressive agent has been shown in several animal models of transplantation. Clinical trials using sirolimus have been performed mainly in kidney transplant patients, with efficacious antirejection effects, and it has been used as rescue therapy for refractory rejection. These trials suggest that sirolimus, used in conjunction with CsA-based regimens, has a synergistic effect on rejection [65]. Studies evaluating the role of sirolimus in cardiac transplant patients offer the prospect of significant improvements in transplant immunosuppression in the form of further reduction of acute rejection, lower immunosuppressive-induced toxicity, and a lower incidence of transplant vasculopathy [66].

H. Antibodies

1. Interleukin-2 Receptor Antibody

To test the hypothesis that the specific blockade of the high-affinity interleukin-2 receptor with the human IgG1 monoclonal antibody daclizumab may prevent rejection of allografts after cardiac transplantation without inducing global immunosuppression, 55 nonsensitized patients undergoing a first cardiac transplantation were randomly assigned to receive either induction therapy with daclizumab or generalized immunosuppressive therapy. Concomitant immunosuppression was achieved in both groups with cyclosporine, mycophenolate mofetil, and prednisone. The primary end points were the incidence and severity of acute rejection and the length of time to a first episode of biopsy-confirmed rejection. During induction therapy, the mean frequency of acute rejection episodes was 0.64 per patient in the control group and 0.19 per patient in the daclizumab group ($P = 0.02$). Acute rejection developed in 17 of 27 patients in the control group (63%), as compared with 5 of 28 patients in the daclizumab group (18%; relative risk, 2.8; 95% confidence interval, 1.1 to 7.4; $P = 0.04$). Throughout follow-up, there were 9 patients with episodes of acute rejection of histologic grade 3 in the control group, as compared with 2 in the daclizumab group ($P = 0.03$), and the time to a first episode of rejection was significantly longer in the daclizumab group ($P = 0.04$). There were no adverse reactions to daclizumab and no significant differences between the groups in the incidence of infection or cancer during follow-up. The authors concluded that induction therapy with daclizumab safely reduces the frequency and severity of cardiac allograft rejection during the induction period [67].

I. Photopheresis

Photopheresis is a leukopheresis-based form of immune modulatory therapy in which lymphocytes treated with 8-methoxypsoralen are irradiated with ultraviolet-A light *ex vivo* and reinfused into the patient (68, 69). Photopheresis has been shown to be effective in a number of disease states such as cutaneous T-cell lymphoma, scleroderma, pemphigus vulgaris, systemic lupus erythematosus, and rheumatoid arthritis, all conditions partially mediated by expanded populations of unregulated effector T cells. Early experimental work in a primate model of cardiac transplantation demonstrated that photochemotherapy in conjunction with CsA and glucocorticoids suppressed the cellular immune response and formation of cytotoxic antibodies against the transplanted antigens [70, 71]. Clinical studies showed that the low toxicity and potential efficacy of photopheresis indicated a role in the prevention and treatment of cardiac transplant rejection [72]. In a study reported by Barr et al., 60 consecutive cardiac transplant patients were randomly assigned to receive either standard triple-drug immunosuppression (CsA, azathioprine, glucocorticoids) alone or in combination with photopheresis. The photopheresis group received a total of 24 photopheresis treatments, each pair given on two consecutive days, during the first 6 months after transplantation. This study concluded that the addition of photopheresis to a triple-drug regimen significantly decreased the risk of cardiac rejection. There was, however, no significant difference in the time to a first rejection episode, incidence of rejection associated with hemodynamic compromise, or survival at 6 and 12 months. There was no difference in the rates or types of infections, although cytomegalovirus DNA was detected less frequently in the photopheresis group [68, 69]. In another randomized single-center study, Barr et al. reported that the addition of prophylactic photopheresis to standard CsA-based triple-drug immunosuppression resulted in significantly decreased coronary artery intimal thickness both at 1- and 2-year follow-up. Further, the photopheresis group had a significant reduction in panel-reactive antibodies levels within the first 6 months post-transplant. These results are indeed exciting, and further studies are needed to assess whether the application of photopheresis to cardiac allograft recipients will result in sustained decrease in the progression of intimal hyperplasia and translate into improved graft and patient survival [73].

III. REJECTION MANAGEMENT

A. Rejection Diagnosis

1. *Reliability of the ISHLT Grading System*

The endomyocardial biopsy has long been the preferred technique for monitoring the rejection status of the cardiac allograft. Since 1973, published reports addressed important issues concerning the endomyocardial biopsy, including the reliability of the International Society of Heart and Lung Transplantation (ISHLT) grading system and other problem areas. No technique developed to date has been shown to have the sensitivity or specificity needed to replace the endomyocardial biopsy as a diagnostic tool, although gene array-based peripheral blood tests have recently shown promising results [74]. In addition, studies of endomyocardial biopsy specimens have furthered our understanding of the pathobiology of rejection and other transplant-related conditions [75]. During the ISHLT Scientific Sessions 2004, San Francisco, a revised ISHLT grading system was proposed [76].

B. Induction Therapy

1. Induction Therapy with Polyclonal Anti-Thymocyte and Monoclonal Anti-CD3-Antibodies

Induction therapy has long been thought to be of great importance in minimizing the risk of acute rejection, and standard regimens in the past have included induction agents. Whether benefits are obtained from the routine use of induction phase agents in heart transplantation is controversial, however. It has been shown that acute rejection episodes adversely affect short-term survival following cardiac transplantation. Rejection is known to occur most frequently during the first three months after transplantation, with the incidence decreasing exponentially thereafter. Repeated or severe episodes of allograft rejection may lead to the development of cardiac allograft vasculopathy, which is the main cause of death after the first year in these patients. The rationale for induction therapy in the perioperative period is to decrease the frequency and severity of early acute rejection. The success obtained with the use of these agents has varied [77, 78, 79].

The two main types of induction agents have been either polyclonal anti-lymphocyte or anti-thymocyte globulins or murine monoclonal antibody OKT3. Randomized trials failed to show a significant difference in survival. Further, several trials comparing the relative efficacy of polyclonal antilymphocyte preparations and monoclonal antibody OKT3 have failed to show any difference in efficacy. While these agents have been shown to be effective in terminating acute allograft rejection and treating refractory rejection, the results of studies that compare outcomes with and without monoclonal induction therapy have varied, with most studies demonstrating that the effect on rejection is maintained only while antibody therapy is ongoing. Without repeated administration, these agents only delay the time to a first rejection episode without decreasing the overall frequency or severity of rejection. More importantly, their use has been associated with an increased risk of short-term complications (infections) and long-term complications (lympho-proliferative disorders) (80). A large, multicenter analysis reported that the use of anti-lymphocyte antibody therapy, specifically OKT3, is associated with an increased incidence of non-fatal cytomegalovirus infections. Swinnen et al. reported a high incidence of post-transplant lymphoproliferative disease in patients receiving perioperative or rescue OKT3 [77]. Other large series using OKT3 have not reported as high an incidence of post-transplant lymphoproliferative disease (PTLD), however, suggesting that the risk of PTLD is more likely dependent on the overall degree of immunosuppression rather than the use of a specific agent [81, 82]. A side effect specific to OKT3 is the development of a "flu-like syndrome" characterized by fever, chills, and mild hypotension, typically seen with the first dose [83].

Since anti-lymphocyte antibodies are produced in non-human species, their use is associated with the phenomenon of sensitization, leading to decreased effectiveness with repeated use, as well as the possibilty of serum sickness. The development of sensitization has been linked to increased risk of acute vascular rejection.

Despite the lack of consistent data supporting the routine use of induction therapy with anti-lymphocyte-antibody agents, there is a role for these agents in certain situations. Specifically, patients with early postoperative renal or hepatic dysfunction may benefit, especially by the avoidance of cyclosporine therapy while using these induction agents. Anti-lymphocyte-antibody therapy can provide effective immunosuppression for at least 10 to 14 days without CsA or tacrolimus therapy. It has also been suggested that patients with overwhelming postoperative bacterial infections or diabetics with severe postoperative hyperglycemia may benefit from the comparatively low doses of glucocorticoids required during anti-lymphocyte induction therapy.

In conclusion, despite the widespread use of induction therapy using anti-lymphocyte antibody in solid organ transplantation, its precise role is unclear. There is no doubt that routine use of these agents is not warranted because the generalized immunosuppression they induce increases the risk of infections and malignancy. Until recently, they were particularly useful in the early postoperative period in patients with renal or hepatic dysfunction in whom CsA could not be used. With the recent success achieved by interleukin-2 receptor blockade in these situations [67], the role of anti-lymphocyte agents as induction agents may be even further minimized.

2. Induction Therapy with Interleukin-2 Receptor Inhibition

The high-affinity IL2 receptor is present on nearly all activated T cells but not on resting T cells. *In vivo* activation of the high-affinity IL2 receptor by IL2 promotes the clonal expansion of the activated T-cell population [67, 84]. A variety of rodent monoclonal antibodies directed against the α chain of the receptor has been used in animals and humans to achieve selective immunosuppression by targeting only T-cell clones responding to the allograft [85, 86]. A fully humanized anti-IL2R monoclonal antibody, daclizumab, and a chimeric anti-IL-2R monoclonal antibody, basiliximab, have undergone successful phase III trials demonstrating their efficacy in the immunoprophylaxis of patients undergoing renal transplantation [86, 87, 88].

Daclizumab is a molecularly engineered human IgG1 monoclonal antibody that binds but does not activate the high-affinity IL2 receptor. Because it consists of 90% human immunoglobulin sequences, daclizumab has a low immunogenicity; its serum half-life is 21 days. Flaventi et al. studied the administration of daclizumab to cadaveric renal transplantation recipients and showed a decrease in the number of episodes of allograft rejection and an increase in the time to a first rejection episode, without a concomitant increase in the incidence of infection or cancer [87]. Beniaminovitz et al. showed that as compared to conventional triple-drug immunosuppressive therapy, induction with daclizumab decreased the frequency of rejection, prolonged the time to a first rejection episode in the first 3 months after cardiac transplantation, and decreased the overall severity of rejection. In this study, treatment with daclizumab resulted in a significant reduction in the frequency and severity of rejection in the treatment period, but after the cessation of therapy, the frequency of rejection increased to a level similar to the control group [67]. This finding suggests that daclizumab has an immunomodulatory effect that is similar to that of other monoclonal antibody-based therapies (i.e., it induces clonal anergy rather than clonal deletion). Daclizumab has several advantages over other induction agents, however. Given its unique composition, its use is not functionally immunogenic. Its effective serum half-life is 21 days; 5 doses thus provide saturation for at least 3 months, which covers the period of highest incidence of cardiac allograft rejection. Moreover, this lack of immunogenicity makes possible prolonged courses and may permit repeated use of this agent for more than 3 months. Furthermore, rejection that occurred after the cessation of daclizumab therapy was preceded by the development of circulating anti-HLA antibodies. Therefore, careful immunologic screening may identify patients who require prolonged, higher dose, or repeated daclizumab therapy. Daclizumab therapy also produced a marked reduction in the formation of anti-HLA antibodies, a reduction that was sustained even after therapy was stopped. This suggests that the drug has a prominent effect on the indirect pathway of recognition. Whereas primary rejection appears to be accompanied by recognition by the recipient's T cells of a dominant HLA-DR allopeptide presented by self-antigen-presenting cells, recurrent episodes of rejection and the development of transplant-related coronary artery disease appear to result from the activation of antigen-specific B cells by soluble HLA-DR molecules. Since the development of anti-HLA IgG antibodies to the graft has been associated with the development of cellular rejection and graft atherosclerosis, effective inhibition by IL2 receptor blockade may thus favorably influence both the development of transplant-related coronary artery disease and long-term survival [89].

The short-term safety profile of daclizumab appears to be superior to that of other therapies based on monoclonal or polyclonal antibodies. The administration of daclizumab was not associated with any detectable signs of the cytokine release syndrome or allergic responses. Furthermore, the incidence of infection or cancer was not higher in the daclizumab group as compared to the control group [67].

The chimeric anti-CD25 mAb basiliximab has been studied as an immunoprophylactic agent against acute rejection in patients undergoing renal transplantation. Patients treated with this agent had a significant reduction in acute rejection and did not have an increased incidence of infections or malignancy. In keeping with the chimeric structure, the half-life of basiliximab was approximately 7 days, considerably shorter than that of either human IgG or daclizumab [90, 91].

In conclusion, daclizumab appears to be an effective adjuvant immunomodulating agent in cardiac allograft recipients. It has advantages over conventional induction therapy as it is more selective and can be used for prolonged and potentially repeated periods. Studies with larger cohorts are needed to further study the short-term and long-term survival benefits for patients following cardiac transplantation; these studies should determine the optimal dosing schedules of daclizumab. Studies using basiliximab in cardiac transplantation are needed to study its efficacy and safety profile.

C. Glucocorticoid Withdrawal

Glucocorticoids are routinely used in almost all immunosuppressive protocols after solid organ transplantation. The metabolic side effects of glucocorticoids are well known and lead to significant morbidity in the post-transplant period. Since the first report by Yacoub and colleagues, there is growing evidence to suggest that glucocorticoids may not be a requirement for post-transplant immunosuppression [92]. Despite these data, almost 90% of patients continue to receive prednisone at 1 year post-transplant and 70% at three years after cardiac transplant. A recent review of over 1800 patients from a combined registry outlined the morbid complications that patients suffer within the first year after transplantation. Many of these complications are known side effects of prednisone, including hypertension (16%), diabetes mellitus (16%), hyperlipidemia (26%), bone disease (5%), and cataracts (2%) [93]. It is thereby obvious that avoidance of glucocorticoids may decrease morbidity and mortality after heart transplantation [94]. Two general approaches are used to institute prednisone-free immunosuppression: early and late withdrawal.

Withdrawal of prednisone during the first month post-transplant has resulted in long-term success of glucocorticoid withdrawal in 50–80% of patients. In these studies, the use of anti-lymphocyte antibody induction therapy appears to increase the likelihood of glucocorticoid withdrawal. Several centers have reported their results with immunosuppressive regimens that did not include steroids in the early post-transplant period

[95]. Studies reporting high success rates of 80% have used specific enrolment criteria, such as excluding women or patients with recurrent acute rejections. In a series of nonrandomized patients, Katz et al. showed that 61% of patients could be treated without glucocorticoids immediately post-transplant; these patients had similar survival, infection, and rejection rates, but a lower incidence of diabetes when compared to patients with triple-drug immunosuppression. Keogh et al. reported 5-year follow-up on over 100 patients prospectively randomized to triple-drug therapy or double-drug therapy with CsA and azathioprine [96]. Patients with significant renal dysfunction or with acute rejection (>3 episodes) were converted to maintenance glucocorticoids. Almost half (47%) the patients required conversion to triple-drug therapy. There was no difference in actuarial survival between the 2 groups of patients. Rejection in the first 3 months was lower with triple-drug therapy but did not differ between the 2 groups beyond 3 months. Patients on triple-drug therapy had higher serum cholesterol levels and increased requirement for anti-hypertensive medication, however. These studies clearly demonstrate that glucocorticoid-free maintenance immunosuppression is possible in at least 50% of patients, is as safe as triple-drug therapy, and may reduce some of the long-term complications of glucocorticoids.

Because the majority of acute rejection episodes occur in the first 3 months post-transplant, glucocorticoid withdrawal is practical after this time period, resulting in long-term success in about 80% of patients [97]. Generally, there is no need for conventional induction agents when late withdrawal of glucocorticoids is done. Using center-specific indications for glucocorticoid withdrawal, Taylor et al. reported successful discontinuation in 30% of patients [98]. Both early and long-term mortality was significantly lower in patients in whom successful early withdrawal from glucocorticoids was achieved. There was also a trend towards decreased transplant vasculopathy in patients from whom glucocorticoids were withdrawn. Olivari et al. found that the degree of post-transplantation weight gain, lipid abnormalities, and incidence of hypertension were not modified by glucocorticoid tapering, whereas the incidence of cataracts and compression fractures and the degree of bone loss were significantly reduced [99].

Successful weaning from glucocorticoids may require a patient subgroup that is immunologically privileged. Kobashigawa et al. reported higher success rates from glucocorticoid withdrawal in patients who had two or three HLA-DR matches [97]. Felkel et al. revealed that being a black recipient was a negative predictive factor for both successful glucocorticoid withdrawal and survival, after adjusting for potential predictors for survival [100]. This raises the question of whether it is the avoidance of glucocorticoid toxicity or immunological privilege due to a favorable donor–recipient match that is contributory to the improved survival reported.

We believe that there is a role for glucocorticoid withdrawal after the first six months following cardiac transplantation. In most patients, glucocorticoids should be administered during the period of greatest risk of rejection, namely the first three to six months, with a determined attempt to withdraw subsequently. There is significant room for improvement in this area of immunosuppression, based on recent data from the ISHLT database revealing 70% of patients to be on long-term prednisone treatment [101].

D. Sensitization Therapy

1. Rejection Prophylaxis in Sensitized Patients

To identify patients at risk of having donor-specific alloreactivity, cardiac transplantation candidates are screened for antibodies reactive with lymphocytes from a panel of volunteers representative of the major HLA allotypes. These antibodies are collectively referred to as panel-reactive antibodies (PRA). Patients with high PRA levels are considered to be sensitized to various alloantigens and require donor-specific T-cell cross-matches before transplantation to exclude the presence of lymphocytotoxic IgG antibodies against donor HLA class I antigens, which can cause early graft failure as a result of complement-mediated humoral rejection [102, 103]. Because a positive donor-specific T-cell cross-match is a contraindication to transplantation, sensitized candidates have longer waiting times and higher mortality rates while waiting for an organ [104, 105, 106]. In addition, the presence of preformed anti-HLA antibodies predicts poorer long-term outcome, including increased cellular rejections, earlier onset of TCAD, and decreased long-term graft survival compared with nonsensitized patients treated with standard triple immunosuppressive regimens. These complications seem to be related primarily to the presence of preformed antibodies against allogeneic HLA class II molecules and may reflect an underlying state of CD4 T-cell allosensitization to class II antigens [107, 108, 109, 110].

The proportion of highly sensitized patients on cardiac transplant waiting lists has been increasing as a result of both widespread use of left ventricular assist devices (LVADs) and more patients undergoing retransplantation [105, 106]. Whereas alloreactivity in retransplant candidates, recipients of blood products, and multiparous women is a result of repeated B- and T-cell exposure to alloantigens, the high frequency of alloreactivity in LVAD recipients seems to result additionally from polyclonal B-cell activation attributable to selective loss of Th1-type cells through activation-induced cell death and unopposed production of Th2-type cytokines [16, 111]. Interventions in sensitized recipients have focused on therapies aimed predominantly at immunoglobulin depletion and B-cell suppression [112, 113, 114, 115, 116, 117].

Recent studies have suggested that pooled human intravenous immunoglobulin (IVIg) is an effective modality to reduce allosensitization [118, 119]. Postulated mechanisms include the presence in IVIg of anti-idiotypic antibodies [119, 120], antibodies against membrane-associated immunologic molecules such as CD4 or CD5 [121, 122], or soluble forms of HLA molecules [123, 124]. We investigated the effects of IVIg on serum reactivity to HLA class I molecules in LVAD recipients and compared these effects to plasmapheresis, an alternative modality for reduction of alloreactive antibodies [106]. Waiting time to transplantation was significantly reduced by IVIg therapy and subsequently approximated that in nonsensitized patients. Side effects of IVIg (2 g/kg) were minimal and related primarily to immune complex disease. Although plasmapheresis caused a similar reduction in alloreactivity to IVIg, this effect was achieved after longer treatment. Moreover, plasmapheresis was associated with an unacceptably high frequency of infectious complications. These results indicate that IVIg is an effective and safe modality for sensitized recipients awaiting cardiac transplantation, reducing serum anti-HLA alloreactivity and shortening the duration to transplantation. The therapeutic and safety profile of IVIg would appear to be superior to plasmapheresis [106].

2. Post-Transplant Rejection Prophylaxis in Sensitized Patients

The post-transplant induction of immunologic markers of allograft rejection were next compared in sensitized cardiac allograft recipients who were treated with cyclosporine–glucocorticoid-based triple immunosuppressive regimens incorporating either intravenous cyclophosphamide pulses or oral mycophenolate mofetil. In comparison with mycophenolate mofetil, treatment for 4–6 months with intravenous pulses of cyclophosphamide protected against IL2-receptor positive T-cell outgrowth from biopsy sites during the first post-transplant year as well as the post-transplant induction of IgG antibodies against HLA class II, but not class I, antibodies.

Immunosuppression using intravenous pulses of cyclophosphamide in sensitized recipients for 4–6 months post-transplantation significantly prolonged the rejection-free interval compared with mycophenolate mofetil and reduced the number of high-grade rejections within the first post-transplant year. Moreover, treatment with cyclophosphamide reduced the cumulative annual rejection frequency by 63%. The only significant protective factor against development of high-grade cellular rejection in sensitized patients was treatment with cyclophosphamide. In comparison with cyclophosphamide, mycophenolate mofetil treatment conferred a 3.7-fold higher risk of rejection ($p = 0.009$) [125].

Treatment with intravenous cyclophosphamide has proved to be extremely safe. The incidence of cytomegalovirus (CMV) disease was lower in cyclophosphamide-treated patients (12%) than in those treated with mycophenolate mofetil (19%). No other viral, bacterial, or fungal infections were seen in patients treated with cyclophosphamide. Intravenous pulse therapy with cyclophosphamide was frequently (>80%) accompanied by transient nausea and vomiting which responded to antiemetic therapy. Mesna (sodium 2-mercaptoethane sulfonate) co-administered with cyclophosphamide may have contributed to the absence of any cases of hemorrhagic cystitis. No malignancies have developed after 540 patient months of follow-up. IVIg therapy was associated with clinical manifestations of immune complex disease in 4/27 (15%) of monthly courses, as evidenced by fever, arthralgia, and maculopapular rashes. Reversible renal insufficiency (defined as >50% increase in serum creatinine level) occurred in 4 cases, all of which resolved spontaneously over the ensuing 3 weeks post-infusion.

These results demonstrate that intravenous pulse cyclophosphamide therapy together with IVIg pretransplantation as part of a cyclosporine–steroid-based regimen in sensitized cardiac allograft recipients is effective and safe for decreasing recipient serum and cellular alloreactivity, shortening transplant waiting time, and reducing allograft rejection.

Presently, we advocate that all patients at risk for sensitization before transplantation be specifically screened for the presence of antibodies against both HLA class I and II antibodies. On the basis of our results, immunosuppressive therapy for sensitized patients should commence before transplantation, because initiation of a standard triple-therapy regimen is not effective at preventing recurrent allograft rejection. Initiation of an immunosuppressive protocol using intravenous cyclophosphamide pulses before and after transplantation is a safe and effective modality for reducing donor-specific B- and T-cell alloreactivity.

REFERENCES

1. Liu, Z., Sun, Y.K., Xi, Y.P., Maffei, A., Reed, E., Harris, P., Suciu-Foca, N. (1993). Contribution of direct and indirect recognition pathways to T cell alloreactivity. *J Exp Med.* 177:1643–1650.
2. Harris, P.E., Cortesini, R., Suciu-Foca, N. (1999). Indirect allorecognition in solid organ transplantation. *Rev Immunogenet.* 1:297–308.
3. Womer, K. L., Sayegh, M.H., Auchincloss, H., Jr. (2001). Involvement of the direct and indirect pathways of allorecognition in tolerance induction. *Philos Trans R Soc London B Biol Sci.* 356(1409):639.
4. Krieger, N.R., Yin, D.P., Fathman, C.G. (1996). CD4+ but not CD8+ cells are essential for allorejection. *J Exp Med.* 184:2013–2018.
5. Zeevi, A., Pavlick, M., Lombardozzi, S., Banas, R., Pappo, O., Rao, A.S., Fontes, P., Demetris, J., Shapiro, R., Dodson, F., et al. (1995). Immune status of recipients following bone marrow-augmented solid organ transplantation. *Transplantation.* 59:616–620.
6. Itescu, S., Tung, T., Burke, E., et al. (1998). Preformed IgG antibodies against major histocompatibility class II antigens are major risk factors for high-grade cellular rejection in recipients of heart transplantation. *Circulation.* 98:786–793.
7. Chang, C.C., Ciubotariu, R., Manavalan, J.S., Yuan, J., Colovai, A.I., Piazza, F., Lederman, S., Colonna, M., Cortesini, R., Dalla-Favera, R., Suciu-Foca, N. (2002). Tolerization of dendritic cells by T(S) cells: the crucial role of inhibitory receptors ILT3 and ILT4. *Nat Immunol.* 3:237–243.
8. Ermann, J., Fathman, C.G. (2003). Costimulatory signals controlling regulatory T cells. *Proc Natl Acad Sci U S A.* 100:15292–15293.
9. Wood, K.J., Sakaguchi, S. (2003). Regulatory T cells in transplantation tolerance. *Nat Rev Immunol.* 3:199–210.

10. Bluestone, J.A., Abbas, A.K. (2003). Natural versus adaptive regulatory T cells. *Nat Rev Immunol.* 3:253–257.
11. Bonnaud, E. N., Lewis, N.P., Masek, M.A., Billingham, M.E. (1995). Reliability and usefulness of immunofluorescence in heart transplantation. *J Heart Lung Transplant.* 14:163.
12. Michaels, P.J., Fishbein, M.C., Colvin, R.B. (2003). Humoral rejection of human organ transplants. *Springer Semin Immunopathol.* 25:119–140.
13. Baldwin, W.M. 3rd, Samaniego-Picota, M., Kasper, E.K., Clark, A.M., Czader, M., Rohde, C., Zachary, A.A., Sanfilippo, F., Hruban, R.H. (1999). Complement deposition in early cardiac transplant biopsies is associated with ischemic injury and subsequent rejection episodes. *Transplantation.* 68:894–900.
14. Baldwin, W.M., Ota, H., Rodriguez, E.R. (2003). Complement in transplant rejection: diagnostic and mechanistic considerations. *Springer Semin Immunopathol.* 25:181–197.
15. Racusen, L.C. (2003). Pathology and the allo-immune response. *Am J Transplant.* 3:1461–1462.
16. Mamula, M.J. and Janeway, C.A. Jr. (1993). Do B cells drive the diversification of immune responses. *Immunol Today.* 14:151–154.
17. Murphy, K.M., Ouyang, W., Farrar, J.D., Yang, J., Ranganath, S., Asnagli, H., Afkarian, M., Murphy, T.L. (2000). Signaling and transcription in T-helper development. *Annu Rev Immunol.* 18:451–494.
18. Hertz, M., Taylor, D., Trulock, E., Boucek, M., Mohacsi, P., Edwards, L., Keck, B. (2003). The registry of the international society for heart and lung transplantation: Twentieth official adult heart transplant report-2003. *J Heart Lung Transplant.* 22:616.
19. Deng, M.C., Baba, H.A., Plenz, G., Erren, M., Wilhelm, M.J., Moennig, G., Scheld, H.H. (2000). Prediction of morbidity and mortality from cardiac allograft vasculopathy. *Z Kardiol.* 89(Suppl 9):IX-63–IX-65.
20. Rickenbacher, P.R., Pinto, F.J., Lewis, N.P., Hunt, S.A., Alderman, E.L., Schroeder, J.S., Stinson, E.B., Brown, B.W., Valantine, H.A. (1995). Prognostic importance of intimal thickness as measured by intracoronary ultrasound after cardiac transplantation. *Circulation.* 92:3445–3452.
21. Bumgardner, G.L., Orosz, C.G. (1999). Transplantation and cytokines. *Semin Liver Dis.* 19:189–204.
22. Orosz, C.G., VanBuskirk, A.M. (1998). Immune mechanisms of acute rejection. *Transplant Proc.* 30:859–861.
23. Toungouz, M., Donckier, V., Goldman, M. (2003). Tolerance induction in clinical transplantation: The pending questions. *Transplantation.* 75:58S–60S.
24. Taylor, D.O. (2000). Immunosuppressive therapies after heart transplantation: best, better, and beyond. *Current Opin Cardiol.* 15:108–114.
25. Billingham, R.E., Brent, L., Medawar, P.B. (1953). "Actively acquired tolerance" of foreign cells. *Nature.* 172:603–606.
26. Opelz, G., Mickey, M.R., Sengar, DPS, et al. (1973). Effect of blood transfusions on subsequent kidney transplants. *Transplant Proc.* 5:253.
27. Salvatierra, O., Vincenti, F., Amend, W., et al. (1982). Deliberate donor-specific blood transfusions prior to living related renal transplantation: A new approach. *Ann Surg.* 192:543.
28. Mazariegos, G.V., Reyes, J., Marino, I.R., et al. (1997). Weaning of immunosuppression in liver transplant recipients. *Transplantation.* 63:243.
29. Starzl, T.E., Demetris, A.J., Trucco, M., et al. (1993). Cell migration and chimerism after whole organ transplantation: The basis of graft acceptance. *Hepatology.* 17:1127.
30. Rifle, G., Mousson, C. (2003). Donor-derived hematopoietic cells in organ transplantation: A major step toward allograft tolerance. *Transplantation.* 75:3S-7S.
31. Hunt, S.A. (2000). New immunosuppressive agents in clinical use: mycophenolate mofetil and tacrolimus. *Cardiol Rev.* 8:180–184.

32. Ho, N. (1996). Activation protein 1-dependent transcriptional activation of interleukin 2 gene by CA2+/calmodulin kinase type IV/Gr. *J Exp Med.* 184:101.
33. Cheung, A., Menkis, A.H. (1998). Cyclosporine heart transplantation. *Transplant Proc.* 30:1881–1884.
34. Sarris, G.E., Moore, K.A., Schroeder, J.S., et al. (1994). Cardiac transplantation: the Stanford experience in the cyclosporine era. *J Thorac Cardiovasc Surg.* 108:240–251.
35. Olivari, M.T., Kubo, S.H., Braunlin, E.A., Bolman, R.M., Ring, W.S. (1990). Five-year experience with triple-drug immunosuppressive therapy in cardiac transplantation. *Circulation.* 82;IV 276-280.
36. DeCampli, W.M., Luikart, H., Hunt, S., Stinson, E.B. (1995). Characteristics of patients surviving more than 10 years after cardiac transplantation. *J Thorac Cardiovasc Surg.* 109:1103–1114.
37. John, R., Rajasinghe, H.A., Chen, J.M., et al. (2001). Long term outcomes following cardiac transplantation: An experience based on different eras of immunosuppression. *Ann Thorac Surg.* 72:440–449.
38. John, R., Rajasinghe, H.A., Itescu, S., et al. (2001). Factors affecting long term survival (>10 years) after cardiac transplantation in the cyclosporine era. *J Am Coll Cardiol.* 37:189–194.
39. Costanzo, M.R. (2001). New immunosuppressive drugs in heart transplantation. *Curr Control Trials Cardiovasc Med.* 2:45–53.
40. Kahan, B.D., Welsh, M., Schoenburg, L., et al. (1996). Variable absorption of cyclosporine: a biological risk factor for chronic renal allograft rejection. *Transplantation.* 62:599–606.
41. Valantine, H. (2000). Neoral use in the cardiac transplant recipient. *Transplant Proc.* 32:27S-44S.
42. Eisen, H.J., Hobbs, R.E., Davis, S.F., et al. (1999). Safety, tolerability and efficacy of cyclosporine microemulsion in heart transplant recipients: a randomized, multicenter, double-blind comparison with the oil-based formulation of cyclosporine – results at six months after transplantation. *Transplantation.* 68:663–671.
43. Lerut, J.P. (2003). Avoiding steroids in solid organ transplantation. *Transpl Int.* 16:213–224.
44. Allison, A.C., Eugui, E.M. (1993). Immunosuppressive and other effects of mycophenolic acid and an ester prodrug, mycophenolate mofetil. *Immuno Rev.* 136:5.
45. Ensley, R.D., Bristow, M.R., Olsen, S.L., et al. (1993). The use of mycophenolate mofetil (RS-61443) in human heart transplant recipients. *Transplantation.* 13:571.
46. Kobashigawa, J.A., Miller, L., Renlund, D., et al. (1998). A randomized active-controlled trial of mycophenolate mofetil in heart transplant recipients. *Transplantation.* 66:507–515.
47. Kobashigawa, J.A. (1998). Mycophenolate mofetil in cardiac transplantaion. *Curr Opin Cardiol.* 13:117–121.
48. Lietz, K., John, R., et al. (2002). IgM to IgG anti-HLA class II antibody switching in cardiac transplant recipients is associated with increased risk of cellular rejection and coronary artery disease and is prevented by mycophenolic acid. *Transplant Proc.* 34 (5):1828.
49. Renlund, D.G., Gopinathan, S.K., Kfoury, A.G., Taylor, D.O. (1996). Mycophenolate mofetil (MMF) in heart transplantation; rejection prevention and treatment. *Clin Transplant.* 10:13.
50. Yamani, M.H., Starling, R.C., Goormastic, M., Van Lente, F., Smedira, N., McCarthy, P., Young, J.B. (2000). The impact of routine mycophenolate mofetil drug monitoring on the treatment of cardiac allograft rejection. *Transplantation.* 69:2326–2330.
51. Rose, M.L., Smith, J., Dureau, G., et al. (2002). Mycophenolate mofetil decreases antibody production after cardiac transplantation. *J Heart Lung Transplant.* 21:282–285.
52. Mele, T.S., Halloran, P.F. (2000). The use of mycophenolate mofetil in transplant recipients. *Immunopharmacology.* 47:215–245.

53. Taylor, D.O., Barr, M.L., Meiser, B.M., et al. (2001). Suggested guidelines for the use of tacrolimus in cardiac transplant recipients. *J Heart Lung Transplant.* 20:734–738.
54. Kino, T., Hataraka, H., Miyata, S., et al. (1987). FK 506, a novel immunosuppression isolated from a streptomyces: immunosuppressive effect of FK 506 in vitro. *J Antibiotics.* 40:1256–1260.
55. Pham, S.M., Kormos, R.L., Hattler, B.G., et al. (1996). A prospective trial of tacrolimus (FK 506) in clinical heart transplantation: intermediate-term results. *J Thorac Cardiovasc Surg.* 111:764–772.
56. Reichart, B.R., Meiser, B.M., Vigano, M., et al. (1998). European multi-center tacrolimus (FK 506) heart pilot study: one-year results—European Multicenter Heart Study Group. *J Heart Lung Transplant.* 17:775–781.
57. Taylor, D.O., Barr, M.L., Radovancevic, B., et al. (1999). Randomized, multicenter, comparison of tacrolimus and cyclosporine immunosuppressive regimens in cardiac transplantation: decreased hyperlipidemia and hypertension with tacrolimus. *J Heart Lung Transplant.* 18:336–345.
58. Meiser, B.M., Pfeiffer, M., Schmidt, D., et al. (1999). Combination therapy with tacrolimus and mycophenolate mofetil following cardiac transplantation: importance of mycophenolic acid therapeutic drug monitoring. *J Heart Lung Transplant.* 18:143–149.
59. Mentzer, R.M. Jr, Jahania, M.S., Lasley, R.D. (1998). Tacrolimus as a rescue immunosuppressant after heart and lung transplantation. The US Multicenter FK506 Study Group. *Transplantation.* 65:109–113.
60. Baran, D.A., Segura, L., Kushwaha, S., et al. (2001). Tacrolimus monotherapy in adult cardiac transplant receipients: intermediate-term results. *J Heart Lung Transplant.* 20:59–70.
61. Gummert, J.F., Ikonen, T., Morris, R.E. (1999). Newer immunosuppressive drugs: a review. *J A Soc Nephrol.* 10:1366–1380.
62. Ingle, G.R., Sievers, T.M., Holt, C.D. (2000). Sirolimus: continuing the evolution of transplant immunosuppression. *Ann Pharmacother.* 34:1044–1055.
63. Poston, R.S., Billingham, M., Hoyt, E.J., et al. (1999). Rapamycin reverses chronic graft vascular disease in a novel cardiac allograft model. *Circulation.* 100:67–74.
64. Ikonen, T.S., Gummert, J.F., Honda, Y., et al. (1999). Sirolimus (rapamycin) blood levels correlate with prevention of graft vascular disease (GVD) in monkey aortic transplants as monitored by graft ultrasound. *J Heart Lung Transplant.* 18:72.
65. Groth, C.G., Backman, L., Morales, J.L., et al. (1999). Sirolimus(rapamycin)-based therapy in human renal transplantation: similar efficacy and different toxicity compared with cyclosporine. *Transplantation.* 67:1036–1042.
66. Eisen, H.J., Tuzcu, E.M., Dorent, R., Kobashigawa, J., Mancini, D., Valantine-von Kaeppler, H.A., Starling, R.C., Sorensen, K., Hummel, M., Lind, J.M., Abeywickrama, K.H., Bernhardt, P.; RAD B253 Study Group. (2003). Everolimus for the prevention of allograft rejection and vasculopathy in cardiac-transplant recipients. *N Engl J Med.* 349:847–858.
67. Beniaminovitz, A., Itescu, S., Lietz, K., et al. (2000). Prevention of the rejection in cardiac transplantation by blockade of the interleukin-2 receptor with a monoclonal antibody. *N Engl J Med.* 342:613–619.
68. Barr, M.L., Meiser, B.M., Roberts, R.F., et al. (1998). Photopheresis for the prevention of rejection in cardiac transplantation. Photopheresis Transplantation Study Group. *N Engl J Med.* 339:1744–1751.
69. Barr, M.L. (1998). Photopheresis in transplantation: future research and directions. *Transplant Proc.* 30:2248–2250.
70. Pepino, P., Berger, C.L., Fuzesi, L., et al. (1989). Primate cardiac allo- and xenotransplantation: modulation of the immune response to chemotherapy. *Eur Sur Res.* 21:105–113.
71. Rose, E., Barr, M., Xu, H., et al. (1992). Photochemotherapy in human heart transplant recipients at high risk for fatal rejection. *J Heart Lung Transplant.* 11:746–750.

72. Costanzo-Nordin, M.R., Hubell, E.A., O'Sullivan, E.J., et al. (1992). Photopheresis versus corticosteroids in the therapy of heart transplant rejection. Preliminary clinical report. *Circulation*. 86:II242-250.
73. Barr, M.L., Baker, C.J., Schenkel, F.A., et al. (2000). Prophylactic photopheresis and chronic rejection: effects on graft intimal hyperplasia in cardiac transplantation. *Clin Transplantation*. 14:162–166.
74. Deng, M.C., Mehra, M.C., Eisen, H.J., et al. (2003). Cardiac allograft monitoring using a novel clinical algorithm based on peripheral leukocyte gene expression profiling. Circulation 108:IV 398.
75. Winters, G.L. (1997). The challenge of endomyocardial biopsy interpretation in assessing cardiac allograft rejection. *Curr Opin Cardiol*. 12:146–152.
76. Stewart, S., et al. JHLT 2004, in press.
77. Swinnen, L.J., Costanzo-Nordin, M.R., Fisher, S.J., et al. (1990). Increased incidence of lymphoproliferative disorder after immunosuppression with the monoclonal antibody OKT3 in cardiac-transplant recipients. *N Engl J Med*. 323:1723–1728.
78. Kirklin, J.K., Naftel, D.C., Levine, T.B., et al. (1994). Cytomegalovirus after heart transplantation. Risk factors for infection and death: a multiinstitutional study. The Cardiac Transplant Research Database Group. *J Heart Lung Transplant*. 13:394–404.
79. John, R., Rajasinghe, H.A., Chen, J.M., et al. (2000). Impact of current management practices on early and late mortality in over 500 consecutive heart transplant recipients. *Ann Surg*. 232:302–311.
80. Johnson, M.R., Mullen, G.M., O'Sullivan, E.J., et al. (1994). Risk/benefit ration of perioperative OKT3 in cardiac transplantation. *Am J Cardiol*. 74:261–266.
81. O'Connell, J.B., Bristow, M.R., Hammond, E.H., et al. (1991). Antimurine antibody to OKT3 in cardiac transplantation: implications for prophylaxis and retreatment of rejection. *Transplant Proc*. 23:1157–1159.
82. Taylor, D.O., Kfoury, A.G., Pisani, B., Hammond, E.H., Renlund, D.G. (1997). Antilymphocyte-antibody prophylaxis: Review of the adult experience in heart transplantation. *Transplant Proc*. 29:13S-15S.
83. Ma, H., Hammond, E.H., Taylor, D.O., et al. (1996). *Transplantation*. 62:205.
84. Taniguchi, T., Minami, Y. (1993). The IL-2/IL-2 receptor system:a current overview. *Cell*. 73:8.
85. Reed, M.H., Shapiro, M.E., Strom, T.B., et al. (1989). Prolongation of primate renal allograft survival by anti-Tac, an anti-human IL-2 receptor monoclonal antibody. *Transplantation*. 47:55–59.
86. Kirkman, R.L., Shapiro, M.E., Carpenter, C.B., et al. (1991). A randomized prospective trial of anti-Tac monoclonal antibody in human renal transplantation. *Transplantation*. 51:107–113.
87. Flaventi, F., Kirkman, R., Light, S., et al. (1998). Interleukin-2 receptor blockade with daclizumab to prevent acute rejection in renal transplantation. *N Engl J Med*. 338:161–165.
88. Vincenti, F. (1999). Daclizumab in solid organ transplantation. *Biodrugs*. 11:333–341.
89. Lietz, K., John, R., Beniaminovitz, A., Burke, E., Mancini, D., Edwards, N., Itescu, S. (2003). A randomized study of interleukin-2 receptor blockade in cardiac transplantation: influence of HLA-DR locus incompatibility on treatment efficacy. *Transplantation*. 75:781–787.
90. Nashan, B., Moore, R., Amlot, P., CHIP 201 International Study Group, et al. (1997). Randomized trial of basiliximab versus placebo for control of acute cellular rejection in renal allograft recipients. *Lancet*. 350:1193–1198.
91. Kahan, B.D., Rajagopalan, P.R., Hall, M., U. S. Simulect Renal Study Group. (1999). Reduction of the occurrence of acute cellular rejection among renal allograft recipients treated with basiliximab, a chimeric anti-interleukin-2 receptor monoclonal antibody. *Transplantation*. 67:276–284.

92. Yacoub, M.A., Khaghani, P., Mitchell, A. (1985). The use of cyclosporine, azathioprine, and antithymocyte globulin with or without low dose steroids for immunosuppression of cardiac transplant patients. *Transplant Proc.* 17:221–222.
93. Brann, W.M., Bennett, L.E., Keck, B.M., Hosenpud, J.D. (1998). Morbidity, functional status, and immunosuppressive therapy after heart transplantation; an analysis of the joint international society for heart and lung transplantation/united network for organ sharing thoracic registry. *J Heart Lung Transplant.* 17:374–382.
94. Esmore, D.S., Spratt, P.M., Keogh, A.M., Chang, V.P. (1989). Cyclosporine and azathioprine immunosuppression without maintenance steroids: a randomized prospective trial. *J Heart Lung Transplant.* 8:194–199.
95. Oaks, T.E., Wannenberg, T., Close, S.A., et al. (2001). Steroid-free maintenance immunosuppression after heart transplantion. *Ann Thorac Surgery.* 72:102–106.
96. Keogh, A., Macdonald, P., Mundy, J., et al. (1992). Five-year follow up of a randomized double-drug versus triple drug therapy immunosuppressive trial after heart transplantation. *J Heart Lung Transplant.* 11:550–555.
97. Kobashigawa, J.A., Stevenson, L.W., Brownfield, E.D., Gleeson, M.P., Moriguchi, J.D., Kawata, N., Minkley, R., Drinkwater, D. C., Laks, H. (1995). Corticosteroid weaning late after heart transplantation: relation to HLA-DR mismatching and long-term metabolic effects. *J Heart Lung Transplant.* 14:963–967.
98. Taylor, D.O., Bristow, M.R., O'Connell, J.B., et al. (1996). Improved long-term survival after heart transplantation predicted by successful early withdrawal from maintenance corticosteroid therapy. *J Heart Lung Transplant.* 15:1039–1046.
99. Olivari, M.T., Jessen, M.E., Baldwin, B.J., et al. (1995). Triple-drug immunosuppression with steroid discontinuation by six months after heart transplantation. *J Heart Lung Transplant.* 14:127–135.
100. Felkel, T.O., Smith, A.L., Reichenspurner, H.C., et al. (2002). Survival and incidence of acute rejection in heart transplant recipients undergoing successful withdrawal from steroid therapy. *J Heart Lung Transplant.* 21:530–539.
101. Hosenpud, J.D., Bennett, L.E., Keck, B.M., et al. (2000). The registry of the International Society for Heart and Lung Transplantation: seventeenth official report-2000. *J Heart Lung Transplant.* 19:909–931.
102. Ratkovec, R.M., Hammond, E.H., O'Connell, J.B., et al. (1992). Outcome of cardiac transplant recipients with a positive donor-specific crossmatch—preliminary results with plasmapheresis. *Transplantation.* 54(4): 651–655.
103. Smith, J.D., Danskine, A.J., Laylor, R.M., Rose, M.L., Yacoub, M.H. (1993). The effect of panel reactive antibodies and the donor specific crossmatch on graft survival after heart and heart-lung transplantation. *Transpl Immunol.* 1(1): 60–65.
104. Itescu, S., Tung, T.C., Burke, E.M., Weinberg, A.D., Mancini, D., Michler, R.E., Suciu-Foca, N.M., Rose, E.A. (1998). An immunological algorithm to predict risk of high-grade rejection in cardiac transplant recipients. *Lancet.* 352:263–270.
105. John, R., Chen, J.M., Weinberg, A., et al. (1999). Long-term survival after cardiac retransplantation: a twenty-year single center experience. *J Thorac Cardiovasc Surg.* 117:543–555.
106. John, R., Lietz, K., Burke, E., et al. (1999). Intravenous immunoglobulin reduces anti-HLA alloreactivity and shortens waiting time to cardiac transplantation in highly sensitized left ventricular assist device recipients. *Circulation.* 100:II229–235.
107. Liu, Z., Colovai, A.I., Tugulea, S., et al. (1996). Indirect recognition of donor HLA-DR peptides in organ allograft rejection. *J Clin Invest.* 98:1150–1157.
108. Vanderlugt, C.J., Miller, S.D. (1996). Epitope spreading. *Curr Opin Immunol.* 8:831–836.
109. Tugulea, S., Ciubotariu, R., Colovai, A.I., et al. (1997). New strategies for early diagnosis of heart allograft rejection. *Transplantation.* 64:842–847.
110. Ciubotariu, R., Liu, Z., Colovai, A.I., Ho, E., Itescu, S., Ravalli, S., Hardy, M.A., Cortesini, R., Rose, E.A., Suciu-Foca, N. (1998). Persistent allopeptide reactivity and epitope spreading in chronic rejection of organ allografts. *J Clin Invest.* 101:398–405.

111. Reed, E.F., Hong, B., Ho, E., et al. (1996). Monitoring of soluble HLA alloantigens and anti-HLA antibodies identifies heart allograft recipients at risk of transplant associated coronary artery disease. *Transplantation.* 61:556–572.
112. Glotz, D., Haymann, J., Sansonetti, N., et al. (1993). Suppression of HLA-specific alloantibodies by high-dose intravenous immunoglobulins (IVIg). *Transplantation.* 56:335–337.
113. Tyan, T.B., Li, V.A., Czer, L., et al. (1994). Intravenous immunoglobulin suppression of HLA alloantibody in highly sensitized transplant candidates and transplantation with a histoincompatible organ. *Transplantation.* 57:553–562.
114. Peraldi, M., Akposso, K., Haymann, J., et al. (1996). Long-term benefit of intravenous immunoglobulins in cadaveric kidney retransplantation. *Transplantation.* 62:1670–1673.
115. McIntyre, J.A., Higgins, N., Britton, R., et al. (1996). Utilization of intravenous immunoglobulin to ameliorate alloantibodies in a highly sensitized patient with a cardiac assist device awaiting cardiac transplantation. *Transplantation.* 62:691–693.
116. De Marco, T., Damon, L.E., Colombe, B., et al. (1997). Successful immunomodulation with intravenous immunoglobulin and cyclophosphamide in an alloimmunized heart transplant recipient. *J Heart Lung Transplant.* 16:360–365.
117. John, R., Lietz, K., Naka, Y., et al. (2003). Immunologic sensitization in recipients of left ventricular assist devices. *J Thorac Cardiovasc Surg.* 125:578–591.
118. Dwyer, J.M. (1992). Manipulating the immune system with immune globulin. *N Engl J Med.* 326:107–116.
119. Dietrich, G., Algiman, M., Sultan, Y., Nydegger, U.E., Kazatchkine, M.D. (1992). Origin of anti-idiotypic activity against anti-factor VIII autoantibodies in pools of normal human immunoglobulin G (IVIg). *Blood.* 79:2946–2951.
120. Rossi, F., Kazatchkine, M.D. (1989). Antiidiotypes against autoantibodies in pooled normal human polyspecific Ig. *J Immunol.* 143:4104–4109.
121. Hurez, V., Kaveri, S.V., Mouhoub, A., et al. (1993). Anti-CD4 activity of normal human immunoglobulins for therapeutic use (IVIg). *Ther Immunol.* 1:269–278.
122. Vassilev, T., Gelin, C., Kaveri, S.V., et al. (1993). Antibodies to the CD5 molecule in normal human immunoglobulins for therapeutic use (IVIg). *Clin Exp Immunol.* 92: 369–372.
123. Blasczyk, R., Westhoff, U., Grossewilde, H. (1993). Soluble CD4, CD8, and HLA molecules in commercial immunoglobulin preparations. *Lancet.* 341:789–790.
124. Lam, L., Whitsett, C.F., McNicholl, J.M., Hodge, T.W., Hooper, J. (1993). Immunologically active proteins in intravenous immunoglobulin. *Lancet.* 342:678.
125. Itescu, S., Burke, E., Lietz, K., et al. (2002). Intravenous pulse administration of cyclophosphamide is an effective and safe treatment for sensitized cardiac allograft recipients. *Circulation.* 105:1214–1219.
126. Avery, R.K. (2003). Cardiac-allograft vasculopathy. *N Engl J Med.* 349:829–830.

CHAPTER 2

Bone Biology: Bone Structure and Remodeling

Lawrence G. Raisz, MD
University of Connecticut Health Center
Farmington, CT

I. INTRODUCTION

The skeleton is a remarkable organ that provides the body with a frame that is strong enough for protection, light enough for mobility, and adaptable for changing structural needs. The skeleton also serves metabolic functions as a storehouse for calcium and phosphorus, a buffering site for hydrogen ion excess, and a binding site for toxic ions such as lead and aluminum. When skeletal tissues are required to fulfill these latter functions, this may occur at the cost of structural integrity and lead to fractures. Once the adult skeleton has been formed, both the structural and metabolic functions are carried out largely by remodeling—removal and replacement of bone tissue at the same site in so-called bone multicellular units (BMU)—rather than modeling, which is formation of bone at sites where no prior resorption has occurred. Both processes do continue throughout life, however. In particular, modeling in the form of new periosteal apposition can occur with aging as a compensatory mechanism to the weakening of bone by the trabecular and endosteal loss and cortical porosity that occurs with increased resorption and inadequate formation in BMUs [1]. This brief overview of bone biology will provide selected references, particularly of recent studies. More detailed information is available in texts and reviews [2, 3, 4, 5].

II. BONE STRUCTURE

Our skeletons are made up of hollow bones in which a dense cortical shell encases a marrow space containing varying amounts of trabecular bone.

The vertebrae, pelvis, skull, and scapulae are filled with a continuous trabecular network, while trabecular bone is found only at the ends of the long bones of the appendicular skeleton. Cortical bone is distributed along lines of stress, with greater amounts of bone in areas under compression or subject to impact loading [6]. Trabecular bone is similarly distributed to maximize strength, with the thicker trabeculae along lines of stress. The cross-struts connecting these trabeculae are of great importance in adding strength to trabecular structure. If these cross-struts are lost, relatively modest losses of bone mass may result in great increases in skeletal fragility.

During development, skeletal structures are first formed as a cartilage template, which is then gradually replaced by bone. Until the end of puberty, a cartilage growth plate remains at the ends of the bone to allow for linear growth. A large number of genes have now been identified that determine skeletal structure through their effects on cartilage as well as their regulation of the conversion of cartilage to bone. These genes determine the extent to which the skeleton achieves optimal peak bone mass and strength.

Chemically, bone is a composite material made up of a collagenous matrix, upon which crystals of calcium and phosphate are laid down in an orderly manner. The mineral resembles, but is not identical to, hydroxyapatite. In addition to collagen and mineral, a large number of non-collagenous proteins are present in the skeleton. These proteins play a role in signaling between cells and matrix as well as in determining the distribution of mineral on the collagen scaffold.

III. BONE REMODELING

The bone remodeling process is vital for maintaining both the structural and metabolic functions of skeletal tissue. Remodeling is needed to repair skeleton damage that occurs with repeated stresses, and it also helps maintain the viability of the skeleton by replacing dying cells. The resorption phase of remodeling, particularly in trabecular bone, can maintain the supply of calcium and phosphate when the diet is deficient in these minerals. On the other hand, when dietary supplies are ample, the formation phase can take up these minerals and make them available for future use.

The bone remodeling cycle is a tightly coupled sequence of events that occurs within a defined time and in a defined space, as illustrated in Figure 1. Remodeling is most active on the surface of trabecular bone where resorption forms the shallow irregular pits called Howship's lacunae. Remodeling also occurs in cortical bone, at sites where resorption produces a cylindrical cutting cone; this cone is then filled in with new bone to form an osteon. Recent studies suggest that bone remodeling occurs within compartments limited by cells of the osteoblastic lineage, similar to the lining cells that cover the inactive surfaces of bone [7, 8, 9]. If this is correct, the extracellular milieu of the BMU may be quite different from that of the

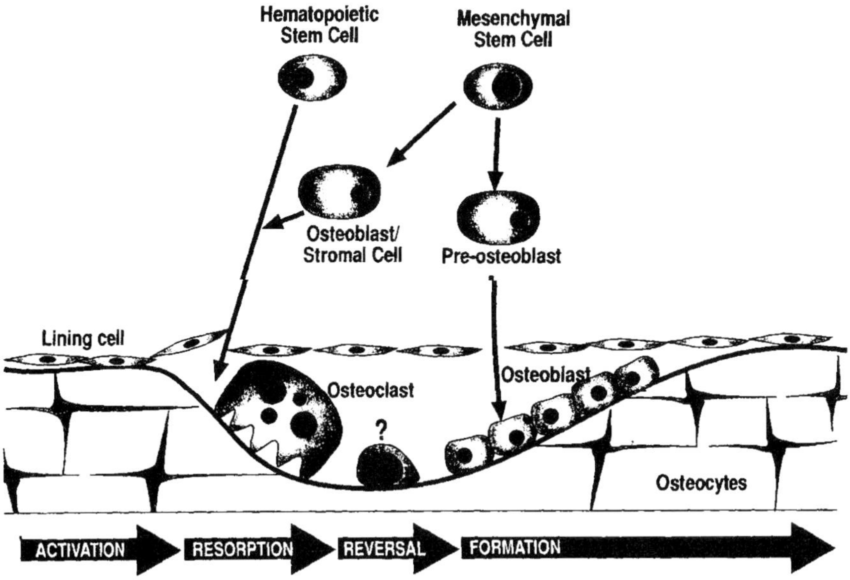

FIGURE 1 The bone remodeling cycle. The activation step probably requires an interaction between cells of the osteoblast lineage and hematopoietic cells as well as a change in the lining cells to facilitate access to the bone surface. This may also involve removal of a protein coat on the bone by secretion of metalloproteinases. In this figure the "compartmentalization" of the BMU is indicated in the form of a continuous sheet of lining cells. The reversal phase is carried out by a cell which may be of either monocyte-macrophage or mesenchymal origin. An alternative way to initiate the formation phase might be to convert lining cells to active osteoblasts.

general circulation. This compartmentalization might result in increased concentrations of ions and other regulatory factors in the BMU.

The remodeling cycle has been divided into four phases: *activation*, *resorption*, *reversal*, and *formation*. The activation step involves an interaction between osteoblasts or their precursors and the hematopoietic cells which differentiate into osteoclasts. Although this interaction was proposed many years ago, the specific proteins responsible were identified only recently (see Figure 2) [10, 11]. Osteoblasts respond to a variety of local and systemic factors by altering their production of the specific proteins. One of these, macrophage colony stimulating factor (M-CSF or CSF-1), appears to be critical to the replication of osteoclast precursors and acts on a specific receptor called c-Fms [12, 13]. The osteoblasts and their precursors also express a ligand called Receptor Activator of Nuclear Factor κB Ligand (RANKL), which interacts with RANK on the osteoclast precursors to stimulate the formation and maintain the activity of osteoclasts. A third protein, osteoprotegerin (OPG), inhibits this interaction by acting as a decoy receptor for RANKL. The rate of bone breakdown appears to be determined by the relative amounts of RANKL and OPG that are produced. Thus mice lacking OPG show severe osteoporosis [14]. This finding led to an exploration of the possibility that OPG deficiency was the cause of osteoporosis, but in fact OPG levels appear to increase in patients

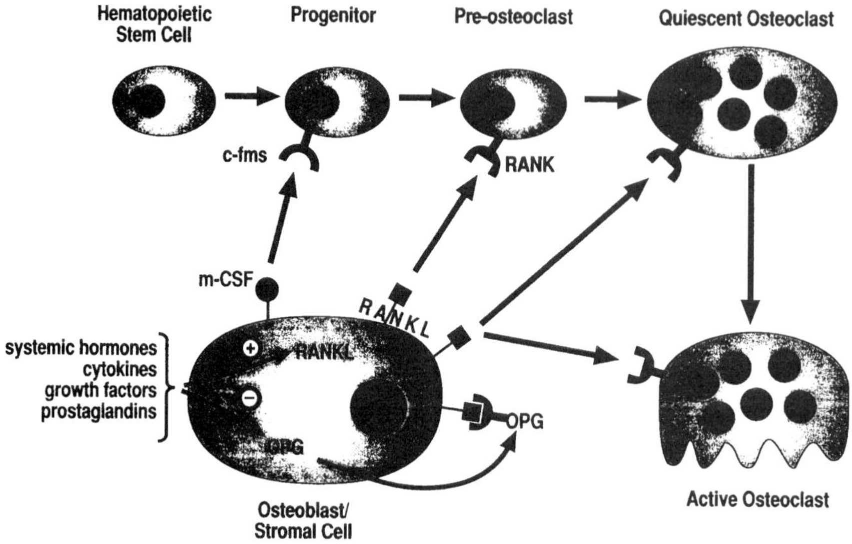

FIGURE 2 The osteoblast-osteoclast interaction. The hormones and local factors that stimulate bone resorption act largely on osteoblasts or stromal cells to increase production of RANKL and decrease production of OPG, thus favoring osteoclastogenesis. As noted in the text, cytokines may also act directly on the hematopoietic lineage. As shown here, the interaction between RANKL and RANK is not only important for formation of osteoclasts but for maintaining their activity and survival.

with high rates of bone breakdown, probably as a compensatory mechanism [15]. While OPG deficiency does not appear to be pathogenetic in osteoporosis, OPG or other compounds that block the RANKL–RANK interaction are effective in inhibiting bone resorption and may be useful therapeutic agents [16]. The driving forces for increased bone resorption are largely the hormones and local factors that act on the osteoblasts, including parathyroid hormone (PTH), calcitriol, and thyroid hormone among the systemic hormones, and interleukins, prostaglandins, and tumor necrosis factor alpha (TNFα) among the local hormones. In addition, the many growth factors that can stimulate bone formation, such as insulin-like growth factor-1 (IGF-1) and fibroblast growth factor-2 (FGF-2), may also stimulate osteoclastic bone resorption [17, 18].

Resorption is accomplished by fully differentiated osteoclasts, which fasten onto the bone with a large circular sealing zone, within which a ruffled border is formed that secretes hydrogen ions to dissolve the mineral and enzymes to break down the matrix. Matrix breakdown is accomplished by a concert of enzymes. Cathepsin K appears to be the most important of these, but other critical enzymes include tartrate resistant acid–phosphatase (TRAP) and metalloproteinases [19, 20]. Because of the complex machinery involved in cell adhesion—the secretion of hydrogen ions and enzymes and the transfer of the products of bone resorption across the osteoclast—these cells require a large number of interacting and relatively specific components of cell machinery. A number of inhibitors of these processes have been developed and might be used as drugs to block osteoclastic bone breakdown [21, 22].

It is not clear what makes osteoclastic bone resorption stop. Local products of bone resorption, such as transforming growth factor β (TGFβ) released from the matrix or calcium itself, may block further activity. The osteoclast probably has a finite lifespan, and its nuclei appear to be programmed to undergo early apoptosis [23]. This rate of apoptosis is another site of regulation by both systemic and local factors. For example, RANKL inhibits this process, and TGFβ and estradiol (E2) accelerate it [24]. Another largely unknown phenomenon is the mechanism for the migration of osteoclasts along the bone surface. The pathway is well defined in Haversian remodeling, in which the cutting cone is usually linear and of relatively uniform size, but it is quite irregular in trabecular remodeling, in which the size and shape of the Howship's lacunae vary greatly in size and shape.

Once the osteoclasts have completed resorbing at a specific site, a reversal phase involves cells that have not been well characterized [25, 26]. They may be lining cells or macrophages. They probably complete the resorption process by removing residual matrix. They may also prepare the surface by secreting a mucopolysaccharide-rich matrix material, the so-called cement line, which facilitates attachment of the packet of new bone that completes the BMU.

The final phase is bone formation. Osteoblastic precursors migrate to the cell surface and differentiate into polygonal cells that produce large amounts of collagen. The collagenous matrix is not mineralized immediately, but undergoes a number of extracellular modifications including hydroxylation of lysines, the formation of crosslinks between collagen molecules, and the deposition and removal of non-collagen proteins at specific sites that regulate mineralization. Mineralization begins several microns away from the osteoblasts. Because formation takes months, compared to the weeks required for resorption, any increase in the rate of resorption will weaken the bone by producing multiple Howship's lacunae or Haversian canals that have not been filled in. These irregularities in bone structure probably produce fragility beyond what might be expected from the amount of bone lost. When osteoblasts complete their work of depositing new bone, they undergo one of three fates: A few osteoblasts become flattened lining cells, a larger number become buried inside the bone as osteocytes, and some undergo apoptosis [23].

The osteoblasts, lining cells, and osteocytes form a syncytium in which thin extensions of these cells are carried through small canaliculi within the bone and connect to each other through gap junctions. This network is able to sense mechanical forces when small strains are placed upon the bone, probably through the fluid shear stress that occurs in the canaliculi and around the osteocytes [27]. The skeleton can then respond to these forces with appropriate changes in formation and resorption. The osteocytes can produce signaling molecules, such as nitric oxide (NO) and prostaglandin E_2 (PGE_2), which may mediate these changes. Loading may also stimulate production of IGF-1 by osteocytes [28]. The interaction of local and systemic factors in the regulation of this system may be critical in the pathogenesis of osteoporosis [29, 30].

IV. SYSTEMIC REGULATORS OF BONE GROWTH AND REMODELING

A large number of systemic hormones act on bone cells (see Table 1). They can be classified into calcium-regulating hormones, such as PTH, calcitriol, and calcitonin, and general growth-regulating hormones, such as thyroid hormone, the growth hormone (GH) IGF-1 system, glucocorticoids, and sex hormones. Other hormones have recently been implicated in the regulation of bone metabolism, such as leptin, amylin, and neuropeptides [31, 32, 33], but their specific roles in human bone metabolism have not been defined.

While the primary role of PTH is considered to be the maintenance of serum calcium concentration, this hormone is also critical in maintaining bone turnover [34, 35]. PTH stimulates both resorption and formation and increases bone remodeling. The remarkable fact that the stimulation of bone formation predominates when small doses of PTH are given intermittently has led to its therapeutic use. PTH also acts on the kidney to increase phosphate excretion, which is critical for calcium regulation. Without this action of PTH, bone resorption would result in increased concentrations of both calcium and phosphate in the blood, which in turn could cause soft-tissue calcification. PTH also increases the activation of vitamin D to calcitriol, thus indirectly increasing intestinal absorption of calcium and phosphate.

The PTH receptor responds to a second hormone, parathyroid hormone–related protein (PTHRP), which is a local hormone that

TABLE 1 Systemic hormones affecting bone cells

Calcium-regulating hormones	Bone resorption	Bone formation
Parathyroid hormone	↑↑↑	↑↑↑
Calcitriol	↑↑	↑*
Calcitonin	↓↓	?
Other systemic hormones		
Growth hormone		
Insulin-like growth factor	↑	↑↑↑
Thyroid hormone	↑↑	↑↑
Cortisol	↑*	↓↓↓
Estradiol	↓↓	↑
Testosterone	↓	↑↑

Up arrows represent stimulation; down arrows represent inhibition. The number of arrows indicates the strength of the effect.

* These may be indirect effects (see text).

regulates cartilage and bone development [34]. PTHRP also has multiple sites of action, for example in mammary tissue, the pancreas, and the nervous system.

The vitamin D hormone system is remarkable for the complex steps involved in the formation of the active hormone calcitriol or 1,25 dihydroxyvitamin D [36, 37]. The precursor, vitamin D, is synthesized from the cholesterol in the skin through the action of ultraviolet light, hydroxylated in the liver to the circulating form, 25 hydroxyvitamin D, then converted to the active hormone by 1α-hydroxylase in the kidney. This system is regulated by calcium and phosphate as well as PTH. There are multiple actions on different tissues of the body. The most important action of calcitriol is to increase the absorption of calcium and phosphate in the intestine. It also stimulates bone resorption, which may be an emergency mechanism that supplies calcium and phosphate from skeletal stores when there is marked calcium and phosphate deficiency in the diet. Bone formation is increased indirectly by vitamin D increasing the supply of mineral, but there may also be some direct effects on bone formation.

The vitamin D system is essential for formation of hair follicles and probably plays a role in regulation of the immune system. Animals lacking the vitamin D receptor can have relatively normal bones if they are supplied with adequate amounts of calcium and phosphate in the diet or by injection. They may still show non-genomic responses to calcitriol [38]. However, they still have alopecia and abnormal immune responses that cannot be reversed by supplying calcium and phosphorus [39, 40, 41].

Calcitonin is the most recently discovered of the calcium-regulating hormones [42]. Its late discovery may be due to the fact that it does not play an important role in calcium regulation in human adults. C-cells in the thyroid gland secrete calcitonin in response to high calcium concentrations, and calcitonin then blocks bone breakdown by inactivating osteoclasts. Its effects on osteoclasts are relatively transient, perhaps because the receptors are rapidly down-regulated. Hence patients with medullary carcinoma of the thyroid who have extremely high serum levels of calcitonin can still remodel bone. Surprisingly, knockout of the calcitonin gene in mice produced a phenotype with increased bone formation and bone mass [43]. Thus calcitonin or its alternative transcript, calcitonin gene-related peptide, may also play a role in bone formation.

The GH–IGF-1 system is the key regulator of skeletal growth during childhood and adolescence. IGF-II, which is not under GH control, is a critical regulator of skeletal growth during fetal life. GH secretion is under neural control. The hypothalamus produces growth hormone–releasing hormone (GHRH), a stimulator, and somatostatin, an inhibitor. In addition, the gastric hormone ghrelin can affect growth hormone release [44]. The extent to which IGF-I is a systemic or local hormone remains uncertain. Knockout of hepatic IGF-I production, which is the major source of the circulating form, causes only minimal impairment of growth in mice [45]. Thus IGF-1 production by osteoblasts may be more important than circulating IGF-1 in maintaining skeletal growth [46]. The GH–IGF-I system can control the size of the skeleton. Excessive production results in gigantism before puberty and acromegaly after puberty. Any impairment of the GH–IGF-I system will result in dwarfism [47].

Thyroid hormones increase the activity of all the cells of the body, including bone cells. Thus thyroid hormone excess results in increased bone turnover and may increase fracture risk [48, 49]. Recent data also suggest that thyroid stimulating hormone (TSH) may have a direct effect on bone metabolism [50].

Cortisol, the major hormone of the adrenal gland in humans, and its rodent counterpart corticosterone, are critical regulators of bone metabolism [51]. The major effect of cortisol on the skeleton is to inhibit bone formation, but a certain amount of this hormone is necessary for normal differentiation of osteoblasts [52]. The diurnal rhythm of cortisol secretion, with low levels in the afternoon and evening, is probably critical for bone growth. Low cortisol and high GH at night may increase osteoblastic replication and activity. Cortisol can also have indirect effects on the skeleton through its effects on the pituitary, muscle, and the intestine. These tend to increase bone resorption.

Sex hormones are critical regulators of skeletal growth and remodeling [53]. Since Fuller Albright proposed that estrogen deficiency was the cause of postmenopausal osteoporosis more than 60 years ago, many studies of estrogen action on bone have been conducted. The precise effects of estrogen are still not fully understood, however, perhaps because estrogen has many different effects on bone cells. Moreover, estrogen may be synthesized in bone cells by local aromatase [54]. Estrogen effects on bone may be mediated by different pathways than those for classic targets since they require much lower doses [55, 56].

There is evidence that estrogen inhibits bone resorption by acting on hematopoietic cell precursors to decrease formation of osteoclasts as well as by acting on osteoblasts to increase the production of OPG [53]. Estrogen may act directly on differentiated osteoclasts to accelerate apoptosis [24]. Some of the effects of estrogen on bone are probably mediated by cytokines. A number of these have been implicated as mediators of estrogen action in animal models, including interleukin-1 (IL-1), IL-7, IL-11, TNFα, and TGFβ [57, 58]. Estrogen slows bone remodeling by decreasing the activation of new BMUs, resulting in an overall decrease in bone formation. Estrogen probably has a direct anabolic effect on osteoblasts, however. For example, the ability of mechanical loading to stimulate bone formation is impaired in animals lacking an estrogen receptor [59]. Also, studies using biochemical markers of bone turnover suggest that estrogen may have a direct effect to increase bone formation [60]. Thus, in estrogen deficiency there is not only an increase in bone remodeling, but also a failure of bone formation to keep pace, so that bone mass decreases.

It is now well established that estrogen regulates bone turnover in men in much the same way it does in women. This was first recognized from observations in men with defects in the estrogen receptor or in the aromatase gene, which is responsible for converting testosterone to estrogen [61]. These individuals had osteoporosis with high bone turnover. More recently, studies of men in whom both testosterone and estrogen production are blocked by treatment with gonadotrophin-releasing hormone agonists and aromatase inhibitors have shown that estrogen is a more effective inhibitor of bone resorption than testosterone [60]. Thus while testosterone has effects on bone similar to the effects of estrogen, it appears to produce a greater stimulation of bone formation than inhibition of bone resorption [62]. Testosterone may also act indirectly on bone by stimulating muscle growth and increasing the stress put on the skeleton.

Despite considerable study, there is still no clear evidence that progesterone has a direct effect on skeletal tissue in adult humans. Effects on fetal skeletal growth have been demonstrated [63], but studies in postmenopausal women have shown no significant effect of progestins on bone turnover [64].

V. LOCAL REGULATORS OF BONE REMODELING

The first potential local regulator of bone remodeling to be identified was prostaglandin E_2, more than 30 years ago [65]. Subsequently, cytokines that regulate immune responses were shown to stimulate bone resorption and inhibit formation [66]. Cells of the osteoblastic lineage produce their own growth factors, which can regulate replication, differentiation, and lifespan [67, 68]. These factors are critical to the ability of bone to adapt to changes in mechanical loading and to repair both microdamage and fractures. There is also increasing evidence that the effects of systemic hormones are mediated to a greater or lesser degree by their ability to alter the production of these local factors. There are now numerous studies suggesting that the effects of estrogen are mediated by changes in one or more of the cytokines that stimulate bone resorption, including IL-1, IL-6, IL-7, and IL-11 as well as TNFα [57, 58, 69]. Most of these studies are based on knockout or inhibition studies in rodent models, however. The role of these cytokines in human bone disease has not been established. One likely possibility is that cytokines and other local factors such as prostaglandins act in concert to produce additive or synergistic effects on bone remodeling [70]. In this case, removal or inhibition of one cytokine might cause substantial effects even though several other cytokines were important in the skeletal response.

Prostaglandins and nitric oxide have complex effects on bone [71, 72]. They can be produced both by bone cells themselves and by adjacent endothelial and hematopoietic cells. The major prostaglandin produced in bone is PGE_2, a potent stimulator of bone resorption and formation [73]. Many of the systemic and local factors that stimulate bone resorption and formation also increase prostaglandin production in bone cells by initiating the synthesis of the inducible form of cyclo-oxygenase (COX-2) [74, 75, 76, 77]. This induction appears to be critical to the late anabolic response that occurs after brief episodes of impact loading [78, 79]. Prostaglandin production is increased not only by hormones and cytokines, but also by high calcium concentrations and by prostaglandins themselves [80, 81]. The latter provide an amplification system that can enhance the skeletal response to mechanical loading, as well as the response to inflammation. In addition to the factors produced by cells of the osteoblast lineage, hematopoietic cells probably play multiple roles as producers of and responders to cytokines in bone remodeling. There is evidence for interaction between T-cells and osteoclast precursors, presumably of the monocyte-macrophage lineage. T-cells can produce inhibitors of osteoclastogenesis, such as IL-4, IL-12, and possibly IL-3 [82, 83]. T-cells may also activate hematopoietic osteoclastogenesis by producing RANKL [84] and may also have a direct effect on osteoblasts [85]. Additional T-cell mechanisms involving TNF-α have been proposed as mediators of the effect of estrogen on bone remodeling [58]. IL-7 may be a stimulus for this T-cell pathway [86], although it also can have a direct inhibitory effect on osteoclastogenesis [87].

Bone cells produce a number of growth factors, perhaps the most of important of which is IGF-1. In addition, fibroblast growth factor (FGF-2), platelet-derived growth factor (PDGF), and vascular endothelial growth factor (VEGF) can be produced by osteoblasts and may regulate their function. The TGFβ family includes not only this agonist, but also a series of bone morphogenetic proteins (BMPs) [88]. These are potent stimulators of bone formation and also act on the growth and differentiation of many other body tissues. In addition to the TGFβ/BMP family, a new regulatory pathway determining bone mass has recently been defined. This discovery was based on analysis of a family with unusually high bone mass and normal skeletal architecture. These individuals were found to have an activating mutation of Lipoprotein Receptor Related Protein-5 (LRP-5) gene, a component of the Wnt signaling pathway [89, 90]. Activation of LRP-5 results in increased bone mass, and deletion of this receptor causes marked osteoporosis in the so-called "osteoporosis-pseudoglioma syndrome" [91].

VI. CONCLUSION

This brief overview is intended to provide a framework for a discussion of the many different pathogenetic mechanisms by which bone loss might occur after transplantation. The recent discovery of new regulators represents the beginning of an explosion of new genetic information concerning bone metabolism. The challenge will be to identify the role of these regulators in the skeletal changes that occur after transplantation and in other metabolic disorders of bone.

REFERENCES

1. Seeman, E. (2003). Periosteal bone formation—a neglected determinant of bone strength. *N Engl J Med.* 349(4):320–3.
2. Favus, M.J., ed. *Primer on the Metabolism Bone Diseases and Disorders of Universial Metabolism,* 4th ed. (1999). Philadelphia: Lipincott Williams & Wilkins.
3. Bilezikian, J.P., Raisz, L.G., and Rodan, G.A., ed. *Principles of Bone Biology*, 2nd ed. (2001). San Diego: Academic Press.
4. Marcus, R., Feldman, D., and Kelsey, J. *Osteoporosis*, 2nd ed. (2001). San Diego: Academic Press.
5. Raisz, L.G. and G.A. Rodan. (2003). Pathogenesis of osteoporosis. *Endocrinol Metab Clin North Am.* 32(1):15–24.
6. Kontulainen, S., et al. (2003). Effect of long-term impact-loading on mass, size, and estimated strength of humerus and radius of female racquet-sports players: a peripheral quantitative computed tomography study between young and old starters and controls. *J Bone Miner Res.* 18(2):352–9.
7. Hauge, E.M., et al. (2001). Cancellous bone remodeling occurs in specialized compartments lined by cells expressing osteoblastic markers. *J Bone Miner Res.* 16(9):1575–82.
8. Parfitt, A.M. (2001). The bone remodeling compartment: a circulatory function for bone lining cells. *J Bone Miner Res.* 16(9):1583–5.
9. Compston, J.E. (2002). Bone marrow and bone: a functional unit. *J Endocrinol.* 173(3):387–94.
10. Rodan, G.A. and T.J. Martin. (1982). Role of osteoblasts in hormonal control of bone resorption—a hypothesis. *Calcif Tissue Int.* 34(3):311.
11. Khosla, S. (2001). Minireview: the OPG/RANKL/RANK system. *Endocrinology.* 142(12):5050–5.
12. Yao, G.Q., et al. (1998). The cell-surface form of colony-stimulating factor-1 is regulated by osteotropic agents and supports formation of multinucleated osteoclast-like cells. *J Biol Chem.* 273(7):4119–28.
13. Van Wesenbeeck, L., et al. (2002). The osteopetrotic mutation toothless (tl) is a loss-of-function frameshift mutation in the rat Csf1 gene: Evidence of a crucial role for CSF-1 in osteoclastogenesis and endochondral ossification. *Proc Natl Acad Sci U S A.* 99(22):14303–8.
14. Bucay, N., et al. (1998). Osteoprotegerin-deficient mice develop early onset osteoporosis and arterial calcification. *Genes Dev.* 12(9):1260–8.
15. Khosla, S., et al. (2002). Correlates of osteoprotegerin levels in women and men. *Osteoporos Int.* 13(5):394–9.
16. Cheng, X., et al. (2004). Disabling of receptor activator of nuclear factor-Kappa B (RANK) receptor complex by novel osteoprotegerin-like peptidomimetics restores bone loss in vivo. *J Biol Chem.* 279(9):8269–8277.
17. Guicheux, J., et al. (1998). Growth hormone stimulatory effects on osteoclastic resorption are partly mediated by insulin-like growth factor I: an in vitro study. *Bone.* 22(1):25–31.
18. Hurley, M.M., et al. (1998). Basic fibroblast growth factor induces osteoclast formation in murine bone marrow cultures. *Bone.* 22(4):309–16.
19. Hollberg, K., et al. (2002). Osteoclasts from mice deficient in tartrate-resistant acid phosphatase have altered ruffled borders and disturbed intracellular vesicular transport. *Exp Cell Res.* 279(2):227–38.

20. Delaisse, J.M., et al. (2003). Matrix metalloproteinases (MMP) and cathepsin K contribute differently to osteoclastic activities. *Microsc Res Tech.* 61(6):504–13.
21. Zaidi, M., et al. (2001). Cathepsin K, osteoclastic resorption, and osteoporosis therapy. *J Bone Miner Res.* 16(10):1747–9.
22. Teti, A., S. Migliaccio, and R. Baron, (2002). The role of the alphaVbeta3 integrin in the development of osteolytic bone metastases: a pharmacological target for alternative therapy? *Calcif Tissue Int.* 71(4):293–9.
23. Manolagas, S.C. (2000). Birth and death of bone cells: basic regulatory mechanisms and implications for the pathogenesis and treatment of osteoporosis. *Endocr Rev.* 21(2):115–37.
24. Hughes, D.E., et al. (1996). Estrogen promotes apoptosis of murine osteoclasts mediated by TGF-beta. *Nat Med.* 2(10):1132–6.
25. Everts, V., et al. (2002). The bone lining cell: its role in cleaning Howship's lacunae and initiating bone formation. *J Bone Miner Res.* 17(1):77–90.
26. Domon, T., et al. (2001). The nature and function of mononuclear cells on the resorbed surfaces of bone in the reversal phase during remodeling. *Ann Anat.* 183(2):103–10.
27. Klein-Nulend, J., et al. (1997). Pulsating fluid flow stimulates prostaglandin release and inducible prostaglandin G/H synthase mRNA expression in primary mouse bone cells. *J Bone Miner Res.* 12(1):45–51.
28. Lean, J.M., et al. (1996). Osteocytic expression of mRNA for c-fos and IGF-I: an immediate early gene response to an osteogenic stimulus. *Am J Physiol.* 270(6 Pt 1):E937–45.
29. Jagger, C.J., J.W. Chow, and T.J. Chambers. (1996). Estrogen suppresses activation but enhances formation phase of osteogenic response to mechanical stimulation in rat bone. *J Clin Invest.* 98(10):2351–7.
30. Lanyon, L. and T. Skerry. (2001). Postmenopausal osteoporosis as a failure of bone's adaptation to functional loading: a hypothesis. *J Bone Miner Res.* 16(11):1937–47.
31. Cornish, J., et al. (2000). Systemic administration of a novel octapeptide, amylin-(1–8), increases bone volume in male mice. *Am J Physiol Endocrinol Metab.* 279(4):E730–5.
32. Cornish, J., et al. (2002). Leptin directly regulates bone cell function in vitro and reduces bone fragility in vivo. *J Endocrinol.* 175(2):405–15.
33. Elefteriou, F., et al. (2003). Monosodium glutamate–sensitive hypothalamic neurons contribute to the control of bone mass. *Endocrinology.* 144(9):3842–7.
34. Stewart, A.F. (2002). Hyperparathyroidism, humoral hypercalcemia of malignancy, and the anabolic actions of parathyroid hormone and parathyroid hormone-related protein on the skeleton. *J Bone Miner Res.* 17(5):758–62.
35. Rubin, M.R., et al. (2002). The anabolic effects of parathyroid hormone. *Osteoporos Int.* 13(4):267–77.
36. Norman, A.W., et al. (2002). Update on biological actions of 1alpha,25(OH)(2)-vitamin D(3) (rapid effects) and 24R,25(OH)(2)-vitamin D(3). *Mol Cell Endocrinol.* 197(1–2):1–13.
37. Christakos, S., et al. (2003). New insights into the mechanisms of vitamin D action. *J Cell Biochem.* 88(4):695–705.
38. Boyan, B.D., et al. (2003). Membrane actions of vitamin D metabolites 1alpha,25(OH)2D3 and 24R,25(OH)2D3 are retained in growth plate cartilage cells from vitamin D receptor knockout mice. *J Cell Biochem.* 90(6):1207–23.
39. Panda, D.K., et al. (2001). Targeted ablation of the 25-hydroxyvitamin D 1alpha-hydroxylase enzyme: evidence for skeletal, reproductive, and immune dysfunction. *Proc Natl Acad Sci U S A.* 98(13):7498–503.
40. Sakai, Y., J. Kishimoto, and M.B. Demay. (2001). Metabolic and cellular analysis of alopecia in vitamin D receptor knockout mice. *J Clin Invest.* 107(8):961–6.
41. O'Kelly, J., et al. (2002). Normal myelopoiesis but abnormal T lymphocyte responses in vitamin D receptor knockout mice. *J Clin Invest.* 109(8):1091–9.
42. Sexton, P.M., D.M. Findlay, and T.J. Martin. (1999). Calcitonin. *Curr Med Chem.* 6(11):1067–93.

43. Hoff, A.O., et al. (2002). Increased bone mass is an unexpected phenotype associated with deletion of the calcitonin gene. *J Clin Invest.* 110(12):1849–57.
44. Merriam, G.R., R.S. Schwartz, and M.V. Vitiello. (2003). Growth hormone–releasing hormone and growth hormone secretagogues in normal aging. *Endocrine.* 22(1):41–8.
45. Sjogren, K., et al. (1999). Liver-derived insulin-like growth factor I (IGF-I) is the principal source of IGF-I in blood but is not required for postnatal body growth in mice. *Proc Natl Acad Sci U S A.* 96(12):7088–92.
46. Yakar, S. and C.J. Rosen. (2003). From mouse to man: redefining the role of insulin-like growth factor-I in the acquisition of bone mass. *Exp Biol Med (Maywood).* 228(3):245–52.
47. Maheshwari, H.G., et al. (2003). The impact of congenital, severe, untreated growth hormone (GH) deficiency on bone size and density in young adults: insights from genetic GH-releasing hormone receptor deficiency. *J Clin Endocrinol Metab.* 88(6):2614–8.
48. Akalin, A., et al. (2002). Bone remodelling markers and serum cytokines in patients with hyperthyroidism. *Clin Endocrinol (Oxf).* 57(1):125–9.
49. Vestergaard, P. and L. Mosekilde. (2002). Fractures in patients with hyperthyroidism and hypothyroidism: a nationwide follow-up study in 16,249 patients. *Thyroid.* 12(5):411–9.
50. Abe, E., et al. (2003). TSH is a negative regulator of skeletal remodeling. *Cell.* 115(2):151–62.
51. Canalis, E. and A.M. Delany. (2002). Mechanisms of glucocorticoid action in bone. *Ann NY Acad Sci.* 966:73–81.
52. Harrison, J.R., H.W. Woitge, and B.E. Kream. (2002). Genetic approaches to determine the role of glucocorticoid signaling in osteoblasts. *Endocrine.* 17(1):37–42.
53. Riggs, B.L., S. Khosla, and L.J. Melton, 3rd ed. (2002). Sex steroids and the construction and conservation of the adult skeleton. *Endocr Rev.* 23(3):279–302.
54. Compston, J. (2002). Local biosynthesis of sex steroids in bone. *J Clin Endocrinol Metab.* 87(12):5398–400.
55. Prestwood, K.M., et al. (2003). Ultralow-dose micronized 17beta-estradiol and bone density and bone metabolism in older women: a randomized controlled trial. *JAMA.* 290(8):1042–8.
56. Manolagas, S.C., S. Kousteni, and R.L. Jilka. (2002). Sex steroids and bone. *Recent Prog Horm Res.* 57:385–409.
57. Horowitz, M.C. (1993). Cytokines and estrogen in bone: anti-osteoporotic effects. *Science.* 260(5108):626–7.
58. Roggia, C., et al. (2001). Up-regulation of TNF-producing T cells in the bone marrow: a key mechanism by which estrogen deficiency induces bone loss in vivo. *Proc Natl Acad Sci U S A.* 98(24):13960–5.
59. Lee, K., et al. (2003). Endocrinology: bone adaptation requires oestrogen receptor-alpha. *Nature.* 424(6947):389.
60. Falahati-Nini, A., et al. (2000). Relative contributions of testosterone and estrogen in regulating bone resorption and formation in normal elderly men. *J Clin Invest.* 106(12):1553–60.
61. Herrmann, B.L., et al. (2002). Impact of estrogen replacement therapy in a male with congenital aromatase deficiency caused by a novel mutation in the CYP19 gene. *J Clin Endocrinol Metab.* 87(12):5476–84.
62. Leder, B.Z., et al. (2003). Differential effects of androgens and estrogens on bone turnover in normal men. *J Clin Endocrinol Metab.* 88(1):204–10.
63. Manzi, D.L., C.C. Pilbeam, and L.G. Raisz. (1994). The anabolic effects of progesterone on fetal rat calvaria in tissue culture. *J Soc Gynecol Investig.* 1(4):302–9.
64. Azizi, G., A. Hansen, and K.M. Prestwood. (2003). Effect of micronized progesterone on bone turnover in postmenopausal women on estrogen replacement therapy. *Endocr Res.* 29(2):133–40.
65. Klein, D.C. and L.G. Raisz. (1970). Prostaglandins: stimulation of bone resorption in tissue culture. *Endocrinology.* 86(6):1436–40.

66. Raisz, L.G., et al. (1975). Effect of osteoclast activating factor from human leukocytes on bone metabolism. *J Clin Invest*. 56(2):408–13.
67. Montero, A., et al. (2000). Disruption of the fibroblast growth factor-2 gene results in decreased bone mass and bone formation. *J Clin Invest*. 105(8):1085–93.
68. Woitge, H.W. and B.E. Kream. (2000). Calvariae from fetal mice with a disrupted Igf1 gene have reduced rates of collagen synthesis but maintain responsiveness to glucocorticoids. *J Bone Miner Res*. 15(10):1956–64.
69. Lorenzo, J.A., et al. (1998). Mice lacking the type I interleukin-1 receptor do not lose bone mass after ovariectomy. *Endocrinology*. 139(6):3022–5.
70. Tai, H., et al. (1997). Transcriptional induction of cyclooxygenase-2 in osteoblasts is involved in interleukin-6-induced osteoclast formation. *Endocrinology*. 138(6):2372–9.
71. Chow, J.W., et al. (1998). Role of nitric oxide and prostaglandins in mechanically induced bone formation. *J Bone Miner Res*. 13(6):1039–44.
72. Raisz, L.G. (1999). Prostaglandins and bone: physiology and pathophysiology. *Osteoarthritis Cartilage*. 7(4):419–21.
73. Zhou, H., et al. (2001). Lumbar vertebral cancellous bone is capable of responding to PGE2 treatment by stimulating both modeling and remodeling-dependent bone gain in aged male rats. *Calcif Tissue Int*. 68(3):179–84.
74. Kawaguchi, H., et al. (1994). Regulation of the two prostaglandin G/H synthases by parathyroid hormone, interleukin-1, cortisol, and prostaglandin E2 in cultured neonatal mouse calvariae. *Endocrinology*. 135(3):1157–64.
75. Okada, Y., et al. (2000). Prostaglandin G/H synthase-2 is required for maximal formation of osteoclast-like cells in culture. *J Clin Invest*. 105(6):823–32.
76. Chikazu, D., et al. (2002). Bone morphogenetic protein 2 induces cyclo-oxygenase 2 in osteoblasts via a Cbfal binding site: role in effects of bone morphogenetic protein 2 in vitro and in vivo. *J Bone Miner Res*. 17(8):1430–40.
77. Pilbeam, C.C., et al. (1997). Regulation of inducible prostaglandin G/H synthase by interleukin-1, transforming growth factors-alpha and -beta, and prostaglandins in bone cells. *Adv Exp Med Biol*. 400B:617–23.
78. Wadhwa, S., et al. (2002). Fluid flow induction of cyclo-oxygenase 2 gene expression in osteoblasts is dependent on an extracellular signal-regulated kinase signaling pathway. *J Bone Miner Res*. 17(2):266–74.
79. Forwood, M.R. (1996). Inducible cyclo-oxygenase (COX-2) mediates the induction of bone formation by mechanical loading in vivo. *J Bone Miner Res*. 11(11):1688–93.
80. Choudhary, S., et al. (2003). Extracellular calcium is a potent inducer of cyclo-oxygenase-2 in murine osteoblasts through an ERK signaling pathway. *J Bone Miner Res*. 18(10):1813–24.
81. Pilbeam, C.C., et al. (1995). Autoregulation of inducible prostaglandin G/H synthase in osteoblastic cells by prostaglandins. *J Bone Miner Res*. 10(3):406–14.
82. Mirosavljevic, D., et al. (2003). T-cells mediate an inhibitory effect of interleukin-4 on osteoclastogenesis. *J Bone Miner Res*. 18(6):984–93.
83. Khapli, S.M., et al. (2003). IL-3 acts directly on osteoclast precursors and irreversibly inhibits receptor activator of NF-kappa B ligand-induced osteoclast differentiation by diverting the cells to macrophage lineage. *J Immunol*. 171(1):142–51.
84. Udagawa, N., et al. (2002). The molecular mechanism of osteoclastogenesis in rheumatoid arthritis. *Arthritis Res*. 4(5):281–9.
85. Rifas, L., S. Arackal, and M.N. Weitzmann. (2003). Inflammatory T cells rapidly induce differentiation of human bone marrow stromal cells into mature osteoblasts. *J Cell Biochem*. 88(4):650–9.
86. Toraldo, G., et al. (2003). IL-7 induces bone loss in vivo by induction of receptor activator of nuclear factor kappa B ligand and tumor necrosis factor alpha from T cells. *Proc Natl Acad Sci U S A*. 100(1):125–30.
87. Lee, S.K., et al. (2003). Interleukin-7 is a direct inhibitor of in vitro osteoclastogenesis. *Endocrinology*. 144(8):3524–31.

88. Canalis, E., A.N. Economides, and E. Gazzerro. (2003). Bone morphogenetic proteins, their antagonists, and the skeleton. *Endocr Rev.* 24(2):218–35.
89. Little, R.D., et al. (2002). A mutation in the LDL receptor-related protein 5 gene results in the autosomal dominant high-bone-mass trait. *Am J Hum Genet.* 70(1):11–9.
90. Boyden, L.M., et al. (2002). High bone density due to a mutation in LDL-receptor-related protein 5. *N Engl J Med.* 346(20):1513–21.
91. Gong, Y., et al. (2001). LDL receptor-related protein 5 (LRP5) affects bone accrual and eye development. *Cell.* 107(4):513–23.

CHAPTER 3

Skeletal Effects of Glucocorticoids: Basic and Clinical Aspects

Ernesto Canalis, MD
Department of Research, Saint Francis Hospital and Medical Center, Hartford, CT, and
The University of Connecticut School of Medicine, Farmington, CT

I. INTRODUCTION

The number and function of cells present in the bone microenvironment determine skeletal homeostasis, which is regulated by hormones, factors present in the bone microenvironment, and intracellular proteins [1, 2]. Glucocorticoids have unique actions in skeletal cells, and continued exposure of skeletal tissue to these steroids leads to severe osteoporosis [3, 4]. Following the initial exposure of skeletal tissue to glucocorticoids, there is significant bone loss and glucocorticoids, even at modest doses frequently considered to be in the physiological range, increase the risk of osteoporotic fractures [5]. The mechanisms involved are complex since glucocortocoids have direct and indirect effects on the skeleton and cause increased bone resorption and decreased bone formation [6]. Recent discoveries have provided new insights on the cellular events leading to the bone loss of glucocorticoid-induced osteoporosis (GIO). Advances in the management of GIO and availability of effective therapeutic alternatives offer possible solutions to patients affected by this condition.

II. MECHANISMS OF GLUCOCORTICOID ACTION IN BONE

Bone biopsies from patients exposed to glucocorticoids reveal increased bone resorption and decreased bone formation [7]. The initial loss of bone is probably secondary to an increase in bone resorption, but patients with GIO eventually develop a state of decreased bone remodeling. The increased bone resorption is secondary to effects of glucocorticoids on mineral metabolism and skeletal cells (see Table 1). In addition, patients receiving glucocorticoids often have an underlying inflammatory disease that by itself carries a risk of osteoporosis, and the mechanisms often involve the secretion of bone-resorbing cytokines.

Glucocorticoids decrease calcium absorption in the gastrointestinal system, causing resistance to vitamin D, and they increase the urinary excretion of calcium [8]. This may result in a degree of secondary hyperparathyroidism. This concept has been challenged, however, since the serum levels of parathyroid hormone (PTH) are modestly elevated and are not in the hyperparathyroid range in patients exposed to glucocorticoids [9]. Furthermore, examination of biopsies from patients with GIO and patients with hyperparathyroidism reveal different skeletal disorders. In hyperparathyroidism there is increased remodeling, whereas in GIO there is decreased remodeling.

Patients exposed to glucocorticoids may develop hypogonadism, and some of the bone loss observed in GIO may be due to estrogen or androgen deficiency. In estrogen deficiency, there is increased resorption secondary to the excessive secretion of cytokines, such as interleukin 6 and tumor necrosis factor α, by T lymphocytes [10, 11]. These cytokines may play a role in the enhanced bone resorption observed following glucocorticoid exposure. Although the indirect effects of glucocorticoids on bone resorption are important, their direct actions on skeletal cells may be more significant with respect to the observed bone loss. Glucocorticoids regulate the receptor activator of nuclear factor-κB ligand (RANK-L) and osteoprotegerin axis. RANK-L is an osteoblastic secreted protein that, following binding to its receptor in cells in the osteoclast lineage, induces osteoclastogenesis in the presence of colony stimulating factor–1 (CSF-1) [12]. Osteoprotegerin is a decoy receptor for RANK-L and prevents RANK-L binding to its signaling receptor, precluding osteoclastogenesis. Glucocorticoids increase the expression of RANK-L and CSF-1 and decrease osteoprotegerin expression

TABLE 1 Mechanisms of glucocorticoid action in bone

- Indirect effects
  - -Decreased intestinal calcium absorption
  - -Hypercalciuria
  - -Hypogonadism
- Direct effects: Cells of the osteoclast lineage
  - -Increased osteoclastogenesis
  - -Changes in osteoclast life span
- Direct effects: Cells of the osteoblast lineage
  - -Shift cell differentiation from osteoblasts to adipocytes
  - -Shortened life span of mature osteoblasts and osteocytes
  - -Decreased osteoblastic function and IGF I transcription

in osteoblasts and stromal cells [13, 14]. These effects may explain the increased osteoclastogenesis and bone resorption observed following exposure of skeletal tissue to glucocorticoids. It is important to note that RANK-L and CSF-1 are osteoblastic signals. Consequently, as glucocorticoids deplete the osteoblastic cell population, the signals are lost with a consequent decrease in osteoclastogenesis and bone remodeling. Glucocorticoids also regulate osteoclast apoptosis, although both increased and decreased apoptosis have been reported [15, 16]. Glucocorticoids oppose the effects of bisphosphonates on osteoclast cell death, prolonging the life of the osteoclast and possibly contributing to the bone resorption observed. The enhanced osteoclastic apoptosis and decreased osteoclastogenesis explain the eventual decrease in bone remodeling.

In addition to their effects on osteoclastic bone resorption, glucocorticoids regulate the expression of collagenases, matrix metalloproteinases (MMP) that cleave collagen fibrils at neutral pH. Collagenases regulate matrix breakdown. Three collagenases have been described: collagenase 1 (MMP-1), collagenase 2 (MMP-8), and collagenase 3 (MMP-13). Osteoblasts synthesize collagenase 1 and 3, which cleave type I collagen fibrils and the activity of which is required for bone resorption [17]. Cortisol increases collagenase 3 synthesis by post-transcriptional mechanisms, prolonging the half-life of collagenase 3 mRNA in osteoblasts [18]. mRNA regions responsible for transcript stabilization are located in the 3′ untranslated region (UTR) of the RNA, which contains AU-rich elements (AREs) responsible for mRNA stabilization. Glucocorticoids enhance the formation of protein-3′ UTR complexes to the AREs and as such modify the half-life of the collagenase transcript.

Studies on the actions of glucocorticoids in bone consistently reveal direct inhibitory effects on osteoblastogenesis, osteoblast function, and bone formation. These are central to the mechanisms of glucocorticoid action in bone. Glucocorticoids have significant effects on cells of the osteoblastic lineage, dependent on the stage of cell differentiation [19, 20, 21]. Some investigators have reported that glucocorticoids induce osteoblastic cell differentiation, an effect that is dependent on specific culture conditions and inconsistent with the loss of cells of the osteoblastic lineage occurring after glucocorticoid exposure. Recently, we have shown that glucocorticoids impair the differentiation of stromal cells toward cells of the osteoblastic lineage and prevent the terminal differentiation of quasi-mature osteoblastic cells, resulting in a decreased pool of mature osteoblasts [20, 21]. Glucocorticoids also induce apoptosis of mature osteoblasts and osteocytes, which, in association with the impaired cell differentiation, results in a reduced number of bone-forming cells [22].

Glucocorticoids shift the differentiation of stromal cells away from the osteoblastic and toward the adipocytic lineage. This shift involves the regulation of nuclear factors of the CCAAT/enhancer binding protein (C/EBP) family and peroxisome proliferator activated receptor $\gamma 2$ (PPAR$\gamma 2$) [20]. Six C/EBPs have been identified. Recently, we confirmed that glucocorticoids induce adipogenesis and enhance the expression of

C/EBP α, β, and δ in osteoblasts. C/EBPs contain a highly conserved DNA binding domain and a leucine dimerization domain through which they form homo- and hetero-dimers [23]. These dimers bind to specific DNA sequences and regulate transcription directly or by interacting with other nuclear factors. C/EBP α, β, and δ play essential roles in adipogenesis, and mice with null mutations of these genes have defective adipocyte formation [24]. Because these C/EBPs are essential for adipogenesis, their induction by cortisol in association with a shift in cellular differentiation suggests that C/EBP α, β, and δ play a role in the effect of glucocorticoids directing mesenchymal cells away from the osteoblastic and toward the adipocytic pathway. In addition, glucocorticoids regulate PPARγ2, which plays a role in their adipogenic effect [25].

The shift of osteoblast toward adipocyte differentiation caused by glucocorticoids involves complex cellular signals, including the induction of Notch1 mRNA [26, 27]. Notch1 to 4 are closely related, conserved transmembrane receptors that mediate signaling mechanisms controlling cell fate decisions [28, 29]. The ligands for Notch, Delta 1 through 4, and Serrate/Jagged 1 and 2 are single-pass transmembrane proteins, which bind and are required for the activation of the Notch receptor on neighboring cells. Notch1 and 2 and their ligands, Delta 1 and Jagged 1, are expressed by osteoblasts, whereas Notch3 and 4 are not [26, 30]. Like glucocorticoids, activated Notch1 receptors prevent osteoblast differentiation and chondrocyte maturation favoring adipogenesis. Consequently, Notch1 and cortisol have common effects in cell differentiation, and the induction of Notch 1 by glucocorticoids may play a role in the shifting of cell differentiation away from osteoblasts.

Glucocorticoids also inhibit the function of differentiated cells. They inhibit the synthesis of type I collagen by transcriptional and posttranscriptional mechanisms [31]. Collagen is the main component of the extracellular matrix, and its decrease results in less bone matrix available for mineralization. In addition to the direct actions of glucocorticoids on the fate, function, and life span of cells of the osteoblastic lineage, glucocorticoids regulate the synthesis, receptor binding, and binding proteins of growth factors present in the bone microenvironment. Bone cells secrete a variety of growth factors, but glucocorticoids affect primarily insulin-like growth factor (IGF I) [32]. Glucocorticoids and IGF I have opposite effects on skeletal metabolism. IGF I increases the function of mature osteoblasts, increasing bone collagen synthesis and bone formation rates *in vitro* and *in vivo*. Consequently, it is not surprising that glucocorticoids suppress *Igf1* gene transcription. The rat *Igf1* gene consists of six exons with clusters of transcription initiation sites in exon 1 and 2. Our laboratory established that cortisol suppresses transcription from *Igf1* exon 1 [32]. Mutation analysis and electrophoretic mobility shift analysis revealed that a C/EBP binding site adjacent to the third start site of transcription abrogated the inhibitory effect of cortisol on *Igf1* transcription. It was also demonstrated that C/EBP α, β, and δ interact with the *Igf1* promoter and play a role in the down-regulation by cortisol. The studies on the regulation of the *Igf1* gene by cortisol reveal commonality in the mechanisms of glucocorticoid action in bone converging on the regulation of C/EBPs in cells of the osteoblastic lineage.

Although IGF I activity can be modulated by changes in receptor binding, glucocorticoids do not alter IGF I receptor number or affinity in osteoblasts. They decrease IGF II receptor number, but the function of the IGF II receptor has remained elusive. The activity of IGFs is regulated by six classic IGF binding proteins (IGFBPs), all of which are expressed by the osteoblast. Of the six IGFBPs, IGFBP-5 was postulated to have anabolic effects for skeletal cells, and its transcription is suppressed by glucocorticoids. The inhibition of IGFBP-5 synthesis by glucocorticoids is probably not important to the ultimate effect of glucocorticoids on osteoblastic function, because transgenic mice overexpressing IGFBP-5 in the bone environment exhibit decreased, not increased, bone formation [33].

III. CLINICAL ASPECTS OF GLUCOCORTICOID-INDUCED OSTEOPOROSIS

Patients exposed to glucocorticoids frequently develop clinical osteoporosis. Although the entire skeleton is affected, trabecular bone loss prevails over cortical bone loss, and about 30–50% of patients develop fractures of the spine or hip (see Table 2) [4]. The degree of bone loss is related to the amount of glucocorticoids taken and the duration of glucocorticoid exposure, but most of the bone loss occurs in the first 6 months of exposure [4, 5]. Following an initial phase of rapid bone loss, there is a slower, continued loss of bone mass, and long-term exposure of the skeleton to glucocorticoids, even at what are considered physiological doses, carries an increased risk of vertebral fractures. The minimal dose of glucocorticoids required to cause osteoporosis is not known with certainty, but a review of the General Practice database in the United Kingdom revealed that doses of prednisolone of 2.5 to 7.5 mg daily resulted in a two- to three-fold increase in the risk of fractures of the spine and hip [5].

It is important to note that there are individual variations in patient sensitivity to glucocorticoid therapy. This might be due to variations in the interconversion of hormonally active cortisol and inactive cortisone by 11 β-hydroxysteroid dehydrogenases (11 β-HSD) type 1 and 2 [34, 35]. These

TABLE 2 Clinical features of glucocorticoid-induced osteoporosis

- Most bone loss occurs in the first six months
- Trabecular bone loss prevails over cortical bone loss
- Dose- and time-dependent bone loss
- Variation in individual sensitivity to glucocorticoids
- Skeletal impact of underlying disease

two isoenzymes catalyze the interconversion of hormonally active and inactive steroids, and can regulate glucocorticoid activity. 11 β-HSD type 1 (11 β-HSD1), a low-affinity nicotinamide adenine dinucleotide phosphate (NADP)(H)-dependent enzyme, is bidirectional (dehydrogenase–reductase), although it displays mostly reductase activity converting cortisone to cortisol. 11 β-HSD type 2 (11 β-HSD2), a high-affinity NAD-dependent enzyme, has exclusively dehydrogenase activity and converts cortisol to cortisone. 11 β-HSD2 is expressed in aldosterone target tissues and inactivates glucocorticoids, and mutations of the 11 β-HSD2 gene cause a syndrome of apparent mineralocorticoid excess. 11 β-HSD2 is expressed by fetal but not adult bone. 11 β-HSD1 is widely expressed by glucocorticoid target tissues, including adult bone, and these steroids enhance the activity of this isoenzyme in human osteoblasts [36]. The mechanisms involved have not been explored, but the effect could be the amplification of the cellular actions of glucocorticoids in skeletal tissue, and auto-regulation of glucocorticoid actions in bone. Differences among individuals in the levels or activity of 11 β–HSD1 may explain their different sensitivity to glucocorticoids.

It is important to note that the underlying disease for which patients receive glucocorticoid therapy carries a risk of osteoporosis [3]. Patients with inflammatory bowel disease, rheumatoid arthritis, and systemic lupus erythematosus (SLE), for example, have additional risk factors for osteoporosis, such as disease chronicity, poor nutrition, and secretion of cytokines that can enhance bone resorption and suppress bone formation. Patients with SLE may develop myopathy, impaired renal function, and immobilization, and they may receive immunosuppressive therapy, all of which can contribute to the development of osteoporosis [37]. They may also develop vitamin D deficiency due to sun avoidance, which can add an osteomalacic component to the skeletal disease. Postmenopausal women are at a greater risk of developing fractures following exposure to glucocorticoids than are premenopausal women, since estrogens offer a degree of protection from the deleterious effects of glucocorticoids in bone. This protective effect is lost in patients who develop hypogonadism as a result of the suppression of gonadotropin hormone secretion by glucocorticoids.

GIO in children is a more complex clinical problem than GIO in adults, since glucocorticoids affect not only bone cell function, causing osteoporosis, but also cartilage, causing a delay in longitudinal growth. This delay is a result of a decrease in basal and growth hormone– and IGF-I–induced chondrocyte cell replication [38]. The mechanism involves a decrease in growth hormone or IGF I receptors and levels in chondrocytes. From a practical point of view, children exposed to glucocorticoids should be evaluated for changes in longitudinal growth.

Accelerated bone loss is a significant clinical problem in patients undergoing kidney, liver, and heart and lung transplantation [39]. Glucocorticoids and other immunosuppressive agents are contributory factors to the bone disorder. Hypogonadism, vitamin D deficiency, malnutrition, reduced physical exercise, impaired renal function, and preexisting bone disease also play a role in the pathogenesis of osteoporosis after organ transplantation. The highest rates of bone loss are observed during the first few months after transplantation, with a tendency for bone mass to recover subsequently. Fractures occur most frequently at the hip and spine.

Bone mineral density (BMD) of the spine and hip is the diagnostic tool of choice in GIO. The diagnostic criteria of the World Health Organization (WHO) for the diagnosis of postmenopausal osteoporosis do not apply to GIO, however (see Table 3). Patients with comparable T scores are at a greater risk of fractures in the context of GIO than in that of postmenopausal osteoporosis. The American College of Rheumatology recommends therapeutic intervention in patients with GIO and T scores of ≤ -1, emphasizing that one should not rely on criteria established for the diagnosis of postmenopausal osteoporosis [40]. Biochemical markers of bone turnover, such as collagen crosslinks, are of limited value in the management of GIO. Biochemical markers are influenced by the length of exposure to glucocorticoids and the underlying disease. Serum levels of osteocalcin and alkaline phosphatase are usually reduced, and urinary N-peptide and pyridinoline crosslinks of type I collagen elevated, during the early phases of glucocorticoid exposure, but these levels are decreased after long-term exposure to glucocorticoids.

IV. MANAGEMENT OF GLUCOCORTICOID-INDUCED OSTEOPOROSIS

Since the effect of glucocorticoids on the skeleton is time- and dose-dependent, the dose and duration of glucocorticoid exposure should be kept to a minimum. Whenever possible, glucocorticoids should be discontinued, because a restoration of bone mass occurs following their discontinuation, particularly in young individuals (see Table 4). In patients with bronchopulmonary disorders, such as asthma and chronic obstructive pulmonary disease (COPD), inhaled corticosteroids are an alternative to the use of oral glucocorticoids. The absorption of inhaled steroids is limited, they have a modest effect on BMD, and only at large cumulative doses do they cause osteoporosis. A recent study conducted in premenopausal

TABLE 3 Diagnosis and evaluation of glucocorticoid-induced osteoporosis

- BMD declines rapidly following initial glucocorticoid exposure, then stabilizes.
- Changes in BMD should be interpreted with caution. Diagnostic criteria not established.
- WHO criteria for postmenopausal osteoporosis do not apply to GIO.
- Biochemical markers of bone remodeling are of limited use; they vary with disease stage and underlying disease.

TABLE 4 Prevention and treatment of glucocorticoid-induced osteoporosis

- Discontinue systemic glucocorticoids when possible.
- Modify lifestyle.
- Supplement with calcium, 1.5 gm daily.
- Supplement with vitamin D, 800 IU daily.
- Pursue prevention and treatment with bisphosphonates (use caution in premenopausal women).
- Monitor BMD.
- Monitor for hypogonadism. Consider hormone replacement therapy.

women with asthma demonstrated that prolonged exposure to inhaled triamcinolone resulted in a modest decrease in BMD of the hip, but not at other skeletal sites [41]. Patients with COPD are at greater risk of osteoporosis for a variety of reasons related to the underlying disease, but inhaled steroids are only minor contributing factors to the development of osteoporotic fractures [42].

Patients on glucocorticoids should modify their lifestyle and whenever possible avoid additional risks factors for osteoporosis. Other preventive measures include the use of supplemental calcium and vitamin D [40]. The negative effects of glucocorticoids on calcium absorption can be reversed by administering calcium and either conventional vitamin D or calcitriol. The American College of Rheumatology recommends 1.5 grams of calcium and 800 units of vitamin D daily. Studies on the effectiveness of calcium and vitamin D in fracture prevention in GIO are limited, and these agents are more effective when given in conjunction with antiresorptive therapy.

In GIO, the difference between prevention and treatment is subtle. Since patients on glucocorticoids lose BMD following three to six months of exposure, trials assessing prevention usually examine therapeutic responses in patients exposed to glucocorticoids for three months or less. Trials assessing treatment examine therapeutic responses in patients exposed to glucocorticoids for six months or longer. Hormonal therapy (HT) should be considered in patients who develop estrogen deficiency. Recent data from the Women's Health Initiative Study have demonstrated a favorable effect of estrogens on fracture reduction in postmenopausal osteoporosis [43]. Estrogens stabilize BMD in patients with GIO, but there are no data documenting an effect on fracture reduction in the disease [44]. Raloxifene is indicated for the prevention and treatment of postmenopausal osteoporosis, but data documenting its effectiveness in GIO are lacking. Currently, the only agents widely approved for the management of GIO are bisphosphonates.

The initial effect of glucocorticoids increasing bone resorption justifies the use of antiresorptive therapy. Trials on the use of oral bisphosphonates, such as alendronate, risedronate, and etidronate, have proven their effectiveness for the prevention and treatment of GIO. A recent study demonstrated the effectiveness of alendronate in the management of GIO [45]. Nearly 500 patients exposed to glucocorticoids for periods of <4, 4–12, and >12 months were placed on alendronate or placebo for 1 or 2 years. Alendronate at 5 and 10 mg daily increased BMD after 1 year and decreased the incidence of vertebral fractures after 2 years. The beneficial effect of alendronate was more apparent in postmenopausal women, suggesting that premenopausal women are protected from the deleterious effects of glucocorticoids in bone. Recently, the beneficial effects of risedronate in the prevention and treatment of GIO were documented [46, 47]. Approximately 500 patients receiving glucocorticoids were enrolled in two clinical trials. The prevention study enrolled patients receiving glucocorticoid therapy for 3 months or less, and the treatment study enrolled those receiving glucocorticoid therapy for 6 months or longer. Patients received placebo or risedronate for 1 year while continuing glucocorticoid therapy. In the prevention trial, risedronate stabilized BMD, and in the treatment trial, it significantly increased BMD. A significant reduction in vertebral fractures was observed with risedronate after 1 year when data from the two studies were pooled. In patients unable to receive oral bisphosphonates, their intravenous administration may be considered. Prospective trials on the use of intravenous pamidronate have demonstrated that it prevents vertebral bone loss in patients exposed to glucocorticoids [48].

Bisphosphonates should not be used in pregnant women because they may cross the placenta and reduce fetal skeletal remodeling, and possibly cause other deleterious effects in the developing embryo. Because of their prolonged half-life, bisphosphonates should be used with caution and only when absolutely justified in premenopausal women with severe GIO. These patients should be informed of the potential risks of bisphosphonates if they are to consider pregnancy.

Anabolic agents may be necessary for the treatment of GIO. Data on the use of 1-34 PTH (teriparatide) in postmenopausal osteoporosis and the use of PTH in GIO are encouraging and suggest a potential role for this hormone in the treatment of GIO [49, 50]. PTH increases bone-forming surfaces associated with a stimulation of the differentiated function of the osteoblast, possibly due to an increase in IGF I synthesis [51]. PTH given intermittently increases bone mass. Its impact on GIO was examined in a group of postmenopausal women with rheumatoid arthritis and osteoporosis receiving glucocorticoids and HT. PTH increased vertebral BMD, but the study was not powered to determine its impact on fracture risk in GIO. PTH is indicated for the treatment of severe postmenopausal osteoporosis, but not specifically for GIO.

Management of osteoporosis after transplantation includes optimization of bone health before surgery and prevention of bone loss after transplantation [39]. This should include the use of bisphosphonates, although in this specific patient population, there have been no randomized controlled trials on the use of these agents with fracture prevention as the primary end point. Future studies may prove that modification of immunosuppressive regimens and the use of bisphosphonates or PTH are beneficial in reducing the severity of osteoporosis and its fractures after transplantation.

In conclusion, GIO is a serious disease often overlooked and not treated. Diagnostic and therapeutic alternatives are available and should be considered for the appropriate management of patients receiving glucocorticoids.

ACKNOWLEDGMENTS

Work from the author's laboratory was supported by grant DK 45227 from the National Institute of Diabetes and Digestive and Kidney Diseases. The author thanks Ms. Kimberly Starr and Ms. Nancy Wallach for secretarial assistance.

REFERENCES

1. Bianco, P., and Robey, P.G. (2000). Marrow stromal stem cells. *J Clin Invest.* 105:1663–1668.
2. Canalis, E., Economides, A.N., and Gazzerro, E. (2003). Bone morphogenetic proteins, their antagonists, and the skeleton. *Endocr Rev.* 24:218–235.
3. Canalis, E., and Giustina, A. (2001). Glucocorticoid-induced osteoporosis: summary of a workshop. *J Clin Endocrinol Metab.* 86:5681–5685.
4. Saag, K. (2003). Glucocorticoid-induced osteoporosis. *Endocrinol Metab Clin N Am.* 32:135–157.
5. van Staa, T.P., Leufkens, H.G.M., Abenhaim, L., Zhang, B., and Cooper, C. (2000). Use of oral corticosteroids and risk of fractures. *J Bone Miner Res.* 15:993–1000.
6. Canalis, E. (2003). Mechanisms of glucocorticoid-induced osteoporosis. *Curr Opin Rheumatol.* 15:454–457.
7. Carbonare, L.D., Arlot, M.E., Chavassieux, P.M., Roux, J.P., Portero, N.R., and Meunier, P.J. (2001). Comparison of trabecular bone microarchitecture and remodeling in glucocorticoid-induced and postmenopausal osteoporosis. *J Bone Miner Res.* 16:97–103.
8. Canalis, E. (1996). Mechanisms of glucocorticoid action in bone: implications to glucocorticoid-induced osteroporosis. *J Clin Endocrinol Metab.* 81:3441–3447.
9. Rubin, M.R. and Bilezikian, J.P. (2002). Clinical review 151: The role of parathyroid hormone in the pathogenesis of glucocorticoid-induced osteoporosis: a re-examination of the evidence. *J Clin Endocrinol Metab.* 87:4033–4041.
10. Srivastava, S., Toraldo, G., Weitzmann, M.N., Cenci, S., Ross, F.P., and Pacifici, R. (2001). Estrogen decreases osteoclast formation by down-regulating receptor activator of NF-kappa B ligand (RANKL)-induced JNK activation. *J Biol Chem.* 276:8836–8840.
11. Cenci, S., Toraldo, G., Weitzmann, M.N., Roggia, C., Gao, Y., Qian, W.P., Sierra, O., and Pacifici, R. (2003). Estrogen deficiency induces bone loss by increasing T cell proliferation and lifespan through IFN-{gamma}-induced class II transactivator. *Proc Natl Acad Sci U S A.* 100:10405–10410.
12. Suda, T., Takahaski, N., Udagawa, N., Jimi, E., Gillespie, M.T., and Martin, T.J. (1999). Modulation of osteoclast differentiation and function by the new members of the tumor necrosis factor receptor and ligand families. *Endocr Rev.* 20:345–357.

13. Hofbauer, L.C., Gori, F., Riggs, B.L., Lacey, D.L., Dunstan, C.R., Spelsberg, T.C., and Khosla, S. (1999). Stimulation of osteoprotegerin ligand and inhibition of osteoprotegerin production by glucocorticoids in human osteoblastic lineage cells: potential paracrine mechanisms of glucocorticoid-induced osteoporosis. *Endocrinology*. 140:4382–4389.
14. Rubin, J., Biskobing, D.M., Jadhav, L., Fan, D., Nanes, M.S., Perkins, S., and Fan, X. (1998). Dexamethasone promotes expression of membrane-bound macrophage colony-stimulating factor in murine osteoblast-like cells. *Endocrinology*. 139:1006–1012.
15. Dempster, D.W., Moonga, B.S., Stein, L.S., Horbert, W.R., and Antakly, T. (1997). Glucocorticoids inhibit bone resorption by isolated rat osteoclasts by enhancing apoptosis. *J Endocrinol*. 154:397–406.
16. Weinstein, R.S., Chen, J.R., Powers, C.C., Stewart, S.A., Landes, R.D., Bellido, T., Jilka, R.L., Parfitt, A.M., and Manolagas, S.C. (2002). Promotion of osteoclast survival and antagonism of bisphosphonate-induced osteoclast apoptosis by glucocorticoids. *J Clin Invest*. 109:1041–1048.
17. Zhao, W., Byrne, M.H., Boyce, B.F., and Krane, S.M. (1999). Bone resorption induced by parathyroid hormone is strikingly diminished in collagenase-resistant mutant mice. *J Clin Invest*. 103:517–524.
18. Delany, A.M., Jeffrey, J.J., Rydziel, S., and Canalis, E. (1995). Cortisol increases interstitial collagenase expression in osteoblasts by post-transcriptional mechanisms. *J Biol Chem*. 270:26607–26612.
19. Bellows, C.G., Aubin, J.E., and Heersche, J.N.M. (1987). Physiological concentrations of glucocorticoids stimulate formation of bone nodules from isolated rat calvaria cells in vitro. *Endocrinology*. 212:1985–1992.
20. Pereira, R.C., Delany, A.M., and Canalis, E. (2002). Effects of cortisol and bone morphogenetic protein-2 on stromal cell differentiation: correlation with CCAAT-enhancer binding protein expression. *Bone*. 30:685–691.
21. Pereira, R.M.R., Delany, A.M., and Canalis, E. (2001). Cortisol inhibits the differentiation and apoptosis of osteoblasts in culture. *Bone*. 28:484–490.
22. Weinstein, R.S., Jilka, R.L., Parfitt, A.M., and Manolagas, S.C. (1998). Inhibition of osteoblastogenesis and promotion of apoptosis of osteoblasts and osteocytes by glucocorticoids. *J Clin Invest*. 102:274–282.
23. Ramji, D.P., and Foka, P. (2002). CCAAT/enhancer-binding proteins: structure, function and regulation. *Biochem J*. 365:561–575.
24. Tanaka, T., Yoshida, N., Kishimoto, T., and Akira, S. (1997). Defective adipocyte differentiation in mice lacking the C/EBPβ and/or C/EBPδ gene. *Eur Med Biol Org J*. 16:7432–7443.
25. Wu, Z., Bucher, N.L.R., and Farmer, S.R. (1996). Induction of peroxisome proliferator-activated receptor γ during the conversion of 3T3 fibroblasts into adipocytes is mediated by C/EBPβ, C/EBPδ, and glucocorticoids. *Mol Cell Biol*. 16:4128–4136.
26. Pereira, R.M.R., Delany, A.M., Durant, D., and Canalis, E. (2002). Cortisol regulates the expression of Notch in osteoblasts. *J Cell Biochem*. 85:252–258.
27. Sciaudone, M., Gazzerro, E., Priest, L., Delany, A.M., and Canalis, E. Notch 1 impairs osteoblastic cell differentiation. *Endocrinology*. (In press).
28. Weinmaster, G. (1997). Review: The ins and outs of notch signaling. *Mol Cell Neurosci*. 9:91–102.
29. Mumm, J.S., and Kopan, R. (2000). Notch signaling: from the outside in. *Dev Biol*. 228:151–165.
30. Dallas, D.J., Genever, P.G., Patton, A.J., Millichip, M.I., McKie, N., and Skerry, T.M. (1999). Localization of ADAM10 and Notch receptors in bone. *Bone*. 25:9–15.
31. Delany, A.M., Gabbitas, B., and Canalis, E. (1995). Cortisol down-regulates osteoblast α1 (I) procollagen mRNA by transcriptional and post-transcriptional mechanisms. *J Cell Biochem*. 57:488–494.
32. Delany, A.M., Durant, D., and Canalis, E. (2001). Glucocorticoid suppression of IGF I transcription in osteoblasts. *Mol Endocrinol*. 15:1781–1789.

33. Devlin, R.D., Du, Z., Buccilli, V., Jorgetti, V., and Canalis, E. (2002). Transgenic mice overexpressing insulin-like growth factor binding protein-5 display transiently decreased osteoblastic function and osteopenia. *Endocrinology*. 143:3955–3962.
34. Diederich, S., Quinkler, M., Burkhardt, P., Grossman, C., Bahr, V., and Oelkers, W. (2000). 11β hydroxysteroid dehydrogenase isoforms: tissue distribution and implications for clinical medicine. *Eur J Clin Invest*. 30:21–27.
35. Canalis, E., and Delany, A.M. (2002). 11β-Hydroxysteroid dehydrogenase, an amplifier of glucocorticoid action in osteoblasts. *J Bone Miner Res*. 17:987–990.
36. Cooper, M.S., Rabbitt, E.H., Goddard, P.E., Bartlett, W.A., Hewison, M., and Stewart, P.M. (2002). Autocrine activation of glucocorticoids in osteoblasts increase with age and glucocorticoid exposure. *J Bone Miner Res*. 17:979–986.
37. Franchimont, N., and Canalis, E. (2003). Management of glucocorticoid induced osteoporosis in premenopausal women with arthritis. *Autoimmunity Reviews*. 2:224–228.
38. Jux, C., Leiber, K., Hugel, U., Blum, W., Ohlsson, C., Klaus, G., and Mehls, O. (1998). Dexamethasone impairs growth hormone (GH)-stimulated growth by suppression of local insulin-like growth factor (IGF)-I production and expression of GH- and IGF-I-receptor in cultured rat chondrocytes. *Endocrinology*. 139:3296–3305.
39. Shane, R., Rivas, M., McMahon, D.J., Staron, R.B., Silverberg, S.J., Seibel, M.J., Mancini, D., Michler, R.E., Aaronson, K., Addesso, V., and Lo, S.H. (1997). Bone loss and turnover after cardiac transplantation. *J Clin Endocrinol Metab*. 82:1497–1506.
40. American College of Rheumatology Ad Hoc Committee on Glucocorticoid-Induced Osteoporosis (2001). Recommendations for the prevention and treatment of glucocorticoid-induced osteoporosis. *Arthritis Rheum*. 44:1496–1503.
41. Israel, E., Banerjee, T.R., Fitzmaurice, G.M., Kotlov, T.V., LaHive, K., and LeBoff, M.S. (2001). Effects of inhaled glucocorticoids on bone density in premenopausal women. *N Engl J Med*. 345:941–947.
42. van Staa, T.P., Leufkens, H.G.M., and Cooper, C. (2001). Use of inhaled corticosteroids and risk of fractures. *J Bone Miner Res*. 16:581–588.
43. Rossouw, J.E., Anderson, G.L., Prentice, R.L., LaCroix, A.Z., Kooperberg, C., Stefanick, M.L., Jackson, R.D., Beresford, S.A., Howard, B.V., Johnson, K.C., Kotchen, J.M., and Ockene, J.; Writing Group for the Women's Health Initiative Investigators. (2002). Risks and benefits of estrogen plus progestin in healthy postmenopausal women: principal results from the Women's Health Initiative randomized controlled trial. *J Amer Med Assoc*. 288:321–333.
44. Lukert, B.P., Johnson, B.E., and Robinson, R.G. (1992). Estrogen and progesterone replacement therapy reduces glucocorticoid-induced bone loss. *J Bone Miner Res*. 7:1063–1069.
45. Saag, K.G., Emkey, R., Schnitzer, T.J., Brown, J.P., Hawkins, F., Goemaere, S., Thamsborg, G., Liberman, U.A., Delmas, P.D., Malice, M.P., Czachur, M., and Daifotis, A.G. (1998). Alendronate for the prevention and treatment of glucocorticoid-induced osteoporosis. *N Engl J Med*. 339:292–299.
46. Cohen, S.K., Levy, R.M., Keller, M., Boling, E., Emkey, R.D., Greenwald, M., Zizic, T.M., Wallach, S., Sewell, K.L., Lukert, B.P., Axelrod, D.W., and Chines, A.A. (1999). Risedronate therapy prevents corticosteroid-induced bone loss. A twelve-month, multicenter, randomized, double-blind, placebo-controlled, parallel-group study. *Arthritis Rheum*. 42:2309–2318.
47. Reid, D.M., Hughes, R.A., Laan, R.F.J.M., Sacco-Gibson, N.A., Wenderoth, D.H., Adami, S., Eusebio, R.A., and Devogelaer, J.P. (2000). Efficacy and safety of daily risedronate in the treatment of corticosteroid-induced osteoporosis in men and women: a randomized trial. *J Bone Miner Res*. 15:1006–1013.
48. Boutsen, Y., Jamart, J., Esselinckx, W., and Devogelaer, J.P. (2001). Primary prevention of glucocorticoid-induced osteoporosis with intravenous pamidronate and calcium: a prospective controlled 1-year study comparing a single infusion, an infusion given once every 3 months, and calcium alone. *J Bone Miner Res*. 16:104–112.

49. Neer, R.M., Arnaud, C.D., Zanchetta, J.R., Prince, R., Gaich, G.A., Reginster, J.Y., Hodsman, A.B., Eriksen, E.F., Ish-Shalom, S., Genant, H.K., Wang, O., and Mitlak, B.H. (2001). Effect of parathyroid hormone (1-34) on fractures and bone mineral density in postmenopausal women with osteoporosis. *N Engl J Med.* 344:1434–1441.
50. Lane, N.E., Sanchez, S., Modin, G.W., Genant, H.K., Pierini, E., and Arnaud, C.D. (1998). Parathyroid hormone treatment can reverse corticosteroid-induced osteoporosis. Results of a randomized controlled clinical trial. *J Clin Invest.* 102:1627–1633.
51. Canalis, E., Centrella, M., Burch, W., and McCarthy, T. (1989). Insulin-like growth factor I mediates selective anabolic effects of parathyroid hormone in bone cultures. *J Clin Invest.* 83:60–65.

CHAPTER 4

Transplantation Bone Disease Induced by Non-Steroid Immunosuppressants

Solomon Epstein, MD
Angela M. Inzerillo, MD
Mone Zaidi, MD, PhD
Mount Sinai Bone Program, Department of Medicine, Division of Endocrinology, Mount Sinai School of Medicine, Bronx VA Medical Center, New York, NY

I. INTRODUCTION

The recognition and identification of the role of T lymphocytes and subsets as well as the B lymphocyte in mediating the immune reaction involved in virtually every disease process—including, among others, infection, cancer, cardiovascular disease, and organ transplantation—allowed development of the class of drugs termed immune modulators. These drugs either enhance or suppress the immune reaction depending upon what type of modulation is required to affect the disease outcome. In organ transplantation, the main requirement is to prevent or inhibit donor-organ rejection by the recipient's immune system. In autoimmune diseases, the drugs must inhibit the recognition of self-destructive autoantibodies. In humans, T lymphocyte numbers and subsets are altered and activated T lymphocytes have been associated with increased osteoclast formation and accelerated under inflammatory conditions *in vivo* and *in vitro* [1, 2]. *In vitro* studies have shown that activated T lymphocytes, both CD4+ and CD8+, secrete soluble osteoclastogenic factors including RANK-L (receptor activator of NF-kappaB ligand). However, RANK-L–independent mechanisms accounting for osteoclast formation may also be found.

These immune-modulating drugs have had an enormous impact on prolonging the lifespan of patients. This impact has come at costs, however. One of the costs is the effect of some of these agents on bone. This review will focus on the effect of drugs other than glucocorticoids on bone. These drugs include the calcineurin inhibitors (CIs) cyclosporine and tacrolimus and the non-CIs rapamycin, mycophenolate mofetil, methotrexate, and azathioprine. A number of other immunosuppressive drugs exist, and the list continues to grow, but data on these other drugs' effects on bone are lacking.

II. CALCINEURIN INHIBITORS

Cyclosporine (CsA) and tacrolimus (FK506) are inhibitors of calcineurin. They both require binding to intracellular proteins: CsA to cyclophilins [3, 4, 5] and FK506 to FK binding proteins [6, 7]. These proteins are called immunophilins and are peptidyl-prolyl cis-trans isomerase enzymes [8]. This binding is essential but not sufficient for immunosuppression. The complexes in turn inhibit the intracellular phosphatase calcineurin [3, 4, 9], which prevents transcription of T lymphocyte cytokine genes and genes that control membrane molecules such as CD40 ligand [10, 11]. Calcineurin is a serine–threonine phosphatase that is uniquely regulated by Ca2+ and calmodulin [9]. Calcineurin interacts with NF-AT^{s} (Nuclear Factor of Activated T cells) [12], which constitute a family of transcription factors necessary for activation of genes involved in the inflammatory and immune system. Thus by inhibiting calcineurin [13, 14, 15, 16, 17], CsA and FK 506 prevent activation of NF-AT with consequent inhibition of growth and differentiation critical to the immune response.

CsA and FK506 have made a huge impact on preventing organ rejection and preserving life. One of the drawbacks to their use, however, is their propensity to cause rapid and profound bone loss [18, 19], a propensity best illustrated in experimental models. This bone loss was first observed in the rat model, where administration of immunosuppressive doses to normal, young or old, male or female gonadomized rats produced significant loss of trabecular and cortical bone after weeks. This loss was reversible after stopping the drug and was dose-dependent [20]. Histomorphometry showed this to be an extremely high-turnover bone loss with increases in markers of resorption and formation. Interestingly, serum 1, 25-dihydroxy vitamin D (1,25$(OH)_2$D) increased more with CsA than FK506 [21] as a result of stimulation of the 1α-hydroxylase enzyme in the kidney. This increase in the vitamin D metabolites has not been seen in humans treated with CsA.

To elucidate potential mechanisms by which CsA exerts its effect on bone, various studies have been performed, including those detailed in the following sections.

III. MECHANISMS

A. T Lymphocytes

It has become evident that T cells are implicated in bone remodeling and that T lymphocytes populations are increased in estrogen deficiency. T-cell deficiency per se is not necessarily associated with high-turnover osteopenia [22]. Bone histomorphometry was largely unaffected by CsA when it was administered to T-cell-deficient nude rats, but T-lymphocyte-replete Sprague-Dawley rats displayed the characteristic high-turnover osteopenia. T lymphocytes thus appear to be a prerequisite for the development of CsA-induced osteopenia [23].

B. Transforming Growth Factor Beta (TGF-β)

Transforming Growth Factor Beta (TGF-β) was studied because of its known potential to induce differentiation of osteoblasts and perhaps modify the bone loss associated with CsA. In rat studies, TGF-β administration blocked CsA's effect and increased osteoblast recruitment and activity, as reflected by an increase in the percentage of mineralizing surface and osteoid perimeter, bone formation rate (bone volume referent), and activation frequency. Thus, it appears that TGF-β administration may have a potential in modulating the deleterious bone effects of CsA [24].

C. Parathyroid Hormone Interaction

In post-transplant bone disease in humans, parathyroid hormone (PTH) has been implicated as a major factor promoting bone loss [25, 26]. In *in vivo* studies using parathyroidectomized rats to look at the interaction between CsA and PTH, CsA alone in the intact rats produced a high-turnover osteopenia consistent with previous studies. In the parathyroidectomized, untreated animals, there was an increase in bone mass, which is consistent with human studies [27]. Parathyroidectomy also decreased osteoblast activity and recruitment, and serum $1{,}25(OH)_2D$ levels. Serum levels of osteocalcin were unaffected by parathyroidectomy. The combination group (parathyroidectomy plus CsA) did not differ statistically from the controls in most of the histomorphometric parameters measured, with the exception of reduced mineral apposition and bone formation rates, reflecting the effects of parathyroidectomy [28]. Thus it appears that endogenous PTH does play a role in the CsA-induced bone loss. Ideally, however, this study should have explored the effect of PTH administration to the parathyroidectomized rats treated with CsA to determine whether PTH replacement produces bone loss.

D. Endothelin Receptor

Endothelin-1, a vasoconstrictive peptide, has been implicated in CsA-induced nephrotoxicity and hypertension. Evidence suggests that endothelin plays a pivotal role in bone metabolism [29]. Thus the administration of endothelin receptor antagonist may modify both renal and bone alterations induced by CsA. Both CsA-treated rats and those treated with CsA–endothelin receptor antagonist demonstrated trabecular osteopenia with raised serum osteocalcin, and $1{,}25(OH)_2D$ levels when compared to control animals ($P < 0.05$). Rats given CsA alone developed renal impairment, as shown by increased blood urea nitrogen. The combination group did not develop renal impairment. The results suggest that endothelin may contribute to the development of CsA-induced nephrotoxicity, which was prevented by the endothelin receptor antagonist, but endothelin does not seem to play a role in CsA-induced osteopenia [30].

E. Testosterone

Immunosuppressive doses of CsA, but not FK506, lower serum total and free testosterone both experimentally and clinically [31, 32]. Administration of testosterone pellets to both FK506- and CsA-treated rats failed to prevent bone loss despite low testosterone levels induced by CsA. Thus, hypoandrogenism does not seem to be a major factor in CsA-induced osteopenia, because bone loss occurs despite testosterone replacement [32].

F. Interferon-γ

Interferon (IFN) gamma *in vitro* inhibits both bone resorption and bone formation, producing a net decrease in bone turnover. As CsA produces a high-turnover bone loss, the effect of interferon-γ (IFNγ) on this model was investigated. Bone histomorphometry revealed that treatment with CsA and/or IFN-γ caused an increase in bone resorption surface and a decrease in some parameters of bone formation, resulting in a net loss of bone volume. Thus, IFN-γ failed to influence the osteopenia caused by CsA, and both in combination and on its own, had adverse effects on bone *in vivo* producing a net loss of bone volume [33].

G. Cyclosporine H

Cyclosporine H (CsH), a D-N-MeVal 11 analog of CsA, is not immunosuppressive, and in contrast to CsA, it neither binds to cyclophilin nor alters cytokine activity. This distinction between CsH and CsA provides a means of elucidating whether CsA exerts an effect on bone and 1,25$(OH)_2$D via immune-mediated mechanisms. The results showed that CsH did not produce the biochemical and histomorphometric changes characteristically seen with CsA, thus confirming that CsA exerts effect on bone via immune-modulating mechanisms [34].

The majority of the studies demonstrating the adverse effect of CsA treatment on bone experimentally were derived from the work of Epstein et al. However, confirmatory evidence of this experimentally-produced bone loss was seen in the studies of bisphosphonates in treating CsA-induced bone loss in the rat [35]. In this study, after 30 days of treatment with CsA at 15 mg/kg, a significant reduction in proximal tibia, spine, and whole-femur bone mineral density (BMD) compared to controls was seen [35].

H. Tacrolimus (FK506)

This immunosuppressant, which acts in a similar fashion to CsA except that it binds to specific FK binding proteins, is used frequently as a first-line immunosuppressant in place of CsA or to prevent rejection when CsA has failed. It is reputed to have less nephrotoxicity than CsA. *In vivo* effects of FK506 did not increase 1,25$(OH)_2$vitaminD_3 serum levels as compared to CsAv but did produce the same histomorphometric picture of high-turnover bone loss. The percentage of trabecular area reduction was significantly greater with FK506 than with CsA, however [36].

Similarly, the effects of FK506 have been confirmed in other studies. FK506 immunosuppression in rats to induce bone formation in isogenic and xenogeneic demineralized bone matrix was studied. After 28 days, examination of the tibias showed both bone formation and resorption to be increased, with significant reduction in the relative trabecular area [37].

There have been conflicting studies, however, with results contrary to what has been previously described when CsA is used in *in vitro* systems. Orcel et al. describe an *in vitro* effect using a fetal rat long-bone resorbing assay and CsA administration. CsA inhibited both PTH-stimulated and -unstimulated bone resorption. This inhibitory effect was dose-dependent, and histomorphometry confirmed a decrease in number of osteoclasts per bone section. This study is an isolated one, however, and it lacks systemic factors that may influence bone metabolism, e.g., T lymphocytes [37a]. Another *in vitro* study using a different system [38] confirms inhibition of resorption. This study differed from that of Orcel in that despite the addition of serum-containing T lymphocytes, the inhibition of resorption could not be reversed.

To provide some insights regarding reversal or prevention of CsA bone loss in the clinical setting, several studies were performed. The effect of CsA is reversible. When CsA is withdrawn, normalization of most histomorphometric parameters, with the exception of a reduced bone volume, occurs within two weeks [39]. CsA-induced osteoporosis is ameliorated, or even reversed, by the administration of PGE_2, 1,25$(OH)_2D_3$, salmon calcitonin, 2-pyridinyl ethlidene bisphosphonates (2-PEBP), alendronate, 17β estradiol in estrogen deficiency, and raloxifene [40].

IV. THERAPEUTIC CONSIDERATIONS

A. Bisphosphonates

The antiresorptive drugs such as the bisphosphonates have been extremely successful in treating both primary and secondary osteoporosis [41]. Thus, the effect of bisphosphonates was studied in CsA-treated rats to see whether bone resorption could be prevented or modified. The bisphosphonate 2 PEBP inhibited CsA-induced bone loss, and the FDA approved nitrogen-containing bisphosphonate alendronate prevented CsA's adverse effects, particularly maintaining trabecular bone volume by decreasing turnover [42, 43].

B. Flurbiprofen

Flurbiprofen, a propionic acid derivative NSAID, was demonstrated *in vivo* to reduce osteoclast numbers in normal rats. Flubiprofen administration was unable to prevent the trabecular bone loss induced by CsA therapy, however [44].

C. Calcitonin

This antiresorptive drug acts by inhibition of osteoclasts and is approved by the FDA for treating postmenopausal osteoporosis. Thus it was studied in the CsA rat model to see whether it had any clinical potential. The high-turnover bone loss was attenuated by the combination of CsA and calcitonin to resemble the histomorphometry of the control group. The most plausible mechanism accounting for the prevention of bone loss was the inhibition of osteoclast number by calcitonin [45].

D. Vitamin D

1, $25(OH)_2$ Vitamin D_3, in addition to acting as a $1{,}25(OH)_2D_3$ essential factor in normal bone physiology, also has immune-modifying properties. Consequently, the effect of $1{,}25(OH)_2D_3$ combined with CsA was studied in the rat. $1{,}25(OH)_2D_3$ restored bone volume by increasing the amount of osteoid tissue. Hypercalcemia was also seen in treated rats, however [46].

E. Raloxifene

This selective estrogen receptor modultor (SERM) has been approved for the treatment of osteoporosis and is antiresorptive in action on bone. In *in vivo* studies in rats, treatment with a raloxifene analogue completely prevented the high-turnover osteopenia caused by oophorectomy and was able to attenuate substantially the effects of CsA in the oophorectomized rat [47].

F. Insulin-like Growth Factor 1 (IGF-1)

This growth factor has anabolic actions both *in vivo* and *in vitro* on trabecular and cortical bone. This study examined whether systemic IGF-1 can modify CsA's deleterious effects. CsA caused severe trabecular bone loss which was not prevented by IGF-1. IGF-1 even further increased the bone eroded surface. CsA and IGF-1 had little effect on cortical bone volume or marrow area [48].

G. Estrogen

Postmenopausal osteoporosis is characterized by estrogen deficiency and accelerated bone loss soon after menopause. Postmenopausal women are also candidates for organ transplantation. CsA-treated rats exhibit rapid bone loss, so it is important to determine whether estrogen replacement can reverse the effects of CsA in the oophorectomized rat, thus providing some insight into postmenopausal women who undergo transplantation. 17β-estradiol administration prevented osteopenia in the oophorectomized rat treated with CsA and in fact reversed the changes compared to that seen in control rats [49].

V. CLINICAL STUDIES SUPPORTING THE ROLE OF CALCINEURIN INHIBITORS IN BONE LOSS AFTER TRANSPLANTATION

Clinically, there are studies directly implicating calcineurin inhibitors in bone loss after organ transplantation [50, 51], which confirm the experimental evidence. The first study linking CsA to bone abnormality was published in 1988 [52]. In this study, histology in renal transplant patients revealed unexpected high bone turnover unlike that seen with glucocorticoid administration or secondary hyperparathyroidism [53]. In fact, the turnover resembled that observed in experimental studies in the rat. A clinical study in heart transplant recipients also attributed the bone loss seen after cardiac transplantation to CsA, and again the biochemical findings revealed a high-turnover osteoporosis [50]. These studies were all confounded by triple immunosuppression, and the role of one drug as the culprit cannot be ascertained. Studies with CsA monotherapy in transplanted patients compared to other CsA-containing regimens showed that after 12 months, lumbar BMD did not decrease or even increased after 18 months [54, 55, 56, 57]. The most convincing study was a comparison of CsA monotherapy with a non-CsA (prednisone and azathioprine) regimen to isolate the effects of CsA alone in renal transplant patients [53]. This study utilized BMD as well as bone histomorphometry as targets of immunosuppression. The results showed that both regimens decreased bone at the distal radius and less significantly at the lumbar spine with no differences in the degree of bone loss. Histological analysis showed increased osteoclast number and, surprisingly, a decrease in osteoblast number and mineral apposition and bone formation rates, again with no differences between the groups. The findings also did not support a role for PTH both biochemically and histomorphometrically, despite the fact that PTH has been considered by some investigators to be pivotal for bone loss after transplantation. The surprising decrease in bone formation may be related in this study to the time post transplant, as the subjects were 140 ± 75 months since transplantation.

Similarly, the role of FK506 has been hard to separate from the other immunosuppressives used to prevent rejection, despite animal studies showing equal or more severe loss of bone with FK506 than with CsA, with a high-turnover remodeling state similar to CsA [58]. Studies to resolve the role of FK506 were done with patients receiving low-dose prednisone and FK506 compared to normal-dose glucocorticoids and CsA [59]. These studies showed that when the cumulative dose of steroids was adjusted for both groups, the FK506 patients after 1 year did not lose bone compared to the CsA and low-dose prednisone group. There was no relationship to PTH levels.

A prospective, longitudinal, randomized, double blind 2-year-long study was undertaken to assess the effects of FK506, glucocorticoids, azathioprine, or mycophenalate mofetil (instead of azathioprine) and 1,25$(OH)_2D_3$ against the same immunosuppressive regimen without 1,25$(OH)_2D_3$ (placebo group) [60]. The objective was to determine whether tacrolimus produced bone loss and whether 1,25$(OH)_2D_3$ could modify or prevent this bone loss. Results showed that BMD decreased in both groups after transplantation compared to normal age-matched subjects. However, the BMD increased significantly in the lumbar spine in the group receiving 1,25$(OH)_2D_3$, although significant differences between groups could not be shown. In the femoral neck region, the BMD was maintained, but the placebo group lost bone significantly. Again, no between-group significance could be shown. The conclusion of the study was that FK506 is associated with rapid bone loss comparable to CsA, which can be modified by low-dose calcitriol therapy over two years. A more convincing study would compare FK506 against CsA in comparable post-transplant patients not receiving glucocorticoids to determine whether a difference in their effects on bone mass exists between the two CIs.

VI. OTHER IMMUNE-MODIFYING DRUGS

A. Rapamycin

Rapamycin (sirolimus) is also used to prevent organ rejection after transplantation. It is a macrolide and a product of *Streptomyces hygroscopicus*. It does not inhibit the production of interleukins resulting from antigen T-cell activation, but it does inhibit the cellular proliferation stimulated by growth factor signal transduction in response to alloantigens [61, 62]. Rapamycin binds to the same intracellular protein immunophilin FKBP12 to form a complex, which does not target calcineurin but instead targets mTor (mammalian target of rapamycin). mTor inhibits translation of mRNAs that encode for cell cycle regulators and T-cell proliferation [62]. *In vitro* studies have shown that in bone marrow stromal cells, rapamycin, like CsA and FK506, decreases osteoprotegerin (OPG) mRNA and protein levels and increases RANKL, which potentially can induce bone loss [63]. Rapamycin may, in addition, act via TGF-β to enhance osteoclastogenesis by inducing monocyte–macrophage cell differentiation into osteoclasts [64]. Conversely, in *in vivo* rats, rapamycin does not cause bone loss but may interfere with longitudinal bone growth and, at high doses, decrease cortical bone in young rats, which are still rapidly growing [61]. An effect on gonadal function has also been described with rapamycin [61]. In human subjects, studies of rapamycin therapy without glucocorticoids and calcineurin inhibitors, investigating bone density to ascertain an effect has not been reported, and may not be feasible in a transplant population. There is the possibility, however, that the bone loss with calcineurin inhibitors may be mitigated by combining rapamycin with low-dose CsA, which has been shown in rats to prevent bone loss and not compromise the immune suppression [65]. Everolimus, which is a derivative of rapamycin, has a similar mechanism of action to that of rapamycin, but its effect on bone has not been studied [66].

B. Mycophenolate Mofetil

Mycophenolate mofetil, another addition to the immune-modifying drug armamentarium, is now becoming the choice to replace azathioprine as part of triple therapy, together with CsA or FK506 and glucocorticoids, to prevent organ rejection. Mycophenolate mofetil is converted *in vivo* to mycophenolic acid. This natural product of penicillium fungi selectively inhibits the proliferation of T and B cells as well as arterial wall smooth muscle cells. Most other tissues are resistant to the action of mycophenolate mofetil because of alternate nucleotide synthesis. It also causes less bone marrow suppression than azathioprine. Experimentally *in vivo*, there is no evidence of alteration in bone metabolism and no loss of bone volume [67]. Recently it was reported that prednisone and mycophenolate mofetil in the absence of CsA may also be associated with a high-turnover bone loss on bone histomorphometry [68]. This requires further study.

C. Azathioprine

Azathioprine has long been an essential part of therapy in combination with CsA and glucocorticoids to prevent organ rejection. It is also a purine antagonist and therefore inhibits rapidly proliferating cells, which include T and B lymphocytes and bone marrow hematopoietic cells [69]. However, in rats given azathioprine, albeit for a short period, no effect on bone except on bone formation markers was seen [69]. How this would translate with long-term use into clinically relevant outcomes is at present unknown.

D. Chemotherapeutic Agents

The effects of chemotherapeutic agents on bone have largely been neglected because they are often used in combination with other toxic agents and because the patients have diseases, which themselves affect bone loss irrespective of the drugs. Radiological lucencies, lytic and sclerotic lesions, periosteal elevations, osteopenia, and fracture have been described at diagnosis in children with acute lymphoblastic leukemia [70, 71, 72]. In a study of 40 consecutive children treated with a "cocktail" of prednisone, vincristine, L-asparaginase, methotrexate, and 6-mercaptopurine, 39% developed fractures during treatment over 24 months [73]. It is difficult to separate out the contribution of each of the drugs separately and individually, however. Clinically and in experimental animals, both methotrexate and adriamycin have been reported to cause bone loss of a low-turnover variety after relatively short-term administration (14 days) [74].

In children treated with methotrexate for leukemia, an increased incidence of fracture has been reported [73]. Despite its widespread use, no long-term effects of methotrexate on bone had been described until recently, when it was shown that in rats given 2×5 day courses of methotrexate, at 80 and 170 days post treatment there was depressed cancellous and longitudinal bone growth with decreased bone volume, bone formation, and osteoblast activity with increased osteoclast activity [75]. This demonstrates the adverse longitudinal effect of methotrexate long after cessation of treatment. Despite all these negative findings, there was no difference on biomechanical testing between treated animals and controls. Thus, the cause of increased fracture incidence in these patients is still unclear.

E. T-Cell Subset Specific Antigen Receptor Blockade

Various antibodies against lymphocytes have been used as adjunct or rescue therapy in patients with acute rejection or as prophylaxis against rejection.

Muromonab-CD3 (OKT3) is a monoclonal antibody against the CD3 component of the T-cell antigen receptor. Recently the CD40:CD40 ligand pathway has been recognized as having a major role in T-cell activation pathways [2, 10]. The CD40 ligand is expressed on activated CD4 T cells. Stimulation of CD40 is also important in providing signals for antibody production by B cells, which underscores the cross-reactivity between T and B cells. A recombinant fusion protein consisting of the extracellular domain of CTLA-4 (a molecule that binds ligands on activated antigen presenting cells) linked to the constant region of IgG1 has been shown to be useful in preventing an immune response to pancreatic islets and prolonging the survival of cardiac allografts in animals. Given that CsA inhibits CD40 ligand expression in T lymphocytes from transplant populations, it would be important to study a role for these T cell subset antigen-blocking antibodies in bone metabolism. At present, there is little or no knowledge of such a role.

F. Malononitrilamides

Another class of compounds under development is the malononitrilamides, which represent a low-molecular-weight immunosuppressive agent. These are derivatives of leflunomide. These compounds can block both B- and T-cell proliferation and suppress IgG and IgM antibody production [76]. The effect on bone is yet unknown and may need to be studied. The real potential of these agents, if indeed they are found to be "bone-safe" or at least bone-sparing, is that their use may allow decreased doses or even elimination of immunosuppressant agents that cause bone loss, while not compromising the organ transplant.

VII. CANCER THERAPIES AND HYPOGONADISM

Although it is not within the scope of this chapter, bone loss associated with chemotherapeutic agents is an expanding area. Although these agents are not classified as immune modulators, they do have an impact on the immune precursor cells present in the bone marrow. Use of these bone marrow suppressants to treat malignant diseases, either of the bone marrow itself or due to metastatic spread of the primary tumor (e.g., in breast and prostate cancer chemotherapy with adjunct therapy), results in bone loss and sometimes an increased incidence of fracture [77, 78, 79]. The bone loss in these patients may well be the result of sex steroid deficiency due to chemical or surgical ablation. This may result in bone loss similar to that seen with acute loss of sex steroid production, e.g., after acute ovarian sex steroid production inhibition. Unfortunately, long-term, randomized, controlled trials examining the consequences of these drugs on bone loss and fracture incidence, as well as the effect of the covariants (e.g., immobilization, polypharmacy, and poor nutrition) affecting bone mineral metabolism in such a sick population, are lacking.

The reader is advised to refer to other texts dealing with this topic in more detail. See references 80–82.

VIII. CONCLUSION

The non-steroidal immunosuppressants belonging to the calcineurin inhibiting family have been shown experimentally and clinically to produce severe and rapid high-turnover bone loss. In the clinical setting, however, these drugs are often used with glucocorticoids, which are also known to produce severe and rapid bone loss. Despite the production of a low-turnover bone loss by glucocorticoids, bone histomorphometry in the combination treatment (see references 50–52) reveals a high-turnover state. The end result of this combination of drugs is rapid and severe bone loss with a very high rate of fractures. Other immunosuppressants, such as sirolimus, azathioprine, and mycophenolate mofetil, have not yet been clearly demonstrated experimentally to have adverse effects on bone. These more recent immunomodulators have not been well studied in regard to bone loss and fracture in clinical trials. The ability to separate the contribution of an individual drug as the culprit for producing adverse skeletal effects is extremely difficult given the clinical situation and the other confounding variables found in patients awaiting and post transplantation. Development of immunosuppressant drugs that can prevent organ rejection and other adverse side effects including bone loss would be a major advancement in the field of organ transplantation.

IX. ACKNOWLEDGMENTS:

The work described was supported by the National Institutes of Health (AG 14917-08, DK-70526-09 and AG-23176-02) and the Department of Veteran Affairs (Merit Review) to M.Z.

REFERENCES

1. John, V., Hock, J.M., Short, L.L., Glasebrook, A.L., Galvin, R.J. (1996). A role for CD8+ T lymphocytes in osteoclast differentiation in vitro. *Endocrinology*. 137:2457–2463.
2. Weitzmann, M., Cenci, S., Rifas, L., Haug, J., Dipersio, J., Pacifici, R. (2001). T cell activation induces human osteoclast formation via receptor activator of nuclear factor B ligand-dependent and -independent mechanisms. *J Bone Miner Res*. 16:328–337.
3. Walsh, C.T., Zydowsky, L.D., McKeon, F.D. (1992). Cyclosporine A, the cyclophilin class of peptidylprolyl isomerases, and blockade of T cell signal transduction. *J Biol Chem*. 267:13115–13118.

4. Handschumacher, R.E., Harding, M.W., Rice, J., Drugge, R.J., Speicher, D.W. (1984). Cyclophilin: a specific cytosolic binding protein for cyclosporin A. *Science.* 226:544–547.
5. Cardenas, M.E., Muir, R.S., Breuder, T., Heitman, J. (1995) Targets of immunophilin-immunosuppressant complexes are distinct highly conserved regions of calcineurin A. *EMBO J.* 14:2772–2783.
6. Dolinski, K., Muir, S., Cardenas, M., Heitman, J. (1997). All cyclophilins and FK506 binding proteins are, individually and collectively, dispensable for viability in Saccharomyces cerevisiae. *Proc Natl Acad Sci.* 94:13,093–13,098.
7. Liu, J., Albers, M.W., Wandless, T.J., Luan, S., Alberg, D.G., Belshaw, P.J., Cohen, P., MacKintosh, C., Klee, C.B., Schreiber, S.L. (1992). Inhibition of T cell signaling by immunophilin-ligand complexes correlates with loss of calcineurin phosphatase activity. *Biochemistry.* 31:3896–3901.
8. Gothel, S.F., Marahiel, M.A. (1999). Peptidyl-prolyl cis-trans isomerases, a superfamily of ubiquitous folding catalysts. *Cell Mol Life Sci.* 55:423–436.
9. Siekierka, J.J., Sigal, N.H. (1992). FK-506 and cyclosporin A: immunosuppressive mechanism of action and beyond. *Curr Opin Immunol.* 4:548–552.
10. Fuleihan, R., Ramesh, N., Horner, A., Ahern, D., Belshaw, P.J., Alberg, D.G., Stamenkovic, I., Harmon, W., Geha, R.S. (1994). Cyclosporin A inhibits CD40 ligand expression in T lymphocytes. *J Clin Invest.* 93:1315–1320.
11. Shaw, K.T., Ho, A.M., Raghavan, A., Kim, J., Jain, J., Park, J., Sharma, S., Rao, A., Hogan, P.G. (1995). Immunosuppressive drugs prevent a rapid dephosphorylation of transcription factor NFAT1 in stimulated immune cells. *Proc Natl Acad Sci U S A.* 92:11205–11209.
12. Mages, H.W., Baag, R., Steiner, B., Kroczek, R.A. (1998). Utilization of an NF-ATp binding promoter element for EGR3 expression in T cells but not fibroblasts provides a molecular model for the lymphoid cell specific effect of cyclosporin A. *Mol Cell Biol* 18:7157–7165.
13. Zhang, B.W., Zimmer, G., Chen, J., Ladd, D., Li, E., Alt, F.W., Wiederrecht, G., Cryan, J., O'Neill, E.A., Seidman, C.E., Abbas, A.K., and Seidman, J.G. (1996). T cell responses in calcineurin A alpha-deficient mice. *J Exp Med.* 183:413–420.
14. Hodge, M.R., Ranger, A.M., Charles de la Brousse, F., Hoey, T., Grusby, M.J., Glimcher, L.H. (1996) Hyperproliferation and dysregulation of IL-4 expression in NF-ATp-deficient mice. *Immunity.* 4:397–405.
15. Xanthoudakis, S., Viola, J.P., Shaw, K.T., Luo, C., Wallace, J.D., Bozza, P.T., Luk, D.C., Curran, T., Rao, A. (1996). An enhanced immune response in mice lacking the transcription factor NFAT1. *Science.* 272:892–895.
16. Yoshida, H., Nishina, H., Takimoto, H., Marengere, L.E., Wakeham, A.C., Bouchard, D., Kong, Y.Y., Ohteki, T., Shahinian, A., Bachmann, M., Ohashi, P.S., Penninger, J.M., Crabtree, G.R., Mak, T.W. (1998). The transcription factor NF-ATc1 regulates lymphocyte proliferation and Th2 cytokine production. *Immunity.* 8:115–124.
17. Ranger, A.M., Hodge, M.R., Gravallese, E.M., Oukka, M., Davidson, L., Alt, F.W., de la Brousse, F.C., Hoey, T., Grusby, M., Glimcher, L.H. (1998). Delayed lymphoid repopulation with defects in IL-4-driven responses produced by inactivation of NF-ATc. *Immunity.* 8:125–134.
18. Movsowitz, C., Epstein, S., Fallon, M., Ismail, F., Thomas, S. (1988). Cyclosporin-A in vivo produces severe osteopenia in the rat: effect of dose and duration of administration. *Endocrinology.* 123:2571–2577.
19. Movsowitz C, Epstein S, Ismail F, Fallon M, Thomas S. (1989). Cyclosporin A in the oophorectomized rat: unexpected severe bone resorption. *J Bone Miner Res.* 4:393–398.
20. Schlosberg, M., Movsowitz, C., Epstein, S., Ismail, F., Fallon, M.D., Thomas, S. (1989). The effect of cyclosporin A administration and its withdrawal on bone mineral metabolism in the rat. *Endocrinology.* 124:2179–2184.

21. Stein, B., Halloran, B.P., Reinhardt, T., Engstrom, G.W., Bales, C.W., Drezner, M.K., Currie, K.L., Takizawa, M., Adams, J.S., Epstein, S. (1991). Cyclosporin-A increases synthesis of 1,25-dihydroxyvitamin D3 in the rat and mouse. *Endocrinology*. 128:1369–1373.
22. Buchinsky, F.J., Ma, Y., Mann, G.N., Rucinski, B., Bryer, H.P., Paynton, B.V., Jee, W.S., Hendy, G.N., Epstein, S. (1995). Bone mineral metabolism in T lymphocyte-deficient and -replete strains of rat. *J Bone Miner Res*. 10:1556–1565.
23. Buchinsky, F.J., Ma, Y., Mann, G.N., Rucinski, B., Bryer, H.P., Romero, D.F., Jee, W.S., Epstein, S. (1996). T lymphocytes play a critical role in the development of cyclosporin A–induced osteopenia. *Endocrinology*. 137:2278–2285.
24. Goodman, G.R., Dissanayake, I.R., Bowman, A.R., Pun, S., Ma, Y., Jee, W.S., Bryer, H.P., Epstein, S. (2001). Transforming growth factor-beta administration modifies cyclosporine A-induced bone loss. *Bone*. 28:583–588.
25. Guo, C.Y., Johnson, A., Locke, T.J., Eastell, R. (1998). Mechanisms of bone loss after cardiac transplantation. *Bone*. 22:267–271.
26. Cohen, A., Shane, E. (2003). Osteoporosis after solid organ and bone marrow transplantation. *Osteoporos Int*. 14:617–630.
27. Jiang, Y., Zhao, J.J., Mitlak, B.H., Wang, O., Genant, H.K., Eriksen, E.F. (2003). Recombinant human parathyroid hormone (1-34) [teriparatide] improves both cortical and cancellous bone structure. *J Bone Miner Res*. 18:1932–1941.
28. Epstein, S., Dissanayake, I.R., Goodman, G.R., Bowman, A.R., Zhou, H., Ma, Y., Jee, W.S. (2001). Effect of the interaction of parathyroid hormone and cyclosporine A on bone mineral metabolism in the rat. *Calcif Tissue Int*. 68:240–247.
29. Stern, P.H., Tatrai, A., Semler, D.E., Lee, S.K., Lakatos, P., Strieleman, P.J., Tarjan, G., Sanders, J.L. (1995). Endothelin receptors, second messengers, and actions in bone. *J Nutr*. 125 (7 Suppl):2028S–2032S.
30. Sodam, B.R., Awumey, E.M., Sampson, W.H., Epstein, S. (2001). The endothelin receptor antagonist, L-754,142 does not prevent cyclosporine A-induced osteopenia in rats. *Calcif Tissue Int*. 68:117–121.
31. Shane, E., Rivas, M., McMahon, D.J., Staron, R.B., Silverberg, S.J., Seibel, M.J., Mancini, D., Michler, R.E., Aaronson, K., Addesso, V., Lo, S.H. (1997). Bone loss and turnover after cardiac transplantation. *J Clin Endocrinol Metab*. 82:1497–1506.
32. Bowman, A.R., Sass, D.A., Dissanayake, I.R., Ma, Y.F., Liang, H., Yuan, Z., Jee, W.S., Epstein, S. (1997). The role of testosterone in cyclosporine-induced osteopenia. *J Bone Miner Res*. 12:607–615.
33. Mann, G.N., Jacobs, T.W., Buchinsky, F.J., Armstrong, E.C., Li, M., Ke, H.Z., Ma, Y.F., Jee, W.S., Epstein, S. (1994). Interferon-gamma causes loss of bone volume in vivo and fails to ameliorate cyclosporin A–induced osteopenia. *Endocrinology*. 135:1077–1083.
34. Rucinski, B., Liu, C.C., Epstein, S. (1994). Utilization of cyclosporine H to elucidate the possible mechanisms of cyclosporine A–induced osteopenia in the rat. *Metabolism*. 43:1114–1118.
35. Zeni, S.N., Gregorio, S., Gomez, A.C., Somoza, J., Mautalen, C. (2002). Olpadronate prevents the bone loss induced by cyclosporine in the rat. *Calcif Tissue Int*. 70:48–53.
36. Cvetkovic, M., Mann, G.N., Romero, D.F., Liang, X.G., Ma, Y., Jee, W.S., Epstein, S. (1994). The deleterious effects of long-term cyclosporine A, cyclosporine G, and FK506 on bone mineral metabolism in vivo. *Transplantation*. 57:1231–1237.
37. Voggenreiter, G., Assenmacher, S., Kreuzfelder, E., Wolf, M., Kim, M.R., Nast-Kolb, D., Schade, F.U. (2000). Immunosuppression with FK506 increases bone induction in demineralized isogeneic and xenogeneic bone matrix in the rat. *J Bone Miner Res*. 15:1825–1834.
37a. Orcel, P., Denne, M.A., de Vernejoul, M.C. (1991). Cyclosporin-A in vitro decrease bone resorption, osteoclast formation, and the fusion of cells of the monocyte-macrophage lineage. *Endocrinology*. 128:1638–1646.
38. Awumey, E.M., Moonga, B.S., Sodam, B.R., Koval, A.P., Adebanjo, O.A., Kumegawa, M., Zaidi, M., Epstein, S. (1999). Molecular and functional evidence for calcineurin-A

alpha and beta isoforms in the osteoclast: novel insights into cyclosporin A action on bone resorption. *Biochem Biophys Res Commun.* 254:248–252.
39. Schlosberg, M., Movsowitz, C., Epstein. S., Ismail, F., Fallon, M.D., Thomas, S. (1989). The effect of cyclosporin A administration and its withdrawal on bone mineral metabolism in the rat. *Endocrinology.* 124:2179–2184.
40. Epstein, S., Shane, E., Bilezikian, J.P. (1995). Organ transplantation and osteoporosis. *Curr Opin Rheumato.* 7:255–261.
41. Watts, N.B. (2003). Bisphosphonate treatment of osteoporosis. *Clin Geriatr Med.* 19:395–414.
42. Movsowitz, C., Epstein, S., Fallon, M., Ismail, F., Thomas, S. (1990). The bisphosphonate 2-PEBP inhibits cyclosporin A induced high-turnover osteopenia in the rat. *J Lab Clin Med.* 115:62–68.
43. Sass, D.A., Bowman, A.R., Yuan, Z., Ma, Y., Jee, W.S., Epstein, S. (1997). Alendronate prevents cyclosporin A-induced osteopenia in the rat. *Bone.* 21:65–70.
44. Sass, D.A., Rucinski, B., Bryer, H.P., Mann, G.N., Yuan, Z., Ma, Y., Jee, W.S., Epstein, S. (1996). Combined flurbiprofen and cyclosporin-A does not attenuate bone loss and exaggerates renal impairment. *Bone.* 19:381–386.
45. Stein, B., Takizawa, M., Katz, I., Joffe, I., Berlin, J., Fallon, M., Epstein, S. (1991). Salmon calcitonin prevents cyclosporin-A-induced high turnover bone loss. *Endocrinology.* 129:92–98.
46. Epstein, S., Schlosberg, M., Fallon, M., Thomas, S., Movsowitz, C., Ismail, F. (1990). 1, 25 Dihydroxyvitamin D3 modifies cyclosporine-induced bone loss. *Calcif Tissue Int.* 47:152–157.
47. Bowman, A.R., Sass, D.A., Marshall, I., Ma, Y.F., Liang, H., Jee, W.S., Epstein, S. (1996). Raloxifene analog (LY117018 HCL) ameliorates cyclosporin A–induced osteopenia in oophorectomized rats. *J Bone Miner Res.* 11:1191–1198.
48. Mann, G.N., Sass, D.A., Chen, H.K., Buchinsky, F.J., Bryer, H.P., Ma, Y.F., Jee, W.S., Rucinski, B., Epstein, S. (1996). Short-term systemic insulin-like growth factor-1 is unable to prevent cyclosporin A–induced osteopenia in the rat. *Calcif Tissue Int.* 59:38–44.
49. Joffe, I., Katz, I., Jacobs, T., Stein, B., Takizawa, M., Liu, C., Berlin, J., Epstein, S. (1992). 17 beta-estradiol prevents osteopenia in the oophorectomized rat treated with cyclosporin-A. *Endocrinology.* 130:1578–1586.
50. Thiebaud, D., Krieg, M.A., Gillard-Berguer, D., Jacquet, A.F., Goy, J.J., Burckhardt, P. (1996). Cyclosporine induces high bone turnover and may contribute to bone loss after heart transplantation. *Eur J Clin Invest.* 26:549–555.
51. Rich, G.M., Mudge, G.H., Laffel, G.L., LeBoff, M.S. (1992). Cyclosporine A and prednisone-associated osteoporosis in heart transplant recipients. *J Heart Lung Transplant.* 11:950–958.
52. Aubia, J., Masramon, J., Serrano, S., Lloveras, J., Marinosa, L.L. (1988). Bone histology in renal transplant patients receiving cyclosporine. *Lancet.* 1:1048.
53. Cueto-Manzano, A.M., Konel, S., Crowley, V., France, M.W., Freemont, A.J., Adams, J.E., Mawer, B., Gokal, R., Hutchison, A.J. (2003). Bone histopathology and densitometry comparison between cyclosporine a monotherapy and prednisolone plus azathioprine dual immunosuppression in renal transplant patients. *Transplantation.* 75:2053–2058.
54. Ponticelli, C., Aroldi, A. (2001). Osteoporosis after organ transplantation. *Lancet.* 357:1623.
55. Grotz, W., Mundinger, A., Gugel, B., Exner, V., Reichelt, A., Schollmeyer, P. (1994). Missing impact of cyclosporine on osteoporosis in renal transplant recipients. *Transplant Proc.* 26:2652–2653.
56. McIntyre, H.D., Menzies, B., Rigby, R., Perry-Keene, D.A., Hawley, C.M., Hardie, I.R. (1995). Long-term bone loss after renal transplantation: comparison of immunosuppressive regimens. *Clin Transplant.* 9:20–24.

57. Moreno, A., Torregrosa, J.V., Pons, F., Campistol, J.M., Martinez de Osaba, M.J., Oppenheimer, F. (1999). Bone mineral density after renal transplantation: long-term follow-up. *Transplant Proc.* 31:2322–2323.
58. Abdelhadi, M., Ericzon, B.G., Hultenby, K., Sjoden, G., Reinholt, F.P., Nordenstrom, J. (2002). Structural skeletal impairment induced by immunosuppressive therapy in rats: cyclosporine A vs tacrolimus. *Transpl Int.* 15:180–187.
59. Goffin, E., Devogelaer, J.P., Depresseux, G., Squifflet, J.P., Pirson, Y., van Ypersele de Strihou, C. (2003). Evaluation of bone mineral density after renal transplantation under a tacrolimus-based immunosuppression: a pilot study. *Clin Nephrol.* 59:190–195.
60. Stempfle, H.U., Werner, C., Siebert, U., Assum, T., Wehr, U., Rambeck, W.A., Meiser, B., Theisen, K., Gartner, R. (2002). The role of tacrolimus (FK506)-based immunosuppression on bone mineral density and bone turnover after cardiac transplantation: a prospective, longitudinal, randomized, double-blind trial with calcitriol. *Transplantation.* 73:547–552.
61. Romero, D.F., Buchinsky, F.J., Rucinski, B., Cvetkovic, M., Bryer, H.P., Liang, X.G., Ma, Y.F., Jee, W.S., Epstein, S. (1995). Rapamycin: a bone sparing immunosuppressant? *J Bone Miner Res.* 10:760–768.
62. Kuo, C.J., Chung, J., Fiorentino, D.F., Flanagan, W.M., Blenis, J., Crabtree, G.R. (1992). Rapamycin selectively inhibits interleukin-2 activation of p70 S6 kinase. *Nature.* 358:70–73.
63. Hofbauer, L.C., Shui, C., Riggs, B.L., Dunstan, C.R., Spelsberg, T.C., O'Brien, T., Khosla, S. (2001). Effects of immunosuppressants on receptor activator of NF-kappaB ligand and osteoprotegerin production by human osteoblastic and coronary artery smooth muscle cells. *Biochem Biophys Res Commun.* 280:334–339.
64. Shui, C., Riggs, B.L., Khosla, S. (2002). The immunosuppressant rapamycin, alone or with transforming growth factor-beta, enhances osteoclast differentiation of RAW264.7 monocyte-macrophage cells in the presence of RANK-ligand. *Calcif Tissue Int.* 71:437–446.
65. Goodman, G.R., Dissanayake, I.R., Sodam, B.R., Gorodetsky, E., Lu, J., Ma, Y.F., Jee, W.S., Epstein, S. (2001). Immunosuppressant use without bone loss—implications for bone loss after transplantation. *J Bone Miner Res.* 16:72–78.
66. Eisen, H.J., Tuzcu, E.M., Dorent, R., Kobashigawa, J., Mancini, D., Valantine-von Kaeppler, H.A., Starling, R.C., Sorensen, K., Hummel, M., Lind, J.M., Abeywickrama, K.H., Bernhardt, P., RAD B253 Study Group. (2003). Everolimus for the prevention of allograft rejection and vasculopathy in cardiac-transplant recipients. *N Engl J Med.* 349:847–858.
67. Dissanayake, I.R., Goodman, G.R., Bowman, A.R., Ma, Y., Pun, S., Jee, W.S., Epstein, S. (1998). Mycophenolate mofetil: a promising new immunosuppressant that does not cause bone loss in the rat. *Transplantation.* 65:275–278.
68. Hamdy, N.A.T., Mallat, M.J.K., Bravenboer, N., Lips, P., de Fijter, J.W. (2003). Factors Determining the Prevalence of Osteoporosis and Fractures a Year after Successful Kidney Transplantation. 25th Annual Meeting ASBMR September 19–23, Minneapolis, Minnesota:S174.
69. Bryer, H.P., Isserow, J.A., Armstrong, E.C., Mann, G.N., Rucinski, B., Buchinsky, F.J., Romero, D.F., Epstein, S. (1995). Azathioprine alone is bone sparing and does not alter cyclosporin A–induced osteopenia in the rat. *J Bone Miner Res.* 10:132–138.
70. Nesbit, M., Krivit, W., Heyn, R., Sharp, H. (1976). Acute and chronic effects of methotrexate on hepatic, pulmonary, and skeletal systems. *Cancer.* 37:1048–1057.
71. Schwartz, A.M., Leonidas, J.C. (1984). Methotrexate osteopathy. *Skeletal Radiol.* 11:13–16.
72. Ragab, A.H., Frech, R.S., Vietti, T.J. (1970). Osteoporotic fractures secondary to methotrexate therapy of acute leukemia in remission. *Cancer.* 25:580–585.

73. Atkinson, S.A., Fraher, L., Gundberg, C.M., Andrew, M., Pai, M., Barr, R.D. (1989). Mineral homeostasis and bone mass in children treated for acute lymphoblastic leukemia. *J Pediatr.* 114:793–800.
74. Friedlaender, G.E., Tross, R.B., Doganis, A.C., Kirkwood, J.M., Baron, R. (1984). Effects of chemotherapeutic agents on bone. I. Short-term methotrexate and doxorubicin (adriamycin) treatment in a rat model. *J Bone Joint Surg.* 66:602–607.
75. Wheeler, D.L., Vander Griend, R.A., Wronski, T.J., Miller, G.J., Keith, E.E., Graves, J.E. (1995). The short- and long-term effects of methotrexate on the rat skeleton. *Bone.* 16:215–221.
76. Bilolo, K.K., Ouyang, J., Wang, X., Zhu, S., Jiang, W., Qi, S., Xu. D., Hebert, M.J., Bekersky, I., Fitzsimmons, W.E., Chen, H. (2003). Synergistic effects of malononitrilamides (FK778, FK779) with tacrolimus (FK506) in prevention of acute heart and kidney allograft rejection and reversal of ongoing heart allograft rejection in the rat. *Transplantation.* 75:1881–1887.
77. Hadji, P., Maskow, C., Gottschalk, M., Ziller, V., Fischer, F. (2003). Influence of Chemotherapy (AC) on Bone Mineral Density (BMD) and Bone Ultrasonometry (QUS) in Women with Breast Cancer. 25th Annual Meeting ASBMR September 19-23, Minneapolis, Minnesota:S198.
78. Eastell, R. (2003). Effect of Anastrozole on Bone Mineral Density: 2-year Results of the 'Arimidex' (anastrozole), Tamoxifen, Alone or in Combination (ATAC) Trial, 25th Annual Meeting ASBMR September 19–23, Minneapolis, Minnesota:S312.
79. Chen, Z., Maricic, M., Bassford, T.L., Ritenbaugh, C., Lopez, A.M., Leboff, M.S., Gass, M., Barad, D.H. (2003). Increased Fracture Risk among Breast Cancer Survivors - Results from the Women's Health Initiative Presentation. 25th Annual Meeting ASBMR September 19–23, Minneapolis, Minnesota:S22.
80. Epstein, S. (1996). Post-transplantation bone disease: the role of immunosuppressive agents and the skeleton. *J Bone Miner Res.* 11:1–7.
81. Shane, E., Epstein, S. (2001). Transplantation Osteoporosis. *Transplantation Reviews.* 15:11–32.
82. Cohen, A., Shane, E. (2003). Osteoporosis after solid organ and bone marrow transplantation. *Osteoporos Int.* 14:617–630.

CHAPTER 5

Molecular Effects of Calcineurin Inhibitors

Adina E. Schneider, MD
Mone Zaidi, MD, PhD, FRCP
Solomon Epstein, MD
Mount Sinai Bone Program, Department of Medicine, Division of Endocrinology, Diabetes and Bone Diseases, Mount Sinai School of Medicine, Bronx VA Medical Center, New York, NY

I. INTRODUCTION

Calcineurin inhibitors are widely used in the management of autoimmune disorders and have revolutionized organ transplantation. These agents block T-cell proliferation by inhibiting the Ca^{++}-calmodulin–sensitive phosphatase, calcineurin. Unfortunately, these drugs have been shown to cause high-turnover bone loss in both human and animal studies. Bone loss and increased rates of fracture have also been described in transplant recipients. A 3-year prospective study of cardiac transplant recipients demonstrated a rapid high-turnover bone loss in the first year post transplantation [1]. 44% of patients undergoing heart transplant with CsA and prednisone develop clinical fractures [2]. Similar findings have been observed in patients undergoing kidney [3], lung [4], and liver [5] transplantation.

A direct causative role for calcineurin inhibitors has been difficult to demonstrate in clinical studies as a result of the concomitant use of glucocorticoids. A recent study found that patients who received CsA monotherapy had a lower incidence of osteoporosis than patients treated with glucocorticoid-containing regimens [6]. In the aforementioned study by Shane et al., increased doses of prednisone in cardiac transplant patients were associated with greater rates of bone loss, while no relationship between CsA doses or serum levels and rates of bone loss were found [1]. Thus, there is compelling clinical evidence that bone loss ensues not only with glucocorticoids, but also with calcineurin inhibitors.

This chapter will review the cellular and molecular mechanisms that have recently been discovered regarding the bone loss associated with calcineurin inhibitors.

II. CYCLOSPORIN A

A. Effects of CsA on Bone Mass and Metabolism

In vitro and *in vivo* data have revealed paradoxical effects of CsA on bone metabolism. CsA inhibits bone resorption in bone organ cultures [7, 8, 9] and decreases osteoclast formation in bone marrow cultures [10]. We have demonstrated similarly that bone resorption by isolated osteoclasts in the pit assay is inhibited profoundly by CsA [11].

In contrast, *in vivo* data reveal that use of CsA leads to significant high-turnover bone loss, with a greater impact on trabecular than cortical bone. The first reports of increased bone resorption *in vivo* were by Movsowitz et al., who found a dramatic and unexpected increase in bone turnover after the administration of CsA to rats [12]. This effect was dependent on dose and duration. In a separate study, the administration of CsA to both young and old rats caused a 44% and 20% decrease in trabecular bone, respectively, compared to controls [13]. CsA has also been shown to exacerbate the high turnover osteopenia associated with oophorectomy [14]. Of note, osteocalcin levels appear to rise in response to CsA administration [15]. CsA is also associated with increased 1,25-dihydroxy vitamin D_3 (1,25$(OH)_2D_3$) levels in animals via stimulation of 1α-hydroxylase [16].

Interestingly, the effects of CsA on rat trabecular bone appear to be reversible [17]. We found that both estrogen [18] and a raloxifene analog [19] ameliorated the CsA-induced bone loss seen in oophorectimized rats. Thus, the high turnover bone loss induced by CsA was at one point attributed to changes in sex hormone levels, and this may be true to some extent. In fact, CsA inhibits testosterone biosynthesis in Leydig cells [20]. Although free testosterone levels have been shown to decrease with CsA treatment, estrogen and estrogen receptor expression are not decreased [21]. Despite the reported change in testosterone levels, testosterone replacement has failed to prevent CsA-induced bone loss in rats, indicating that hypoandrogenemia was not a major determinant of CsA-induced bone disease [22].

Other agents that have been found to attenuate the effects of CsA-induced bone loss include alendronate [23], calcitonin [24], and 1,25$(OH)_2D_3$ [25]. IGF-1 has also been used *in vivo* to attempt to prevent CsA-induced bone loss. Administration of IGF-1 to male Sprague-Dawley rats failed to prevent the severe trabecular bone loss associated with CsA [26]. Transforming growth factor beta (TGFβ), a stimulator of osteoblastic bone formation and inhibitor of bone resorption, blocked CsA effects on bone [27].

B. Effect of CsA on Osteoblast Function

Although osteoblast function seems to increase *in vivo* as part of the high remodeling induced by CsA, limited data are available on its direct effects on osteoblasts and bone mineralization. An *in vitro* study found that low-dose CsA (0.1μM) and SDZ 220-384, a nonimmunosuppressant derivative of CsA that does not effect calcineurin, inhibited mineralization in rat marrow stromal cell cultures under dexamethasone stimulation [28]. High-dose CsA, however, was not found to inhibit mineralization. The mechanism of the observed effects of low-dose CsA and SDZ is likely via their ability to bind a mitochondrial membrane peptidyl propyl cis-trans isomerase (PPI), which controls permeability transition pores. It was demonstrated subsequently that the effects of CsA on mineralization may be mediated through Src's non-kinase actions [29]. The differential effects of high-dose CsA and SDZ thus warrant further investigation. A more recent study found, however, that CsA decreased osteoblast numbers, type I collagen mRNA expression, and protein accumulation in MC3T3-E1 osteoblast cells [30]. We have demonstrated, in line with this observation, that bone formation is reduced in mice in which the Aα isoform of calcineurin is genetically ablated (see below).

C. Role of T Cells and RANK-L in CsA-Induced Bone Loss

Receptor activator of NF-kB ligand (RANKL), which is produced by osteoblasts, is sufficient and necessary for osteoclast differentiation. RANKL is also produced by bone marrow stromal cells and T cells. Osteoprotogerin (OPG) is a soluble decoy receptor that neutralizes the stimulatory effects of RANKL. *In vitro* data suggest that calcineurin inhibitors decrease OPG mRNA expression and increase RANKL gene expression by human osteoblasts, which would suggest increased bone resorption [31]. A recent human study found that OPG levels declined in patients treated with immunosuppressive therapy, and changes in OPG accounted for 67% of the variance in bone mineral density in the 6 months after cardiac transplantation [32]. Very interestingly, Buchinsky et al. found that 28 days of CsA administration caused high-turnover bone loss in Sprague-Dawley rats, while no effect on bone mass was seen in Rowett athymic nude rats [33]. Of note, body mass, iPTH, 1,25$(OH)_2D_3$, and calcium levels were similar between the two groups of rats. It was hypothesized thereafter that the presence of lymphocytes *in vivo* might explain the contradictory *in vitro* and *in vivo* effects of CsA. The anti-resorptive effects of CsA *in vitro* have not been reversed by the presence of lymphocytes, however [11]. The role of T cells in CsA-induced bone loss thus requires urgent exploration.

III. FK506

FK506, or tacrolimus, a fungal macrolide produced by *Streptomyces tskubaensis*, is a more recently developed calcineurin inhibitor that appears to be more potent than CsA, but has less impact on bone metabolism. It binds to the immunophilin FK binding protein (FKBP), which then inhibits calcineurin, thereby decreasing cytokine production from T lymphocytes [34, 35].

FK506 decreases both cortical and trabecular bone mass in rats [36]. *In vivo* data suggest that this agent causes a much less dramatic decrease in BMD than CsA does, however [37]. A possible explanation for the difference between these two agents may be an increase in IGF-1 levels in normal rats treated with FK506 [36]. Another study, however, using higher doses of FK506, found that this agent caused marked trabecular bone loss in rats [38]. The same was found in humans, although preliminary data show significant bone loss after heart transplantation in patients using tacrolimus-based immunosuppression [39]. A prospective study published in abstract form only demonstrated less severe bone loss in patients treated with FK506 than those treated with CsA [40]. This observation may, however, be related to the lower doses of glucocorticoids used in FK506-treated patients [41].

The direct effect of FK506 on the osteoblast that likely translates into enhanced bone remodeling is discussed in the next section. It has been surmised, however, that another potential mechanism for the *in vivo* effects of tacrolimus on bone turnover is through the possible induction of hypogonadism. However, short-term administration of FK506 did not adversely affect rat Leydig cell function. Moreover, Bowman et al. found that, unlike CsA, rats treated with FK506 for 28 days did not experience a decrease in serum testosterone levels [42]. Thus, the hypogonadism hypothesis remains to be proven.

A. Effects of FK506 on Osteoblast Differentiation and Function

FK506 has been shown to cause a dose- and time-dependent increase in alkaline phosphatase in mesenchymal cells, indicating a profound effect on osteoblastic differentiation. The drug also potentiates the prodifferentiation effects of bone morphogenetic protein-4 (BMP-4). In contrast, no increase in ALP activity was seen with CsA, and alkaline phosphatase decreased with rapamycin administration [43]. Likewise, it has been demonstrated that FK506 promotes bone formation in cultured allogenic bone [44]. Systemic administration of FK506 to rats implanted with demineralized bone matrix led to increased bone volume. Histomorphometry of the tibia revealed a significant increase in bone resorption and formation [45]. In a separate study, short-term administration of FK506 promoted osteoinduction by recombinant human BMP-2, while long-term administration led to decreased bone formation [46]. Of note, Voggenreiter et al. found a positive correlation between parameters of bone turnover and the $CD4^+/CD8^+$ T-cell ratio, thus lending support to the hypothesis that T lymphocytes may play a crucial role in mediating the effects of FK506 on bone metabolism [45]. Finally, in support of the prodifferentiation action of FK506, we find marked increases in osteoblast precursors in cultures of bone marrow. Importantly, however, we also find that this effect is not exerted via calcineurin, as calcineurin $A\alpha^{-/-}$ cells show an equally profound increase in progenitor number [47].

IV. MECHANISM OF BONE LOSS WITH CALCINEURIN INHIBITION

CsA and FK506 have been best studied in T cells, where their effects are exerted through the inhibition of calcineurin, a calcium-dependent phosphatase. After entering cells via passive diffusion, CsA binds to the cyclophylin (CyP) family of proteins, thereby forming a CsA-CyP complex that inhibits calcineurin activity [48]. In contrast, FK506 binds with a protein, FK-binding protein-12, and the complex activates calcineurin's phosphatase activity. Activated calcineurin interacts with the transcription factor NFAT (nuclear factor for activated T cells) in lymphoid cells.

A. Calcineurin and NFATc1

Calcineurin, discovered as a neural phosphatase, is a heterodimeric enzyme with two subunits. The catalytic subunit A has an active site dinuclear metal center and three functional (calcineurin B-binding, calmodulin-binding, and auto-inhibitory) domains. The regulatory subunit B has four Ca^{2+} binding sites. The calcineurin isoforms ($A\alpha$, $A\beta$, $A\gamma$, B1, and B2) have highly conserved amino acid sequences, except at the amino and carboxyl termini. Calcineurins regulate cellular processes such as T-cell activation, apoptosis, endocytosis, muscle development, Ca^{2+} channel activation, and cell cycling. They have possible roles in the genesis of hypertension, Alzheimer's disease, brain ischemia, and muscle hypertrophy.

The primary target for calcineurin is NFAT. NFAT has three isoforms (c1-c4), each with a highly conserved DNA binding domain. Each isoform also has an amino-terminal NFAT homology region approximately 400 amino acids in length for calcineurin binding with clusters of short-repeating SP motifs. In response to its activation by calmodulin and Ca^{2+}, calcineurin dephosphorylates NFAT, causing its nuclear import and enhanced DNA affinity. Translocated NFAT activates a wide array of genes, including the IL-2, IL-4, TNF-α, and interferon-γ genes. It binds a 9-bp consensus element containing a core GGAAA sequence next to a 7–8-bp AP1, CREB/ATF, or bZIP binding domain. It also binds certain κB-like sites. Crystal studies reveal that NFAT forms a ternary complex with *c-fos*/*c-jun* dimers and the NFAT–AP1 domain. Signals such as protein kinase C and A, and GTPases (*Rho, Rac, Raf,* and *Ras*) influence both NFAT activation and function.

B. Calcineurin and Osteoclast Formation

Initially discovered as a T-cell transcriptional regulator, new functions of NFAT have continued to unravel. The c1 isoform is critical for cardiac valve and skeletal myofiber formation, rendering $c1^{-/-}$ mice embryonic lethal. NFATc2 regulates vascular endothelial cell, skeletal myotube, chondrocyte, adipocyte, and pancreatic acinar cell differentiation. Likewise, NFATc3 and c4 control perivascular tissue and keratinocyte development. Recent studies suggest that NFATc1 mediates osteoclast formation as a master molecule responsive to RANKL. Thus, $NFATc1^{-/-}$ ES cells and antisense-transfected RAW cells fail to produce osteoclasts when exposed to RANKL. In our hands, constitutively active and dominant-negative NFATs stimulate and inhibit, respectively, RANK-L-induced osteoclast differentiation (unpublished). Further, the c1 isoform is up-regulated during osteoclastogenesis, and its expression and function are both *c-fos*-dependent.

The interaction of RANKL with its receptor, RANK, on the osteoclast precursor results in the binding of TNF receptor-associated factors (TRAFs), mainly TRAF-6, to its intracellular domain and the subsequent activation of MAP kinases (JNK, ERK, and p38), NFκB, and Akt. JNK, by phosphorylating *c-jun* at the N-terminus, causes its nuclear import followed by *c-jun–c-fos* binding to AP-1 sites on gene promoters. The three NFkB subunits, p65, p50, and *c-Rel*, are similarly osteoclastogenic, but their nuclear import is inhibited by IkBa. Thus, overexpression of a persistently dephosphorylated mutant, Y42-IkBa, abrogates osteoclast formation. Likewise, osteoclast formation could potentially be inhibited through calcineurin-induced IkB dephosphorylation, which we have shown in preliminary studies. Indeed, it makes biological sense for a single molecular switch (calcineurin) that enhances osteoclast formation (via NFATc1) to simultaneously activate an inhibitory signal (IkBa). This should prevent excessive osteoclastogenesis and bone loss.

C. Calcineurin in Osteoclast Formation and Function

We characterized the skeletal phenotype of the calcineurin $A\alpha^{-/-}$ mouse. We first confirmed the absence of the Aα protein in $A\alpha^{-/-}$ mouse bones by Western immunoblotting. Seven of 10 week-old $A\alpha^{-/-}$ mice had severe low-turnover osteoporosis at both cancellous and cortical sites. A marked reduction in cortical bone thickness and a modest reduction in trabecular bone were noted on histological examination. Tetracycline labeling indicated an approximately 60% reduction in the mineral apposition rate, indicative of attenuated bone formation. Although there was little difference in resorbed surfaces, likely due to compensation, $A\alpha^{-/-}$ osteoclast precursors showed a pronounced reduction in their responsiveness to RANKL *ex vivo*. RANKL-induced osteoclastogenesis was thus attenuated by approximately 50%, consistent with a similar reduction seen with the calcineurin inhibitors, CsA and

FK506, in bone marrow cultures. Thus, there are phenotypic similarities between the knockout mouse and those treated with CsA and FK506. Nonetheless, the knockout mouse that displays low turnover osteoporosis represents a model for chronic deficiency of only one isoform of the enzyme. Acute inhibition with cyclosporine inhibitors, in contrast, leads to high turnover osteoporosis, and this may be due to an additional effect exerted via T cells. Further studies are required to clarify this apparent difference.

Finally, to perform gain-of-function experiments, we attempted to transduce osteoclast precursors with calcineurin with high efficiency. We created fusion proteins with TAT, an HIV-derived, Arg-rich sequence of 12 amino acids. TAT fusion proteins traverse cell membranes in a receptorless fashion and refold within the cytosol with minimal efflux. We synthesized and purified TAT-calcineurin Aα and TAT-hemaglutinnin (TAT-HA, control). We incubated purified TAT-Aα with isolated rat osteoclasts and RAW cells. Confocal microscopy revealed a solely cytosolic localization of TAT-calcineurin Aα with virtually no nuclear penetration. Surprisingly, TAT-calcineurin Aα inhibited osteoclastic bone resorption.

Thus, the mechanism responsible for the bone loss observed in clinical and animal studies has been difficult to elucidate in molecular terms. As previously mentioned, *in vitro* data have demonstrated an inhibition of bone resorption with CsA administration, an effect that was thought to result from calcineurin inhibition [11]. TAT-calcineurin Aα transduction, however, also inhibits bone resorption [49]. It is thus likely that CsA has additional effects to those exerted via calcineurin. The phenotype of the osteoporotic knockout mouse is also characterized by reduced osteoclast formation *ex vivo*, and this is mimicked by CsA and FK506. However, although the mouse displays a bone formation defect, FK506 stimulates osteoblast differentiation and does not mimic the effects of enzyme deletion in this respect. Thus, it appears that both drugs have effects on bone cells that are distinguishable to calcineurin inhibition. The molecular basis of these effects merits further characterization.

An interesting recent study comparing the effects of CsA to tamoxifen, a known calmodulin antagonist, on osteoclast activity again demonstrates nonparallel effects of calcineurin–calmodulin inhibition and the ensuing reduction in bone resorption. CsA inhibited osteoclast calcineurin activity by 70%, but reduced resorption by only 12% without affecting acid transport. In contrast, tamoxifen inhibited calcineurin activity by 25%, but caused a 60% inhibition of bone resorption and significantly inhibited acid transport activity [50]. This suggested modes of action of the two drugs other than those involving calcineurin.

V. RAPAMYCIN

Rapamycin is a novel immunosuppressant that binds to FK binding protein, which then binds to the FKBP-rapamycin associated protein. This tertiary complex inhibits activation of p70 S6, thereby inhibiting T-cell activation and proliferation [51]. Unlike rats treated with FK506 or CsA, no loss in trabecular bone volume was demonstrated in a study of rats treated with rapamycin for 28 days [52]. Rapamycin did, however, stimulate both modeling and remodeling and decreased the longitudinal growth rate of rat tibias.

In vitro, rapamycin, in the presence of RANKL, has been shown to increase TRAP activity and mRNA expression, indicating increased osteoclastogenesis [52]. Like CsA and FK506, however, rapamycin decreases OPG and increases RANKL production [53]. In contrast, CsA and high-dose FK506 inhibit TRAP mRNA expression and osteoclast formation. Rapamycin also appears to act synergistically with TGFβ when the latter stimulates osteoclast differentiation [54]. This effect may be exerted via the demonstrated weak affinity of rapamycin to the TGFβ receptor [55]. The significance of this finding remains unclear.

Rapamycin stimulates osteoblast differentiation *in vitro*. It has been shown to be more potent than FK506, for example in stimulating alkaline phosphatase activity that was only moderately increased by FK506 and was decreased by CsA. Moreover, rapamycin had the most potent positive effect on expression of osteopontin and osteocalcin, markers of osteoblastic differentiation [56].

VI. SUMMARY

The rapid and severe bone loss that occurs after organ transplant is likely to be attributable not only to glucocorticoids, but also to calcineurin inhibitors, CsA, and FK506 [57]. Animal studies have demonstrated acute increases in bone remodeling, consisting of both osteoclast activation and, in some circumstances, increases in osteoblastic bone formation. These changes are not exactly recapitulated following the genetic ablation of the calcineurin Aα isoform in mice, suggesting alternative mechanisms through which these drugs act. There is limited but persuasive evidence that T cells may mediate the action of both CsA and FK506, but again, this needs further confirmation. Likewise, the molecular mechanism underlying the proremodeling action of rapamycin, an apparently "safe" immunosuppressant, needs investigation.

REFERENCES

1. Shane, E., Rivas, M., McMahon, D.J., Staron, R.B., Silverberg, S., Seibel, M.J., Mancini, D., Michler, R.E., Aaronson, K., Addesso, V. (1997). Bone loss and bone turnover after cardiac transplantation. *J Clin Endocrinol Metab.* 82:1497–1506.
2. Rich, G.M., Mudge, G.H., Laffel, G.L., LeBoff, M.S. (1992). CsA and prednisone associated osteoporosis in heart transplant recipients. *J Heart Lung Transplant.* 11:950–8.

3. Durieux, S., Mercadal, L., Orcel, P., Dao, H., Rioux, C., Bernard, M., Rozenberg, S., Barrou, B., Bourgeois, P., Deray, G., Bagnis, C.I. (2002). Bone mineral density and fracture prevalence in long term kidney graft recipients. *Transplantation*. 74:496–500.
4. Shane, E., Papadopoulos, A., Staron, R.B., Addesso, V., Donovan, D., McGregor, C., Schulman, L.L. (1999). Bone loss and fracture after lung transplantation. *Transplantation*. 68(2):220–7.
5. Ninkovic, M., Skingle, S.J., Bearcroft, P.W., Bishop, N., Alexander, G.J., Compston, J.E. (2000). Incidence of vertebral fractures in the first three months after orthotopic liver transplantation. *Eur J Gastroenterol Hepatol*. 12(8):931–5.
6. Montagnino, G., Tarantino, A., Segoloni, G.P., Cambi, V., Rizzo, G., Altie, P., Castagneto, M., Salvador, M., Cossu, M., Pisani, F., Carmellini, M., Mastrangelo, F., Ferrara, R., Ponticelli, C. (2001). Long term results of a randomized study comparing three immunosuppressive schedules with cyclosporine in cadaveric kidney transplantation. *J Am Soc Nephrol*. 12:2163–9.
7. Stewart, P.J., Green, O.C., Stern, P.H., (1986). Cyclosporine A inhibits calcemic hormone induced bone resorption in vitro. *J Bone Miner Res*. 1:285–291.
8. Klaushofer, K., Hoffman, O., Stewart, P.J. et al. (1987). Cyclosporine A inhbits bone resorption in cultured neonatal mouse calvaria. *J Pharmacol Exp Ther*. 241:584–590.
9. Stewart, P.J., Stern, P.H. (1989). Interaction of cyclosporine A and calcitonin on bone resorption in vitro. *Horm Metab Res*. 21:194–197.
10. Orcel, P., Denne, M.A., DeVernejoul, M.C. (1991). Cyclosporine A in vitro decreases bone resorption, osteoclast formation, and fusion of cells of the moncyte-macrophage lineage. *Endocrinology*. 128:1638–1646.
11. Awumey, E., Moonga, B.S., Sodam, B., Koval, A.P., Adebanjo, O.A., Kumegawa, M., Zaidi, M., Epstein, S. (1999). Molecular and functional evidence for calcineurin A_ and _ isoforms in the osteoclast. Novel insights into the mode of action of cyclosporin A. *Biochem Biophys Res Commun*. 254:248–252.
12. Movsowitz, C., Epstein, S., Ismail, F., Fallon, M., Thomas, S. (1989). Cyclosporin A in the oophorectomized rat: unexpected severe bone resorption. *J Bone Miner Res*. 4(3):393–8.
13. Katz, I., Li, M., Joffe, I., Stein, B., Jacobs, T., Liang, X.G., Ke, H.Z., Jee, W., Epstein, S. (1994). Influence of age on cyclosporin A-induced alterations in bone mineral metabolism in the rat in vivo. *J Bone Miner Res*. 9(1):59–67.
14. Marshall, I., Isserow, J., Buchinsky, F., Paynton, B., and Epstein, S. (1995). Expression of interleukin-1 and interleukin-6 in bone from normal and cyclosporin A-treated rats. The XII International Conference on Calcium Regulating Hormones 16, 1, suppl.
15. Movsowitz, C., Epstein, S., Fallon, M., Ismail, F., and Thomas, S. (1988). Cyclosporin-A in vivo produces severe osteopenia in the rat: effect of dose and duration of administration. *Endocrinology*. 123:2571–7.
16. Stein, B., Halloran, B.P., Reinhardt, T., Engstrom, G.W., Bales, C.W., Drezner, M.K., Currie, K.L., Takizawa, M., Adams, J.S., Epstein, S. (1991). Cyclosporin-A increases synthesis of 1,25-dihydroxyvitamin D3 in the rat and mouse. *Endocrinology*. 128(3):1369–73.
17. Schlosberg, M., Movsowitz, C., Epstein, S., Ismail, F., Fallon, M.D., Thomas, S. (1989). The effect of cyclosporin A administration and its withdrawal on bone mineral metabolism in the rat. *Endocrinology*. 124:2179–2184.
18. Joffe, I., Katz, I., Jacobs, T., Stein, B., Takizawa, M., Liu, C., Berlin, J., Epstein, S. (1992). 17 beta-estradiol prevents osteopenia in the oophorectomized rat treated with cyclosporin-A. *Endocrinology*. 130(3):1578–86.
19. Bowman, A.R., Sass, D.A., Marshall, I., Ma, Y.F., Liang, H., Jee, W.S., Epstein, S. (1996). Raloxifene analog (LY117018 HCL) ameliorates cyclosporin induced osteopenia in oopherectomized rats. *J Bone Miner Res*. 11:1191–8.
20. Seethalakshmi, L., Flores, C., Malhotra, R.K., Pallias, J.D., Tharakan, D., Khauli, R.B., Menon, M. (1992). The mechanism of cyclosporine's action in the inhibition of testosterone biosynthesis by rat Leydig cells in vitro. *Transplantation*. 53(1):190–5.

21. Shin, W.Y., Li, S.Z., Chung, S.S., Lee, H.C., Huh, K.B., Lim, S.K. (2000). Effects of cyclosporin A on sex hormone and estrogen receptor in male rat with special reference to cyclosporin A induced osteoporosis. *Yonsei Med J.* 41:61–7.
22. Bowman, A.R., Sass, D.A., Dissanayake, I.R., Ma, Y.F., Liang, H., Yuan, Z., Jee, W.S., Epstein S. (1997). The role of testosterone in cyclosporin induced osteopenia. *J Bone Miner Res.* 12:607–615.
23. Sass, D.A., Bowman A.R., Yuan, Z., Ma, Y., Jee, W.S.S., Epstein, S. (1997). Alendronate prevents cylosporine A induced osteopenia in the rat. *Bone.* 21:65–70.
24. Stein, B., Takizawa, M., Katz, I., Joffe, I., Berlin, J., Fallon, M., and Epstein, S. (1991). Salmon calcitonin prevents cyclosporin-A-induced high turnover bone loss. *Endocrinology.* 129:92–8.
25. Epstein, S., Schlosberg, M., Fallon, M., Thomas, S., Movsowitz, C., Ismail, F. (1990). 1,25 dihydroxyvitamin D3 modifies cyclosporine induced bone loss. *Calcif Tissue Int.* 47:152–7.
26. Mann, G.N., Sass, D.A., Chen, H.K., Buchinsky, F.J., Bryer, H.P., Jee Rucinski, B., Epstein S. (1996). Short term systemic insulin like growth factor-1 is unable to prevent cyclosporin A-induced osteopenia in the rat. *Calcif Tissue Int.* 59:38–44.
27. Goodman, G.R., Dissanayake, I.R., Bowman, A.R., Pun, S., Ma, Y., Jee, W.S.S., Bryer, H.P., Eptsein, S. (2001). Transforming growth factor beta administration modifies cyclosporine A-indcued bone loss. *Bone.* 28:583–588.
28. Klein, B.Y., Gal, I., Mosheiff, R., Liebergall, M., Ben-Bassat, H. (1997). Cyclosporin A and its non-immunosuppressive derivative exhibit a differential effect on cell mediated mineralization in culture. *J Cell Biochom.* 65:209–216.
29. Stekelenburg, J., Klein, B.Y., Ben-Bassat, H., Rojansky, N. (1998). Opposing effects of CsA and tyrphostin AG 1478 indicate a role for Src protein in cellular control of mineralization. *J Cell Biochem.* 71:116–126.
30. Fornoni, A., Cornacchia, F., Howard, G.A. , Roos, B.A., Strike, G.E., Striker, L.J. (2001). Cyclosporin A affects extracellular matrix synthesis and degradation by mouse MC3T3-E1 osteoblasts in vitro. *Nephrol Dial Transplant.* 16:500–505.
31. Hofbauer, L.C., Shui, C., Riggs, B.L., Dunstan, C.R., Spelsberg, T.C., O'Brien, T., Khosla, S. (2001). Effects of immunosuppressants on receptor activator of NF-kappB ligand and osteoprotegerin production by smooth muscle cells. *Biochem Biophys Res Commun.* 280:334–9.
32. Fahrleitner, A., Prenner, G., Leb, G., Tscheliessnigg, K.H., Piswanger-Solkner, C., Obermayer-Pietsch, B., Portugaller, H.R., Berghold, A., Dobnig H. (2003). Serum osteoprotegerin is a major determinant of bone density development and prevalent vertebral fracture status following cardiac transplantation. *Bone.* 32:96–106.
33. Buchinsky, F.J., Ma, Y., Mann, G.N., Rucinski, B., Bryer, H.P., Romero, D.F., Jee, W.S., Epstein S. (1996). T lymphocytes play a critical role in the development of cyclosporin A-induced osteopenia. *Endocrinology.* 137(6):2278–85.
34. Liu, J., Farmer, J.D., Lane, W.S. (1991). Calcineurin is a common target of cyclophilin-cyclosporine A and FJBP-FK506 complexes. *Cell.* 66:807.
35. Clipstone, N.A., Crabtree, G.R. (1992). Identification of calcineurin as a key signaling enzyme in T lymphocyte activation. *Nature.* 357:692.
36. Abdelhadi, M., Ericzon, B.G., Hultenby, K., Sjoden, G., Reinhold, F.P., Nordenstrom J. (2002). *Transpl Int.* 14:180–187.
37. Inoue, T., Kawamura, I., Aketa, M., Mabuchi, M., Seki, J., Got, T. (2000). Lesser reduction of bone mineral density by the immunosuprressant, Fk506, compared with cyclosporine in rats. *Tranplantation.* 15:774–779.
38. Cvetkovic, M., Mann, G.N., Romero, D.F., Liang, X.G., Ma, Y., Jee, W.S., Epstein, S. (1994). The deleterious effects of long-term cyclosporine A, cyclosporine G, and FK506 on bone mineral metabolism in vivo. *Transplantation.* 57(8):1231–7.
39. Stempfle, H.U., Werner, C., Echtler, S., Assum, T., Meiser, B., Angermann, C.E., Theisen, K., Gartner, R. (1998). Rapid trabecular bone loss after cardiac transplantation using FK506 (Tacrolimus) based immunosuppression. *Transplantation Proc.* 30:1132–1133.

40. Apostolinas, S., Sheiner, P., Genyk, Y., O'Rourke, M., Wallenstein, S., Luckey, M. (1997). Prospective comparison of bone loss with tacrolimus and cyclosporin A after organ transplantion. *J Bone Miner Res.* 12(suppl):S402.
41. Monegal, A., Navasa, M., Guanabens, N., Peris, P., Pons, F., Martinez de Os, M.J., Rodes, J., Munoz-Gomez, J. (2001). Bone mass and mineral metabolism in liver transplant patients treated with FK506 and cyclosporine A. *Calcif Tissue Int.* 68:83–6.
42. Bowman, A.R, Sass, D.A., Dissanayake, I.R., Ma, Y.F., Liang, H., Yuan, Z., Jee, W.S., Epstein, S. The role of testosterone in cyclosporine-induced osteopenia. *J Bone Miner Res.* 12(4):607–15.
43. Tang, L., Evara, S., Kawasaki, S., Wakabayashi, S., Nikaido, T., Takaoka, K. (2002). FK506 enhanced osteoblastic differentiation in mesenchymal cells. *Cell Biol Internat.* 26:75–84.
44. Yoshikawa, T., Nakajima, H., Yamada, E., Akahane, M., Dohi, Y., Oghushi, H., Tamai, S., Ichijima, K. (2000). In vivo osteogenic capability of cultured allogenic bone in porous hydroxyappetite: immunosuppressive and osteogenic potential of FK506 in vivo. *J Bone Miner Res.* 15:1147–57.
45. Voggenreiter, G., Assenmacher, S., Kreuzfelder, E., Wolf, M., Kim, M.R., Na Kolb, D., Schade, F.U. (2000). Immunosuppression with FK506 increases bone induction in demineralized isogeneic and xenogeneic bone matrix in the rat. *J Bone Miner Res.* 15:1825–1834.
46. Shinji, K., Kazuhisa, B., Yasunori, O., Junya, S., Kenji, K,, Yutaka, O. and Tadahiko, I. (2002). Effect of FK506 on osteoinduction by recombinant human bone morphogenetic protein-2. *Life Sciences.* 72:247–256.
47. Sun, L., Zaide, M., et al. (2004).
48. Walsh, C.T., Zydowsky, L.D., McKeon, F.D., (1992). Cyclosporin A, the cyclophilin class of peptidyl isomerases, and blockade of T cell transduction. *J Biol Chem.* 267:13115–8.
49. Sun, L., Moongo, B.S, Lu, M., Zaidi, N., Iqbal, J., Blair, H., Epstein, S., Abe, E., Troen, B., Huang, C.L.H., Zaidi, M. (2003). Molecular cloning, expression, and function of osteoclastic calcineurin A. *Am J Physiol Renal Physiol.* 284:F575-F583.
50. William, J.P., Mckenna, M.A., Thames III, A.M., McDonald, J.M. (2003). Effects of cyclosporine on osteoclast activity: inhibition of calcineurin activity with minimal effects on bone resorption and acid transport activity. *J Bone Miner Res.* 18:451–457.
51. Kuo, C.J., Chung, J., Fiorentino, D.F., Flanagan, W.M., Crabtree G.R. (1992). Rapamycin selectively inhibits interleukin-2 activation of p70 S6 kinase. *Nature.* 358:70–3.
52. Romero, D.F., Buchinsky, F.J., Rucinski, B., Cvetkovic, M., Bryer, H.P., Liang, X.G., Ma, Y.F., Jee, W.S., Epstein, S. (1995). *J Bone Miner Res.* 10:760–768.
53. Shui, Riggs, B.L., Khosla, S. (2002). The immunosuppressant rapamycin, alone or with transforming growth factor-b, enhances osteoclast differentiation of RAW264.7 monocyte-macrophage cells in the presence of RANK-ligand. *Calcif Tiss Int.* 71:437–446.
54. Quinn, J.M., Itoh, K., Udagawa, N., Hausler, K., Yasuda, H., Shima, N., Mizuno, A., Higashio, K., Takahashi, N., Suda, T., Martin, T.J., Gillepsie, M.T. (2001). Transforming growth factor affects osteoclast differentiation via direct and indirect actions. *J Bone Miner Res.* 16:1787–1794.
55. Chen, Y.G., Liu, F., Massague, J. (1997). Mechanism of TGF-β receptor inhibition by FKBP12. *EMBO J.* 16:3866–3876.
56. Ogawa, T., Tokuda, M., Tomizawa, K., Matsui, H., Itano, T., Konishi, R., Na, S., Hatase, O. (1998). Osteoblastic differentiation is enhanced by rapamycin in rat osteoblast-like osteosarcoma cells. *Biochem Biophys Res Commun.* 249:226–30.
57. Epstein, S., Inzerillo, A.M., Caminis, J., Zaidi, M. (2003). Disorders associated with acute rapid and severe bone loss. *J Bone Miner Res.* 18(12):2083–94.

CHAPTER 6

Bone and the Immune System

M. Neale Weitzmann, PhD
Roberto Pacifici, MD
Division of Endocrinology, Metabolism and Lipids, Emory University School of Medicine, Atlanta, GA

I. INTRODUCTION

Post transplant bone disease (PTBD) is a common complication of solid organ transplantation and bone marrow transplantation (BMT) and is characterized by abnormal bone turnover leading to rapid bone loss and increased fracture incidence [1, 2]. The pathogenesis of this condition is complex and poorly understood. The main causes of PTBD are listed in Table 1.

Although glucocorticoids and immunosuppressants play a pivotal role in inducing PTBD, bone loss and fractures frequently occur in patients subjected to autologous BMT who are not routinely treated with these agents. This observation suggests that additional pathogenetic factors play a key role in PTBD. Among them, and of particular importance, is sex steroid deficiency, which often ensues as a complication of bone marrow ablation, total irradiation, pharmacological interventions, and the disease state itself [3]. Thus, the pathogenesis of PTBD may be, in part, similar to that of the bone disease induced by estrogen deficiency. The main mechanism by which sex steroid deficiency leads to bone loss is augmentation of the production of osteoclastogenic and inflammatory cytokines by T cells, bone marrow macrophages (BMM), and bone cells. Indeed, recent studies have shown the presence of increased osteoclastogenic cytokine levels in patients with PTBD [4, 5, 6], hence the main osteoclastogenic cytokines presently known to regulate bone mass are extremely relevant for PTBD, and current knowledge pertaining to their effects and mechanisms of regulation will be reviewed in detail in this chapter.

TABLE 1 Main causes of transplant-induced osteoporosis

- Glucocorticoids
- Immunosuppressive therapy
- Myeloablative therapy
- Irradiation
- Inflammation
- Sex-Steroid deficiency

II. CELLS AND CYTOKINES THAT REGULATE OSTEOCLAST FORMATION

Osteoclasts arise by cytokine-driven proliferation and differentiation of hematopoietic precursors of the monocytic lineage [7]. This process is facilitated by bone marrow stromal cells (see Figure 1), a population that provides a physical support for nascent osteoclasts and produces soluble and membrane-associated factors essential for the proliferation and/or differentiation of osteoclast precursors. Lymphocytes of both T- and B-cell lineage also contribute to the regulation of osteoclastogenesis, especially in stimulated conditions.

T cells have the capacity to secrete a wide variety of cytokines, some pro-osteoclastogenic and some anti-osteoclastogenic. Inactive T cells appear to repress osteoclast formation [8], but the relevance of this phenomenon *in vivo* has not been established. In contrast, naïve and activated T cells play a key role in the regulation of osteoclast formation through increased production of Receptor Activator of NFκB Ligand (RANKL) [8, 9, 10, 11, 12], and its decoy receptor osteoprotegerin (OPG) [8]. Activated T cells also produce IFNα and IFNγ [13] which limit, in part, RANKL-induced bone resorption by repressing NFκB and JNK signaling pathways. The net effect

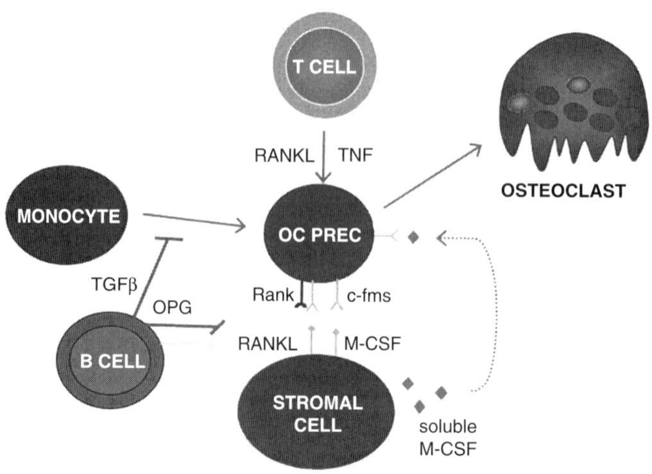

FIGURE 1 Cells and cytokines critical for osteoclast formation.

of T cells on osteoclast formation may consequently represent the prevailing balance of anti- and pro-osteoclastogenic T-cell cytokine secretion. It appears, however, that during stimulated conditions such as inflammation [9] and during estrogen deficiency [14, 15, 16, 17], pro-osteoclastogenic cytokines prevail.

B cells have been reported to have complex and controversial effects on osteoclastogenesis. For example, preliminary data demonstrate that B-cell-deficient mice display decreased trabecular area and increased bone resorption, as compared to B-cell-replete mice of the same strain, suggesting that B cells inhibit bone resorption and osteoclastogenesis. This is consistent with *in vitro* studies demonstrating that B cells may secrete OPG [18], an anti-osteoclastogenic factor. In addition, human B cells inhibit osteoclast formation as they are an important source of transforming growth factor beta (TGFβ), a factor with complex actions on osteoclastogenesis. TGFβ inhibits osteoclast formation directly by inducing apoptosis of early and late osteoclast precursors and mature osteoclasts [19, 20] as well as by suppressing osteoblastic transcription of the key osteoclastogenic cytokine RANKL [21]. TGFβ has also been reported to be capable of augmenting RANKL-induced osteoclast formation, however [21]. In contrast to the inhibitory actions of B cells on osteoclast formation, activated B cells have been reported to produce RANKL and thus may potentially stimulate osteoclast formation [22]. In addition, estrogen deficiency up-regulates B-lymphopoiesis in the bone marrow, suggesting that cells of the B lineage may contribute to the increased osteoclast production characteristic of estrogen-deficient animals [23]. Although the *in vitro* actions of B cells may appear to be contradictory, ultimately, the final balance and concentrations of stimulatory and inhibitory B-cell-derived cytokines *in vivo* will determine the final outcome on osteoclastogenesis under the prevailing environmental conditions, be they physiological or pathological.

Among the cytokines involved in the regulation of osteoclast formation are RANKL and macrophage colony stimulating factor (M-CSF). These factors are produced primarily by bone marrow stromal cells [24, 25, 26], osteoblasts [25, 27], and activated T cells [10, 12, 28, 29]. A member of the TNF superfamily, RANKL exists in both membrane-bound and soluble forms. RANKL binds to the transmembrane receptor RANK, which is expressed on the surface of osteoclasts and osteoclast precursor cells of the monocytic lineage. RANKL also binds to OPG, a soluble decoy receptor produced by numerous hematopoietic cells. Thus, by sequestering RANKL and preventing its binding to RANK, OPG functions as a potent anti-osteoclastogenic cytokine [7, 26].

In physiological conditions, M-CSF and RANKL are the only factors produced in the bone marrow in an amount sufficient to induce osteoclast formation. Thus, M-CSF and RANKL are regarded as the true essential physiologic osteoclastogenic cytokines. The critical role of each of these cytokines in the osteoclastogenic process is demonstrated by the finding that deletion of either gene prompts osteopetrosis due to the absence of osteoclasts [29, 30], a circumstance reversed by administration of the relevant cytokine [24, 30].

M-CSF induces the proliferation of early osteoclast precursors, the differentiation of more mature osteoclasts, and the fusion of mononucleated pre-osteoclasts, and it increases the survival of mature osteoclasts. RANKL does not induce cell proliferation, but promotes the differentiation of osteoclast precursors from an early stage of maturation to fully mature multinucleated osteoclasts. RANKL is also capable of activating mature osteoclasts, thus stimulating the capacity of these cells to resorb bone.

III. MECHANISM OF ACTION OF ESTROGEN IN BONE

The antiresorptive activity of estrogen is a result of multiple genomic and nongenomic effects on bone marrow (BM) and bone cells which lead to decreased osteoclast formation, increased osteoclast apoptosis, and decreased capacity of mature osteoclasts to resorb bone [31]. Although it is now recognized that stimulation of bone resorption in response to estrogen deficiency is mainly due to cytokine-driven increased osteoclast formation [32, 33], the responsible factors are not completely understood. Osteoclast formation occurs when BMM are costimulated by RANKL and M-CSF [29, 33, 34], but additional cytokines, including IL-1, IL-6, IL-7, IL-11, and TNF, are responsible for the up-regulation of osteoclast formation observed in a variety of conditions such as inflammation, hyperparathyroidism, and estrogen deficiency [35, 36, 37].

One of the cytokines responsible for the augmented osteoclastogenesis of estrogen deficiency is TNF [34], a factor that enhances osteoclast formation by up-regulating the stromal cell production of RANKL and M-CSF [38, 39] and by augmenting the responsiveness of osteoclast precursors to RANKL [14, 40]. The ability of TNF to increase the osteoclastogenic activity of RANKL is due to synergistic interactions between TNF and RANKL at the level of NFκB and JNK signaling.

The relevance of TNF to the mechanism by which estrogen causes bone loss has been demonstrated using multiple animal models. For example, ovariectomy fails to induce bone loss in TNF knockout mice [16], transgenic mice insensitive to TNF due to the overexpression of a soluble TNF receptor [41], and mice treated with the TNF inhibitor, TNF binding protein [42].

The presence of increased levels of TNF in the BM of ovariectomized animals and in the conditioned media (CM) of peripheral blood cells of postmenopausal women is well documented [43, 44, 45, 46, 47, 48]. The cells responsible for this phenomenon have not been conclusively identified, however. Earlier studies revealed that estrogen deficiency increases TNF production by monocyte-enriched peripheral blood mononuclear cells and unfractionated human and murine BM cells [45, 46]. Based on these data, the source of up-regulated TNF production was ascribed to BMM. Recent studies on highly purified cells, however, have revealed that ovariectomy increases the production of TNF by T cells, but not by BMM [14]. These conflicting results are due in part to the fact that adherent BM cells contain T cells (approximately 10% of total cells) and that ovariectomy approximately doubles T-cell content. Thus, the ovariectomy-induced increase in TNF levels is likely to be a result of T-cell TNF production. These findings in the mouse are concordant with those of others [49] in humans, which demonstrated that adherent mononuclear blood cells contain $CD3^+$ $CD56^+$ lymphocytes, a TNF-producing subset of adherent T cells. In that study, the number of $CD3^+$ $CD56^+$ T cells was decreased by estrogen treatment and inversely correlated with bone density. Thus, earlier findings in BM and adherent cell cultures are consistent with the stimulatory effect of estrogen deficiency on the T-cell production of TNF observed in more recent studies.

IV. T CELL–PRODUCED CYTOKINES AND BONE LOSS

Recently, evidence has accumulated suggesting that activated T cells play a pivotal role in the bone wasting induced by estrogen deficiency [14]. T cells are a major source of TNF, and ovariectomy enhances the production of T-cell-derived TNF. TNF acts through the TNF receptor p55, to augment RANKL-induced osteoclastogenesis and osteoclast activity [50].

Attesting to the relevance of TNF in estrogen deficiency–induced bone loss *in vivo*, athymic T cell–deficient nude mice are completely protected against the bone loss and increase in bone turnover induced by ovariectomy (see Figure 2) [14, 16]. Reconstitution studies in nude mice have subsequently shown that the relevant T-cell subpopulation is $CD4^+$ cells. In fact, nude ovariectomized mice lose bone like Wild Type (WT) ovariectomized mice after adoptive transfer of $CD4^+$ cells. In contrast, adoptive transfer of $CD8^+$ cells does not reinduce the capacity of ovariectomy to cause bone loss and elevate bone turnover. Together these data establish $CD4^+$ T cells as essential mediators of the bone-wasting effect of estrogen deficiency *in vivo*.

T cells play a key role as inducers of bone wasting because ovariectomy increases T-cell production of TNF to a level sufficient to augment RANKL-induced osteoclastogenesis [14]. Although T cells are also a significant source of soluble RANKL, T cell–derived RANKL alone appears to be insufficient to drive estrogen deficiency–induced osteoporosis. One explanation for this is that RANKL-induced osteoclastogenesis may be compensated for by an increase in the production of OPG, hence counteracting the effect of increased RANKL. Alternatively, enhanced RANKL-induced bone resorption may be compensated for by an increase in the rate of bone formation, a direct consequence of coupling between osteoclasts and osteoblasts. Thus, despite a higher rate of total bone turnover, no net loss of bone may occur.

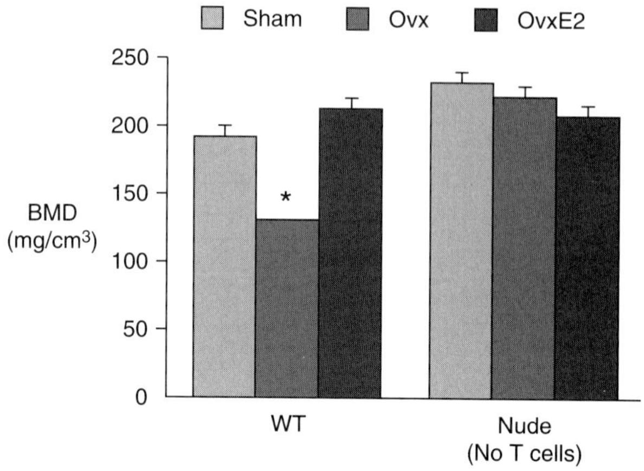

FIGURE 2 Nude mice are completely protected against ovariectomy-induced bone loss.

The data suggest, however, that elevated T cell–derived TNF may be pivotal to disrupting the coupling between bone resorption and bone formation, not only by synergizing with RANKL to potently stimulate bone resorption, but also by repressing the compensatory increase in bone formation. During estrogen deficiency, bone formation, although actually increased, fails to reach the magnitude necessary to compensate for elevated levels of bone resorption. This imbalance in formation rate relative to resorption ultimately leads to net bone loss. The mechanism of uncoupling is poorly understood, but TNF has long been recognized as a repressor of bone formation *in vivo*, as TNF neutralization in ovariectomized rats leads not only to a suppression of osteoclastic bone resorption, but also to a stimulation of bone formation [51]. *In vitro*, TNF inhibits osteocalcin production and mineralization of osteoblastic cell lines [52]. Consistent with these observations, TNF has been reported to repress the differentiation of osteoblast precursors into mature osteoblasts [53] by inhibiting the critical osteoblastic transcription factor Runx2. TNF blocks the expression of Runx2 at multiple levels, including destabilization of its mRNA and suppression of its transcription [54]. Thus TNF appears to be a critical cytokine in the etiology of osteoporosis resulting from estrogen deficiency.

Although TNF may be derived from many sources in the bone marrow, the specific relevance of T cell–produced TNF *in vivo* was demonstrated by the finding that while reconstitution of nude recipient mice with T cells from WT mice restores the capacity of ovariectomy to induce bone loss, reconstitution with T cells from TNF-deficient mice does not [16]. It should be noted that nude mice reconstituted with TNF −/− T cells were protected against ovariectomy-induced bone loss even though they possess BMM and other TNF-producing cells, a finding that establishes a specific role for T cell–derived TNF. TNF has been reported to stimulate RANKL in osteoblasts. Thus, the possibility that T cell–produced TNF further augments bone loss by stimulating T-cell production of RANKL cannot be formally excluded, although TNF has not been reported to induce RANKL production by murine T cells.

Evidence is beginning to accumulate to suggest that T cells play a relevant role in regulating bone resorption not only in rodents but also in humans. For example, it has been shown that RANKL expression in T cells is up-regulated by estrogen deficiency and correlates directly with increases in bone resorption markers and inversely with serum 17ß-estradiol [55].

In summary, up-regulated T-cell production of TNF appears to be a key mechanism by which ovariectomy induces bone loss for the following reasons: first, ovariectomy increases T-cell TNF production in the BM. Second, TNF increases the responsiveness of osteoclast precursors to RANKL (produced by either stromal cells/osteoblasts or T cells), while simultaneously suppressing the magnitude of the compensatory increase in bone formation. Third, mice lacking or insensitive to TNF are completely protected against ovariectomy-induced bone loss. Finally, WT T-cell reconstitution in nude mice restores the capacity of ovariectomy to induce bone loss, while reconstitution of nude mice with TNF −/− T cells fails to do so.

V. MECHANISMS OF ESTROGEN REGULATION OF T-CELL PRODUCTION OF TNF

Ovariectomy up-regulates T-cell TNF production by increasing the number of TNF-producing T cells without altering the amount of TNF produced by each T cell [16]. This is the result of a complex pathway, summarized in Figure 3. Ovariectomy causes an expansion of the T-cell pool in the BM, spleen, and lymph nodes by increasing T-cell activation, a phenomenon that results in increased T-cell proliferation and life span. Ovariectomy increases T-cell activation by enhancing antigen presentation by BMM; this is a result of the ability of estrogen deficiency to up-regulate the expression of major histocompatibility complex II (MHCII). Although the mechanism of T-cell activation elicited by estrogen deficiency is similar to that triggered by infections, the intensity of the events that follow estrogen withdrawal is significantly less severe. This process should be envisioned as a partial increase in T-cell autoreactivity to self-peptides, resulting in a doubling of the pool of effector $CD4^+$ cells. Modulation of antigen presentation by estrogen is BMM- and dendritic cell-specific because no changes are induced by ovariectomy in B cells and dendritic cells, the other two populations of professional antigen-presenting cells (APCs) [15].

The relevance of this mechanism *in vivo* was established by using DO11.10 mice, a strain in which all T cells recognize a single peptide epitope of chicken albumin (ovalbumin), which is not expressed in mice. In the absence of ovalbumin, APC of DO11.10 mice are unable to induces T-cell activation. If APC are a relevant target of estrogen, therefore, these

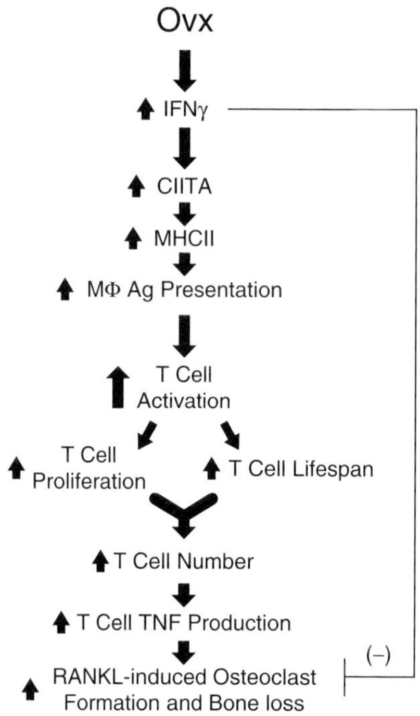

FIGURE 3 Summary of mechanism by which estrogen deficiency increases the T cell production of TNF.

mice should be protected from the increased T-cell proliferation, the suppression of activation-induced T-cell death, and the bone loss that follows ovariectomy. As predicted, ovariectomy fails to increase T-cell proliferation and lifespan in DO11.10 mice. As a result, ovariectomy fails to increase the pool of T cells and to induce bone loss in these mice [15]. In addition, injection of ovalbumin, which permits the generation of the appropriate MHC-peptide antigen for these T cells, restores the capacity of ovariectomy to expand the T-cell pool by targeting proliferation and apoptosis and inducing bone loss. These data demonstrate that antigen presentation, specifically the generation of appropriate peptide–MHC complexes, is critical to the process by which ovariectomy increases T-cell proliferation and lifespan and leads to bone loss. Furthermore, the finding that T cells from ovariectomized mice exhibit an increased response to ovalbumin (an antigen not present in mammals) demonstrates that ovariectomy increases the reactivity of APC to endogenous antigens, rather than stimulating the production of a new antigen or modulating antigen levels.

The mechanism just described hinges on the ability of APCs to present antigenic peptides bound to MHCII molecules to T cells. The question thus arises about the source of the involved antigens. Estrogen deficiency is likely to increase the reactivity of T cells to a pool of self and foreign antigens physiologically present in healthy animals. This is consistent with the fact that clones of T cells expressing T-cell receptor (TCR) directed against self antigens not expressed in the thymus survive negative selection during T-cell maturation [56, 57, 58, 59]. Such clones are known as autoreactive or self-reactive T cells and reside in peripheral lymphatic organs of adult individuals [60]. In addition, foreign antigens of bacterial origin are physiologically absorbed in the gut. As these peptides come in contact with immune cells locally and systemically, they induce a low-grade T-cell activation [60]. Thus, a moderate immune response is constantly in place in healthy humans and rodents due to presentation by MHCII and MHCI molecules of both self and foreign peptides to $CD4^+$ and $CD8^+$ T cells [61]. This autoreactive response is thought to be essential for immune-cell survival and renewal [62]. In summary, according to our hypothesis, ovariectomy would increase T-cell autoreactivity by up-regulating antigen presentation by BMM.

The effects of ovariectomy on antigen presentation and the resulting changes in T-cell activation, proliferation, and lifespan are explained by a stimulatory effect of ovariectomy on the expression of the gene encoding Class II Transactivator (CIITA). The product of the CIITA gene is a non-DNA binding factor that functions as a transcriptional coactivator when recruited to the MHCII promoter by interaction with promoter-bound factors [63, 64]. CIITA expression is, indeed, required and sufficient for the stimulation of antigen presentation in BMM.

CIITA expression is regulated by four distinct promoters that direct the transcription of four separate first exons spliced to a common second exon [65]. While initial studies revealed that IFNγ-inducible expression in murine BMM is regulated exclusively by promoter IV [65, 66], it is now recognized that both promoter I and IV account for IFNγ-induced CIITA in BMM *in vitro* and *in vivo* [67, 68].

CIITA is constitutively expressed in B cells and dendritic cells, but not in BMM. The physiologic inducer of CIITA in BMM is IFNγ. Increased CIITA expression in BMM from ovariectomized mice is a result of the ability of ovariectomy to increase both the T-cell production of IFNγ and the responsiveness of the CIITA gene to IFNγ in BMM [15]. This second regulatory mechanism is revealed by the greater expression of CIITA and MHCII by BMM from ovariectomized mice as compared to BMM harvested from estrogen-replete animals, in response to an equal stimulation with IFNγ [15].

That ovariectomy increases T-cell production of IFNγ was demonstrated both by measuring the level of the cytokine in the culture media of purified T cells cultured for 24 hours and by FACS analysis of unfractionated BM. IFNγ production by T cells is induced by either a cyclosporin-A-sensitive T cell receptor (TCR)–dependent mechanism, mediated by T-cell activation or by the cytokines IL-12 and IL-18 through activation of the MAP kinase p38. The increased production of IFNγ by T cells from ovariectomized mice is suppressed by *in vitro* treatment with the selective p38 inhibitor SB203580, but not by the activation inhibitor cyclosporin-A, indicating that increased IFNγ production by $CD4^+$ cells in ovariectomized mice is cytokine-driven. The expression of the IL-12 and IL-18 genes in BMM is induced by NFκB and AP-1, nuclear proteins whose transcriptional activity is directly repressed by estrogen [69, 70, 71]. Unstimulated BMM such as those from estrogen-replete mice are known to express low or undetectable levels of NFκB and AP-1 [72]. Accordingly, ELISAs revealed that sham BMM express minimal levels of IL-12 and IL-18, and ovariectomy potently increases secretion of IL-12 and IL-18 while *in vitro* treatment with 17β estradiol represses it. Thus, one mechanism by which estrogen represses CIITA is by decreasing IFNγ production via an inhibitory effect on the BMM production of IL-12 and IL-18.

It should also be noted that because CIITA expression in T cells stimulates IFNγ production [73], and IFNγ stimulates both its own inducers, IL-18 and IL-12, and IL-12 receptor expression [74, 75], ovariectomy triggers an amplification loop leading to a further increase in the level of IFNγ and the resulting induction of CIITA.

VI. ESTROGEN REGULATION OF IFNγ PRODUCTION AND *IN VIVO* EFFECTS OF IFNγ IN BONE

IFNγ is a key upstream factor in a complex pathway by which ovariectomy leads to increased T-cell proliferation and T-cell TNF production. We found ovariectomy to up-regulate IFNγ production *in vivo*, despite reports that estrogen exerts a direct stimulatory effect on IFNγ gene expression *in vitro* [76]. Together, the data suggest that *in vivo,* the indirect repressive effect of estrogen is more potent than the direct stimulatory effect of sex steroid previously observed *in vitro*. Similarly, IFNγ has been shown to repress osteoclast formation *in vitro* via a direct effect on maturing osteoclasts [77]. In contrast, we found IFNγ to indirectly stimulate osteoclast formation via augmentation of T-cell TNF production *in vivo*. IFNγ receptor knockout mice are entirely protected against ovariectomy-induced bone loss (see Figure 4). Furthermore, ovariectomy fails to increase CIITA expression in IFNγ receptor knockout mice [15]. Thus, the data strongly suggest that during *in vivo* conditions of estrogen deficiency, the indirect proresorptive effect of IFNγ prevails over the direct repressive effect on osteoclastogenesis. This is consistent with previous reports showing increased bone resorption and/or bone loss *in vivo* in models of IFNγ overexpression [78, 79]. Although other studies have found that IFNγ decreases bone resorption *in vivo*, such investigations have been carried out in T cell–deficient mice [80, 81], thus further demonstrating that the T cell–mediated indirect effects of IFNγ are more potent than the direct repressive effects. In one study, IFNγ has been shown to repress bone resorption *in vivo* in a T cell–replete model, but the only *in vivo* data presented were obtained in the calvarias of newborn mice [13]. Thus the significance of these observations in mature bone remains unknown.

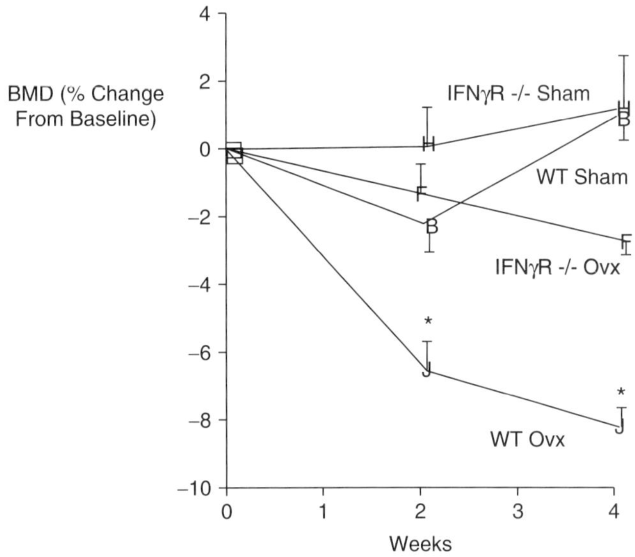

FIGURE 4 IFNγR −/− mice are completely protected against ovariectomy-induced bone loss.

VII. THE ROLE OF IL-7 IN PTBD AND POSTMENOPAUSAL BONE LOSS

Another cytokine now implicated as a potential key player in osteoporosis induced by estrogen deficiency is IL-7 [82]. Following solid organ and BMT transplantation, the production of IL-7 increases sharply in response to both marrow ablation and estrogen deficiency [17].

IL-7 is a powerful lymphopoietic cytokine that has previously been recognized as a potent inducer of bone destruction *in vivo* [83]. How IL-7 leads to bone loss is controversial, and its mechanisms of action are only now beginning to be elucidated. IL-7 is a stimulator of both B- and T-cell lineages, and it has been suggested that IL-7 induces bone loss by a mechanism involving the expansion of cells of the B lineage, in particular $B220^{+}IgM^{-}$ B cell precursors [23, 83, 84, 85], as estrogen deficiency has been reported to potently induce the expansion of these cells [23, 83]. How B lineage cells may lead to bone destruction is not presently understood but may involve overexpression of RANKL, a property of activated B cells [22]. Alternatively, early $B220^{+}IgM^{-}$ precursor cells have been found to be capable of differentiating into OCs in response to M-CSF and/or RANKL *in vitro* [84, 86, 87], hence IL-7 may increase the pool of early osteoclast precursors. Other studies, however, have reported that IL-7 inhibits the differentiation of $B220^{+}$ cells into OCs *in vitro* in the presence of saturating concentrations of RANKL and M-CSF (87). IL-7 is also established to regulate multiple stages of T-cell metabolism [88]. IL-7 knockout mice are severely lymphopenic [89] and have been reported to display increased bone volume and bone mineral density [83]. In contrast, IL-7 transgenic mice have expanded bone marrow cavities with focal osteolysis of cortical bone and eroded bone surfaces [90]. These data suggest that IL-7 may induce bone loss by a T cell–mediated mechanism. Indeed, IL-7 has been reported to induce production of RANKL by human T cells [91], and injection of IL-7 into mice *in vivo* induces bone destruction [83, 86] by eliciting the secretion by T cells of the key osteoclastogenic cytokines RANKL and TNF [86]. In addition, levels of IL-7 are significantly elevated following ovariectomy. Attesting to the key role of IL-7 in the bone destruction associated with estrogen deficiency, *in vivo* IL-7 blockade, using neutralizing antibodies, is effective in preventing ovariectomy-induced bone destruction [17]. Furthermore, IL-7–induced osteoclastogenesis and bone loss is compounded by suppression of bone formation leading to uncoupling of bone formation from resorption.

As described previously, IFNγ is a powerful inducer of macrophage CIITA, a transcription factor required for MHCII expression and antigen presentation [15]. IL-7 in turn is a potent stimulator of IFNγ production [92]. This suggests that the elevated levels of IL-7 during estrogen deficiency may be responsible for driving the T-cell proliferation that expands the TNF-producing T-cell population, by direct stimulatory and trophic effects on T cells, as well as by indirectly stimulating IFNγ and APC activity. The elevated response of BMMs and antigen presentation to T cells further drives and sustains T-cell activation, proliferation, and osteoclastogenic cytokine secretion. Finally, as IL-7 and TGFβ are reported to inversely regulate each others' production [93, 94, 95], the reduction in TGFβ signaling, characteristic of estrogen deficiency, may serve to further stimulate IL-7 production, thus driving the cycle of osteoclastogenic cytokine production and ultimately of bone destruction.

VIII. CONCLUSIONS

The mechanism leading to PTBD appears to be particularly complex as it involves the regulated production of multiple cytokines from hematopoietic cells and bone cells and the altered responsiveness of target cells to these cytokines. In addition, the contribution of specific factors to PTBD appears to vary as the system adapts over time to the hormonal withdrawal, pharmacological treatment, and disease recovery. Although many details of this process remain to be defined, it is now clearly established that sex steroid and myeloablative treatments play a pivotal role in PTBD, as they regulate the production of pro-osteoclastogenic and anti-osteoclastogenic factors by targeting several bone and bone marrow cells. This complex interplay of cytokines and cell populations is summarized in Figure 5.

The recent data pointing to a causal role of TNF and IL-7 in both PTBD and ovariectomy-induced bone loss are consistent with previous published evidence demonstrating the relevance of other estrogen-regulated cytokines such as IL-1, IL-6, M-CSF, and OPG [32]. Cytokines are, in fact, under reciprocal control and organized in a cascade fashion.

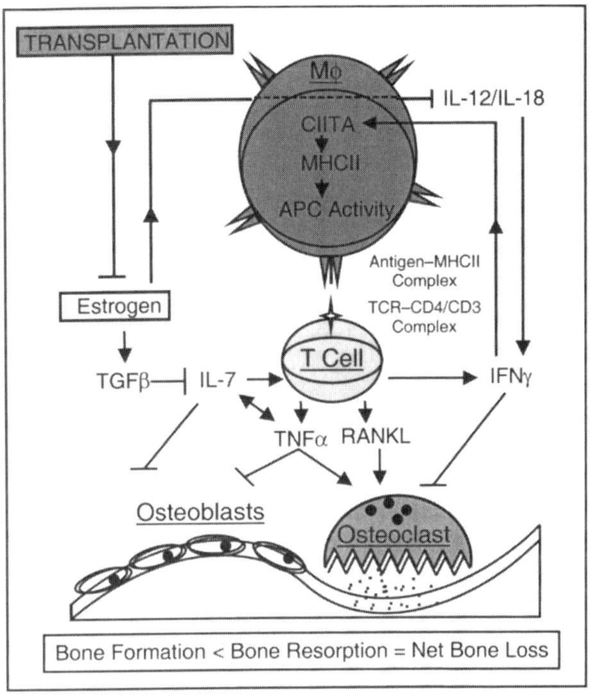

FIGURE 5 Model mechanism by which estrogen leads to PTBD.

Thus, blockade of either upstream or downstream factors in the same cascade is effective in preventing bone loss in ovariectomized mice. Furthermore, cytokines are recognized for their synergistic interactions. Thus, the neutralization of a single factor may achieve the same effect as the neutralization of the sister cytokine or both factors. For example, the report that ovariectomy fails to induce bone loss in TNF–/– mice [16] is consistent with previous studies demonstrating that mice lacking IL-6 [96] or IL-1R [97] are also protected against ovariectomy-induced bone loss. In addition, the well-defined synergies between IL-1 and TNF [98] and between TNF and RANKL [14, 40, 86, 99] are well documented.

Together, the data provide evidence of a novel regulatory link between the immune system and bone homeostasis, and contribute to our understanding of the immune targets of estrogen. Remarkable progress has been accomplished in clarifying the mechanism of the bone-sparing effect of estrogen in animal models. A more challenging task will be to demonstrate the relevance of the mechanisms described above in human subjects.

REFERENCES

1. Epstein, S., Shane, E., and Bilezikian, J.P. (1995). Organ transplantation and osteoporosis. *Current Opinion in Rheumatology*. 7:255–261.
2. Shane, E., Rivas, M., Staron, R.B., Silverberg, S.J., Seibel, M.J., Kuiper, J., Mancini, D., Addesso, V., Michler, R.E., and Factor-Litvak, P. (1996). Fracture after cardiac

transplantation: a prospective longitudinal study. *Journal of Clinical Endocrinology & Metabolism*. 81:1740–1746.

3. Ebeling, P.R., Thomas, D.M., Erbas, B., Hopper, J.L., Szer, J., and Grigg, A.P. (1999). Mechanisms of bone loss following allogeneic and autologous hemopoietic stem cell transplantation. *J Bone Miner Res*. 14:342–350.
4. Min, C.K., Lee, W.Y., Min, D.J., Lee, D.G., Kim, Y.J., Park, Y.H., Kim, H.J., Lee, S., Kim, D.W., Lee, J.W., et al. (2001). The kinetics of circulating cytokines including IL-6, TNF-alpha, IL-8 and IL-10 following allogeneic hematopoietic stem cell transplantation. *Bone Marrow Transplant*. 28:935–940.
5. Lee, W.Y., Kang, M.I., Oh, E.S., Oh, K.W., Han, J.H., Cha, B.Y., Lee, K.W., Son, H.Y., Kang, S.K., and Kim, C.C. (2002). The role of cytokines in the changes in bone turnover following bone marrow transplantation. *Osteoporos Int*. 13:62–68.
6. Withold, W., Wolf, H.H., Kollbach, S., Heyll, A., Schneider, W., and Reinauer, H. (1996). Relationship between bone metabolism and plasma cytokine levels in patients at risk of post-transplantation bone disease after bone marrow transplantation. *European Journal of Clinical Chemistry & Clinical Biochemistry*. 34:295–299.
7. Teitelbaum, S.L. (2000). Bone resorption by osteoclasts. *Science*. 289:1504–1508.
8. Grcevic, D., Lee, S.K., Marusic, A., and Lorenzo, J.A. (2000). Depletion of CD4 and CD8 T lymphocytes in mice In vivo enhances 1, 25-dihydroxyvitamin D(3)-stimulated osteoclast-like cell formation In vitro by a mechanism that is dependent on prostaglandin synthesis [In Process Citation]. *J Immunol*. 165:4231–4238.
9. Kong, Y.Y., Feige, U., Sarosi, I., Bolon, B., Tafuri, A., Morony, S., Capparelli, C., Li, J., Elliott, R., McCabe, S., et al. (1999). Activated T cells regulate bone loss and joint destruction in adjuvant arthritis through osteoprotegerin ligand. *Nature*. 402:304–309.
10. Horwood, N.J., Kartsogiannis, V., Quinn, J.M., Romas, E., Martin, T.J., and Gillespie, M.T. (1999). Activated T lymphocytes support osteoclast formation in vitro. *Biochem Biophys Res Commun*. 265:144–150.
11. Teng, Y.T., Nguyen, H., Gao, X., Kong, Y.Y., Gorczynski, R.M., Singh, B., Ellen, R.P., and Penninger, J.M. (2000). Functional human T-cell immunity and osteoprotegerin ligand control alveolar bone destruction in periodontal infection. *J Clin Invest*. 106:R59-67.
12. Weitzmann, M.N., Cenci, S., Rifas, L., Haug, J., Dipersio, J., and Pacifici, R. (2001). T cell activation induces human osteoclast formation via receptor activator of nuclear factor kappaB ligand-dependent and -independent mechanisms. *J Bone Miner Res*. 16:328–337.
13. Takayanagi, H., Ogasawara, K., Hida, S., Chiba, T., Murata, S., Sato, K., Takaoka, A., Yokochi, T., Oda, H., Tanaka, K., et al. (2000). T-cell-mediated regulation of osteoclastogenesis by signalling cross-talk between RANKL and IFN-gamma. *Nature*. 408:600–605.
14. Cenci, S., Weitzmann, M.N., Roggia, C., Namba, N., Novack, D., Woodring, J., and Pacifici, R. (2000). Estrogen deficiency induces bone loss by enhancing T-cell production of TNF-alpha. *J Clin Invest*. 106:1229–1237.
15. Cenci, S., Toraldo, G., Weitzmann, M.N., Roggia, C., Gao, Y., Qian, W.P., Sierra, O., and Pacifici, R. (2003). Estrogen deficiency induces bone loss by increasing T cell proliferation and lifespan through IFN-gamma-induced class II transactivator. *Proc Natl Acad Sci U S A* 100:10405–10410.
16. Roggia, C., Gao, Y., Cenci, S., Weitzmann, M.N., Toraldo, G., Isaia, G., and Pacifici, R. (2001). Up-regulation of TNF-producing T cells in the bone marrow: A key mechanism by which estrogen deficiency induces bone loss in vivo. *Proc Natl Acad Sci U S A* 98:13960–13965.
17. Weitzmann, M.N., Roggia, C., Toraldo, G., Weitzmann, L., and Pacifici, R. (2002). Increased production of IL-7 uncouples bone formation from bone resorption during estrogen deficiency. *J Clin Invest*. 110:1643–1650.
18. Bengtsson, A.K., and Ryan, E.J. (2002). Immune function of the decoy receptor osteoprotegerin. *Crit Rev Immunol*. 22:201–215.

19. Weitzmann, M.N., Cenci, S., Haug, J., Brown, C., DiPersio, J., and Pacifici, R. (2000). B lymphocytes inhibit human osteoclastogenesis by secretion of TGFbeta. *J Cell Biochem.* 78:318–324.
20. Hughes, D.E., Dai, A., Tiffee, J.C., Li, H.H., Mundy, G.R., and Boyce, B.F. (1996). Estrogen promotes apoptosis of murine osteoclasts mediated by TGF-beta. *Nature Medicine.* 2:1132–1136.
21. Quinn, J.M., Itoh, K., Udagawa, N., Hausler, K., Yasuda, H., Shima, N., Mizuno, A., Higashio, K., Takahashi, N., Suda, T., et al. (2001). Transforming growth factor beta affects osteoclast differentiation via direct and indirect actions. *J Bone Miner Res.* 16:1787–1794.
22. Manabe, N., Kawaguchi, H., Chikuda, H., Miyaura, C., Inada, M., Nagai, R., Nabeshima, Y., Nakamura, K., Sinclair, A.M., Scheuermann, R.H., et al. (2001). Connection between B lymphocyte and osteoclast differentiation pathways. *J Immunol.* 167:2625–2631.
23. Masuzawa, T., Miyaura, C., Onoe, Y., Kusano, K., Ohta, H., Nozawa, S., and Suda, T. (1994). Estrogen deficiency stimulates B lymphopoiesis in mouse bone marrow. *J Clin Invest.* 94:1090–1097.
24. Lacey, D.L., Timms, E., Tan, H.L., Kelley, M.J., Dunstan, C.R., Burgess, T., Elliott, R., Colombero, A., Elliott, G., Scully, S., et al. (1998). Osteoprotegerin ligand is a cytokine that regulates osteoclast differentiation and activation. *Cell.* 93:165–176.
25. Yasuda, H., Shima, N., Nakagawa, N., Yamaguchi, K., Kinosaki, M., Mochizuki, S., Tomoyasu, A., Yano, K., Goto, M., Murakami, A., et al. (1998). Osteoclast differentiation factor is a ligand for osteoprotegerin/osteoclastogenesis-inhibitory factor and is identical to TRANCE/RANKL. *Proc Natl Acad Sci U S A.* 95:3597–3602.
26. Khosla, S. (2001). Minireview: the OPG/RANKL/RANK system. *Endocrinology.* 142:5050–5055.
27. Rifas, L., Arackal, S., and Weitzmann, M.N. (2003). Inflammatory T cells rapidly induce differentiation of human bone marrow stromal cells into mature osteoblasts. *J Cell Biochem.* 88:650–659.
28. Anderson, D.M., Maraskovsky, E., Billingsley, W.L., Dougall, W.C., Tometsko, M.E., Roux, E.R., Teepe, M.C., DuBose, R.F., Cosman, D., and Galibert, L. (1997). A homologue of the TNF receptor and its ligand enhance T-cell growth and dendritic-cell function. *Nature.* 390:175–179.
29. Kong, Y.Y., Yoshida, H., Sarosi, I., Tan, H.L., Timms, E., Capparelli, C., Morony, S., Oliveira-dos-Santos, A.J., Van, G., Itie, A., et al. (1999). OPGL is a key regulator of osteoclastogenesis, lymphocyte development and lymph-node organogenesis. *Nature.* 397:315–323.
30. Felix, R., Cecchini, M.G., and Fleish, H. (1990). Macrophage colony-stimulating factor restores in vivo bone resorption in the op/op osteopetrotic mouse. *Endocrinology.* 127:2592–2597.
31. Manolagas, S.C., Kousteni, S., and Jilka, R.L. (2002). Sex steroids and bone. *Recent Prog Horm Res.* 57:385–409.
32. Pfeilschifter, J., Koditz, R., Pfohl, M., and Schatz, H. (2002). Changes in Proinflammatory Cytokine Activity after Menopause. *Endocr Rev.* 23:90–119.
33. Hofbauer, L.C., Khosla, S., Dunstan, C.R., Lacey, D.L., Boyle, W.J., and Riggs, B.L. (2000). The roles of osteoprotegerin and osteoprotegerin ligand in the paracrine regulation of bone resorption. *J Bone Miner Res.* 15:2–12.
34. Suda, T., Takahashi, N., Udagawa, N., Jimi, E., Gillespie, M.T., and Martin, T.J. (1999). Modulation of osteoclast differentiation and function by the new members of the tumor necrosis factor receptor and ligand families. *Endocr Rev.* 20:345–357.
35. Grey, A., Mitnick, M.A., Masiukiewicz, U., Sun, B.H., Rudikoff, S., Jilka, R.L., Manolagas, S.C., and Insogna, K. (1999). A role for interleukin-6 in parathyroid hormone-induced bone resorption in vivo. *Endocrinology.* 140:4683–4690.
36. Pacifici, R. (1998). Cytokines, estrogen and postmenopausal osteoporosis. The second decade. *Endocrinology.* 139:2659–2661.

37. Manolagas, S.C., Bellido, T., and Jilka, R.L. (1995). Sex steroids, cytokines and the bone marrow: new concepts on the pathogenesis of osteoporosis. [Review]. *Ciba Foundation Symposium*. 191:187–196; discuss.
38. Hofbauer, L.C., Lacey, D.L., Dunstan, C.R., Spelsberg, T.C., Riggs, B.L., and Khosla, S. (1999). Interleukin-1beta and tumor necrosis factor-alpha, but not interleukin-6, stimulate osteoprotegerin ligand gene expression in human osteoblastic cells. *Bone*. 25:255–259.
39. Sherman, M.L., Weber, B.L., Datta, R., and Kufe, D.W. (1990). Transcriptional and post-transcriptional regulation of macrophage-specific colony stimulating factor gene expression by tumor necrosis factor. *J. Clin. Invest*. 85:442–447.
40. Lam, J., Takeshita, S., Barker, J.E., Kanagawa, O., Ross, F.P., and Teitelbaum, S.L. (2000). TNF-alpha induces osteoclastogenesis by direct stimulation of macrophages exposed to permissive levels of RANK ligand. *J Clin Invest*. 106:1481–1488.
41. Ammann, P., Rizzoli, R., Bonjour, J.P., Bourrin, S., Meyer, J.M., Vassalli, P., and Garcia, I. (1997). Transgenic mice expressing soluble tumor necrosis factor-receptor are protected against bone loss caused by estrogen deficiency. *J. Clin. Invest*. 99:1699–1703.
42. Kimble, R., Bain, S., and Pacifici, R. (1997). The functional block of TNF but not of IL-6 prevents bone loss in ovariectomized mice. *JBMR*. 12:935–941.
43. Pacifici, R., Brown, C., Puscheck, E., Friedrich, E., Slatopolsky, E., Maggio, D., McCracken, R., and Avioli, L.V. (1991). Effect of surgical menopause and estrogen replacement on cytokine release from human blood mononuclear cells. *Proc. Natl. Acad. Sci*. 88:5134–5138.
44. Ralston, S.H. (1994). Analysis of gene expression in human bone biopsies by polymerase chain reaction: evidence for enhanced cytokine expression in postmenopausal osteoporosis. *J. Bone Miner. Res*. 9:883–890.
45. Kitazawa, R., Kimble, R.B., Vannice, J.L., Kung, V.T., and Pacifici, R. (1994). Interleukin-1 receptor antagonist and tumor necrosis factor binding protein decrease osteoclast formation and bone resorption in ovariectomized mice. *J. Clin. Invest*. 94:2397–2406.
46. Kimble, R.B., Srivastava, S., Ross, F.P., Matayoshi, A., and Pacifici, R. (1996). Estrogen deficiency increases the ability of stromal cells to support murine osteoclastogenesis via an interleukin-1and tumor necrosis factor-mediated stimulation of macrophage colony-stimulating factor production. *J Biol Chem*. 271:28890–28897.
47. Ralston, S.H., Gallacher, S.J., Patel, U., Fraser, W.D., Dryburgh, F.J., and Boyle, I.T. (1990). Use of bisphosphonates in hypercalcaemia due to malignancy [letter]. *Lancet*. 335:737.
48. Shanker, G., Sorci-Thomas, M., and Adams, M.R. (1994). Estrogen modulates the expression of tumor necrosis factor alpha mRNA in phorbol ester-stimulated human monocytic THP-1 cells. *Lymphokine Cytokine Res*. 13:377–382.
49. Abrahamsen, B., Bendtzen, K., and Beck-Nielsen, H. (1997). Cytokines and T-lymphocyte subsets in healthy post-menopausal women: estrogen retards bone loss without affecting the release of IL-1 or IL-1ra. *Bone*. 20:251–258.
50. Fuller, K., Murphy, C., Kirstein, B., Fox, S.W., and Chambers, T.J. (2002). TNFalpha potently activates osteoclasts, through a direct action independent of and strongly synergistic with RANKL. *Endocrinology*. 143:1108–1118.
51. Kimble, R.B., Matayoshi, A.B., Vannice, J.L., Kung, V.T., Williams, C., and Pacifici, R. (1995). Simultaneous block of interleukin1 and tumor necrosis factor is required to completely prevent bone loss in the early post-ovariectomy period. *Endocrinology*. 136:3054–3061.
52. Taichman, R.S., and Hauschka, P.V. (1992). Effects of interleukin-1 beta and tumor necrosis factor-alpha on osteoblastic expression of osteocalcin and mineralized extracellular matrix in vitro. *Inflammation*. 16:587–601.
53. Gilbert, L., He, X., Farmer, P., Boden, S., Kozlowski, M., Rubin, J., and Nanes, M.S. (2000). Inhibition of osteoblast differentiation by tumor necrosis factor-alpha. *Endocrinology*. 141:3956–3964.

54. Gilbert, L., He, X., Farmer, P., Rubin, J., Drissi, H., van Wijnen, A.J., Lian, J.B., Stein, G.S., and Nanes, M.S. (2002). Expression of the osteoblast differentiation factor RUNX2 (Cbfa1/AML3/Pebp2alpha A) is inhibited by tumor necrosis factor-alpha. *J Biol Chem.* 277:2695–2701.
55. Eghbali-Fatourechi, G., Khosla, S., Sanyal, A., Boyle, W.J., Lacey, D.L., and Riggs, B.L. (2003). Role of RANK ligand in mediating increased bone resorption in early postmenopausal women. *J Clin Invest.* 111:1221–1230.
56. Robey, E.A., Ramsdell, F., Gordon, J.W., Mamalaki, C., Kioussis, D., Youn, H.J., Gottlieb, P.D., Axel, R., and Fowlkes, B.J. (1992). A self-reactive T cell population that is not subject to negative selection. *Int Immunol.* 4:969–974.
57. Tanchot, C., and Rocha, B. (1997). Peripheral selection of T cell repertoires: the role of continuous thymus output. *J Exp Med.* 186:1099–1106.
58. Grossman, Z. (1993). Cellular tolerance as a dynamic state of the adaptable lymphocyte. *Immunol Rev.* 133:45–73.
59. Ahmed, R., and Gray, D. (1996). Immunological memory and protective immunity: understanding their relation. *Science.* 272:54–60.
60. Rammensee, H.G., Falk, K., and Rotzschke, O. (1993). Peptides naturally presented by MHC class I molecules. *Annu Rev Immunol.* 11:213–244.
61. Grossman, Z., and Paul, W.E. (2000). Self-tolerance: context dependent tuning of T cell antigen recognition. *Semin Immunol.* 12:197–203; discussion 257–344.
62. Tanchot, C., Lemonnier, F.A., Perarnau, B., Freitas, A.A., and Rocha, B. (1997). Differential requirements for survival and proliferation of CD8 naive or memory T cells. *Science.* 276:2057–2062.
63. Boss, J.M., and Jensen, P.E. (2003). Transcriptional regulation of the MHC class II antigen presentation pathway. *Curr Opin Immunol.* 15:105–111.
64. Nagarajan, U.M., Bushey, A., and Boss, J.M. (2002). Modulation of gene expression by the MHC class II transactivator. *J Immunol.* 169:5078–5088.
65. Muhlethaler-Mottet, A., Otten, L.A., Steimle, V., and Mach, B. (1997). Expression of MHC class II molecules in different cellular and functional compartments is controlled by differential usage of multiple promoters of the transactivator CIITA. *EMBO J.* 16:2851–2860.
66. O'Keefe, G.M., Nguyen, V.T., Ping Tang, L.L., and Benveniste, E.N. (2001). IFN-gamma regulation of class II transactivator promoter IV in macrophages and microglia: involvement of the suppressors of cytokine signaling-1 protein. *J Immunol.* 166:2260–2269.
67. Waldburger, J.M., Suter, T., Fontana, A., Acha-Orbea, H., and Reith, W. (2001). Selective abrogation of major histocompatibility complex class II expression on extrahematopoietic cells in mice lacking promoter IV of the class II transactivator gene. *J Exp Med.* 194:393–406.
68. Pai, R.K., Askew, D., Boom, W.H., and Harding, C.V. (2002). Regulation of class II MHC expression in APCs: roles of types I, III, and IV class II transactivator. *J Immunol.* 169:1326–1333.
69. An, J., Ribeiro, R.C., Webb, P., Gustafsson, J.A., Kushner, P.J., Baxter, J.D., and Leitman, D.C. (1999). Estradiol repression of tumor necrosis factor-alpha transcription requires estrogen receptor activation function-2 and is enhanced by coactivators. *Proc Natl Acad Sci U S A.* 96:15161–15166.
70. Shevde, N.K., Bendixen, A.C., Dienger, K.M., and Pike, J.W. (2000). Estrogens suppress RANK ligand-induced osteoclast differentiation via a stromal cell independent mechanism involving c-Jun repression. *Proc Natl Acad Sci U S A.* 97:7829–7834.
71. Galien, R., and Garcia, T. (1997). Estrogen receptor impairs interleukin-6 expression by preventing protein binding on the NF-kappaB site. *Nucleic Acids Res.* 25:2424–2429.
72. Muegge, K., and Durum, S. (1990). Cytokines and transcription factors. [Review]. *Cytokine.* 2:1–8.
73. Gourley, T., Roys, S., Lukacs, N.W., Kunkel, S.L., Flavell, R.A., and Chang, C.H. (1999). A novel role for the major histocompatibility complex class II transactivator CIITA in the repression of IL-4 production. *Immunity.* 10:377–386.

74. Murphy, K.M., Ouyang, W., Farrar, J.D., Yang, J., Ranganath, S., Asnagli, H., Afkarian, M., and Murphy, T.L. (2000). Signaling and transcription in T helper development. *Annu Rev Immunol.* 18:451–494.
75. Kim, Y.M., Im, J.Y., Han, S.H., Kang, H.S., and Choi, I. (2000). IFN-gamma up-regulates IL-18 gene expression via IFN consensus sequence-binding protein and activator protein-1 elements in macrophages. *J Immunol.* 165:3198–3205.
76. Fox, H.S., Bond, B.L., and Parslow, T.G. (1991). Estrogen regulates the IFN-gamma promoter. *J Immunol.* 146:4362–4367.
77. Fox, S.W., and Chambers, T.J. (2000). Interferon-gamma directly inhibits TRANCE-induced osteoclastogenesis. *Biochem Biophys Res Commun.* 276:868–872.
78. Mann, G.N., Jacobs, T.W., Buchinsky, F.J., Armstrong, E.C., Li, M., Ke, H.Z., Ma, Y.F., Jee, W.S., and Epstein, S. (1994). Interferon-gamma causes loss of bone volume in vivo and fails to ameliorate cyclosporin A-induced osteopenia. *Endocrinology.* 135: 1077–1083.
79. Baker, P.J., Dixon, M., Evans, R.T., Dufour, L., Johnson, E., and Roopenian, D.C. (1999). CD4 (+) T cells and the proinflammatory cytokines gamma interferon and interleukin-6 contribute to alveolar bone loss in mice. *Infect Immun.* 67:2804–2809.
80. Sato, K., Satoh, T., Shizume, K., Yamakawa, Y., Ono, Y., Demura, H., Akatsu, T., Takahashi, N., and Suda, T. (1992). Prolonged decrease of serum calcium concentration by murine gamma-interferon in hypercalcemic, human tumor (EC-GI)-bearing nude mice. *Cancer Res.* 52:444–449.
81. Tohkin, M., Kakudo, S., Kasai, H., and Arita, H. (1994). Comparative study of inhibitory effects by murine interferon gamma and a new bisphosphonate (alendronate) in hypercalcemic, nude mice bearing human tumor (LJC-1-JCK). *Cancer Immunol Immunother.* 39:155–160.
82. Ross, F.P. (2003). Interleukin 7 and estrogen-induced bone loss. *Trends Endocrinol Metab.* 14:147–149.
83. Miyaura, C., Onoe, Y., Inada, M., Maki, K., Ikuta, K., Ito, M., and Suda, T. (1997). Increased B-lymphopoiesis by interleukin 7 induces bone loss in mice with intact ovarian function: similarity to estrogen deficiency. *Proc Natl Acad Sci U S A.* 19:9360–9365.
84. Sato, T., Shibata, T., Ikeda, K., and Watanabe, K. (2001). Generation of bone-resorbing osteoclasts from B220+ cells: its role in accelerated osteoclastogenesis due to estrogen deficiency. *J Bone Miner Res.* 16:2215–2221.
85. Onoe, Y., Miyaura, C., Ito, M., Ohta, H., Nozawa, S., and Suda, T. (2000). Comparative effects of estrogen and raloxifene on B lymphopoiesis and bone loss induced by sex steroid deficiency in mice. *J Bone Miner Res.* 15:541–549.
86. Toraldo, G., Roggia, C., Qian, W.P., Pacifici, R., and Weitzmann, M.N. (2003). IL-7 induces bone loss in vivo by induction of receptor activator of nuclear factor kappa B ligand and tumor necrosis factor alpha from T cells. *Proc Natl Acad Sci U S A.* 100:125–130.
87. Lee, S.K., Kalinowski, J.F., Jastrzebski, S.L., Puddington, L., and Lorenzo, J.A. (2003). Interleukin-7 is a direct inhibitor of in vitro osteoclastogenesis. *Endocrinology.* 144:3524–3531.
88. Fry, T.J., and Mackall, C.L. (2001). Interleukin-7: master regulator of peripheral T-cell homeostasis? *Trends Immunol.* 22:564–571.
89. von Freeden-Jeffry, U., Vieira, P., Lucian, L.A., McNeil, T., Burdach, S.E., and Murray, R. (1995). Lymphopenia in interleukin (IL)-7 gene-deleted mice identifies IL-7 as a nonredundant cytokine. *J Exp Med.* 181:1519–1526.
90. Valenzona, H.O., Pointer, R., Ceredig, R., and Osmond, D.G. (1996). Prelymphomatous B cell hyperplasia in the bone marrow of interleukin-7 transgenic mice: precursor B cell dynamics, microenvironmental organization and osteolysis. *Exp Hematol.* 24: 1521–1529.
91. Weitzmann, M.N., Cenci, S., Rifas, L., Brown, C., and Pacifici, R. (2000). Interleukin-7 stimulates osteoclast formation by up-regulating the T-cell production of soluble osteoclastogenic cytokines. *Blood.* 96:1873–1878.

92. van Roon, J.A., Glaudemans, K.A., Bijlsma, J.W., and Lafeber, F.P. (2003). Interleukin 7 stimulates tumour necrosis factor alpha and Th1 cytokine production in joints of patients with rheumatoid arthritis. *Ann Rheum Dis.* 62:113–119.
93. Huang, M., Sharma, S., Zhu, L.X., Keane, M.P., Luo, J., Zhang, L., Burdick, M.D., Lin, Y.Q., Dohadwala, M., Gardner, B., et al. (2002). IL-7 inhibits fibroblast TGF-beta production and signaling in pulmonary fibrosis. *J Clin Invest.* 109:931–937.
94. Dubinett, S.M., Huang, M., Dhanani, S., Economou, J.S., Wang, J., Lee, P., Sharma, S., Dougherty, G.J., and McBride, W.H. (1995). Down-regulation of murine fibrosarcoma transforming growth factor-beta 1 expression by interleukin 7. *J Natl Cancer Inst.* 87:593–597.
95. Tang, J., Nuccie, B.L., Ritterman, I., Liesveld, J.L., Abboud, C.N., and Ryan, D.H. (1997). TGF-beta down-regulates stromal IL-7 secretion and inhibits proliferation of human B cell precursors. *J Immunol.* 159:117–125.
96. Poli, V., Balena, R., Fattori, E., Markatos, A., Yamamoto, M., Tanaka, H., Ciliberto, G., Rodan, G.A., and Costantini, F. (1994). Interleukin-6 deficient mice are protected from bone loss caused by estrogen depletion. *EMBO J.* 13:1189–1196.
97. Lorenzo, J.A., Naprta, A., Rao, Y., Alander, C., Glaccum, M., Widmer, M., Gronowicz, G., Kalinowski, J., and Pilbeam, C.C. (1998). Mice lacking the type I interleukin-1 receptor do not lose bone mass after ovariectomy. *Endocrinology.* 139:3022–3025.
98. Dinarello, C.A., Okusawa, S., and Gelfand, J.A. (1989). Interleukin-1 induces a shock-like state in rabbits: synergism with tumor necrosis factor and the effect of ibuprofen. *Prog. Clin. Biol Res.* 299:203–215.
99. Zhang, Y.H., Heulsmann, A., Tondravi, M.M., Mukherjee, A., and Abu-Amer, Y. (2001). Tumor necrosis factor-alpha (TNF) stimulates RANKL-induced osteoclastogenesis via coupling of TNF type 1 receptor and RANK signaling pathways. *J Biol Chem.* 276:563–568.

PART II

Pathogenesis of Transplantation-Related Bone Disease

CHAPTER 7

Fracture Prevalence and Incidence in Solid Organ Transplant Recipients

Bart L. Clarke, MD
Division of Endocrinology, Metabolism, Diabetes, and Nutrition, Mayo Clinic, Rochester, MN

Gudrun Leidig-Bruckner, MD
Department of Nuclear Medicine, Klinikum Ludwigshafen, Ludwigshafen, Germany

I. INTRODUCTION

Post-transplantation bone disease is a major complication of successful organ transplantation. It has gained clinical importance as survival rates after solid-organ transplantation have improved over the last several decades, and complications independent of graft function are of increasing relevance to the long-term outcome of these patients.

Post-transplantation bone disease is a generic term referring to the summation of transplantation-related disorders of bone metabolism and function. The most important of these disorders are the development of osteoporosis and related fractures, aseptic bone necrosis, and diffuse bone pain predominantly located in the lower limbs. The clinical significance of bone loss is related to the occurrence of insufficiency and fragility fractures, while loss of bone mass, as determined by bone mineral density (BMD) measurement, is asymptomatic and does not cause pain or dysfunction by itself. In patients with postmenopausal osteoporosis, it is well documented that osteoporotic fractures, especially of the hip, but also vertebral fractures, cause an enormous burden to patients by causing pain, limitations in activities of daily living, and emotional stress, as well as a significant burden on the public health system by costs related to direct and indirect fracture consequences.

The clinical importance of bone-related complications after organ transplantation was directly assessed by Navasa et al. [1], who evaluated quality of life and major complications in patients after liver transplantation due to primary biliary cirrhosis. In this group of 26 patients, bone pain was present in 12% and fractures in 8% before transplantation; these numbers increased to 58% and 31%, respectively, within the first year after transplantation. In the same study it was shown that in those patients with unscheduled outpatient visits after transplantation, the incidence of bone pain was significantly higher than in those who did not require unscheduled visits (81% versus 18%). These results dramatically underline the clinical and socio-economic significance of osteoporosis after solid-organ transplantation.

The occurrence of osteoporotic fractures and the resulting consequences for affected patients were recognized relatively soon after establishment of organ transplantation as a standard intervention for severe end-stage disease, but this knowledge was not readily applied to the clinical management of patients before and after organ transplantation. This deficiency seems to have been a result mainly of the non-life-threatening character of osteoporosis, in contrast to other complications such as rejection or infection, especially in the perioperative time period. Furthermore, the care of patients before and after transplantation was, and predominantly still is, performed by specialists who focus on the well-being of the transplanted organs (e.g., cardiology or gastroenterology), rather than specialists in metabolic bone disease or chronic diseases such as osteoporosis. Meanwhile, it became evident that development of osteoporosis after organ transplantation is not a slowly evolving process resulting in clinical consequences years after transplantation, but rather a rapidly developing complication that occurs around the time of organ transplantation. This understanding of post-transplantation osteoporosis developed mainly as the result of several studies documenting changes in bone mass within several months after transplantation. While there are multiple studies on the time course of changes in bone mass after transplantation of different solid organs, only a limited number of studies have evaluated the occurrence of osteoporotic fractures using prospective and standardized protocols for fracture ascertainment.

The aim of this chapter is to summarize the available data on the prevalence of osteoporotic fractures before transplantation, and the incidence or prevalence of fractures after transplantation, in patients undergoing liver, cardiac, lung, kidney, or kidney–pancreas transplantation. Available information about type of fracture, time of fracture occurrence, and predictors or risk factors for post-transplantation fracture will be reviewed. Risk factors for development of bone loss and fracture can be divided into those that influence bone health before transplantation and those that affect bone loss after transplantation. Pre-transplantation risk factors include general risk factors for osteoporosis such as age, gender, weight or body mass index, underlying end-stage disease, comorbidities, and medications known to cause bone loss. The main post-transplantation factors are immunosuppressive medications (glucocorticoids, cyclosporine, tacrolimus, and others), duration of immobilization after transplantation, and transplantation-related complications such as rejection, time to recovery, gonadal hormone status, and other factors. The frequency of osteonecrosis as another related bone complication after organ transplantation will also be described, where this is known.

II. LIVER TRANSPLANTATION

A. Pre-Transplantation Bone Loss and Fracture Prevalence

Abnormalities of bone metabolism and clinically inapparent low bone density are a common finding in patients with various chronic liver diseases [2–8]. The etiology of osteopenia or osteoporosis in patients with chronic liver diseases is multifactorial and includes impaired vitamin D metabolism, hypogonadism, immobilization, and malnutrition. Development of osteoporotic fractures has been a recognized clinical complication in cholestatic liver diseases such as primary biliary cirrhosis for many years, although the pathophysiological mechanism(s) are still not completely understood [9–14]. In several studies BMD was measured before transplantation to assess the risk of osteoporosis. In a recent study [15], including 243 consecutive patients with chronic liver diseases prior to liver transplantation, the prevalence of osteoporosis defined by WHO criteria (T-score less than −2.5) was 37%, the prevalence of osteopenia (T-score between −1.0 and −2.5) was 48%, and a normal BMD (T-score greater than −1.0) was found in only 15% of these patients. In two other studies, decreased BMD (defined by Z-score less than −2.0, or greater than 2.0 standard deviations below the mean for age- and sex-matched controls) was found in 26% and 29%, respectively [5, 6].

In spite of knowledge of decreased BMD in patients with chronic liver diseases, there are only a few studies in which transplanted patients were investigated with respect to bone fractures before liver transplantation. Therefore, in some cross-sectional studies performed after transplantation, it is not possible to differentiate clearly between fractures that occurred pre-transplantation and those that occurred post-transplantation, especially for vertebral fractures, as most studies did not include pre-transplantation spine X-rays. Porayko et al. [16] reported that in a cohort of 146 patients who underwent liver transplantation between 1985 and 1996, 3.5% of the patients had clinically diagnosed fractures before transplantation. This study reported that the prevalence of fractures before liver transplantation was markedly higher in those patients with cholestatic diseases (6%) than in those with hepatitis or other liver diseases (1%), but pre-transplant screening spine X-rays were not performed, suggesting an underestimation of true fracture prevalence. In several other studies, where pre-transplant spine X-rays were obtained, the rate of prevalent fractures before transplantation was relatively constant in the range of 7% to 13% [17–21], while in one study a higher proportion of vertebral fractures (22%) was found in patients waiting for liver transplantation [22].

B. Post-Transplantation Fracture Prevalence and Incidence

The occurrence of osteoporotic fractures within a relatively short time period after liver transplantation was noticed soon after establishment of liver transplantation [23]. Several studies on change of bone mass after liver transplantation agreed with the observation that bone loss after transplantation predominantly occurs during the first 6 months after transplantation [7, 12, 20, 24–29], with a more variable course afterwards, resulting in some recovery of bone mass [30, 31]. However, in subsequent clinical studies, mostly retrospective or cross-sectional, the rate of fractures reported has varied widely, ranging from about 4 to 65%. Most of these studies reported a fracture incidence between 20 to 30% during the first year [12, 16, 17, 18, 24, 32–37], while a few studies found lower fracture rates [27, 38, 39, 40] (see Table 1).

Because of this variation in reported fracture incidence, the clinical significance of bone loss and fractures remained unclear and was ignored for a long time. Part of this variation in reported fracture incidence after transplantation is a result of the methods used for fracture identification, as only in a few studies were spine X-rays performed routinely after transplantation, and in others, only clinically evident fractures were recorded. Furthermore, the composition and selection of patients with respect to underlying diseases, follow-up examinations, and immunosuppressive regimens varied remarkably among the studies, and these factors contribute significantly to the different fracture rates reported after liver transplantation. The importance of patient selection and underlying diseases is shown by one of the first studies on osteoporotic fractures after liver transplantation, by Porayko et al. [16], who found an overall prevalence of vertebral or rib fractures in 22% of the transplanted patients. There were impressive differences in fracture incidence according to the type of underlying liver disease, however: incident fractures occurred in 43% of the patients with primary biliary cirrhosis (PBC), 31% of the patients with primary sclerosing cholangitis (PSC), and only 4% of patients with chronic active hepatitis (CAH) and other liver diseases. While Porayko et al. [16] did not report any nonvertebral fractures, they found that 8% of all transplanted patients suffered from bone necrosis, with a distribution similar to osteoporotic fractures, indicating a higher rate in cholestatic diseases (9.5% in PBC and 19% in PSC), and a lower rate of only 4% in those with noncholestatic diseases. The reported fractures occurred predominantly within a short time period after transplantation: 57% of the fractures occurred within the first 6 months, 24% between 6 and 12 months, and only 19% more than 12 months after transplantation. This pattern of fracture development, with fractures occurring predominantly within the first year after transplantation, has been confirmed in several other studies [12, 17, 18, 24, 32, 33, 35, 36, 41].

A remarkably high rate of incident fractures was reported by Eastell et al. [12] in a subgroup of 20 patients transplanted because of primary biliary cirrhosis. Thirteen of these 20 patients had fractures (65%). The occurrence of fractures was accompanied by increased loss of BMD during the first 3 months at the lumbar spine, but an increase of BMD afterwards, resulting in bone density increase to the pre-transplantation range after 12 months,

(Text continues on p. 133)

TABLE 1A: Summary of studies on fracture prevalence and incidence after liver, cardiac, and lung transplantation (TX)

	Study type [Reference]	Mean number of patients/study (min–max, Σ patients)	Prevalence of fractures before TX (% pat.)	Prevalence of fractures after TX (% pat.)	Incidence of: Vertebral fractures after TX (% pat.)	Incidence of: Other fractures after TX (% pat.)	Incidence of: Necrosis of bone after TX (% pat.)	Special findings in respect to fractures and bone mass (BMD)
Liver	Cross sectional (10 studies; some only pretransplantation) [15,18, 19,22,27,31, 32,37,38,44]	70 (37–120; Σ 564 patients)	4–35	17–38	–	–	–	• Fractures and loss of BMD occurred predominantly during the first 6–12 months after transplantation. • Multiple fractures were common. • Cholestatic diseases had a higher fracture risk than non-cholestatic.
	Longitudinal (14 studies; some with intervention) [1,12,16,17,20, 21,24,29,34,36, 39,41,42,45]	52 (20–130; Σ 736 patients)		–	8–38	7–40	5–10	• BMD before TX did not clearly predict fractures. • Prevalent fractures before TX were associated with a higher fracture risk after TX.
Cardiac	Cross sectional (8 studies; some only pretransplantation) [40,48,55,58, 59,60,61,64]	49 (16–123; Σ 390 patients)	4–14	15–56				• Fractures and loss of BMD occurred predominantly during the first 6–12 months after transplantation. • Multiple fractures were common. • Trend for lower pre-transplantation BMD in fracture patients.
	Longitudinal (9 studies; some with intervention) [21,49,50, 51,52,54,56,62,63]	49 (25–105; Σ 437 patients)			8–36	0–8	2–6	

(Continues)

TABLE 1 *(Continued)*

	Study type [Reference]	Mean number of patients / study (min-max, Σ patients)	Prevalence of fractures before TX (% pat.)	Prevalence of fractures after TX (% pat.)	Incidence of: Vertebral fractures after TX (% pat.)	Incidence of: Other fractures after TX (% pat.)	Incidence of: Necrosis of bone after TX (% pat.)	Special findings in respect to fractures and bone mass (BMD)
Lung	Cross sectional (3 studies; some only pre-transpla-ntation) [66,69,74]	55 (21–71; Σ 220 patients)	5–32	–				• BMD before transplantation and glucocorticoid treatment before transplantation are risk factors for fractures after transplantation • Up to 80% of patients were osteoporotic or osteopenic before transplantation
	Longitudinal (6 studies; some with intervention) [68,70–73,75]	30 (12–34; Σ 183 patients)			4–23	4–33	?	

TABLE 1B: Prevalence and incidence of fractures, bone necrosis, and changes in bone mineral density (BMD) after solid organ transplantation

Liver transplantation

Reference	Patients (n)	Prevalence of fractures before TX (% pat.)	Prevalence of fractures after TX (% pat.)	Incidence of: Vertebral fractures after TX (% pat.)	Incidence of: Other fractures after TX (% pat.)	Necrosis of bone after TX (% pat.)	Special findings in respect to fractures	BMD before TX	BMD – change after TX
Haagsma et al. [41]	36	–		38			-fractures occurred within the first 6 months -no predictors for fractures		

Porayko et al. [16]	146	4		22 (Vertebrae or ribs)	–	8	57% of fractures occurred within the first 6 months; higher fracture rate in cholestatic diseases		
Eastell et al. [12]	20 (primary biliary cirrhosis)	?		35	*n-fractures:* 35 ribs 10 hip 5 radius 35 various stress fractures	5 (humerus)	65% suffered any fracture (13/20 pat) Fractures occurred predominantly during the first and second year after TX	7% lower than in age matched normal women	Decrease during the first 3 months after TX, increase afterwards
Mc Donald et al. [24]	29			17	3 (1 wrist)	10 (3 pat. with hip or knee necrosis)	Fractures were diagnosed in a mean duration of 6 months after TX		24% loss of spinal BMD in the first 3 months
Arnold et al. [17]	80 pre-TX 48 with follow up after TX	10 (8/80)		31 (15/48)	–	–			
Meys et al. [18]	31 pat. 1 yr after TX vs. 33 pat. pregraft	8.4 (pre-graft group)	29	–	–	–			
Navasa M et al. [32]	91	–	24				Multiple fractures (a total of 56 fractures in 22 patients)		
Hawkins et al. [38]	82	–		–	–	–		No correlation between BMD or loss of BMD and underlying disease, immunosuppression, acute rejections	

(*Continues*)

TABLE 1 *(Continued)*

Liver transplantation *(Continued)*

Reference	Patients (n)	Fractures before TX (% pat.)	Prevalence of fractures after TX	Incidence of: Vertebral fractures after TX (% pat.)	Incidence of: Other fractures after TX (% pat.)	Incidence of: Necrosis of bone after TX (% pat.)	Special findings in respect to fractures	BMD before TX	BMD – loss after TX
Valero et al. [19]	120 (cross sectional) 40 (longitudinal + treatment)	10	–	–	–	–			36% (of 120 pat. at various time intervals after TX) had a BMD z-score <–2 SD
Navasa et al. [1]	26			*First year:* 31 *Second year:* 8			58% of the patients had bone pain during the 1. year, which caused additional unscheduled outpatient visits		
Riemens et al. [20]	53 (therapy study)	6 (vertebral) 8 (rib)	–	25 (in the first year after TX)	–	None	Pat. with retransplantation n = 7 had an increased risk for fractures: 3/7 (=43%)		
Monegal et al. [22]	58 (BMD + X-rays prior liver TX)	22 vertebral fractures	–	–	–	–	Fractures or low BMD were found in 43% (25/58)		

Reeves et al. [37]	29 Intervention vs. historical control	–	*Since 1995* 0 (0 / 13 pat. with low BMD) *Before 1995* 38% (6/16 pat. with low BMD)				*Since 1995:* Prophylactic pamidronate therapy to patients with low BMD before and every 3 months after TX -No systematic fracture assessment, no follow up BMD *Before 1995:* No intervention	
Park et al. [45]	25 pts. 13 tacrolimus, 12 cyclosporin	–	–	28 (during the first year)			*Cyclosporin:* 8% (1/12; 1 vertebra, 1 rib) *Tacrolimus:* 46% (6/13; 5 vertebrae, 1 clavicle)	
Hussaini et al. [27]	56	–	–	–	–	–	–	L–BMD: decreases up to 12 months after TX, recovery until 24 months F-BMD decreases up to 9 months after TX without recovery
Ninkovic et al. [34]	37	35	–	27			Incident fractures were more common in pat. with prevalent fractures	t-score <–2.5 SD in 39%

(Continues)

TABLE 1 *(Continued)*

Liver transplantation *(Continued)*

Reference	Patients (n)	Fractures before TX (% pat.)	Prevalence of fractures after TX	Incidence of: Vertebral fractures after TX (% pat.)	Incidence of: Other fractures after TX (% pat.)	Incidence of: Necrosis of bone after TX (% pat.)	Special findings in respect to fractures	BMD before TX	BMD – loss after TX
Giannini et al. [31]	46 in part cross sectional/ in part longitudinal (n=21)			–	–	–		Cholestatic diseases had lower BMD; cumulative GC as a predictor of hip BMD; loss of L-BMD to daily related glucocorticoid dosages	
Ninkovic et al. [15]	243 (cross sectional, BMD and predictors prior liver TX)	–	–	–	–	–	Age and weight were predictors of BMD in women; No predictors of BMD in men	t-score (SD) 37% <-2.5 48% -1- –2.5 15% >–1	–
Monegal A et al. [36]	45	–	–	33 (vertebral + other)			Age and low BMD at transplantation were risk factors for fractures		
Leidig-Bruckner et al. [21]	130	7		1.yr: 14% 2. yr: 21% 3.yr: 30% 4.yr: 31%	7 (2 arms, 4 legs, 1 pelvis 2 others)	none	Multiple fractures: 29% 1 fracture 47% 2–4 fracture 24% > 5 fracture	t-score <–2.5 SD: 34%	

					5 of these 9 pat. had additional vertebral fractures		Prevalent vertebral fractures were the only significant predictor for incident fractures		–
Ninkovic et al. [39]	99		–	8			No difference in fracture rates between pat. with pamidronate treatment before TX and those without;		No significant lumbar but only femoral bone loss
Hommann et al. [29]	33 (liver) 3 (liver + kidney or pancreas) (therapy study)	–	–	–	–	–	No data on baseline BMD and fractures	?	BMD loss after 3–6 months, afterwards constant
Segal et al. [42]	29 (bone status mean 7.5 yrs after TX)		17 (Spinal X-rays only in relation to clinical complaints)		40 hip and others		50% of fractures occured within the first year; *Cyclosporine:* 17 fractures in 9 of 21 patients *Tacrolimus:* 2 fractures in 1 of 8 patients; Fractures occurred up to 5 yrs after TX		
Guthery et al. [44]	109 (children; mean age at TX 4 years)	–	–	–	–	–	Long term follow up of BMD in children (6±6yrs after OLT)	–	Low BMD in n = 8 (7.3%) – related to rejection therapy

(Continues)

TABLE 1 *(Continued)*

Cardiac transplantation

Reference	Patients (n)	Fractures before TX (% pat.)	Prevalence of fractures after TX	Incidence of: Vertebral fractures after TX (% pat.)	Incidence of: Other fractures after TX (% pat.)	Incidence of: Necrosis of bone after TX (% pat.)	Special findings in respect to fractures	BMD before TX	BMD loss after TX
Rich et al. [58]	16 (out of 93 pat. after TX; duration after TX 19–33 months)	–	44 (7/16 had 6 vertebral and 1 hip fracture)	–	–	–			Cumulative GC and cyclosporine dosages were negatively correlated to BMD
Shane et al. [60]	40	–	35	–	–	–	Femoral BMD was significantly lower in patients with fractures; Bio-chemical markers were not different between fracture and non-fracture patients		
Meys et al. [59]	123/203– 6 months follow up; 46 days-2 years follow up (intervention)	– –	31 (6/19)	–	–	–			No decrease in the calcidiol group, increase in the fluoride group

Lee et al. [48]	31 after cardiac TX; 14 before cardiac TX	14 (2/14 vertebral fractures)	26 (8/31 vertebral compression fractures)	–	No femoral neck fractures	6 (2/31 with osteonecrosis of the femoral head)	pts. with fractures had twice as many rejections than those without fractures; LBMD was not sig. different between pat. with and without fractures	
Sambrook et al. [54]	25 (Prospective, longitudinal BMD: 0-12 months after TX)	–	–	8	?	?	–	Change of LBMD: 0–6 mo.: −7.4±4.5% 0–12 mo: −7.8% GC or Cyclosporine dosage were not predictive for bone loss GC predicted L—BMD;
Sambrook et al. [50]	25 Prospective observational study	–	–	–	–	-		Change of LBMD (%) 0–6 mo.: −6.7 (4.8–8.6) 0–12 mo: −8.8 (6.7–10.9) Bone markers and BMD: bone loss is due to accelerated bone turnover and hypogonadism
Berguer et al. [55]	38 Group 1 (no pre-TX BMD) n = 24 Group 2 (longitudinal with pre-TX BMD) n = 14	–	–	–	–	–		*Group 1:* continuous decrease of FN-BMD over 24 months; increase of BMD at the lumbar spine and total hip after 18 /24 months *Group 2:* rapid decrease of BMD within 6 months after TX (6–10%) at L and F; stabilization or slight increase of BMD after 6–12 months

(Continues)

TABLE 1 *(Continued)*

Cardiac transplantation

				Incidence of					
Reference	Patients (n)	Fractures before TX (% pat.)	Prevalence of fractures after TX	Vertebral fractures after TX (% pat.)	Other fractures after TX (% pat.)	Necrosis of bone after TX (% pat.)	Special findings in respect to fractures	BMD before TX	BMD loss after TX
Van Cleemput et al. [52]	33	–	–	16 (clinical evident and radio-logical confirmed)	–	None	Trend for lower BMD in pat. with fractures		1 year after TX: decrease of L-BMD 8.5% and of F-BMD 10.4%
Shane et al. 1996 [62]	47 Prospective observation study	8.5 (4/47; vertebral fracture)	–	36 one or more fractures (7/13 women = 54%, 10/34 men = 29%)	8 (2 hip, 2 ribs)	–	Most fractures occurred during the first 6 months after TX; average time to first fracture 4 months F-BMD in women with fractures sig. lower than in those without; no difference in BMD in men	BMD was not a reliable predictor for fractures	Loss of BMD higher in men with fractures than in those without, no influence in women
Negri et al. [64]	24 (Cross sectional; Mean time after TX 35.4 ± 5.1 months)	–	29	–	4 (n = 1)	–	-L-BMD not different between pat. with and without fractures -F-BMD significantly lower in pat. with fractures	No data	

Van Cleemput et al. [49]	48 (intervention study)	5	–	21 (4/19-Etidronate) 5 (1/22-α-calcidol)	–	1 necrosis of femoral head	-both regimens did not prevent bone loss during the first year; -most significant bone loss during the first six months -bone loss continued at the F during the second year
Shane et al. [51]	70 (3 year follow up of BMD and bone markers)	–	–	–	–	–	Yr 1: −7.3 ± 0.9% L −10.5 ± 1.1% F Yr 2: −0.9 ± 0.9% L −0.1 ± 1.0% F Yr 3: +2.4 ± 0.8% L 0 ± 0.0% F *Radius:* decrease during the 2. and 3.year of −2.1/2.9%
Shane et al. [56]	Intervention *Group A:* 18 pat. (pamidronate + 4 cycles etidronate + 0.25 μg Calcitriol) *Group B:* 52 pat. (calcium and 400 IU vit. D)	?	–	*Group A:* 11 (3 fractures in 2/18 pat) *Group B:* 33 (30 fractures in 17/52 pat)	?	?	*After 1 yr:* In group A no significant loss of L-BMD (0.2 ± 0.9%) vs *group B* (−6.8 ± 1.0%) In *group A* no significant loss of F-BMD (0.2 ± 0.9%) vs *group B* (−6.8 ± 1.0%)

(Continues)

TABLE 1 *(Continued)*

Cardiac transplantation

Reference	Patients (n)	Fractures before TX (% pat.)	Prevalence of fractures after TX	Incidence of: Vertebral fractures after TX (% pat.)	Incidence of: Other fractures after TX (% pat.)	Incidence of: Necrosis of bone after TX (% pat.)	Special findings in respect to fractures	BMD before TX	BMD loss after TX
Ramsey-Goldman et al. [40]	61 months (Mean time since TX 51.6 ± 36)	–	15 (9/61–4 vertebrae 5 limb fractures)	–	–	–	One-third of the pat. had multiple fractures (vertebral and others)	–	–
Leidig-Bruckner et al. [21]	105	5	–	Mean follow up 3years 1.yr: 21% 2. yr: 27% 3.yr: 31% 4.yr: 32%	None	3 (3 pat. avascular necrosis of hip head)	No. of fr. 34% –1 fracture 47% 2–4 fracture 19% > 5 fracture	Osteoporosis (T-score <–2.5 SD): 1 3%	
Fahrleitner et al. [61]	57	–	56	–	–	–	-Serum osteoprotegrin the only significant predictor of BMD in a multivariate model -Prospective bone loss is correlated to the decrease of S-osteoprotegrin		
Ippoliti et al. [63]	64 (intervention)	–	–	Clodronate: 0 Placebo: 6 (2/32)	Clodronate: 0 Placebo: 3 (1/32–hip)			Clodronate: increase of LBMD, sig. higher BMD than placebo	

Lung transplantation

Reference	Patients (n)	Fractures before TX (% pat.)	Prevalence of fractures after TX	Incidence of: Vertebral fractures after TX (% pat.)	Incidence of: Other fractures after TX (% pat.)	Incidence of: Necrosis of bone after TX (% pat.)	Special findings in respect to fractures	BMD before TX	BMD loss after TX
Shane et al. [66]	70 Pre-TX-candidates end stage pulmonary disease	Vertebral fractures in 29% of COPD 25% of cystic fibrosis	–	–	–	–	Pat. with pre-exposure to GC had sig. more vertebral fractures than those without Correlation between GC-duration and BMD (r = – 0.39)	**T-score <–2.5 SD:** 30% L 49% F **T-score –1 to –2.5 SD** 35% L 31% F COPD and cystic fibrosis vs. others had significant lower BMD	
Ferrari et al. [70]	21 before TX; follow up: 6 months, 9 pat. 12 pat. 12 months	14 (3/21)	–	17 (2/12)				30% osteoporosis according to BMD before TX T-score<–2.5SD	Decrease L-BMD 4% after 6 months
Aris et al. [75]	55 pre-TX 45 after TX (3mo-3yrs)	5 (6 fractures in 3/55 pat.: radius, femur, rib, ulna)	–	?	27 (12 fractures in 10/45 pat.: 2 ulna, ischium, 4 spine, –1 meta-carpal, 2 rib, 1 radius)	–	BMD was lower in cystic fibrosis than in COPD than in others Best predictor of pre- and post-TX BMD was BMI (r = 0.5) and cummulative GC dosage (r = 0.5)	Pre-TX: L Z-score (SD) –1.3 ± 1.2 F Z-score (SD) –1.5 ± 1.1	Post-TX: L Z-score (SD) –2.3 ± 1.2 F Z-score (SD) –2.3 ± 1.3

(Continues)

TABLE 1 *(Continued)*

Lung transplantation

Reference	Patients (n)	Fractures before TX (% pat.)	Prevalence of fractures after TX	Incidence of: Vertebral fractures after TX (% pat.)	Incidence of: Other fractures after TX (% pat.)	Incidence of: Necrosis of bone after TX (% pat.)	Special findings in respect to fractures	BMD before TX	BMD – loss after TX
Schulmann et al. [74]	71	?	–	?	4/71 (5.6%) sacrum		Sacrum fractures were missed on X-rays – detected on bone scan!	3 of 4 pat. with fractures had a T-score <–2.5 SD	–
Shane et al. [72]	30	7 (vertebral fractures)	–	23 (7/30) suffered a total of 18 vertebral fractures	8 pat. with a total of 26 rib fract.; 3 pat. with sacrum fr. 2 pat. with hip fract. 1 pat. ankle 3 pat. pelvis 1 pat. sternum		37% of pat. (11/30) sustained a total of 54 fractures in the first year; average time to first fracture: 4.5 ± 1 month *Fracture pat. had:* Significant lower pre-TX BMD, More often GC before TX and duration of GC use was also longer But no differences in respect to age, rates of bone loss, rejection episodes, GC-dosages after TX	Only 6/30 (=20%) had a BMD > –1 SD t-score, the other pat. were osteo-penic or osteoporotic	L-BMD: –1.3 ± 1.2% F-BMD: –2.8 ±1.4% -no predictive variables for increased bone loss High fracture incidence although rate of bone

							Bone turnover was higher in fracture pat.		
Spira et al. [71]	28	–	–	18 (5/28) (4 pat. with vertebral fractures; 1 pat. suffered multiple fractures)	1 ankle	–	–	L-T-score: <−2.5 in 32% F-T-score <−2.5 in 54%	L-BMD: −4.8% T<−2.5SD in 50% FN-BMD: −5.3% t<−2.5SD in 78%
Aris et al. [73]	34 after lung TX Controlled randomized nonblinded trial (16 pamidronate 30 mg every 3 mo + Ca + Vit D vs 18 Ca + vit D)	32 (11/34 pat had a total of 16 vertebral 3 rib fractures)	–	Pamidronate group: 19 (3/16) control group 6 (1/18)	Pamidronate group: 19 (3/16) control group 33 (6/18) long bone fractures	–		Pam. group: T-score <−2.5 at L or F-BMD: 81 (13/16) Control group: T-score<−2.5 at L or FN-BMD: 67 (12/18)	After 2 years Change of L-BMD 8.8 ± 2.5% in the pam. group vs. 2.6±3.2% in the controls Change in FN-BMD 8.2 ± 3.8% in the pam. group vs. 0.3±2.2% in the controls

(Continues)

TABLE 1 *(Continued)*

Lung transplantation

Reference	Patients (n)	Fractures before TX (% pat.)	Prevalence of fractures after TX	Incidence of: Vertebral fractures after TX (% pat.)	Incidence of: Other fractures after TX (% pat.)	Incidence of: Necrosis of bone after TX (% pat.)	Special findings in respect to fractures	BMD before TX	BMD – loss after TX
									Change in FN-BMD 0.3 ± 2.2%
Cahill et al. [68]	**Pre-TX** N= 45 **Post-TX** 34/45 pat were trans-planted-follow up of more than 1 yr in 26 pat, 21/26 had follow up BMD	**29%** vertebral fractures or hip; untreated hypogonadism pre-TX in 50% of men and in 20% of women 15% had hypovita-minosis of Vit D	–	4 (1/21) several vertebral fractures.		?	**Pre-TX:** patients received Ca, Vit D, HRT in cases of hypogo-nadism, and after 7/1998 bisphos-phonates in pat. with T-score <–1 SD (13/21 patients) **Post-TX:** all pat. received 90 mg pamidronate i.v. every 12 weeks independent from BMD	85 % (38/45) had either osteopenia or osteo-porosis -only 15% (7/45) had normal BMD at F and L before TX BMD before TX: BMI and GC dosages as independent factors influencing BMD	BMD was stable or increased in 16/21 (76%) -of those with a significant loss of BMD most had started pamidro-nate therapy after TX
Tschopp et al. [69]	74 (observation before TX)	–	–	–	–	–		LT-score: <–2.5 in 50% FT-score <–2.5 in 61%	–

Abbreviations: GC, glucocorticoid; L, lumbar spine; F, femoral; BMD, bone mineral density; pat., patients.

and in bone density above the pre-transplantation range after 24 months of follow up. This time course of change in BMD, with a characteristic rapid decrease directly after transplantation accompanied by an increased fracture risk and subsequent recovery during long-term follow-up, seems specific for cholestatic liver diseases.

In a longitudinal observational study with a mean follow-up of more than 3 years after transplantation, Leidig-Bruckner et al. [21] showed that the rate of incident vertebral fractures was 21% after two years, and that the rate increased to 30% and 31% after 3 and 4 years, respectively. Among those patients with incident vertebral fractures, 61% had two or more vertebral fractures, which emphasizes the resulting burden of fractures for the affected patients. The distribution of incident vertebral fractures between the fourth thoracic and fifth lumbar vertebra in patients after liver or cardiac transplantation [21] is shown by fracture type in Figure 1. The pattern of fracture distribution is similar to that known from postmenopausal osteoporosis: most wedge fractures were found in the thoracic spine and in the first lumbar vertebrae, and most concavity fractures in the lumbar spine. During follow-up, further vertebral fractures occurred among 46% of the patients with incident fractures after liver transplantation.

Besides the vertebral fractures, 7% of patients experienced nonvertebral fractures, but no bone necrosis was found in this study [21]. A similar rate of nonvertebral fractures was described within a small group of patients after liver transplantation [40], in which 6% (3 of 49 patients) suffered a limb fracture, but only 4% (2 of 49 patients) suffered a vertebral fracture within two years of follow-up after transplantation. One-third of patients with a fracture suffered multiple fractures.

While there are multiple clinical studies that underline the high risk of fractures during the first and second year after liver transplantation, there

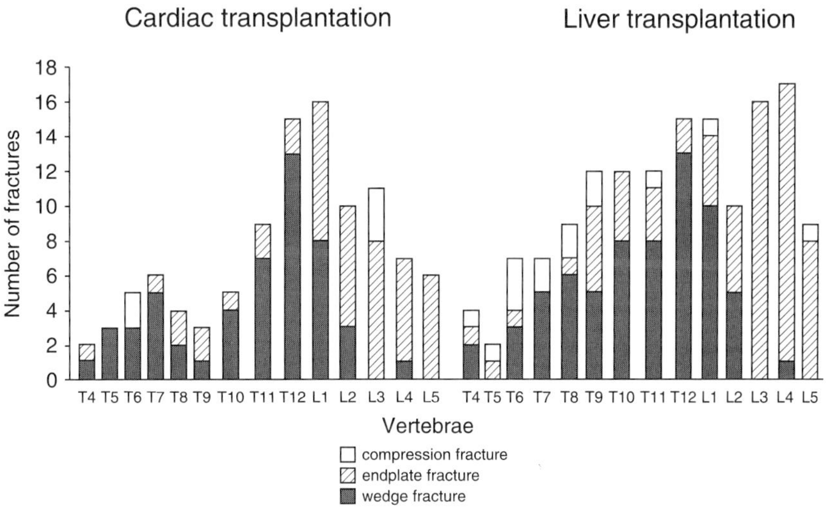

FIGURE 1 Distribution of vertebral fractures by type (wedge, concavity, compression) between the fourth thoracic and fifth lumbar vertebrae in patients with incident fractures after cardiac or liver transplantation [21].

are only a few studies with long-term follow-up data. Leidig-Bruckner et al. [21] reported that there seemed to be a stabilization in fracture incidence after the third year; however, some patients continued to fracture even up to 5 years after transplantation. Similar evidence of continued increased fracture risk is provided in a recent report by Segal et al. [42] on long-term follow-up of liver transplant patients. In this study, long-term follow-up of 29 patients after liver transplantation was reported, indicating that about 50% of post-transplantation fractures had occurred within the first year, while further fractures were observed up to 5 years after transplantation. This study is limited, however, by its cross-sectional design and the fact that X-rays were performed only in relation to clinical complaints, which probably led to underestimation of vertebral fractures in the 17% (5 of 29) of patients reported to have them, compared to nonvertebral fractures (hip and others) in 38% (11 of 29).

As most of the studies on bone loss and fracture occurrence describe patients who were transplanted in the late 1980s or the first half of the 1990s, there is an expected change in fracture incidence in relationship to the progress in transplantation medicine, including criteria for patient selection and changes in immunosuppressive regimens. Ninkovic et al. [34] reported a decrease in incidence of osteoporotic fractures during the first year after transplantation during the last decade, from about 27% in patients recruited between 1993 and 1995, to about 5% in those recruited between 1995 and 1998. Possible reasons for this observed decline in incident fractures are reduced glucocorticoid dosages and introduction of new immunosuppressive agents, as well as a change of criteria for transplantation, including patients with an earlier stage of liver disease who have better bone health before transplantation. Furthermore, a change in the type of underlying liver diseases, with a decrease in cholestatic liver diseases and an increase in patients with viral hepatitis and alcoholic cirrhosis, may have contributed to this changing risk of osteoporotic fractures over time. This observation needs further investigation, however, and the incidence of post-transplantation fractures may be expected to vary somewhat among different transplantation centers, based on variation in patient selection criteria and on center-specific intervention bias.

C. Predictors and Risk Factors for Fracture

From the studies of Porayko et al. [16], Eastell et al. [12], and Navasa et al. [32], it is clear that cholestatic liver diseases are associated with an increased risk of osteoporotic fractures after transplantation in comparison to other underlying liver diseases. While the study population of Porayko et al. [16] included a relatively large group of PBC and PSC patients (78 of 146 patients, 53%), the composition of patients in other transplantation centers is different, and characterized by a lower rate of cholestatic diseases (17 of 130 patients, 13%) [21]. As shown in the Leidig-Bruckner et al. and Carey et al. studies, the relationship between fracture risk and cholestatic diseases was still present, but less evident, and there was also a relatively high risk of fractures in patients with other liver diseases [21, 43]. Furthermore, there was no clear influence of sex or age on post-transplantation fracture risk.

Several studies have assessed the relationship between pre-transplantation BMD and risk of fractures after transplantation. There is a trend for lower BMD in patients with fractures, but no clear threshold above which fractures did not occur. In the Leidig-Bruckner et al. study [21], patients with BMD T-score less than −2.5 had a significantly higher rate of fractures than those above this level, but even patients with normal BMD before transplantation (T-score greater than −1.0) suffered from osteoporotic fractures (about 20% of this group).

Among the various post-transplantation factors likely to contribute to fracture risk, much attention has focused on the immunosuppressive regimens used. In general, daily or cumulative glucocorticoid dosages, as well as cyclosporine dosages, did not differ between patients who fractured and those who did not [12, 16, 21]. In spite of this missing direct relationship between immunosuppression and fracture development, there is strong indirect evidence that glucocorticoid therapy is one of the etiologic factors for development of severe post-transplantation osteoporosis. The first months after transplantation is the time interval with the highest rate of bone loss and highest incidence of fractures, and it is also the time interval in which the highest dosages of glucocorticoids are used. There are a few studies that have found a relationship between glucocorticoid dosages and changes in bone mass [31, 36, 44].

The influence of the new immunosuppressive therapy regimens on fracture incidence is not yet clear. From a small subgroup analysis in one study [21], and another observational study [42] in 29 patients on long-term outcome in respect to osteoporosis, there is some evidence that the rate of incident fractures is lower in liver transplant patients treated with tacrolimus in comparison to cyclosporine A. The study by Park et al. [45], however, reported a higher rate of fractures in 13 patients on tacrolimus, in comparison to 12 patients on cyclosporine. The effect of other newer immunosuppressants, such as sirolimus or mycophenolate mofetil, on fracture incidence has not yet been established.

In one study on long-term outcome after liver transplantation, older age and low BMD before transplantation predicted fractures after transplantation [36], while another study [21] using multivariate regression analysis showed that only the presence of vertebral fractures before transplantation (prevalent fractures) predicted incident post-transplantation fractures, whereas sex, age, underlying disease, and cumulative glucocorticoid dosage did not.

In summary, on the basis of the present data, it is not possible to reliably predict the risk of fracture after liver transplantation in an individual patient. All patients scheduled for liver transplantation must be considered at high risk of developing incident fractures after transplantation.

III. CARDIAC TRANSPLANTATION

A. Pre-Transplantation Bone Loss and Fracture Prevalence

Patients with chronic heart failure have been found to have increased risk of low bone mass or osteoporosis, attributed to multiple reasons such as prolonged immobility, anorexia, hypogonadism, use of diuretics, and vitamin D deficiency. Muchmore et al. [46] reported lower BMD in two-thirds of cardiac patients before transplantation in comparison to age-matched controls. In one study of patients waiting for heart transplantation, 7% met criteria for osteoporosis, defined by a T-score less than −2.5 at the lumbar spine, and 43% met criteria for osteopenia [47]. Leidig-Bruckner et al. [21] found that 13% (8 of 62) of the patients in their study were osteoporotic before transplantation, defined as having a T-score less than −2.5 at the lumbar spine, with a higher proportion of women meeting criteria for osteoporosis (45%, 5 of 11) than men (6%, 3 of 51). Similarly, 34% (21 of 62) of the patients had lumbar spine osteopenia before transplantation, defined as a T-score between −1.0 and −2.5. Fewer women met the criterion for osteopenia (27%, 3 of 11) than men (35%, 18 of 51). Nearly all cohorts of cardiac transplant patients have a strong predominance of men; women account for only about 20% of transplanted patients.

Although many studies have shown decreased BMD before cardiac transplantation, only a few studies are available looking at fracture status before transplantation and reporting pre–cardiac transplant vertebral fracture assessment by systematic spine X-ray analysis.

Lee et al. [48] reported that 2 of 14 men (14.3%) awaiting cardiac transplantation had prevalent vertebral fractures. In a cohort of 47 patients (34 men and 13 women) transplanted between 1991 and 1994, Shane et al. [45] found prevalent vertebral fractures before transplantation in 4 of 47 (8.5%). In two similar cohort studies, in which all patients were evaluated with spine X-rays before cardiac transplantation, prevalent vertebral fractures were found in 4.8% (5 of 105) [21] and 4.9% (2 of 41) [49] of patients, with all fractures found in men.

B. Post-Transplantation Fracture Prevalence and Incidence

Between 1991 and 1996, an increasing number of reports focused on changes in BMD and development of osteoporosis after cardiac transplantation, predominantly triggered by impressive case reports of the rapid occurrence of osteoporotic fractures within a short time interval after cardiac transplantation. Several prospective observational studies on change in bone mass after cardiac transplantation showed a similar pattern to that in liver transplantation, with the most rapid rate of bone loss after transplantation occurring during the first year, and with the highest rates during the first 6 months after transplantation. Bone loss at the lumbar spine during the first year was found to range between 3 and 9%, and at the femoral neck between 6 and 11%, with the highest rate of bone loss found during the first 6 months after transplantation [50–56]. The prevalence rate of osteoporotic fractures reported after cardiac transplantation varies between 15% and 56% [48, 57–61] (see Table 1). A clearer assessment of the magnitude of osteoporotic fractures after cardiac transplantation became evident from the prospective study by Shane et al. [62], who reported that osteoporotic fractures occurred in 36% (17 of 47) of patients (34 men and 13 women) with a higher proportion of fractures among women (54%, 7/13) than in men (29%, 10/34). These patients suffered a total of 34 fractures, which were predominantly vertebral, although there were 2 hip and 2 rib fractures. The most striking finding of this study was that 85% of the patients with fractures had sustained their fractures within the first 6 months after transplantation, with a peak fracture incidence during the first 3 months, and an average time to first fracture of 4 months after transplantation. In this prospective study, BMD before transplantation was not a reliable predictor of post-transplant fractures, as there was a substantial overlap in BMD between patients with and without incident fractures. Loss of femoral neck BMD during the first 6 months was significantly higher in men with fractures compared to those without, but loss of BMD did not predict fracture occurrence in women.

Van Cleemput et al. [52] found clinically evident and radiologically confirmed fractures within 1 year after cardiac transplantation in 5 of 31 men (16%). Within one recent intervention trial [63] comparing the effect of clodronate versus a placebo, the incidence of fractures was low, with no patients with vertebral fractures in the clodronate group and only 6% (2 of 32) in the placebo group, and also a low rate of nonvertebral fractures (none in the clodionate and 3% (1/32) into placebo group). In a single-center cohort study, Ramsey-Goldman et al. [40] reported fracture incidence in 9 of 61 (15%) patients after cardiac transplantation. Half of these patients had vertebral fractures, and the other half had limb fractures. The relatively low rate of vertebral fractures in comparison to nonvertebral fractures suggests an underestimation of vertebral fractures, since spine X-rays were not routinely performed. Multiple fractures were found in one third of these patients.

In an observational study of 105 patients after cardiac transplantation, with mean follow-up of 3 years, Leidig-Bruckner et al. [21] reported that the incidence of at least one fracture was 21% at the end of the first year, and that this increased to 31% at the end of the third year after transplantation. In accordance with the results reported by Shane et al. [62], most patients had vertebral fractures, and more than two-thirds of the patients with incident fractures had two or more vertebral fractures. Fracture distribution in these patients is shown in Figure 1 [21]. During follow-up, 38% of these patients with incident vertebral fractures developed further fractures.

Although the occurrence of osteonecrosis in cardiac transplant patients has been inconsistently reported, there is some evidence that osteonecrosis of the hip is a severe transplantation-related complication in some patients.

Osteonecrosis of the femoral head was reported by Lee et al. [48] in 2 of 31 (6%) male patients, by Van Cleemput et al. [49] in 1 of 48 (2%) patients, and by Leidig-Bruckner et al. [21] in 3 of 105 (3%) patients.

C. Predictors and Risk Factors for Fracture

The study by Shane et al. [62] did not clearly identify risk factors or predictors for the development of osteoporotic fractures after cardiac transplantation. There was a trend for higher fracture risk in women than in men, but the number of women in this study was small. Similar to the study done by Shane et al., Leidig-Bruckner et al. [21] found a comparably high rate of incident vertebral fractures over the first three years after transplantation, but did not find a higher fracture risk in women than in men.

The relationship between pre-transplantation BMD and risk of fractures after transplantation was assessed in several studies [21, 52, 62, 64], which found a trend for lower BMD in patients with fractures but no clear threshold above which fractures did not occur. Leidig-Bruckner et al. [21] found a significantly higher rate of fractures in those patients with a BMD T-score less than −1.0, in comparison to those with a BMD T-score above this level (hazard ratio 3.1 [95% CI, 1.1–8.8]). BMD values between patients with and without fractures still showed remarkable overlap, however, and pre-transplantation BMD did not reliably predict future fracture risk in a single patient. Additionally, there was a nonsignificant trend for a higher rate of incident vertebral fractures among patients with ischemic cardiomyopathy in comparison to those with dilated cardiomyopathy or other cardiac diseases, suggesting that vascular changes due to atherosclerosis may be also related to bone metabolism and somehow increase the risk of osteoporosis.

Among the post-transplantation factors possibly affecting bone loss and fractures, immunosuppressive regimens have been investigated extensively. In general, neither daily nor cumulative glucocorticoid dose, nor cyclosporine dose, have been different between patients who fractured and those who did not. In an observational study using multivariate regression analysis, Leidig-Bruckner et al. [21] found that age (per increase of 5 years) was the only variable associated with increased fracture risk (hazard ratio, 1.34; 95% CI, 1.03–1.75), whereas sex, underlying cardiac disease, vertebral fractures before transplantation, and cumulative glucocorticoid dose did not predict future fracture development.

The influence of new immunosuppressive therapy regimens on fracture incidence in patients after cardiac transplantation is not clear and has not been studied to date. The use of tacrolimus (FK506) did not prevent rapid bone loss in patients after cardiac transplantation in one study [65]. The more rapid reduction of glucocorticoid dose, and possibly the introduction of mycophenolate mofetil and sirolimus into immunosuppressive regimens, should be advantageous to the skeleton, and result in a lower rate of bone loss and lower incidence of fractures after cardiac transplantation. This speculation needs to be further investigated and proven in clinical studies, however, emphasizing the importance of ongoing standardized assessment of bone metabolism and fracture rates after cardiac transplantation.

IV. LUNG TRANSPLANTATION

A. Pre-Transplantation Bone Loss and Fracture Prevalence

During the last two decades, several developments and improvements in solid organ transplantation have led to an increasing number of lung transplantations and the establishment of this procedure as a treatment option in several types of end-stage lung disease. Due to experience with bone complications in patients receiving cardiac and other transplants, as well as the fact that many lung transplant candidates receive long-term glucocorticoid therapy before transplantation, bone loss and risk of osteoporotic fracture have been assessed more intensively before lung transplantation than in other types of organ transplantation.

Patients with chronic lung disease have a significantly increased risk of low bone mass and osteoporosis before transplantation. In several studies, only 15% to 25% of patients had normal BMD before transplantation, defined as a T-score above −1.0 [66, 67, 68]. Most patients before lung transplantation have a BMD in the osteoporotic range, defined as a T-score less than −2.5 (about 30–60%), or within the osteopenic range, defined as a T-score between −1.0 and −2.5 (about 35–50%). In one study in patients who were waiting for lung transplantation, 50% had osteoporosis at the lumbar spine, and 61% had osteoporosis at the femoral neck, defined by a T-score at either site of less than −2.5 [69].

There are only a few studies that have investigated the prevalence of fractures prior to lung transplantation, and the number of patients included in these studies is relatively small. In one cross-sectional study, Shane et al. [66] reported that 29% of those with chronic obstructive pulmonary disease (COPD), and 25% of those with cystic fibrosis, in a group of 70 patients with end-stage pulmonary disease awaiting lung transplantation, had at least one vertebral fracture. In this study, the proportion of patients with BMD less than T-score −2.5 was 30% at the lumbar spine and 49% at the femoral neck, and it was shown that patients with COPD or cystic fibrosis had significantly lower BMD than those with other types of lung disease. Furthermore, it was found that patients with pretransplant exposure to glucocorticoids had significantly more vertebral fractures than those without glucocorticoid use prior to transplantation. Vitamin D deficiency was found in 36% of patients with cystic fibrosis and in 20% of the other lung patients.

Ferrari et al. [70] observed fractures in 10% of patients before lung transplantation, while Spira et al. [71] found no fractures before transplantation within a smaller observational study of 28 patients (16 men, 12 women). In a prospective study by Shane et al. [72], vertebral fractures were present before transplantation in only 2 of 30 (6.7%) patients, while Cahill et al. [68] found a higher rate of prevalent vertebral or hip fractures of 29% (13 of 45) in patients before lung transplantation. A similar high rate of prevalent fractures was described by Aris et al. [73], who found vertebral or rib fractures in 11 of 34 (32%) patients before lung transplantation.

In summary, the rate of pre-transplantation bone loss as determined by low BMD, as well as the rate of prevalent osteoporotic fractures, is remarkably high in patients with end-stage pulmonary disease.

B. Post-Transplantation Fracture Prevalence and Incidence

A small number of prospective studies have evaluated the prevalence and incidence of fractures after lung transplantation (see Table 1). All studies are limited by their relatively small sample size, and differences between studies may result from the variety of underlying lung diseases and differences in the severity of these chronic diseases. Shane et al. [72] followed 30 patients over 1 year after lung transplantation, and measured changes in BMD and assessed for fractures. Of the patients included, 63% (19 of 30) had been on glucocorticoids prior to transplantation. All patients received calcium and vitamin D supplementation, as well as one or several antiresorptive agents, after transplantation. In spite of these interventions, 37% (11 of 30) of the patients sustained a total of 54 fractures in the first year after transplantation. Seven patients had a total of 18 vertebral fractures, 8 patients had a total of 26 rib fractures, 3 patients had sacrum fractures, 2 patients had hip fractures, 3 patients had pelvis fractures, 1 patient had an ankle fracture, and 1 patient had a sternal fracture. This remarkably high incidence of vertebral and non-vertebral fractures occurred despite patients having received antiresorptive treatment, although the rate of bone loss after transplantation was relatively low (lumbar spine, $-1.3 \pm 1.2\%$, and femoral neck, $-2.8 \pm 1.4\%$). There was a relatively wide intra-individual range in change of BMD after 1 year, but there were no significant predictors for increased loss of BMD. Patients with incident fractures had significantly lower pre-transplantation BMD values, but there was still significant overlap with patients who did not have fractures. The average time to first fracture was about 4–5 months after transplantation in this study.

In contrast to the high incidence of fractures found by Shane et al. [72], Cahill et al. [68] reported follow-up of 26 patients observed for more than 1 year after lung transplantation. These patients were all treated with pamidronate 90 mg IV every 3 months, independent of their BMD value before transplantation. All patients received calcium and vitamin D supplementation, and hormone replacement therapy was given in cases of recognized hypogonadism. Some of these patients had also been treated with bisphosphonates before transplantation. Only 1 of the 21 patients (5%) developed incident vertebral fractures after transplantation, and BMD remained stable or increased in 76% (16 of 21) of the patients. Patients with significant loss of BMD started pamidronate therapy predominantly after transplantation, and had not been treated with bisphosphonate therapy before transplantation. The authors concluded that pre-transplantation antiresorptive treatment might be of benefit in preventing bone loss and fractures after transplantation.

In a similar study, Aris et al. [73] followed 34 patients with cystic fibrosis, 16 of whom were treated with pamidronate 30 mg intravenously every 3 months, in comparison to 18 patients treated only with calcium and vitamin D supplementation. Although BMD increased significantly more in the pamidronate group than in the control group over 2 years after transplantation, incident fractures were not different between the two groups. Vertebral fractures occurred in 3 of 16 (19%) patients treated with pamidronate, and only 1 of 18 (6%) control patients. Nonvertebral fractures occurred in 3 of 16 (19%) patients treated with pamidronate, and 6 of 18 (33%) control patients.

C. Predictors and Risk Factors for Fracture

Shane et al. [72] found that patients with incident fractures had lower BMD before transplantation, and had more often used glucocorticoids before transplantation than those without fractures. The mean duration of glucocorticoid use was 4.9 years in fracture patients and 1.3 years in patients without fractures. Furthermore, markers of bone turnover at baseline were higher in patients with fractures. There were no differences in fractures with respect to age, rates of bone loss, rejection episodes, or glucocorticoid dosages after transplantation, however. This study indicates that lung transplantation patients with the highest risk of incident fracture are those with low pre-transplantation BMD, longer glucocorticoid use, and high bone turnover markers before transplantation.

The high rate of incident vertebral and nonvertebral fractures after lung transplantation [72, 74, 75], and prevalent bone loss and increased fracture risk before lung transplantation, highlight the value of pre-transplantation bone loss in predicting post-transplantation fracture risk. In other types of solid organ transplantation, it is also likely true that pre-transplant bone loss and fracture risk correlates with post-transplant fracture risk. To prevent development of post-transplantation osteoporosis, therefore, more attention should be focused on optimizing bone metabolism and bone mass before transplantation.

There is evidence from the Vautour population-based study [76] of renal transplant recipients that long-term risk of fractures remains markedly increased over 10 or more years after transplantation. There are no comparable data on long-term risk in patients after liver, cardiac, or lung transplantation. The study by Leidig-Bruckner et al. [21] demonstrated only a small increase in fractures after four years after liver or heart transplantation, but this was a relatively small cohort study with only a small number of patients under observation. Long-term bone density and fracture outcomes need to be studied, particularly to help evaluate the use of preventive and therapeutic strategies, and to clarify the necessity for long-term therapeutic interventions after transplantation.

V. KIDNEY TRANSPLANTATION

A. Pre-Transplantation Bone Loss and Fracture Prevalence

Patients with severe chronic kidney disease who undergo renal transplantation now have 1-year survival following renal transplantation exceeding 90% [77, 78]. New immunosuppressants introduced over the last 20 years have led to reduced rejection episodes and prolonged graft survival [79]. Improving the long-term quality of life for renal transplant recipients has therefore become very important. Preventing fractures and their adverse clinical consequences is a major goal of post-transplantation patient management.

Fractures may result from multiple disturbances in bone metabolism among patients with chronic kidney disease before transplantation [80, 81]. Patients with chronic kidney disease have renal osteodystrophy, making this the most complex type of bone disease before transplantation [53]. Multiple pathogenetic mechanisms may lead to one or more types of bone disease in patients with chronic renal failure [82]. Secondary hyperparathyroidism typically causes high-turnover hyperparathyroid bone disease, which is manifest in its most severe form as osteitis fibrosa cystica. Low-turnover forms of bone disease in this population include osteomalacia, adynamic bone disease, or aluminum bone disease. Other types of bone disease that may be present include osteoporosis, osteosclerosis, or β_2-microglobulin amyloidosis. Other factors which may contribute to abnormal bone metabolism and/or bone loss in patients with chronic kidney disease include hypogonadotropic hypogonadism, metabolic acidosis, and certain medications, such as loop diuretics, glucocorticoids, cyclosporine, and occasionally heparin.

Chronic kidney disease patients on dialysis typically have low BMD at the lumbar spine, hip, and distal radius. Risk factors for low BMD in the dialysis population include female gender, Caucasian race, amenorrhea, lower body weight or body mass index, increased parathyroid hormone level, duration of hemodialysis, and previous kidney transplantation. The vertebral fracture prevalence in the dialysis population is as high as 21%, and the relative risk of hip fracture is increased from 2- to 14-fold [53]. Fracture risk is increased with older age, female gender, Caucasian race [83], duration of dialysis [84], diabetic nephropathy [85], peripheral vascular disease [83], low lumbar spine BMD, and lower parathyroid hormone levels [86, 87].

Two studies evaluated population-based fracture data on pre-transplant patients from the United States Renal Data System (USRDS). Alem et al. [84] found a significantly increased cumulative incidence of hip fractures in patients with chronic kidney disease, compared to the general population. New Caucasian dialysis patients beginning dialysis between 1989 and 1996 were identified, and 6,542 hip fractures were recorded in 326,464 patients over 643,831 patient-years of follow-up. The overall incidence of hip fracture was 7.45 per 1,000 person-years for men, and 13.63 per 1,000 person-years for women. The relative risk of hip fracture for men was 4.44 (95% CI, 4.16–4.75) for men, and 4.40 (95% CI, 4.17–4.64) for women, compared to persons of the same gender in the general population. The authors concluded that overall risk of hip fracture among Caucasian patients with chronic kidney disease is considerably higher than that in the general population, independent of age and gender. Ball et al. [85] evaluated hip fracture risk in 101,039 patients with end-stage renal disease placed on the renal transplant waiting list between January 1990 and December 1999, and found that hip fractures occurred in 2.9 per 1,000 patients per year before renal transplant, compared to 3.3 per 1,000 patients per year after transplant. A total of 971 hip fractures were identified from Medicare claims data during the follow-up period of 314,767 person-years. The relative risk of hip fracture associated with transplantation was 1.34 when compared to dialysis initially (95% CI, 1.12–1.61), but this decreased by 1% per month until the estimated risk became equal for dialysis and transplantation approximately 630 days after transplantation. Among the transplant recipients, the risk of fracture was relatively higher in patients with a prolonged period of dialysis before transplantation.

B. Post-Transplantation Fracture Prevalence and Incidence

Following renal transplantation, pre-transplant renal osteodystrophy generally improves, with at least partial resolution of high turnover parathyroid bone disease in most patients by the end of the first year after transplantation. Despite this favorable change, however, osteoclast activity remains increased in many patients, and osteoblast activity fails to improve adequately during the first year after transplantation. These changes are thought to be primarily due to the acute and chronic effects of glucocorticoids on bone cells [88], and bone histomorphometry demonstrates decreased osteoblast activity and decreased mineral apposition rate [89]. Hyperphosphaturia may continue for many years after renal transplantation, which may predispose patients to hypophosphatemia and ongoing bone loss. Hyperphosphaturia may be a result of persistent hyperparathyroidism in some patients.

As a consequence of these changes with renal transplantation, BMD decreases rapidly in the first 6–12 months after transplantation [88, 90–99], with rates of loss in the first year after transplant reported to range from 4 to 9% at the lumbar spine and 5 to 8% at the hip. Some studies have shown gender differences in the rate of bone loss at different skeletal sites, with men losing bone more rapidly at the hip [83, 84]. One study showed much less bone loss when patients took alternate-day rather than daily prednisone therapy [100].

Most renal transplant patients have either osteopenia or osteoporosis when their BMD is checked at various times after transplantation. The prevalence of osteoporosis in cross-sectional studies of patients after renal transplantation, using the WHO definition of osteoporosis as a T-score less than −2.5, has been reported to be 17–49% at the lumbar spine, 11–56% at the femoral neck, and 22–52% at the distal radius [88, 92, 93, 95–99, 101, 102–111]. Moreover, patients treated with large doses of glucocorticoids have increased bone loss and fractures [112], so it is logical that kidney transplant patients would also be at increased risk of bone loss.

With renal transplantation, trabecular bone loss is typically rapid [113], and lumbar spine BMD losses of 3–10% have been reported in the first 6 months following renal transplantation [88, 90, 92, 99], with continued slower bone loss thereafter [93]. This transplantation-associated bone loss is superimposed on age-related bone loss characteristic for a patient's age, and will increase fracture risk as renal transplantation patients survive longer [114].

Some longitudinal studies have shown continuing, although less rapid, loss of bone after renal transplantation. Patients evaluated at a mean of seven years after renal transplantation had increased loss of bone at the lumbar spine and hip if they had increased markers of bone turnover [115]. Stopping glucocorticoid therapy after renal transplantation may help BMD improve. Patients evaluated at a mean of ten years after renal transplantation gained BMD at the lumbar spine and femoral neck when they tapered and stopped low-dose glucocorticoid therapy without kidney rejection, and those who stopped glucocorticoid therapy had increased markers of bone formation, but little change in markers of bone resorption, compared to those who continued to take glucocorticoid therapy [116].

Other studies have shown variable changes in BMD after the first few years after renal transplantation. One study showed decreased lumbar spine BMD over time [101], whereas other studies have shown no change or improved BMD [117-122]. One study demonstrated improved BMD in the lumbar spine but a slight decrease at the femoral neck [121]. Two studies have shown variable improvement or worsening, depending on the patient [40, 115], with one study showing that bone loss correlated with increased markers of bone turnover [115]. In spite of the fact that some studies show improvement in BMD in renal transplant recipients over time, most studies show decreased BMD as long as 20 years after transplantation [123, 124].

Fractures in kidney transplant patients appear to be more common in the appendicular skeleton than the axial skeleton [40]. Hip, long bone, ankle, and foot bone fractures may be more common after renal transplantation than vertebral and rib fractures.

Several reports have demonstrated above-average fracture rates in renal transplant patients [101, 125]. Unfortunately, the magnitude of the problem of bone loss and fractures after renal transplantation has not been well quantified. Various clinical series have concluded that fractures, particularly of the axial skeleton, are either very common [101, 107, 126–132] or relatively infrequent [100, 104, 108, 122, 125, 133, 134] (see Table 2). Fracture prevalence after renal transplant has been variably estimated to range between 5 and 21%, with an estimated incidence of 2% per year [113, 127].

One study evaluated population based fracture data on post-renal transplant patients from the United States Renal Data System (USRDS). Abbott et al. [125] studied 33,479 renal transplant patients who received kidney grafts between 1994 and 1997, and documented a 4.59-fold increase (95% CI, 3.29–6.31) in total hospitalized fracture incidence during the first 3 years after transplantation, compared to the general population. Patients hospitalized for hip fracture had decreased all-cause survival by Cox regression analysis (hazard ratio, 1.69; 95% CI 1.13–2.26).

Vautour et al. [76] studied a smaller population-based sample to evaluate long-term fracture risk in renal transplantation patients in Olmsted County, Minnesota. During the period 1965–1995, 86 Olmsted County residents received a first renal transplant at mean age 38.3 ± 14.8 years. The study population included 59 males (69%) and 27 females, 7 of whom were postmenopausal. Ninety-two percent of the patients were Caucasian. Survival in this cohort of Olmsted County patients was greatly reduced, likely reflecting early experience with kidney transplantation and immunosuppressive regimens. After 15 years, 51% of these patients were still alive by actuarial analysis, compared to 92% expected ($p < 0.001$). The 86 patients in the study were followed from their initial renal transplant for 911 person-years (mean, 10.6 ± 7.4 years per subject; range, 25 days to 33 years). Forty-three of the patients (50%) were followed until death, and among survivors, 56% were followed for at least 10 years.

During this period of observation, 49 subjects experienced 117 different fractures, for a crude incidence rate of 128 per 1,000 person-years (95% CI, 106–154). The cumulative incidence of fractures increased steadily over time, but the ratio of observed to expected fractures remained relatively constant. After 15 years, the cumulative incidence of any fracture was 60%, compared with an expected 20% ($p < 0.001$). The overall risk of any fracture was increased almost 5-fold (standardized incidence ratio [SIR], 4.8; 95% CI, 3.6–6.4). The risk of a vertebral fracture was 23 times greater than expected for Olmsted County residents generally. This was also reflected in the cumulative incidence of vertebral fractures in this cohort, which was 20% among 15-year survivors, compared to an expected 1% ($p < 0.001$). The Standardized Incidence Ratio (SIR) for vertebral fractures was as high among the men as among the women. There were statistically

TABLE 2 Osteoporosis after kidney or kidney-pancreas transplantation

Prevalence after transplantation		Incidence after transplantation		
Osteoporosis[a]	Fractures	Bone loss	Fracture incidence	Reference
–	Kidney: 33/432 (8.0%) at 19.7 ± 14.1 months; K-P: 9/58 (15.5%) at 13.6 ± 11.5 months	–	Kidney: 39/1,000 patient-yrs; K-P: 110/1,000 patient-yrs	Ramsay-Goldman [40]
–	All types 49/86 (60%) at 15 years	–	All types 128/1,000 person-years	Vautour [76]
–	–	–	Hip 3.3/1,000 patient-years	Ball [85]
–	–	L spine −6.8 ± 5.6% at 6 months; −8.8 ± 7.0% at 18 months	–	Julian [88]
–	–	L spine −2.8%, FN −4.2% at 6 months	–	Kwan [90]
–	–	L spine −1.6 ± 0.2%/month at 6 months	–	Horber [92]
–	–	L spine −7 ± 10% at 12 months; −1 ± 9% in 2nd and 3rd year	–	Grotz [93]
–	–	L spine −4.3% at 6 months; −5.1% at 12 months	–	Aroldi [95]
–	–	L spine −2.6 ± 5.7%, FN −2.0 ± 3.0% at 12 months	–	Giannini [97]
–	–	L spine −6.2% at 6 months	–	Kovac [98]
–	–	L spine −2.4%, FN 0% at 6 months	–	Mikuls [99]
L-spine 33.3%, FN 10% at 8.1 years	Vertebral 4/70 (5.7%)	−1.7 ± 2.8%/yr over 22 ± 5 months	–	Pichette [101]
Women: L-spine 10%, FN 14%, UDR 44%; Men: L-spine 6.3%, FN 7.4%, UDR 23% at 5.1 years	Vertebral 27/165 (16%)	–	–	Patel [102]
L-spine 23% at 6 months (below fracture threshold of 1.0 g/cm^2)	–	–	–	Wolpaw [103]

L spine 55% at 84 months (below fracture threshold of 0.85 g/cm^2)	Vertebral 1/44 (2%)	–	–	Bagni [104]
L spine 21% at 63 ± 53 months (below fracture threshold of 0.75 g/cm^2)	All types 14% at 103 ± 59 months	–	32 peripheral fractures/ 1,000 patient-years	Grotz [105]
All sites 31/54 (57%) at 8.0 ± 0.8 years	All types 17/54 (32%)	–	–	Parker [108]
L spine 14%, FN 41%, Total Hip 17%, Wrist 22% at 5.82 ± 4.33 years	–	–	–	Cayco [110]
–	–	L spine −15.0% over 2 years	–	Grotz [123]
31/59 (53%) at 8.5 ± 3.1 years	All types 26/59 (44%) at 8.5 ± 3.1 years	–	–	Durieux [124]
–	–	–	All types 7.2/1,000 person-years	Abbott [125]
–	All types 53/204 (26%) at 46 months	–	–	Elmstedt [126]
–	All types 40/180 (22%)	–	–	Takeo [127]
–	All types 18/50 (36%) at 2.85 ± 1.5 years	–	–	Bruce [128]
L spine 7/31 (23%), FN 18/31 (58%) at 40 ± 23 months	All types 14/31 (45%) at 40 ± 23 months	–	–	Smets [129]
–	All types 17/35 (49%) at 49 ± 28 months	–	All types 12.1%/patient-year	Chiu [130]
–	All types 33/193 (17%)	–	–	Nisbeth [131]
–	All types 300/1572 (19.1%) at 6.5 ± 5.4 years	–	–	O'Shaughnessy [132]

[a] Abbreviations: L-spine, lumbar spine; FN, femoral neck; UDR, ultradistal radius; K-P, Kidney-Pancreas.

significant increases in fractures of the ribs (SIR, 15.0; 95% CI, 9.5–22), pelvis (SIR, 17.1; 95% CI, 4.7–44), and foot (SIR, 8.4; 95% CI, 5.1–13). The risk of all lower-limb fractures combined (SIR, 5.0; 95% CI, 3.1–7.5) was increased more than that of all upper-limb fractures combined (SIR, 2.1; 95% CI, 1.1–3.6). Although the risk of a traditional osteoporotic fracture (hip, spine, or distal forearm fracture due to moderate trauma at age ≥ 35 years) was also increased (SIR, 10.7; 95% CI, 5.8–18), this increase was almost entirely accounted for by the vertebral fractures. The relative risk of any fracture was 5.7 (95% CI, 3.9–8.2) within the first five years of follow-up, 5.0 (95% CI, 2.8–8.5) between 5 and 10 years of follow-up, and 2.3 (95% CI, 0.8–5.5) after 10 years of observation.

The 4.8-fold increase in fracture risk in the Vautour et al. study [76] was nearly identical to the 4.6-fold increased risk reported in the Abbott et al. USRDS system study [125], but the fracture incidence rate in the Abbott et al. USRDS study (8.9 per 1,000 person-years) was much lower than seen in the Vautour et al. study (128 per 1,000 person-years). This difference may be due to the inclusion of all fractures in the population (hospitalized and outpatient) with longer-term follow-up in the Vautour et al. study. The Abbott et al. study evaluated only fractures in hospitalized patients within the first 3 years after transplantation in a relatively recent cohort. The Vautour et al. study found that increased fracture risk continues long-term following renal transplantation, even beyond 10 years, so that by 15 years after transplantation the cumulative incidence of fracture is 3 times expected.

Unfortunately, no other population based studies of fracture risk after kidney transplantation have been published. Most studies evaluating bone loss after kidney transplantation have focused on changes in BMD rather than fractures. There is no evidence that BMD T-scores predict fracture risk in the renal transplant population, as documented in postmenopausal women.

C. Predictors and Risk Factors for Fracture

Rates of bone loss after renal transplantation have not been consistently correlated with gender, age, cumulative glucocorticoid dose, rejection episodes, physical activity level, or parathyroid hormone levels. Some studies, but not all, have shown a correlation between daily or cumulative dose of glucocorticoid and BMD. Some studies have identified risk factors for fracture including female gender and patients transplanted due to diabetic nephropathy.

Abbott et al. [125] performed multivariate analysis that revealed that risk factors for fracture included prevalent fractures prior to transplantation, Caucasian ethnicity, female gender, low body weight (<95.9 kg), end-stage renal disease due to diabetes mellitus, or prolonged pre-transplant dialysis. Vautour et al. [76] found that increasing age (hazard ratio [HR] per 10-year increase, 1.3; 95% CI, 1.1–1.6) and diabetes as the cause of end-stage renal disease (HR, 3.6; 95% CI, 1.9–6.6) were independent predictors of overall fracture risk, whereas higher activity status at the time of transplant was protective against fracture (HR, 0.4; 95% CI, 0.2–0.9).

VI. KIDNEY–PANCREAS TRANSPLANTATION

Only a few studies have reported fracture prevalence after kidney–pancreas transplantation in patients with type 1 diabetes mellitus. Patients with type 1 diabetes mellitus undergoing kidney transplantation have been reported to have a higher prevalence of osteoporosis than patients without diabetes. Smets et al. [129] reported that 23% of patients with type 1 diabetes mellitus who had received renal transplants 40 ± 23 months previously had osteoporosis at the lumbar spine, whereas 58% had osteoporosis at the femoral neck. Vertebral and nonvertebral fractures were more prevalent in patients with lumbar spine osteoporosis. Chiu et al. [130] reported a fracture prevalence of 26–49% within several years after transplantation in type 1 diabetics undergoing renal–pancreas transplantation. Vautour et al. [76] found that pancreas transplantation was not an independent predictor of increased fracture risk on multivariate analysis.

VII. SUMMARY AND CONCLUSIONS

This chapter summarizes current understanding of pre-transplantation and post-transplantation bone loss and fractures in patients undergoing solid organ transplantation. Most of the studies described in this review are relatively recent, relatively small, and of short duration, which obviously limits the ability to draw firm conclusions about rates of bone loss or fractures in most types of solid organ transplantation. Nevertheless, impressive progress has been made over the last two decades in more clearly defining the risk of bone loss and fractures before solid organ transplantation, and in clarifying the rate of bone loss and fractures after transplantation.

Due to changes in standard immunosuppressive regimens over the last 20 years, it is difficult to directly compare rates of bone loss and fractures in solid organ transplantation patients over different time periods, but most of the studies reviewed in this chapter reflect clinical experience since 1993, when standard immunosuppressive regimens typically included glucocorticoids, cyclosporine, tacrolimus, and/or azathioprine. This makes it easier to draw conclusions about bone loss and fractures in patients undergoing transplantation within the last decade, but harder to assess fracture risk in patients undergoing transplantation today. Relatively few studies are available in patients treated with the newer immunosuppressive agents mycophenolate mofetil or sirolimus.

While acknowledging these limitations, it is apparent that many, if not most, patients develop significant bone loss and fractures while waiting for solid-organ transplantation. It is reasonable to speculate that the longer patients wait for organ transplantation, the worse the cumulative skeletal effects of pre-transplantation bone disease are likely to be. Glucocorticoids may play a major role in bone loss prior to transplantation in some types of end-stage organ disease, particularly in patients undergoing lung transplantation. Just as different types of end-stage organ disease may cause different rates of bone loss and fracture prior to transplantation, with lung, liver, and heart patients typically more severely affected than kidney or kidney–pancreas patients, different types of end-stage disease affecting the same organ seem to cause variable rates of bone loss and fractures. For example, patients with cholestatic liver disease appear to be more severely affected than patients with autoimmune, viral hepatitis–associated, or alcoholic liver disease.

The importance of pre-transplantation bone disease in predicting post-transplantation fracture risk is evident from lower mean pre-transplantation BMD values in those patients who develop fractures after solid organ transplantation, in comparison to those without incident fractures. It is not possible, however, to predict fracture risk reliably in solid organ transplant patients based just on pre-transplantation BMD measurements, as there is wide overlap of BMD measurements between patients with and without incident fractures. The amount of loss of bone mass after transplantation does not necessarily predict fracture risk.

Bone loss after solid organ transplantation develops rapidly, beginning at the time of organ transplantation, with highest rates of bone loss and incident fractures during the first six months after transplantation. This pattern is very similar in patients after liver, cardiac, and lung transplantation, who suffer predominantly from vertebral fractures, while it appears that patients with kidney transplantation more commonly have fractures of the appendicular skeleton in addition to vertebral fractures, and that these fractures may occur variably after transplantation.

Clinical recognition of the existence of pre- and post-transplantation bone loss and fractures, and better understanding of the pathophysiology leading to bone loss and fractures, has led to interventions likely to have significantly altered the natural history of these pathophysiological processes and events already. Calcium and vitamin D supplementation, alone or in combination with potent antiresorptive agents, are widely used to prevent and treat significant bone loss and fractures in patients before and after transplantation. Targeted immunosuppressive regimens and rapidly tapered glucocorticoid therapy, likely have significantly reduced the risk of bone loss and fractures after transplantation. It is possible that bone loss and fractures before and after transplantation will be easily prevented or treated in the future, or that future anabolic therapies may be able to correct whatever bone loss has occurred around the time of transplantation.

REFERENCES

1. Navasa, M., Forns, X., Sanchez, V., Andreu, H., Marcos, V., Borras, J.M., Rimola, A., Grande, L., Garcia-Valdecasas, J. C., Granados, A., and Rodes, J. (1996). Quality of life, major medical complications and hospital service utilization in patients with primary biliary cirrhosis after liver transplantation. *J Hepatol.* 25:129–134.
2. Long, R.G., Meinhard, E., Skinner, R.K., Varghese, Z., Wills, M.R., and Sherlock, S. (1978). Clinical, biochemical, and histological studies of osteomalacia, osteoporosis, and parathyroid function in chronic liver disease. *Gut.* 19:85–90.
3. Stellon, A.J., Webb, A., Compston, J., and Williams, R. (1986). Lack of osteomalacia in chronic cholestatic liver disease. *Bone.* 7:181–185.
4. Compston, J. (1999). Osteoporosis after liver transplantation. *Liver Transpl.* 9:321–330.
5. Bonkovsky, H.L., Hawkins, M., Steinberg, K., Hersh, T., Galambos, J.T., Henderson, J.M., Millikan, W.J., and Galloway, J.R. (1990). Prevalence and prediction of osteopenia in chronic liver disease. *Hepatology.* 12:273–280.
6. Diamond, T., Stiel, D., Lunzer, M., Wilkinson, M., Roche, J., and Posen, S. (1990). Osteoporosis and skeletal fractures in chronic liver disease. *Gut.* 31:82–87.
7. Abdelhadi, M., Eriksson, S.A., Ljusk Eriksson, S., Ericzon, B.G., and Nordenstrom, J. (1995). Bone mineral status in end-stage liver disease and the effect of liver transplantation. *Scand J Gastroenterol.* 30:1210–1215.
8. Hay, J.E. (1995). Bone disease in cholestatic liver disease. *Gastroenterology.* 108:276–283.
9. Hodgson, S.F., Dickson, E.R., Wahner, H.W., Johnson, K.A., Mann, K.G., and Riggs, B. L. (1985). Bone loss and reduced osteoblast function in primary biliary cirrhosis. *Ann Intern Med.* 103:855–860.
10. Stellon, A.J., Webb, A., Compston, J., and Williams, R. (1987). Low bone turnover state in primary biliary cirrhosis. *Hepatology.* 7:137–142.
11. Hay, J. E., Lindor, K.D., Wiesner, R.H., Dickson, E.R., Krom, R.A., and LaRusso, N. F. (1991). The metabolic bone disease of primary sclerosing cholangitis. *Hepatology.* 14:257–261.
12. Eastell, R., Dickson, E.R., Hodgson, S.F., Wiesner, R.H., Porayko, M.K., Wahner, H. W., Cedel, S.L., Riggs, B.L., and Krom, R.A. (1991). Rates of vertebral bone loss before and after liver transplantation in women with primary biliary cirrhosis. *Hepatology.* 14:296–300.
13. Janes, C.H., Dickson, E.R., Okazaki, R., Bonde, S., McDonagh, A.F., and Riggs, B.L. (1995). Role of hyperbilirubinemia in the impairment of osteoblast proliferation associated with cholestatic jaundice. *J Clin Invest.* 95:2581–2586.
14. Compston, J.E. (2003). Osteoporosis after liver transplantation. *Liver Transpl.* 9: 321–330.
15. Ninkovic, M., Love, S.A., Tom, B., Alexander, G.J., and Compston, J.E. (2001). High prevalence of osteoporosis in patients with chronic liver disease prior to liver transplantation. *Calcif Tissue Int.* 69:321–326.
16. Porayko, M.K., Wiesner, R.H., Hay, J.E., Krom, R.A., Dickson, E.R., Beaver, S., and Schwerman, L. (1991). Bone disease in liver transplant recipients: incidence, timing, and risk factors. *Transplant Proc.* 23:1462–1465.
17. Arnold, J.C., Hauser, D., Ziegler, R., Kommerell, B., Otto, G., Theilmann, L., and Wuster, C. (1992). Bone disease after liver transplantation. *Transplant Proc.* 24: 2709–2710.
18. Meys, E., Fontanges, E., Fourcade, N., Thomasson, A., Pouyet, M., and Delmas, P.D. (1994). Bone loss after orthotopic liver transplantation. *Am J Med.* 97:445–450.
19. Valero, M.A., Loinaz, C., Larrodera, L., Leon, M., Moreno, E., and Hawkins, F. (1995). Calcitonin and bisphosphonates treatment in bone loss after liver transplantation. *Calcif Tissue Int.* 57:15–19.
20. Riemens, S.C., Oostdijk, A., van Doormaal, J.J., Thijn, C.J., Drent, G., Piers, D.A., Groen, E.W., Meerman, L., Slooff, M.J., and Haagsma, E.B. (1996). Bone loss after liver

transplantation is not prevented by cyclical etidronate, calcium and alphacalcidol. The Liver Transplant Group, Groningen. *Osteoporos Int.* 6:213–218.
21. Leidig-Bruckner, G., Hosch, S., Dodidou, P., Ritschel, D., Conradt, C., Klose, C., Otto, G., Lange, R., Theilmann, L., Zimmerman, R., Pritsch, M., and Ziegler, R. (2001). Frequency and predictors of osteoporotic fractures after cardiac or liver transplantation: a follow-up study. *Lancet.* 357:342–347.
22. Monegal, A., Navasa, M., Guanabens, N., Peris, P., Pons, F., Martinez de Osaba, M.J., Rimola, A., Rodes, J., and Munoz-Gomez, J. (1997). Osteoporosis and bone mineral metabolism disorders in cirrhotic patients referred for orthotopic liver transplantation. *Calcif Tissue Int.* 60:148–154.
23. Weaver, G.A., Franck, W.A., Streck, W. F., and Starzl, T.E. (1983). Hepatic osteodystrophy after liver transplantation in a patient with primary biliary cirrhosis. *Am J Gastroenterol.* 78:102–106.
24. McDonald, J.A., Dunstan, C.R., Dilworth, P., Sherbon, K., Sheil, A.G., Evans, R.A., and McCaughan, G.W. (1991). Bone loss after liver transplantation. *Hepatology.* 14:613–619.
25. Floreani, A., Fries, W., Luisetto, G., Burra, P., Fagiuoli, S., Boccagni, P., Della Rovere, G.R., Plebani, M., Piccoli, A., and Naccarato, R. (1998). Bone metabolism in orthotopic liver transplantation: a prospective study. *Liver Transpl Surg.* 4:311–319.
26. Crosbie, O.M., Freaney, R., McKenna, M.J., and Hegarty, J.E. (1999). Bone density, vitamin D status, and disordered bone remodeling in end-stage chronic liver disease. *Calcif Tissue Int.* 64:295–300.
27. Hussaini, S.H., Oldroyd, B., Stewart, S.P., Roman, F., Smith, M.A., Pollard, S., Lodge, P., O'Grady, J.G., and Losowsky, M.S. (1999). Regional BMD after orthotopic liver transplantation. *Eur J Gastroenterol Hepatol.* 11:157–163.
28. Monegal, A., Navasa, M., Guanabens, N., Peris, P., Pons, F., Martinez de Osaba, M.J., Rimola, A., Rodes, J., and Munoz-Gomez, J. (2001). Bone mass and mineral metabolism in liver transplant patients treated with FK506 or cyclosporine A. *Calcif Tissue Int.* 68:83–86.
29. Hommann, M., Abendroth, K., Lehmann, G., Patzer, N., Kornberg, A., Voigt, R., Seifert, S., Hein, G., and Scheele, J. (2002). Effect of transplantation on bone: osteoporosis after liver and multivisceral transplantation. *Transplant Proc.* 34:2296–2298.
30. Guichelaar, M.H.J., Porayko, M., Regan, K., Therneau, T.M., and Wiesner, R. (1999). The long term influence of liver transplantation on BMD of cholestatic patients. *Gastroenterology.* 30:171A.
31. Giannini, S., Nobile, M., Ciuffreda, M., Iemmolo, R. M., Dalle Carbonare, L., Minicuci, N., Casagrande, F., Destro, C., Gerunda, G.E., Sartori, L., and Crepaldi, G. (2000). Long-term persistence of low bone density in orthotopic liver transplantation. *Osteoporos Int.* 11:417–424.
32. Navasa, M., Monegal, A., Guanabens, N., Peris, P., Rimola, A., Munoz-Gomez, J., Visa, J., and Rodes, J. (1994). Bone fractures in liver transplant patients. *Br J Rheumatol.* 33:52–55.
33. Taillandier, J., Alemanni, M., Samuel, D., and Bismuth, H. (1999). Rheumatic complications following liver transplantation. *Transplant Proc.* 31:1717–1718.
34. Ninkovic, M., Skingle, S.J., Bearcroft, P.W., Bishop, N., Alexander, G.J., and Compston, J. E. (2000). Incidence of vertebral fractures in the first three months after orthotopic liver transplantation. *Eur J Gastroenterol Hepatol.* 12:931–935.
35. Hamberg, S.M., van den Berg, A.P., Slooff, M.J.H., Haagsma, E.B. (2000). BMD in the long term after liver transplantation. *Osteoporos Int.* 11:600–606.
36. Monegal, A., Navasa, M., Guanabens, N., Peris, P., Pons, F., Martinez de Osaba, M.J., Ordi, J., Rimola, A., Rodes, J., and Munoz-Gomez, J. (2001). Bone disease after liver transplantation: a long-term prospective study of bone mass changes, hormonal status and histomorphometric characteristics. *Osteoporos Int.* 12:484–492.
37. Reeves, H.L., Francis, R.M., Manas, D.M., Hudson, M., and Day, C.P. (1998). Intravenous bisphosphonate prevents symptomatic osteoporotic vertebral collapse in patients after liver transplantation. *Liver Transpl Surg.* 4:404–409.

38. Hawkins, F.G., Leon, M., Lopez, M.B., Valero, M.A., Larrodera, L., Garcia-Garcia, I., Loinaz, C., and Moreno Gonzalez, E. (1994). Bone loss and turnover in patients with liver transplantation. *Hepatogastroenterology*. 41:158–161.
39. Ninkovic, M., Love, S., Tom, B.D., Bearcroft, P.W., Alexander, G.J., and Compston, J.E. (2002). Lack of effect of intravenous pamidronate on fracture incidence and BMD after orthotopic liver transplantation. *J Hepatol*. 37:93–100.
40. Ramsey-Goldman, R., Dunn, J.E., Dunlop, D.D., Stuart, F.P., Abecassis, M.M., Kaufman, D.B., Langman, C.B., Salinger, M.H., and Sprague, S.M. (1999). Increased risk of fracture in patients receiving solid organ transplants. *J Bone Miner Res*. 14: 456–463.
41. Haagsma, E.B., Thijn, C.J., Post, J.G., Slooff, M.J., and Gips, C.H. (1988). Bone disease after orthotopic liver transplantation. *J Hepatol*. 6:94–100.
42. Segal, E., Baruch, Y., Kramsky, R., Raz, B., Tamir, A., and Ish-Shalom, S. (2003). Predominant factors associated with bone loss in liver transplant patients—after prolonged post-transplantation period. *Clin Transplant*. 17:13–19.
43. Carey, E.J., Balan, V., Kremers, W.K., and Hay, J.E. (2003). Osteopenia and osteoporosis in patients with endstage liver disease caused by hepatitis C and alcoholic liver disease: not just a cholestatic problem. *Liver Transpl*. 9:1166–1173.
44. Guthery, S.L., Pohl, J.F., Bucuvalas, J.C., Alonso, M.H., Ryckman, F.C., Balistreri, W.F., and Heubi, J. E. (2003). BMD in long-term survivors following pediatric liver transplantation. *Liver Transpl*. 9:365–370.
45. Park, K.M., Hay, J.E., Lee, S.G., Lee, Y.L., Wiesner, R.H., Porayko, M.K., and Krom, R.A.F. (1996). Bone loss after orthotopic liver transplantation: FK 506 versus cyclosporine. *Transplant Proc*. 28:1738–1740.
46. Muchmore, J.S., Cooper, D.K., Ye, Y., Schlegel, V., Pribil, A., and Zuhdi, N. (1992). Prevention of loss of vertebral bone density in heart transplant patients. *J Heart Lung Transplant*. 11:959–963; discussion 963–964.
47. Shane, E., Mancini, D., Aaronson, K., Silverberg, S.J., Seibel, M.J., Addesso, V., and McMahon, D. J. (1997). Bone mass, vitamin D deficiency, and hyperparathyroidism in congestive heart failure. *Am J Med*. 103:197–207.
48. Lee, A.H., Mull, R.L., Keenan, G.F., Callegari, P.E., Dalinka, M.K., Eisen, H.J., Mancini, D. M., DiSesa, V. J., and Attie, M. F. (1994). Osteoporosis and bone morbidity in cardiac transplant recipients. *Am J Med*. 96:35–41.
49. Van Cleemput, J., Daenen, W., Geusens, P., Dequeker, P., Van De Werf, F., and VanHaecke, J. (1996). Prevention of bone loss in cardiac transplant recipients. A comparison of biphosphonates and vitamin D. *Transplantation*. 61:1495–1499.
50. Sambrook, P.N., Kelly, P.J., Fontana, D., Nguyen, T., Keogh, A., Macdonald, P., Spratt, P., Freund, J., and Eisman, J. A. (1994). Mechanisms of rapid bone loss following cardiac transplantation. *Osteoporos Int*. 4:273–276.
51. Shane, E., Rivas, M., McMahon, D.J., Staron, R.B., Silverberg, S.J., Seibel, M.J., Mancini, D., Michler, R. E., Aaronson, K., Addesso, V., and Lo, S. H. (1997). Bone loss and turnover after cardiac transplantation. *J Clin Endocrinol Metab*. 82:1497–1506.
52. Van Cleemput, J., Daenen, W., Nijs, J., Geusens, P., Dequeker, J., and Vanhaecke, J. (1995). Timing and quantification of bone loss in cardiac transplant recipients. *Transpl Int*. 8:196–200.
53. Cohen, A., Ebeling, P., Sprague, S., and Shane, E. (2003). Transplantation osteoporosis, in Primer on the Metabolic Bone Diseases and Disorders of Mineral Metabolism, 5th ed., M.J. Favus, ed., pp. 370–379. Washington, D.C.: American Society for Bone and Mineral Research.
54. Sambrook, P.N., Kelly, P.J., Keogh, A.M., Macdonald, P., Spratt, P., Freund, J., and Eisman, J. A. (1994). Bone loss after heart transplantation: a prospective study. *J Heart Lung Transplant*. 13:116–120; discussion 121.
55. Berguer, D.G., Krieg, M.A., Thiebaud, D., Burckhardt, P., Stumpe, F., Hurni, M., Sadeghi, H., Kappenberger, L., and Goy, J.J. (1994). Osteoporosis in heart transplant recipients: a longitudinal study. *Transplant Proc*. 26:2649–2651.

56. Shane, E., Rodino, M.A., McMahon, D.J., Addesso, V., Staron, R.B., Seibel, M.J., Mancini, D., Michler, R.E., and Lo, S.H. (1998). Prevention of bone loss after heart transplantation with antiresorptive therapy: a pilot study. *J Heart Lung Transplant.* 17:1089–1096.
57. Muchmore, J.S., Cooper, D.K., Ye, Y., Schlegel, V.T., and Zuhdi, N. (1991). Loss of vertebral bone density in heart transplant patients. *Transplant Proc.* 23:1184–1185.
58. Rich, G.M., Mudge, G.H., Laffel, G.L., and LeBoff, M. S. (1992). Cyclosporine A and prednisone-associated osteoporosis in heart transplant recipients. *J Heart Lung Transplant.* 11:950–958.
59. Meys, E., Terreaux-Duvert, F., Beaume-Six, T., Dureau, G., and Meunier, P.J. (1993). Bone loss after cardiac transplantation: effects of calcium, calcidiol and monofluorophosphate. *Osteoporos Int.* 3:322–329.
60. Shane, E., Rivas, M.C., Silverberg, S.J., Kim, T.S., Staron, R.B., and Bilezikian, J.P. (1993). Osteoporosis after cardiac transplantation. *Am J Med.* 94:257–264.
61. Fahrleitner, A., Prenner, G., Leb, G., Tscheliessnigg, K.H., Piswanger-Solkner, C., Obermayer-Pietsch, B., Portugaller, H.R., Berghold, A., and Dobnig, H. (2003). Serum osteoprotegerin is a major determinant of bone density development and prevalent vertebral fracture status following cardiac transplantation. *Bone.* 32:96–106.
62. Shane, E., Rivas, M., Staron, R.B., Silverberg, S.J., Seibel, M.J., Kuiper, J., Mancini, D., Addesso, V., Michler, R.E., and Factor-Litvak, P. (1996). Fracture after cardiac transplantation: a prospective longitudinal study. *J Clin Endocrinol Metab.* 81:1740–1746.
63. Ippoliti, G., Pellegrini, C., Campana, C., Rinaldi, M., D'Armini, A., Goggi, C., Aiello, M., and Vigano, M. (2003). Clodronate treatment of established bone loss in cardiac recipients: a randomized study. *Transplantation.* 75:330–334.
64. Negri, A.L., Perrone, S., Gallo, R., Bogado, C.E., and Zanchetta, J.R. (1996). Osteoporosis following heart transplantation. *Transplant Proc.* 28:3321–3324.
65. Stempfle, H.U., Werner, C., Echtler, S., Assum, T., Meiser, B., Angermann, C.E., Theisen, K., and Gartner. R. (1998). Rapid trabecular bone loss after cardiac transplantation using FK506 (tacrolimus)-based immunosuppression. *Transplant Proc.* 30:1132–1133.
66. Shane, E., Silverberg, S.J., Donovan, D., Papadopoulos, A., Staron, R.B., Addesso, V., Jorgesen, B., McGregor, C., and Schulman, L. (1996). Osteoporosis in lung transplantation candidates with end-stage pulmonary disease. *Am J Med.* 101:262–269.
67. Aris, R.M., Stephens, A.R., Ontjes, D.A., Denene Blackwood, A., Lark, R.K., Hensler, M.B., Neuringer, I.P., and Lester, G.E. (2000). Adverse alterations in bone metabolism are associated with lung infection in adults with cystic fibrosis. *Am J Respir Crit Care Med.* 162:1674–1678.
68. Cahill, B.C., O'Rourke, M.K., Parker, S., Stringham, J.C., Karwande, S.V., and Knecht, T.P. (2001). Prevention of bone loss and fracture after lung transplantation: a pilot study. *Transplantation.* 72:1251–1255.
69. Tschopp, O., Boehler, A., Speich, R., Weder, W., Seifert, B., Russi, E. W., and Schmid, C. (2002). Osteoporosis before lung transplantation: association with low body mass index, but not with underlying disease. *Am J Transplant.* 2:167–172.
70. Ferrari, S.L., Nicod, L.P., Hamacher, J., Spiliopoulos, A., Slosman, D.O., Rochat, T., Bonjour, J.P., and Rizzoli, R. (1996). Osteoporosis in patients undergoing lung transplantation. *Eur Respir J.* 9:2378–2382.
71. Spira, A., Gutierrez, C., Chaparro, C., Hutcheon, M.A., and Chan, C.K. (2000). Osteoporosis and lung transplantation: a prospective study. *Chest.* 117:476–481.
72. Shane, E., Papadopoulos, A., Staron, R.B., Addesso, V., Donovan, D., McGregor, C., and Schulman, L. L. (1999). Bone loss and fracture after lung transplantation. *Transplantation.* 68:220–227.
73. Aris, R.M., Lester, G.E., Renner, J.B., Winders, A., Denene Blackwood, A., Lark, R. K., and Ontjes, D.A. (2000). Efficacy of pamidronate for osteoporosis in patients with cystic fibrosis following lung transplantation. *Am J Respir Crit Care Med.* 162: 941–946.

74. Schulman, L.L., Addesso, V., Staron, R.B., McGregor, C.C., and Shane, E. (1997). Insufficiency fractures of the sacrum: a cause of low back pain after lung transplantation. *J Heart Lung Transplant.* 16:1081–1085.
75. Aris, R.M., Neuringer, I.P., Weiner, M.A., Egan, T.M., and Ontjes, D. (1996). Severe osteoporosis before and after lung transplantation. *Chest.* 109:1176–1183.
76. Vautour, L.M., Melton, L.J. 3rd, Clarke, B.L., Achenbach, S.J., Oberg, A.L., and McCarthy, J.T. (2004). Long-term fracture risk following renal transplantation: a population-based study. *Osteoporos Int* 15:160–167.
77. U.S. Renal Data System: USRDS 2000 Annual Data Report. National Institutes of Health, National Institute of Diabetes and Digestive and Kidney Diseases, Bethesda, Maryland, June 2000.
78. Pascual, M., Theruvath, T., Kawai, T., Tolkoff-Rubin, N., and Cosimi, A.B. (2002). Strategies to improve long-term outcomes after renal transplantation. *N Engl J Med.* 346:580–590.
79. Hariharan, S., Johnson, C.P., Bresnahan, B.A., Taranto, S.E., McIntosh, M.J., and Stablein, D. (1996). Improved graft survival after renal transplantation in the United States, 1988 to 1996. *N Engl J Med.* 342:605–612.
80. Gonzalez, E.A., and Martin, K.J. (2001). Renal osteodystrophy. *Rev Endocr Metab Disord.* 2:187–193.
81. Elder, G. (2002). Pathophysiology and recent advances in the management of renal osteodystrophy. *J Bone Miner Res.* 17:2094–2105.
82. Goodman, W.G., Coburn, J.W., Slatopolsky, E., Salusky, I.B., and Quarles, L.D. (2003). Renal osteodystrophy in adults and children, in Primer on the Metabolic Bone Diseases and Disorders of Mineral Metabolism, 5th ed., M.J. Favus, ed., pp. 430-447. Washington, D.C.: American Society for Bone and Mineral Research.
83. Stehman-Breen, C.O., Sherrard, D.J., Alem, A.M., Gillen, D.L., Heckbert, S.R., Wong, C.S., Ball, A., and Weiss, N.S. (2002). Risk factors for hip fracture among patients with end-stage renal disease. *Kidney Int.* 58:2200–2205.
84. Alem, A.M., Sherrard, D.J., Gillen, D.L., Weiss, N.S., Beresford, S.A., Heckbert, S.R., Wong, C., and Stehman-Breen, C. (2000). Increased risk of hip fracture among patients with end-stage renal disease. *Kidney Int.* 58:396–399.
85. Ball, A.M., Gillen, D.L, Sherrard, D., Weiss, N.S., Emerson, S.S., Seliger, S.L., Kestenbaum, B.R., and Stehman-Breen, C. (2002). Risk of hip fracture among dialysis and renal transplant patients. *J Am Med Assn.* 288:3014–3018.
86. Inaba, M., Nagasue, K., Okuno, S., Ueda M., Kumeda, Y., Imanishi, Y., Shoji, T., Ishimura, E., Ohta, T., Nakatani, T., Kim, M., and Nishizawa, Y. (2002). Impaired secretion of parathyroid hormone, but not refractoriness of osteoblast, is a major mechanism of low bone turnover in hemodialyzed patients with diabetes mellitus. *Am J Kidney Dis.* 39:1261–1269.
87. Coco, M., and Rush, H. (2000). Increased incidence of hip fractures in dialysis patients with low serum parathyroid hormone. *Am J Kidney Dis.* 36:1115–1121.
88. Julian, B.A., Laskow, D.A., Dubovsky, J., Dubovsky, E.V., Curtis, J.J., and Quarles, L.D. (1991). Rapid loss of vertebral mineral density after renal transplantation. *N Engl J Med.* 325:544–550.
89. Monier-Faugere, M., Mawad, H., Qi, Q., Friedler, R., and Malluche, H.H. (2000). High prevalence of low bone turnover and occurrence of osteomalacia after kidney transplantation. *J Am Soc Nephrol.* 11:1093–1099.
90. Kwan, J.T., Almond, M.K., Evans, K., and Cunningham, J. (1992). Changes in total body bone mineral content and regional BMD in renal patients following renal transplantation. *Miner Electrolyte Metab.* 18:166–168.
91. Almond, M.K., Kwan, J.T.C., Evans, K., and Cunningham, J. (1994). Loss of regional BMD in the first 12 months following renal transplantation. *Nephron.* 66:52–57.
92. Horber, F.F., Casez, J.P., Steiger, U., Czerniak, A., Montandon, A., and Jaeger, P. (1994). Changes in bone mass early after kidney transplantation. *J Bone Miner Res.* 9:1–9.

93. Grotz, W.H., Mundinger, F.A., Rasenack, J., Speidel, L., Olschewski, M., Exner, V.M., and Schollmeyer P. J. (1995). Bone loss after kidney transplantation: a longitudinal study in 115 graft recipients. *Nephrol Dial Transplant.* 10:2096–2100.
94. Torregrosa, J.V., Campistol, J.M., Montesinos, M., Fenollosa, B., Pons, F., Martinez de Osaba, M.J., and Oppenheimer, F. (1995). Factors involved in the loss of BMD after renal transplantation. *Transplant Proc.* 27:2224–2225.
95. Aroldi, A., Tarantino, A., Montagnino, G., Cesana, B., Cocucci, C., and Ponticelli, C. (1997). Effects of three immunosuppressive regimens on vertebral bone density in renal transplant recipients: a prospective study. *Transplantation.* 63:380–386.
96. Kušec, V., Šmalcelj, R., Cvijeitiæ, S., Rožman, B., and Škreb, F. (2000). Determinants of reduced bone density and increased bone turnover after kidney transplantation: cross-sectional study. *Croat Med J.* 41:396–400.
97. Giannini, S., D'Angelo, A., Carraro, G., Nobile, M., Rigotti, P., Bonfante, L., Marchini, F., Zaninotto, M., Dalle Carbonare, L., Sartori, L., and Crepaldi, G. (2001). Alendronate prevents further bone loss in renal transplant recipients. *J Bone Miner Res.* 16: 2111–2117.
98. Kovač, D., Lindič, J., Kandus, A., and Bren, F.A. (2003). Quantitative ultrasound of the calcaneus and dual x-ray absorptiometry of the lumbar spine in assessment and follow-up of skeletal status in patients after kidney transplantation. *Osteoporosis Int.* 14:166–170.
99. Mikuls, T.R., Julian, B.A., Bartolucci, A., and Saag, K.G. (2003). BMD changes within six months of renal transplantation. *Transplantation.* 75:49–54.
100. Masse, M., Girardin, C., Ouimet, D., Dandavino, R., Boucher, A., Madore, F., Hebert, M.J., Leblanc, M., and Pichette, V. (2001). Initial bone loss in kidney transplant recipients: a prospective study. *Transplant Proc.* 33:1211.
101. Pichette, V., Bonnardeaux, A., Prudhomme, L., Gagne, M., Cardinal, J., and Ouimet, D. (1996). Long-term bone loss in kidney transplant recipients: a cross-sectional and longitudinal study. *Am J Kidney Dis.* 28:105–114.
102. Patel, S., Kwan, J.T., McCloskey, E., McGee, G., Thomas, G., Johnson, D., Wills, R., Ogunremi, L., and Barron, J. (2001). Prevalence and causes of low bone density and fractures in kidney transplant patients *J Bone Miner Res.* 16:1863–1870.
103. Wolpaw, T., Deal, C.L., Fleming-Brooks, S., Bartucci, M.R., Schulak, J.A., and Hricik, D. E. (1994). Factors influencing vertebral bone density after renal transplantation. *Transplantation.* 58:1186–1189.
104. Bagni, B., Gilli, P., Cavallini, A., Bagni, I., Marzola, M.C., Orzincolo, C., and Wahner H.W. (1994). Continuing loss of vertebral mineral density in renal transplant recipients. *Eur J Nucl Med.* 21:108–112.
105. Grotz, W.H., Mundinger, F.A., Gugel, B., Exner, V., Kirste, G., and Schollmeyer, P.J. (1994). Bone fracture and osteodensitometry with dual energy x-ray absorptiometry in kidney transplant recipients. *Transplantation.* 58:912–915.
106. Behnke, B., Altrogge, H., Delling, G., Kruse, H-P., and Müller-Wiefel, D.E. (1996). BMD in pediatric patients after renal transplantation. *Clin Nephrol.* 46:24–29.
107. Cueto-Manzano, A.M., Konel, S., Hutchison, A.J., Crowley, V., France, M.W., Freemont, A.J., Adams, J.E., Mawer, B., and Gokal, R. (1999). Bone loss in long-term renal transplantation: histopathology and densitometry analysis. *Kidney Int.* 55:2021–2029.
108. Parker, C.R., Freemont, A.J., Blackwell, P.J., Grainge, M.J., and Hosking, D.J. (1999). Cross-sectional analysis of renal transplantation osteoporosis. *J Bone Miner Res.* 14: 1943–1951.
109. Caglar, M., and Adeera, L. (1999). Factors affecting BMD in renal transplant patients. *Ann Nucl Med.* 13:141–145.
110. Cayco, A.V., Wysolmerski, J., Simpson, C., Mitnick, M.A., Gundberg, C., Kliger, A., Lorber, M., Silver, D., Basadonna, G., Friedman, A., Insogna, K., Cruz, D., and Bia, M. (2000). Posttransplant bone disease: evidence for a high bone resorption state. *Transplantation.* 70:1722–1728.

111. Carlini, R.G., Rojas, E., Weisinger, J.R., Lopez, M., Martinis, R., Arminio, A., and Bellorin-Font, E. (2000). Bone disease in patients with long-term renal transplantation and normal renal function. *Am J Kidney Dis.* 36:160–166.
112. Tannirandorn, P., and Epstein, S. (2000). Drug-induced bone loss. *Osteoporosis Int.* 11:637–659.
113. Shane, E., and Epstein, S. (2001). Transplantation osteoporosis. *Transplant Rev.* 15:11–32.
114. Melton, L.J., III, and Riggs, B.L. (2003). Epidemiology, classification and history of osteoporosis, in Rheumatology, 3rd ed., M. Hochberg, A. Silman, J. Smolen, M. Weinblatt, and M. Weisman, eds., 2059–2066. London, England: Harcourt Health Services.
115. Cruz, D.N., Wysolmerski, J.J., Brickel, H.M., Gundberg, C.G., Simpson, C.A., Mitnick, M.A., Kliger, A.S., Lorber, M.I., Basadonna, G.P., Friedman, A. L., Insogna, K.L., and Bia, M.J. (2001). Parameters of high bone-turnover predict bone loss in renal transplant patients: a longitudinal study. *Transplantation.* 72:83–88.
116. Farmer, C.K.T., Hampson, G., Vaja, S., Abbs, I.C., Hilton, R.M., Koffman, G., Watkins, J., Sacks, S.H., and Fogelman, I. (2002). Late low dose steroid withdrawal in renal transplant recipients increases bone formation and BMD without altering renal function: a randomized controlled trial. *J Bone Miner Res.* 17:S158 (abstract).
117. Hurst, G., Alloway, R., Hathaway, D., Somerville, T., Hughes, T., and Gaber, A. (1998). Stabilization of bone mass after renal transplant with preemptive care. *Transplant Proc.* 30:1327–1328.
118. Moreno, A., Torregrosa, J.V., Pons, F., Campistol, J.M., Martinez de Osaba, M.J., and Oppenheimer, F. (1999). BMD after renal transplantation: long-term follow-up. *Transplant Proc.* 31:2322–2323.
119. Nowacka-Cieciura, E., Durlik, M., Cieciura, T., Lewandowska, D., Baczkowska, T., Kukula, K., Lao, M., Szmidt, J., and Rowinski, W. (2002). Steroid withdrawal after renal transplantation-risks and benefits. *Transplant Proc.* 34:560–563.
120. Cueto-Manzano, A.M., Konel, S., Freemont, A.J., Adams, J.E., Mawer, B., Gokal, R., and Hutchinson, A.J. (2000). Effect of 1,25-dihydroxyvitmamin D3 and calcium carbonate on bone loss associated with long-term renal transplantation. *Am J Kidney Dis.* 35:227–236.
121. Grotz, W., Rump, A.L., Niessen, H., Schmidt-Gayt, A., Reichelt, G., Kirste, G., Olschewski, G., and Schollmeyer, P. (1998). Treatment of osteopenia and osteoporosis after kidney transplantation. *Transplantation.* 66:1004–1008.
122. Brandenburg, V.M., Ketteler, M., Fassbender, W.J., Heussen, N., Freuding, T., Floege, J., and Ittel, T.H. (2002). Development of lumbar BMD in the late course after kidney transplantation. *Am J Kidney Dis.* 40:1066–1074.
123. Grotz, W. H., Mundinger, F.A., Gugel, B., Exner V.M., Kirste, G., and Schollmeyer, P.J. (1995). BMD after kidney transplantation: a cross-sectional study in 190 graft recipients up to 20 years after transplantation. *Transplantation.* 7:982–986.
124. Durieux, S., Mercadal, L., Orcel, P., Dao, H., Rioux, C., Bernard, M., Rozenberg, S., Barrou, B., Bourgeois, P., Deray, G., and Bagnis, C. I. (2002). BMD and fracture prevalence in long-term kidney graft recipients. *Transplantation.* 74:496–500.
125. Abbott, K.C., Oglesby, R.J., Hypolite, I.O., Kirk, A.D., Ko, C.W., Welch, P.G., Agodoa, L.Y., and Duncan, W.E. (2001). Hospitalizations for fractures after renal transplantation in the United States. *Ann Epidemiol.* 1:450–457.
126. Elmstedt, E., and Svahn, T. (1981). Skeletal complications following renal transplantation. *Acta Orthop Scand.* 52:279–286.
127. Takeo, Y., Tominaga, K., Tsuji, H., Yoh, K., and Nakano, K. (1989). Spontaneous fracture and osteoporosis following renal transplantation. *J Jpn Orthop Assoc.* 63:507–513.
128. Bruce, D.S., Newell, K.A., Josephson, M.A., Woodle, E.S., Piper, J.B., Millis, J.M., Seaman, D.S., Carnrike, Jr., C.L., Huss, E., and Thistlethwaite, Jr., J.R. (1996). Long-term outcome of kidney-pancreas transplant recipients with good graft function at one year. *Transplantation.* 62:451–456.

129. Smets, Y.F.C., van der Pijl, J., de Fijter, J.W., Ringers, J., Lemkes, H.H.P.J., and Hamdy, N. A. T. (1998). Low bone mass and high incidence of fractures after successful simultaneous pancreas-kidney transplantation. *Nephrol Dial Transplant*. 13:1250–1255.
130. Chiu, M.Y., Sprague, S.M., Bruce, D.S., Woodle, E.S., Thistlethwaite, Jr., J.R., and Josephson, M.A. (1998). Analysis of fracture prevalence in kidney-pancreas allograft recipients. *J Am Soc Nephrol*. 9:677–683.
131. Nisbeth, U., Lindh, E., Ljunghall, S., Backman, U., and Fellström, B. (1999). Increased fracture rate in diabetes mellitus and females after renal transplantation. *Transplantation*. 67:1218–1222.
132. O'Shaughnessy, E.A., Dahl, D.C., Smith, C.L., and Kasiske, B.L. (2002). Risk factors for fractures in kidney transplantation. *Transplantation*. 74:362–366.
133. Griffiths, H.J., Ennis, J.T., and Bailey, G. (1974). Skeletal changes following renal transplantation. *Radiology*. 113:621–626.
134. Nielsen, H.E., Melsen, F., and Christensen, M.S. (1979). Spontaneous fractures following renal transplantation. Clinical and biochemical aspects, bone mineral content and bone morphometry. *Miner Electrolyte Metab*. 2:323–330.

CHAPTER 8

Bone Histomorphometry and Its Application to Transplantation Bone Disease

Juliet Compston, MD, FRCP
Department of Medicine, Addenbrooke's Hospital, Cambridge, England

I. INTRODUCTION

Bone histomorphometry provides a unique tool by which static and dynamic indices of bone remodelling and turnover can be quantitatively assessed. Although biochemical markers of bone turnover enable assessment of whole-body turnover, they cannot indicate remodelling balance, and since approximately 80% of the skeleton is composed of cortical bone, they do not always accurately reflect turnover in cancellous bone. Furthermore, biochemical markers do not provide the detailed information about cellular and structural mechanisms of bone loss and gain that can be obtained from bone histomorphometric analysis. Similarly, bone densitometric assessment, while valuable in the assessment of changes in bone mineral density, does not indicate the underlying alterations in bone remodelling and turnover.

The usual site for bone biopsy in humans is the iliac crest; the preferred approach is trans-iliac, in which a core of bone is obtained that contains inner and outer cortices and intervening cancellous bone [1]. The biopsy is taken approximately one inch below and behind the anterior superior iliac spine and, when used for the purpose of bone histomorphometry, should have an internal diameter of 6–8 mm. The procedure has a low morbidity, the commonest adverse effect being haematoma [2]. It is usually performed under local anaesthetic with light sedation.

There are some limitations associated with bone histomorphometry, mainly resulting from sampling and measurement variance. There may be considerable heterogeneity in bone remodelling and turnover between skeletal sites, both in health and disease, so that changes in the iliac crest are not necessarily representative of other parts of the skeleton, for example the spine [3]. Many of the measurements made in bone histomorphometry have a subjective element, and this, together with differences in staining techniques, magnification, and measurement methods, contributes to significant measurement variability, both inter- and intraobserver [4, 5, 6]. Even within a single biopsy there may be considerable variation in remodelling and turnover, depending on the site chosen for sampling. Finally, current histomorphometric techniques are seriously limited by the lack of reliable markers for activation and active resorption [7]. Dynamic indices related to these processes are calculated from bone formation rates, based on the assumptions that bone resorption and formation are coupled in time and space and that bone remodelling is in a steady state; these assumptions may not be tenable in disease states. Notwithstanding these limitations, however, bone histomorphometry has proved a valuable tool for understanding cellular and structural mechanisms of bone loss in health and disease and the means by which therapeutic effects are achieved.

II. PATHOPHYSIOLOGY OF BONE LOSS AFTER TRANSPLANTATION

A. Bone Remodelling

Bone remodelling is a surface-based phenomenon that serves to maintain the mechanical integrity of bone [8]. It occurs in individual bone remodelling units and involves the removal of a quantum of bone by osteoclasts, followed by the formation and mineralisation by osteoblasts of osteoid within the cavity so created. Under normal circumstances, the sequence of events is resorption followed by formation (coupling), and the amounts of bone resorbed and formed are quantitatively similar (remodelling balance). The lifespan of a single bone remodelling unit is approximately 6 months, most of this time being occupied by the formation and mineralisation of osteoid.

B. Increased Bone Turnover and Remodelling Imbalance

Quantitatively the most important mechanism of bone loss in osteoporosis is increased bone turnover, in which the number of remodelling units present on the bone surface at any one time is increased (see Figure 1A). This form of bone loss is potentially reversible, provided that remodelling balance is maintained. The second mechanism is that of remodelling imbalance, in which the amount of bone formed within individual remodelling units is less than that resorbed due to an increase in resorption, a decrease in formation, or a combination of the two (see Figure 1B). This form of

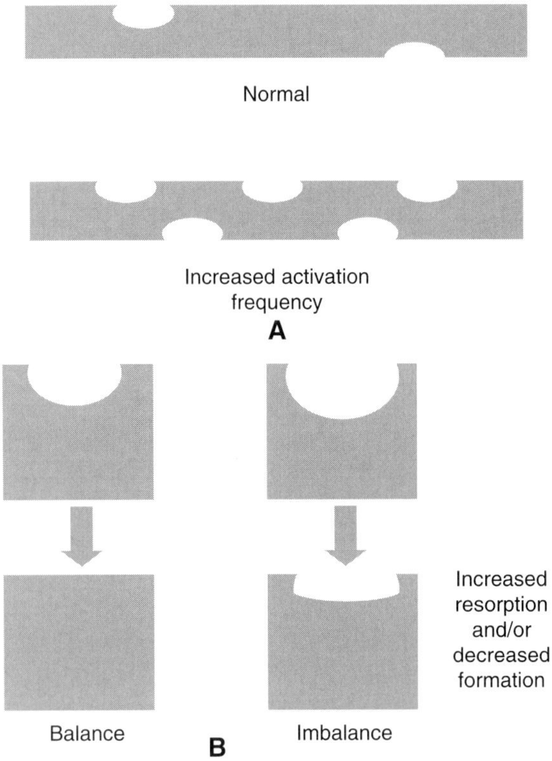

FIGURE 1 Mechanisms of cancellous bone loss. Increased activation frequency (a) results in a greater number of unfilled resorption cavities in a given volume of bone at any one time. This results in bone loss and also weakens the trabecular structure and predisposes it to penetration and erosion by osteoclasts. A negative remodelling imbalance (b) occurs when the amount of bone formed within individual remodelling units is less than than resorbed. Reproduced from Compston, J.: *Endocrine* 2002. 17:21-27, with permission.

bone loss is irreversible once the remodelling cycle has been completed and may co-exist with increased activation frequency.

C. Effects of Bone Loss on Cancellous Bone Microarchitecture

The alterations in bone remodelling responsible for bone loss determine the accompanying changes in bone microarchitecture, an important determinant of the mechanical strength of bone. In cancellous bone, trabecular thinning or trabecular perforation and erosion may occur; these two processes are to some extent interdependent. Trabecular thinning is associated with better preservation of bone architecture than penetration and erosion of trabeculae, the latter having the greater adverse effects on bone strength. Increased activation frequency and/or increased resorption depth predispose to trabecular penetration and erosion, whereas low bone turnover states favor trabecular thinning. As trabecular thinning proceeds, however, the likelihood of trabecular penetration by a resorption cavity of normal size increases (see Figure 2).

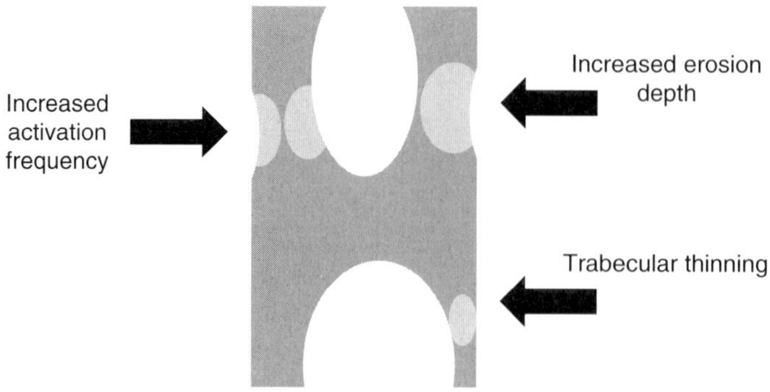

FIGURE 2 Mechanisms of trabecular penetration.

III. HISTOMORPHOMETRIC ASSESSMENT OF BONE REMODELLING AND STRUCTURE

A. Bone Turnover

The administration of two time-spaced doses of a tetracycline prior to bone biopsy enables measurements and calculation of dynamic indices of bone formation and, by extrapolation, bone resorption [9]. Tetracyclines bind to calcium and become incorporated at sites of active mineralisation; when unstained, undecalcified sections are viewed under blue light, and the tetracycline fluoresces. Bone turnover, which describes the tissue level of bone resorption and formation, can be calculated from the surface extent of tetracycline labelling and the rate of mineralisation of the osteoid seams (mineral apposition rate), derived from the gap separating the two tetracycline labels. In the absence of tetracycline labelling, the osteoid perimeter may provide some indication of bone turnover, increased osteoid perimeter being characteristic of high turnover states. Bone resorption rates cannot be directly measured but are assessed indirectly from bone formation rates. In addition, it should be noted that an increase in the eroded surface of bone does not necessarily imply increased resorption (or turnover) but may rather reflect failure of formation to occur in previously resorbed cavities.

Activation frequency is defined as the probability that a new remodelling cycle will be initiated at any point on the bone surface; it is a key determinant of bone mass in the adult skeleton. At present there are no *in situ* markers of activation, and it is therefore calculated indirectly from indices of bone formation [10].

B. Remodelling Balance

The amount of bone formed within individual remodelling units is termed the wall width and is measured as the mean width of completed bone structural units [11]. These can be identified under polarized light or using certain stains, for example toluidine blue. Investigation of short-term effects of a disease or its treatment on wall width necessitates differentiation of those units formed during the period of observation from those formed prior to that time; in practice this can only be achieved by identification of uncompleted bone structural units (which are still covered by osteoid) [12]. If this approach is not adopted, detection of changes in wall width due to disease or its treatment may require periods of two to three years or longer.

Accurate assessment of the amount of bone resorbed during each remodelling cycle is problematic for several reasons [7]. Identification of resorption cavities can be difficult and is to some extent subjective. Although the presence of resorbing cells within the cavity provides a means of identification, they may be missed because of the level of sectioning. Also, histochemical characterization by tartrate-resistant acid phosphatase staining may be unreliable when the biopsy has been embedded in certain resins. Another problem arises from the difficulty in identifying those cavities in which resorption has been completed; the presence of preosteoblastic cells may indicate completion [13], but such cavities are hard to identify and often form only a very small proportion of all the cavities present. Furthermore, the phenomenon of arrested resorption may produce small cavities in which resorption has apparently been completed [14]. Finally, those cavities that have resulted in trabecular perforation cannot be identified, and their omission may lead to underestimation of the true mean cavity depth.

Current methods for assessing erosion cavity size include counting the number of lamellae eroded beneath the trabecular surface after characterization of different cell types within the cavity [13], and computerized or manual reconstruction of the eroded bone surface followed by measurement of cavity depth and area [15, 16]. The former method is technically difficult and may overestimate true resorption depth, whereas the latter produces a mean value for cavities in all stages of completion and thus underestimates the true value for mean erosion depth.

These limitations preclude accurate assessment of remodelling balance by histomorphometric techniques; nevertheless, measurements of wall width and resorption depth provide useful information about changes in remodelling balance in untreated and treated disease, particularly when considered in parallel with changes in cancellous bone microarchitecture.

C. Assessment of Bone Structure

Both cortical and cancellous bone structure are important determinants of bone strength. In cortical bone, thickness and porosity can be measured; an increase in thickness may occur as a result of changes either at the endosteal or periosteal surface, the latter resulting in an increase in bone size. In cancellous bone, trabecular number, separation, and number can be assessed

[17], and several two-dimensional approaches to the assessment of connectivity have been described, including strut analysis [18], marrow star volume [19], and trabecular bone pattern factor [20]. More sophisticated three-dimensional measurements of connectivity, anisotropy, and trabecular shape can also be obtained using techniques such as magnetic resonance imaging and microtron computerized tomography.

IV. BONE HISTOMORPHOMETRIC ANALYSIS OF TRANSPLANTATION BONE DISEASE

Histomorphometric data on transplantation bone disease are sparse and exist only in patients undergoing liver, renal, and cardiac transplantation. Studies of renal transplantation bone disease are considered separately in Chapters 11 and 12. In this chapter, therefore, only the information relating to liver and cardiac transplantation bone disease will be considered. In addition, preexisting abnormalities in bone related to the underlying disease will be discussed for those conditions in which histomorphometric data are available.

A. Pre-Transplantation Bone Disease

Many individuals undergoing solid organ transplantation already have bone disease as a result of their underlying condition and, in some cases, its treatment. This has been best characterized in the case of chronic liver disease and chronic renal failure, for both of which a number of histomorphometric studies have been performed. More recently, the changes in bone remodelling and turnover in patients with cystic fibrosis have also been reported. The nature and severity of preexisting bone disease are important determinants of subsequent post-transplantation bone disease, and preventive measures undertaken early in the course of the disease are therefore appropriate. Because of the presence of preexisting bone disease in many patients, accurate characterization of the mechanisms of bone loss associated with organ transplantation requires knowledge of bone remodelling and turnover prior to transplantation, and prospective studies with paired biopsies are hence most informative.

1. Bone Disease Associated with Chronic Liver Disease

Osteoporosis is the most common skeletal complication of chronic liver disease, although osteomalacia may rarely occur. Histomorphometric studies in patients with chronic liver disease have demonstrated considerable heterogeneity in indices of bone remodelling and turnover. Thus in some studies, the changes were predominantly those of low bone turnover and reduced bone formation at the cellular level [21, 22, 23], while others have also reported evidence of increased turnover and resorption [24–27]. Biochemical markers of bone formation have been reported to be decreased [28] or normal [29], and resorption markers increased [28, 29]. The heterogeneity observed in the histological characteristics is likely to reflect a number of factors including differences in the underlying liver disease and its severity, the prevalence of vitamin D deficiency and secondary hyperparathyroidism, and the presence or absence of glucocorticoid therapy. Overall, the evidence indicates that reduced bone formation at the cellular level is a consistent feature, while increased bone turnover and resorption are more variable findings. In two studies in which bone histomorphometry was assessed prior to liver transplantation, no evidence of increased bone turnover or resorption was demonstrated. Thus McDonald et al. [30] reported low bone turnover in men and normal turnover in women prior to transplantation, with no increase in osteoclast surface or number. In the study done by Vedi et al. [23], pre-transplant biopsies showed low turnover with a trend towards reduced wall width and erosion depth. No mineralisation defect was evident in either of these studies. More recently, Guichelaar et al. [31] reported evidence of increased resorption and decreased formation in iliac crest biopsies from 33 patients with chronic cholestatic liver disease prior to transplantation.

2. *Bone Disease Associated with Cystic Fibrosis*

The severity of bone disease in individuals with cystic fibrosis has only recently received appropriate recognition, and the cellular pathophysiology of bone loss remains incompletely characterized. In autopsy vertebral bone specimens from four patients who had not undergone transplantation, Haworth et al. [32] described a decrease in osteoblastic surface and an increase in the resorption surface in association with an increased number of osteoclasts. In the absence of tetracycline labelling, however, dynamic indices of bone formation and resorption could not be assessed. In the study done by Elkin et al. [33], iliac crest bone biopsies were obtained from 20 patients with cystic fibrosis and low bone density (Z score at the femoral neck and/or lumbar spine of −1.5 or less). In this cohort, bone turnover was significantly reduced, as were wall width and mineral apposition rate, both indices of osteoblast function. Although the eroded bone perimeter was increased, resorption cavities were on average significantly smaller than normal, suggesting that the increase in eroded perimeter reflected the reduction in bone formation. A trend towards reduced connectivity of the cancellous architecture was also observed, although these differences did not attain statistical significance. One patient was found to have osteomalacia.

While both of these studies indicated that reduced bone formation is an important component of bone disease associated with cystic fibrosis, the results differed with respect to bone resorption. The increase in bone resorption demonstrated in the study of Haworth et al. [32] may reflect the severity of illness prior to death and the associated chronic infection and immobility. In addition, it is possible that differential changes occur at different skeletal sites. In contrast, the patients studied by Elkin et al. [33] were in reasonably good health at the time of their bone biopsy; nevertheless, in this study considerable heterogeneity in resorption cavity measurements was noted, indicating that increased resorption does contribute to bone loss in some individuals. This would be consistent with the increase in markers of bone resorption demonstrated in some studies [34, 35]. It is likely that this heterogeneity reflects the differing contributions of multiple pathogenetic factors, such as glucocorticoid therapy, infection, hypogonadism, immobility, and vitamin D deficiency.

B. Post-Transplantation Bone Disease

1. Cardiac Transplantation

Histomorphometric data in patients who have undergone cardiac transplantation are limited to one retrospective cross-sectional study, in which iliac crest bone biopsies were obtained in a subgroup of 6 patients with osteoporosis as defined by densitometric criteria [36]. The time since transplantation in this study ranged from 6 months to 10 years for all individuals, although no specific data are provided for the individuals undergoing bone biopsy. There was considerable variation in the histomorphometric indices obtained, although 5 of the 6 patients showed an increase in osteoid surface, and the eroded surface was also increased in 3. Tetracycline labelling was not given prior to biopsy in this study, thus limiting the information available. The small sample size and lack of relevant clinical information in these individuals makes it difficult to draw conclusions from this study, although the findings in the majority of patients would be consistent with increased bone turnover.

2. Cystic Fibrosis

In the study done by Haworth et al. [37], samples of vertebral bone were obtained at autopsy in 11 patients with cystic fibrosis with a mean time from transplantation to death of 29.2 ± 6.0 (mean ± SD) months. Bone volume was significantly reduced, with an increase in trabecular separation and decreased trabecular thickness; in addition, as in the 4 patients who had not undergone transplantation, indices of bone formation were reduced, and the resorption surface was increased with an increase in the number of osteoclasts. In view of the lack of pre-transplant biopsies in these subjects, however, it is not possible to assess the contribution of transplantation per se to the observed bone disease, although the abnormalities were generally more pronounced in subjects who had undergone transplantation than in those who had not.

3. Liver Transplantation

Four prospective studies have investigated changes in bone histomorphometric indices following liver transplantation. In two of these studies, bone biopsies were performed before and three months after transplantation [30, 38], and in the other two studies, before transplantation and four and six months postoperatively [31, 39].

McDonald et al. [30] performed bone biopsies before and 3 months after liver transplantation in 17 patients. It should be noted that the biopsies were obtained using a Jamshedi needle, which produces only a small biopsy (approximately 1 mm internal diameter). Both osteoid surface and the mineralizing surface were significantly increased after transplantation, and in addition, the surface extent of osteoblasts was significantly increased. Bone formation rate per tissue area also increased; although the magnitude of this increase was large (mean 88 versus 203 $\mu m^2/\mu m^2$), it did not achieve statistical significance because of the large variance in values. Osteoclast number and surface extent were not increased. The authors suggest that the observed increase in bone formation may be a compensatory mechanism to reverse prior bone loss. An alternative explanation is that the increase in tetracycline labelling and bone formation rate reflected increased activation frequency, and the failure to demonstrate increased osteoclast numbers reflected the difficulties associated with tartrate-resistant acid phosphatase staining of osteoclasts in methylmethacrylate-embedded sections. This latter explanation would be consistent with the rapid bone loss demonstrated in the lumbar spine during the first three post-operative months. Resorption cavity size was not assessed in this study, and activation frequency was not calculated.

In another prospective study, bone biopsies were obtained before and 3 months after liver transplantation in 21 patients [23]. Bone turnover, as assessed both by bone formation rate and activation frequency, increased significantly after transplantation (see Figure 3), and resorption cavity size

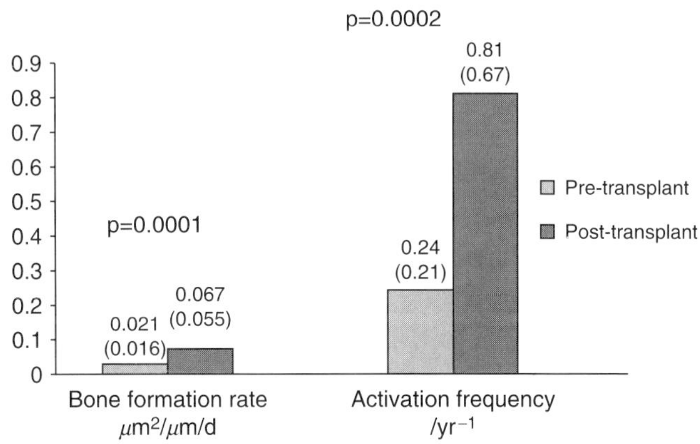

FIGURE 3 Changes in bone turnover rate and activation frequency in 21 patients with chronic liver disease before and 3 months after liver transplantation. The mean ±SD values are shown on top of each column. From reference 23.

also showed a non-significant trend towards an increase; osteoclast number and surface extent were not assessed. Indices of cancellous bone architecture did not change significantly over the study period. Because of the relatively short time period of the study, the values for wall width would mainly reflect those present prior to transplantation, hence no conclusions about this aspect of remodelling balance can be drawn.

Monegal et al. [38] studied bone histomorphometry in 24 patients who underwent bone biopsy within 12 hours of surgery and 6 months after liver transplantation. Tetrracycline labelling was not given prior to bone biopsy, so only static indices of bone resorption and formation could be assessed. There was a significant increase in osteoid surface and osteoblast surface, indicating increased bone formation; eroded surface was slightly increased, although not significantly, and no change in osteoclast number or surface was found. In this study, osteoclasts were presumably identified on morphological grounds alone, since no mention is made of the use of specific osteoclast markers or stains.

In a study of 33 patients with chronic cholestatic liver disease, Guichelaar et al. [31] performed bone biopsies at the time of transplantation and 4 months later. After transplantation, there was a significant increase in bone formation rate at tissue level and an increase in activation frequency from the low values observed pre-transplant to normal levels; indices of bone resorption remained increased. These changes at 4 months were associated with a significant decrease in spine bone mineral density, consistent with increased bone turnover as a mechanism for bone loss in the early post-operative period.

The histomorphometric effects of the bisphosphonate pamidronate in patients undergoing liver transplantation also support a role for increased bone turnover in early post-transplantation bone loss [39]. Bone biopsies were obtained before and 3 months after liver transplantation in 4 males and 8 females who formed a subgroup of a larger randomized, controlled, single-blind study [40]. In untreated patients ($n = 5$), a significant increase in bone formation rate at tissue level was demonstrated at 3 months in comparison to pre-operative values (0.035 ± 0.013 versus 0.161 ± 0.12 $\mu m^2/\mu m/day$; mean $\pm$ SD, $p = 0.003$). In patients treated with pamidronate ($n = 7$), no significant increase in bone formation rate was demonstrated at 3 months, although there was a trend towards an increase in indices of bone turnover. In this group, resorption cavity length was significantly reduced (210.4 ± 63.8 vs 179.8 ± 67.5 μm; $p = 0.03$), and other indices of resorption cavity size were reduced non-significantly. These results indicate that pre-operative administration of pamidronate in patients with chronic liver disease prevents, at least in part, the increase in bone turnover that occurs in untreated patients after transplantation.

Overall, therefore, the available histomorphometric data indicate that increased bone turnover is a major determinant of bone loss early after liver transplantation, probably in association with increased osteoclast activity. These changes are consistent with the rapid bone loss and increase in fracture risk observed early after transplantation [41], and with studies of biochemical markers, which indicate increased bone turnover early after cardiac transplantation [42, 43] and in patients undergoing liver transplantation as studied by Crosbie et al. [44], although the latter finding has not been universal [45]. Subsequent changes in bone remodelling and turnover have not been studied and are an important area for further research in view of the finding, in some studies, of persistence of bone disease [45].

REFERENCES

1. Compston, J.E. Bone histomorphometry, in Vitamin D, D. Feldman, F.H. Glorieux, J.W. Pike, eds., 1997, pp. 573–586. California: Academic Press.
2. Rao, D.S. Practical approach to bone biopsy, in Bone Histomorphometry: Techniques and Interpretation, R.Recker, ed., 1983, pp. 3–11. Boca Raton, Florida: CRC Press.
3. Eventov, I., Frisch, B., Cohen, Z., and Hammel, I. (1991). Osteopenia, hematopoiesis, and bone remodelling in iliac crest and femoral biopsies: a prospective study of 102 cases of femoral neck fractures. *Bone*. 12:1–6.
4. de Vernejoul, M.C., Kuntz, D., Miravet, L., Goutalier, D., and Ryckewaert A. (1981). Histomorphometric reproducibility in normal patients. *Calcif Tissue Int*. 33:369–374.
5. Chavassieux, P.M., Arlot, M.E., and Meunier, P.J. (1985). Intermethod variation in bone histomorphometry. Comparison between manual and computerised methods applied to iliac bone biopsies. *Bone*. 6:211–219.
6. Wright, C.D.P., Vedi, S., Garrahan, N.J., Stanton, M., Duffy, S.W., and Compston, J.E. (1992). Combined inter-observer and inter-method variation in bone histomorphometry. *Bone*. 13:205–208.
7. Compston, J.E., and Croucher, P.I. (1991). Histomorphometric assessment of trabecular bone remodelling in osteoporosis. *Bone Miner*. 14:91–102.
8. Parfitt, A.M. (1984). The cellular basis of bone remodelling. The quantum concept re-examined in light of recent advances in cell biology. *Calcif Tissue Int*. 36:S37–45.
9. Frost, H.M. (1969). Tetracycline-based histological analysis of bone remodeling. *Calcif Tissue Res*. 3:211–237.
10. Parfitt, A.M., Drezner, M.K., Glorieux, F.H., Kanis, J.A., Malluche, H., Meunier, P.J., Ott, S.M., and Recker, R.R. (1987). Bone histomorphometry: standardisation of nomenclature, symbols and units. *J Bone Miner Res*. 2:595–610.
11. Lips, P., Courpron, P., and Meunier, P.J. (1978). Mean wall thickness of trabecular bone packets in the human iliac crest: changes with age. *Calcif Tissue Int*. 26:13–17.
12. Steiniche, T., Eriksen, E.F., Kudsk, H., Mosekilde, L., and Melsen, F. (1992). Reconstruction of the formative site in trabecular bone by a new, quick, and easy method. *Bone*. 13:147–152.
13. Eriksen, E.F., Melsen, F., and Mosekilde L. (1984). Reconstruction of the resorptive site in iliac trabecular bone: a kinetic model for bone resorption in 20 normal individuals. *Metab Bone Dis Rel Res*. 5:235–242.
14. Croucher, P.I., Gilks, W., and Compston, J.E. (1995). Evidence for interrupted bone resorption in human iliac cancellous bone. *J Bone Miner Res*. 10:1537–1543.
15. Garrahan, N.J., Croucher, P.I., and Compston, J.E. (1990). A computerised technique for the quantitative assessment of resorption cavities in bone. *Bone*. 11:241–246.
16. Cohen-Solal, M., Morieux, C., and de Vernejoul, M.C. (1991). Relationship between the number of resorbing cells and the amount resorbed in metabolic bone disorders. *J Bone Miner Res*. 6:915–920.

17. Parfitt, A.M., Mathews, C.H.E., Villanueva, A.R., Kleerekoper, M., Frame, B., and Rao, D.S. (1983). Relationships between surface volume and thickness of iliac trabecular bone in ageing and in osteoporosis. Implications for the microanatomic and cellular mechanisms of bone loss. *J Clin Invest.* 72:1396–1409.
18. Garrahan, N.J., Mellish, R.W.E., and Compston, J.E. (1986). A new method for the two-dimensional analysis of bone structure in human iliac crest biopsies. *J Microsc.* 142:341–349.
19. Vesterby, A. (1990). Star volume of marrow space and trabeculae in iliac crest: sampling procedure and correlation to star volume of first lumbar vertebra. *Bone.* 11:149–155.
20. Hahn, M., Vogel, M., Pompesius-Kempa, M., and Delling, G. (1992). Trabecular bone pattern factor—A new parameter for simple quantification of bone microarchitecture. *Bone.* 13:327–330.
21. Stellon, A.J., Webb, A., Compston, J.E., and Williams, R. (1987). Low bone turnover state in primary biliary cirrhosis. *Hepatology.* 7:137–142.
22. Stellon, A.J., Webb, A., and Compston, J.E. (1988). Bone histomorphometry and studies in corticosteroid treated chronic active hepatitis. *Gut.* 29:378–389.
23. Vedi, S., Greer, S., Skingle, S.J., Garrahan, N.J., Ninkovic, M., Alexander, G.M., and Compston, J.E. (1999). Mechanism of bone loss after liver transplantation: a histomorphometric analysis *J Bone Miner Res.* 14:281–287.
24. Cuthbert, J.A., Pak, C.Y.C., Zerwekh, J.E., Glass, K.D., and Combes, B. (1984). Bone disease in primary biliary cirrhosis: increased bone resorption and turnover in the absence of osteoporosis or osteomalacia. *Hepatology.* 4:1–8.
25. Lalor, B.C., France, M.W., Adams, P.H., and Counihan, T.B.(1986). Bone and mineral metabolism and chronic alcohol abuse. *Quart J Med.* 59:497–511.
26. Hay, J.E., Lindor, K.D., Wiesner, R.H., Dickson, E.R., Krom, R.A.F., and LaRusso, N.F. (1991). The metabolic bone disease of primary sclerosing cholangitis. *Hepatology.* 14:257–261.
27. Hodgson, S.F., Dickson, E.R., Eastell, R., Eriksen, E.F., Bryant, H.U., and Riggs, B.L. (1993). Rates of cancellous bone remodeling and turnover in osteopenia associated with primary biliary cirrhosis. *Bone.* 14:819–827.
28. Monegal, A., Navasa, M., Guanabens, N., Peris, P., Pons, F., Martinez de Osaba, M.J., Rimola, A., Rodes, J., and Munoz-Gomez, J. (1997). Osteoporosis and bone mineral metabolism disorders in cirrhotic patients referred for orthotopic liver transplantation. *Calcif Tissue Int.* 60:148–54.
29. Crosbie, O.M., Freaney, R., McKenna, M.J., and Hegarty, J.E. (1999). Bone density, vitamin D status, and disordered bone remodeling in end-stage chronic liver disease. *Calcif Tissue Int.* 64:295–300.
30. McDonald, J.A., Dunstan, C.R., Dilworth, P., Sherbon, K., Sheil, A.G.R., Evans, R.A., and McCaughan, G.W. (1991). Bone loss after liver transplantation. *Hepatology.* 14:613–619.
31. Guichelaar, M.M.J., Malinchoc, M., Sibonga, J.D. Clarke, B.L., and Hay, J.E. (2003). Bone histomorphometric changes after liver transplantation for chronic cholestatic liver disease. *J Bone Miner Res.* 18:2190–2199.
32. Haworth, C.S., Webb, A.K., Egan, J.J., Selby, P.L., Hasleton, P.S., Bishop, P.W. and Freemont, A.J. (2000). Bone histomorphometry in adult patients with cystic fibrosis. *Chest.* 118:434–439.
33. Elkin, S.L., Vedi, S., Bord, S. Garrahan, N.J., Hodson, M.E., and Compston, J.E. (2002). Histomorphometric analysis of bone biopsies from the iliac crest of adults with cystic fibrosis. *Amer J Resp Crit Care Med.* 75:736–742.
34. Haworth, C.S., Selby, P.L., Webb, A.K., Dodd, M.E., Musson, H., Economou, G., Horrocks, A.W., Freemont, A.J., Mawer, E.B., and Adams, J.E. (1999). Low bone mineral density in adults with cystic fibrosis. *Thorax.* 54:961–967.

35. Aris, R.M., Ontjes, D.A., Buell, H.E., Blackwood, A.D., Lark, R.K., Caminiti, M., Brown, S.A., Renner, J.B., Chalermskulrate, W., and Lester, G.E. (2002). Abnormal bone turnover in cystic fibrosis adults. *Osteoporos Int.* 13:151–157.
36. Glendenning, P., Kent, G.N., Adler, B.D., Matz, L., Watson, I., O'Driscoll, G.J., and Hurley, D.M. (1999). High prevalence of osteoporosis in cardiac transplant recipients and discordance between biochemical turnover markers and bone histomorphometry. *Clin Endocrinol.* 50:347–355.
37. Haworth, C.S., Selby, P.L., Adams, J.E., Mawer, E.B., Horrocks, A.W., and Webb, A.K. (2001). Effect of intravenous pamidronate on bone mineral density in adults with cystic fibrosis. *Thorax.* 56:314–316.
38. Monegal, A., Navasa, M., Guanabens, N., Peris, P., Pons, F., Martinez de Osaba, M.J., Ordi, J., Rimola, A., Rodes, J., and Munoz-Gomez, J. (2001). Bone disease after liver transplantation: a long-term prospective study of bone mass changes, hormonal status and histomorphometric characteristics. *Osteoporos Int.* 12:484–492.
39. Vedi, S., Ninkovic, M., Garrahan, N.J., Alexander, G.J.M., and Compston, J.E. (2002). Effects of a single infusion of pamidronate prior to liver transplantation: a bone histomorphometric study. *Transplant Int.* 15:290–295.
40. Ninkovic, M., Love, S., Tom, B.D., Bearcroft, P.W., Alexander, G.J., and Compston, J.E. (2002). Lack of effect of intravenous pamidronate on fracture incidence and bone mineral density after orthotopic liver transplantation. *J Hepatol.* 37:93–100.
41. Compston, J. (2003). Osteoporosis after liver transplantation. *Liver Transplant.* 9:321–330.
42. Shane, E., Rivas, M., McMahon, D.J., Staron, R.B., Silverberg, S.J., Seibel, M.J., Mancini, D.S., Michler, R.E., Aaronson, K., Addesso, V., and Lo, S.H. (1997). Bone loss and turnover after cardiac transplantation. *J Clin Endocrinol Metab.* 82:1497–1506.
43. Välimäki, M.J., Kinnunen, K., Tähtelä, R., Löyttniemi, E., Laitenen, K., Mäkelä, P., Keto, P., and Nieminen, M. (1999). A prospective study of bone loss and turnover after cardiac transplantation: effect of calcium supplementation with or without calcitonin. *Osteoporos Int.* 10:128–136.
44. Crosbie, O.M., Freaney, R., McKenna, M.J., Curry, M.P., and Hegarty, J.E. (1999). Predicting bone loss following orthotopic liver transplantation. *Gut.* 44:430–434.
45. Giannini, S., Nobile, M., Ciuffreda, M., Iemmolo, R.M., Dalle Carbonare, L., Minicuci, N., Casagrande, F., Destro, C., Gerunda, G.E., Sartori, L., and Crepaldi, G. (2000). Long-term persistence of low bone density in orthotopic liver transplantation. *Osteoporos Int.* 11:417–424.

CHAPTER 9

The Role of Parathyroid Hormone in the Evolution of Bone Loss after Organ Transplantation

Mishaela R. Rubin, MD
Department of Medicine, College of Physicians and Surgeons, Columbia University New York, NY

John P. Bilezikian, MD
Departments of Medicine and Pharmacology, College of Physicians and Surgeons, Columbia University New York, NY

I. INTRODUCTION

Bone loss after organ transplantation has many causes. In this chapter, we evaluate the evidence for parathyroid hormone (PTH) as an important factor in this syndrome. PTH has been implicated because it is believed that the immunosuppressive drugs used after organ transplantation, specifically glucocorticoids and calcineurin inhibitors (cyclosporine and tacrolimus, or FK506) [1], increase the secretion of PTH [2, 3, 4]. If this were to occur with organ transplantation, PTH could be important in the development of post-transplant osteoporosis. We consider other means by which PTH could be etiologically important in this syndrome.

To consider the role of PTH in transplantation osteoporosis, a distinction between the two phases of post-transplantation bone loss has to be made. This distinction is based on the presence or absence of high-dose glucocorticoids. During the first six months after transplantation, when glucocorticoid doses generally are high enough to profoundly suppress bone formation, PTH does not appear to play an important role. The bone loss that occurs, rather, is more reminiscent of that seen in glucocorticoid-induced osteoporosis (GIO). Serum markers of bone formation, particularly osteocalcin, are suppressed and urinary markers of bone resorption are elevated during this period [5]. Calcineurin inhibitors, which are believed to play a less important role at this time, may directly increase bone resorption, although this has not been established definitively in humans [6]. The simultaneous administration of high-dose glucocorticoids and calcineurin inhibitors leads to uncoupling of resorption and formation during this first phase of the post-transplant period [7]. There is therefore a disparity between rates of bone formation and bone resorption, the dominating effect being that of high-dose glucocorticoids, with resultant rapid bone loss and high fracture rates [5, 8, 9].

During the second post-transplant period, after glucocorticoids have typically been reduced, PTH could become a more important contributor to bone loss. Glucocorticoids are typically tapered to levels below 5 mg/d of prednisone or discontinued completely. Osteoblast function recovers, and the suppressive effects on bone formation are reversed. Adverse effects of calcineurin inhibitors remain, however, so bone resorption remains elevated. Skeletal dynamics still demonstrate relative uncoupling and bone loss continues, although at a slower pace [3]. There may even be some recovery during this phase, particularly at the spine, although significant radial loss can occur [5].

II. ISOLATED GLUCOCORTICOID USE AND PTH

A. Glucocorticoid-Induced Osteoporosis (GIO)

Since early post-transplant bone loss is similar to that of GIO, observations about the role of PTH in GIO can be extrapolated to the early post-transplant situation. The cardinal effect of glucocorticoids on skeletal dynamics is a profound reduction in bone formation. Glucocorticoids act directly on osteoblasts to stimulate apoptosis, decrease production of osteoblasts and osteoclasts from progenitors in the bone marrow, decrease numbers of osteoblasts in cancellous bone, and decrease osteoblastic production of type I collagen [10–14]. Biochemical markers of bone formation, osteocalcin and bone-specific alkaline phosphatase, are suppressed; bone resorption, as measured by urinary NTX and pyridinoline cross-link excretion, is accelerated [15, 16]. Osteoclast number and activity increase, as does the fraction of eroded bone surface [17–21]. Glucocorticoid use can therefore be associated with rapid bone loss as a result of both reduced bone formation and accelerated bone resorption. With continued use of glucocorticoids, the rapid rate of osteoclast-mediated bone resorption slows [18], but suppression of bone formation continues as the dominant skeletal dynamic. Thus, bone loss is progressive since bone resorption chronically exceeds bone formation.

One of the proposed mechanisms for the adverse skeletal effects of glucocorticoids is a direct effect on calcium metabolism. At daily doses of prednisone, ≥10 mg, intestinal calcium absorption is reduced [22, 23]. Alterations in vitamin D metabolism, or an independent non-competitive effect to counter the actions of vitamin D [24], could account, in part, for reduced intestinal calcium absorption. When prednisone doses are increased to 20 mg/d or higher, a direct effect to increase renal calcium excretion adds to negative calcium balance [25, 26]. These perturbations have led to the belief that a state of secondary hyperparathyroidism ensues with glucocorticoid use, although evidence to support this is conflicting.

B. Evidence that PTH Contributes to GIO

Older literature has suggested that isolated glucocorticoid use might be associated with increases in PTH. Hahn et al. compared 17 glucocorticoid-treated patients with normal subjects and found increases in PTH, along with decreases in ^{47}Ca absorption and forearm bone mass [27]. Similar findings were noted in other small studies when patients on glucocorticoid therapy were found to have increases in PTH [28, 29]. In a larger study by Suzuki et al., 44 glucocorticoid-treated patients were found to have elevated PTH, nephrogenous cAMP, and fasting urinary calcium excretion [26]. Elevated PTH levels were observed in infant piglets administered dexamethasone for 15 days [30]. This might occur from a direct effect of glucocorticoids on glandular secretion of PTH [31]. For example, dexamethasone administration increases PTH secretion from cultured bovine parathyroid cells and cortisol-stimulated PTH secretion from cultures of rat parathyroid glands in a dose-dependent manner [32, 33]. In human parathyroid cells from hyperplastic parathyroid glands, dexamethasone stimulates PTH release, both time- and dose-dependently [34]. The effects of glucocorticoids on glandular secretion of PTH might occur by effects on gene transcription, a well known molecular action of glucocorticoids [34]. Recently, it was found that higher baseline PTH levels were predictive of vertebral fracture at 1 year in 111 glucocorticoid-treated patients (RR=1.8) [35].

An increase in circulating levels of PTH is therefore one mechanism by which bone loss can occur with glucocorticoid use. Another mechanism by which glucocorticoids might affect the parathyroid-bone axis is by increasing the sensitivity of bone cells to PTH, even if circulating PTH is not elevated. This could occur by a number of different mechanisms. For example, glucocorticoids increase the expression [36, 37, 38] and availability [39] of PTH receptors on osteoblasts. Greater numbers of PTH receptors could thus be associated with enhanced sensitivity to PTH. Alternatively, enhanced sensitivity to PTH could be a result of changes in the affinity of the receptor for PTH without any change in the number of receptors. Beyond the receptor per se, glucocorticoids have been shown to enhance the efficiency of post-receptor PTH signaling [39, 40]. Any or all of the aforementioned mechanisms could help to explain the observation that in isolated bone cells, steroids modulate the PTH sensitivity of osteoblasts and osteoclasts in such a way that lower concentrations of bovine PTH elicit measurable biochemical changes. [41]. In mouse cell cultures, the addition of glucocorticoids synergistically affected PTH-mediated bone resorption [42, 43].

Thus, classic models to explain glucocorticoid-induced bone loss invariably include a compensatory increase in PTH due to these proposed effects of glucocorticoids on various points in the PTH-skeletal-renal-GI axes [19]. It is possible that concomitant vitamin D deficiency or resistance contribute to increased PTH activity [44]. In some GIO trials, when calcium or vitamin D was replaced, the rise in PTH levels was attenuated [27, 29, 45, 46], but this has not been consistently found in other studies [47, 48].

C. Evidence that PTH Does Not Contribute to GIO

As early as 1980, Seeman et al. observed that excess glucocorticoid levels, whether endogenous or exogenous in origin, were not associated with alterations in PTH levels [49]. Similarly, Slovik et al. found normal PTH levels in asthmatic patients on short-term and long-term glucocorticoid treatment [48]. In addition, 22 women with rheumatoid arthritis were found to have the same PTH levels whether or not they were receiving low-dose prednisone (6.6 mg/d) [50]. When women were administered even higher amounts of prednisone chronically (for an average of 13 years), PTH levels were the same as in age-matched controls [51]. Hattersley et al. also found no difference in PTH levels in patients treated with chronic glucocorticoids for obstructive airway disease when compared with controls [52]. Even daily assessment of PTH levels did not reveal any increases when multiple sclerosis patients treated with high-dose glucocorticoids were examined [53]. The expectation that PTH levels should have been elevated in these studies, given increases in urinary calcium excretion and decreases in intestinal calcium absorption is thus not confirmed by the data. It is important to note, however, that the subjects in these trials had underlying medical illnesses, which could conceivably have modified both the secretion of and skeletal response to PTH.

Other data indicating that PTH levels are not changed by glucocorticoid administration come from studies in normal, healthy subjects. In 3 separate investigations examining the effects of a short course (5–14 days) of prednisone (doses ranging from 15 to 40 mg daily) in healthy adults, no significant change in PTH levels was found [47, 52, 54]. In a longer study of 9 healthy men who were administered 50 mg of

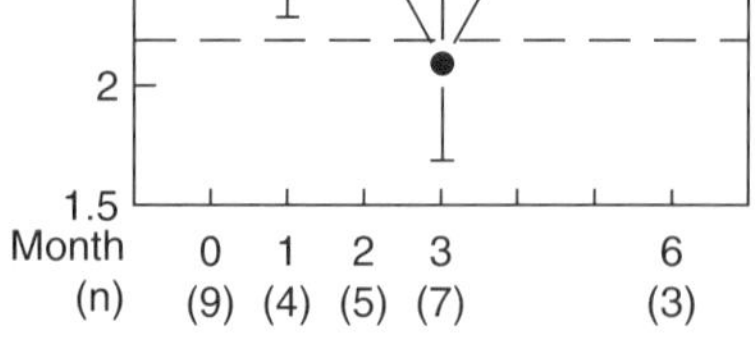

FIGURE 1 Glucocorticoids do not increase parathyroid hormone levels. In 9 healthy men who received 50 mg of prednisolone daily for infertility (due to the presence of antisperm antibodies) for 3.7 ± 0.6 months, PTH did not increase during corticosteroid treatment. The area above the dotted line represents the normal area for PTH. Reprinted with permission from Pearce et al. [55]

prednisolone daily for as long as 6 months, there was no change in PTH levels (see Figure 1) [55]. These observations in normal subjects confirm those in patients with specific medical illnesses, helping to discount any potential confounding effects of underlying illness on circulating PTH levels. It remains possible, however, that skeletal responsiveness to PTH is differentially affected without any change in PTH concentrations when glucocorticoids are present. Thus even a normal PTH level might elicit significant physiologic effects [26, 29].

PTH secretory dynamics have been studied in glucocorticoid-treated men, as compared with normal age- and sex-matched controls [56]. Six men (ages 31–64 years) treated chronically with glucocorticoids (daily dose >7.5 mg of prednisone or equivalent for more than 6 months) and control subjects underwent peripheral blood sampling every 3 minutes for 6 hours. Basal PTH secretory rate was reduced in the glucocorticoid-treated group (4.3 versus 8.8 pg/ml/min, $p=0.017$) despite an increase in amplitude of fractional pulsatile PTH secretion (42 versus 18 pg/ml/min, $p=0.006$) as compared with controls. Chronic glucocorticoid treatment appeared to induce a redistribution of the spontaneous PTH secretory profile by reducing the amount tonically released while increasing the amount released by pulsatile secretion [56]. Although the overall dominant effect was a reduction in PTH secretion, this study could not determine whether tonic or pulsatile secretion was the driving force. If such a distinction could have been made, the principal action of glucocorticoids on PTH, positive or negative, could have been more clearly elucidated. Nevertheless, the implication of the studies in which PTH levels have been measured favor no major effects of glucocorticoids.

If the observations described above are applicable to the first phase of bone loss after organ transplantation, in which glucocorticoid effects are considered to be dominant, one would not expect PTH to play an important role.

III. ISOLATED CALCINEURIN INHIBITOR USE AND PTH

Calicneurin inhibitors become more important in the later post-transplant bone loss phase when glucocorticoids have been tapered. Cyclosporine and tacrolimus inhibit calcineurin, a T-cell phosphatase, and reduce T-cell function [6]. The calcineurin inhibitors have characteristic adverse effects on bone and mineral metabolism that contribute to bone loss after organ transplantation, even in the absence of glucocorticoid use [4, 6, 57]. In direct contrast to the main effect of glucocorticoids, which reduce bone formation, calcineurin inhibitors increase bone turnover [58]. Both resorption and formation are increased, although resorption typically exceeds formation [59]. These observations have been well documented in animals [60]. In the rat, for example, calcineurin inhibitors cause severe bone loss, particularly in cancellous bone, that is associated with marked increases in bone resorption and formation. These effects are prevented by anti-resorptive agents [6]. Elevated levels of bone resorption markers are seen in heart transplant patients who receive both glucocorticoids and calcineurin inhibitors [4, 5, 61, 62], a pattern not observed with isolated, chronic glucocorticoid use [63]. Simultaneous treatment with calcineurin inhibitors and glucocorticoids thus inflicts a dual skeletal insult by increasing resorption while not allowing for adequate compensatory bone formation.

A. Evidence that PTH Contributes to Bone Loss Associated with Calcineurin Inhibitors

Calcineurin inhibitors appear to be associated with increases in PTH. Nephrotoxic effects of this drug class result in measurable declines in renal function and decreased synthesis of 1,25-dihydroxyvitamin D. The ultimate effect is to reduce the efficiency and amount of calcium absorption in the GI tract [6]. Moreover, a renal tubular leak of calcium may occur. In rats treated with cyclosporine A, changes in PTH were not observed [64], although in a different study, cyclosporine A–mediated bone loss was attenuated by parathyroidectomy [60]. FK506, another calcineurin inhibitor, also has been associated with secondary increases in PTH. [65]. Thus, although human data are not available for isolated calcineurin inhibitor use, animal data are not inconsistent with a role for PTH in contributing to bone loss, although the data are not secure.

IV. TRANSPLANT-INDUCED OSTEOPOROSIS AND PTH: DYNAMIC EVIDENCE

A. Evidence that PTH Contributes to Transplant-Induced Osteoporosis

Elevated PTH levels have been observed in numerous patients studied after heart, liver, lung, and kidney transplantation [2, 3, 8, 66–68]. In some cases, these post-transplant increases in PTH have been correlated with declines in renal function [8, 67]. Although a secondary hyperparathyroid state can precede the transplant when patients have preexisting renal dysfunction [69], the focus here is on the data for post-transplant elevations in PTH.

Most of the data relating changes in PTH after organ transplantation are available for heart transplant recipients. Guo et al. found increased bone turnover associated with renal insufficiency and increased PTH in 50 male cardiac transplant patients on prednisone and cyclosporine [2]. The authors postulated that a state of secondary hyperparathyroidism due to renal insufficiency could have contributed to the increased bone turnover. A smaller study of 16 men and women on cyclosporine A and prednisone within 3 years after heart transplant demonstrated slightly elevated PTH levels [57]. In a similar study, half of 32 patients who had undergone cardiac transplant over a prior 10-year period had elevated PTH levels [3]. Similarly, 24 patients after cardiac transplant were found to have a 90% increase in PTH levels 18 months after transplant [4]. Shane et al. have described 70 cardiac transplant patients whose PTH levels did not change over 3 years [5], despite concentrations that were at the very upper end of the normal range. In a secondary analysis, it was found that those whose magnesium and PTH levels were low lost less bone than those with normal magnesium and high PTH levels [70]. A smaller study of 9 adult survivors of adolescent cardiac transplant found that these subjects had mild renal insufficiency and PTH levels that were 3 times higher than in matched controls [71]. Interestingly, the subjects had a greater amount of both biologically inactive and biologically active PTH fragments as compared to controls, raising a point that only a portion of this elevation is caused by biologically active PTH.

In another study of cardiac transplant survivors by Shane et al., PTH was found to increase 6 months after transplant in patients who did or did not receive alendronate (39±4 to 51±4 pg/ml), peaking at 80% above baseline by 6 months (see Figure 2A) [72]. Note that even though the levels increased substantially, they were still within normal limits. In contrast, PTH decreased by 28% in calcitriol-treated patients (44±5 to 29±5 pg/ml), this downward excursion again occurring within the normal range for PTH. In the control group, the PTH level at 6 months was directly related to rates of bone loss at the femoral neck ($r = -0.555$, $p = 0.02$) and total hip ($r = -0.609$, $p = 0.008$) (see Figure 2B), although not at the lumbar spine. In the alendronate-treated patients, the 6-month PTH concentration was directly related to bone loss at the lumbar spine ($r = -0.379$. $p = 0.02$), but not at the hip. There was no relationship between PTH and bone loss in the

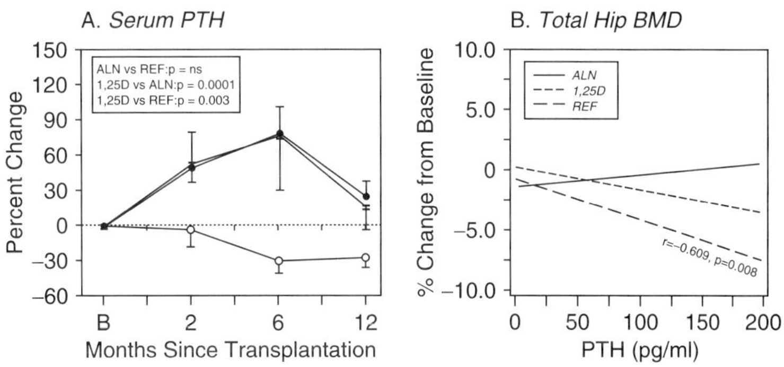

FIGURE 2 **A:** PTH was found to increase 6 months after cardiac transplant in the reference patients (■) and in the alendronate-treated patients (●), peaking at 80% above baseline by 6 months. In contrast, PTH decreased by 28% in patients treated with calcitriol (○). **B:** The PTH level at 6 months in the reference group was inversely and significantly related to the rate of bone loss at the total hip ($r = -0.609$, $p = 0.008$). There was no relationship between PTH levels and total hip bone loss in the alendronate and calcitriol groups. Reproduced with permission from Shane et al. (2004), *N Engl J Med*. 350(8):767–776, and personal communication.

calcitriol-treated group. Presumably, calcitriol suppressed PTH either by its direct actions or via stimulation of intestinal calcium absorption.

Renal transplant recipients may also have elevated PTH levels even in the setting of adequate, but not normal, kidney function. When patients more than 1 year after successful renal transplantation with serum creatinine less than or equal to 2.5 mg/dl were studied, elevated PTH levels were found in all subjects, although to a greater extent in those with osteoporosis and high bone turnover (165.1±46.3 versus 84.3±7.4, normal 10–65 pg/ml) [73]. In a similar cohort of renal transplant survivors, 81% had elevated PTH levels and 88% had a decrease in bone mass [68]. Despite a correlation between PTH and osteocalcin, however, there was no correlation between PTH and BMD or resorption markers, making it harder to fully ascribe the bone loss to hyperparathyroidism.

In patients after liver transplant, increases in PTH have also been observed [74–77]. One study described an early and transient increase in PTH levels after liver transplant which was significant at 1 and 2 months ($p<0.0005$ and 0.001, respectively), but by 3 months levels had returned to the normal preoperative values [76].

In all these studies, several confounding factors limit secure conclusions about PTH being etiologically important in bone loss. These patients invariably develop renal insufficiency. Secondary hyperparathyroidism sometimes occurs as a result of the effect of the calcineurin inhibitor on renal function. In addition, the presence of substantial renal insufficiency raises questions as to the identity of the circulating species of PTH. This setting may lead to increases in biologically inactive fragments as well as authentic full-length PTH.

B. Evidence That PTH Does Not Contribute to Transplant-Induced Osteoporosis

Some studies have failed to document an elevation of PTH in transplanted human subjects. In 25 subjects who underwent cardiac transplant, PTH levels were not increased after 1 year [61]. Other studies have reported similar findings [78, 79]. Meys et al. [80] studied 46 patients who underwent cardiac transplantation and found that PTH was actually reduced 12 months after transplant. Shane et al. reported on 40 cardiac transplant patients in whom an increase in PTH was not observed in the majority of subjects (80%) after at least 8 years of follow-up [8]. Most of these patients were evaluated only once, at an average of 2 years after transplant. In renal transplant survivors, there is also indirect evidence to suggest that PTH is not a major pathophysiologic factor [81]. When renal transplant survivors were treated with 1,25-dihydroxyvitamin D for 1 year, PTH levels fell, yet bone mineral density did not change [81]. Observations after liver transplantation also show that in some studies PTH remains normal [82, 83]. Recently, it was reported that 44 stem-cell transplant recipients followed for

24 months had no change in PTH [84], although the patients did not receive calcineurin inhibitors.

V. TRANSPLANT-INDUCED OSTEOPOROSIS AND PTH: DENSITOMETRIC EVIDENCE

Because PTH is preferentially catabolic at cortical bone, one can infer that cortical loss with cancellous preservation implicates PTH in post-transplant bone loss. In the early post-transplant phase, in fact, preferential cancellous bone loss occurs, consistent with the dominant effect of glucocorticoid effects during this time period. This pattern suggests that an important role for PTH in this phase is unlikely. Soon after transplantation, the vertebral compression fracture is common, reflecting both rate and extent of reductions in BMD at this site. Cross-sectional studies of cardiac transplant recipients treated with both glucocorticoids and calcineurin inhibitors have found remarkably high vertebral fracture prevalence rates of 22–35% [3, 8, 78]. One longitudinal study demonstrated a fracture incidence of 36% during the first year following cardiac transplantation, with the majority of fractures involving the spine [85]. After liver transplantation, ribs and vertebrae are the most common sites for fracture [75, 86–88]. In rats treated with cyclosporine A, rapid and severe preferential cancellous loss ensues [6, 59, 89, 90].

Preferential reduction of spine and hip density, with little if any change in distal radial density, is reminiscent of the typical pattern of bone loss in GIO [91–95]. This would argue against a role for PTH in the early, glucocorticoid-dominated phase after transplant. The observations in primary hyperparathyroidism, a model for PTH-induced bone loss, are in direct contrast to those seen in GIO and in the early stage of transplantation osteoporosis (see Table 1). The preferential action of PTH to be catabolic at cortical sites (e.g., distal 1/3 radius site) is typically seen in primary hyperparathyroidism [96, 97]. In contrast, the lumbar spine, a site of predominantly cancellous bone, is relatively well preserved [98]. This

TABLE 1 Comparison of the densitometric and fracture risk profiles of glucocorticoid-induced osteoporosis and transplantation osteoporosis as compared to primary hyperparathyroidism

Skeletal site	GIO	Transplantation osteoporosis	Primary hyper-parathyroidism
Cancellous bone density (lumbar spine)	Decreased	Decreased initially, then recovery	Maintained or increased
Cortical bone density (distal forearm)	No change or mild decrease in GIO	No change initially, then decrease	Decreased
Site of likely enhanced fracture risk	Thoraco-lumbar spine and hip	Thoraco-lumbar spine and appendicular sites	Distal radius

pattern is seen in patients whose primary hyperparathyroidism is characterized as mild, with elevated PTH within two times the upper limit of normal. Although epidemiological data on site-specific fracture incidence are incomplete, it would appear that forearm fractures are much more likely to occur in primary hyperparathyroidism than vertebral fractures [99, 100]. With more severe disease and prolonged PTH exposure, admittedly, this pattern can be altered and skeletal loss at all sites can occur. Nevertheless, preservation of cancellous bone in mild primary hyperparathyroidism is overall in direct contrast to the pattern of bone loss in GIO and in early post-transplant osteoporosis, where cancellous bone loss is commonly seen.

In the later stage of post-transplant bone loss, however, a decrease in cortical bone can be seen [5, 71]. In fact, cortical bone loss can occur in GIO as well [93, 101]. In a large survey of survivors of solid organ transplants, more appendicular than vertebral fractures were observed [102]. Fifty-Six of 600 (9.3%) patients had at least one fracture following 1,221 person-years of observation; the sites were: foot (n = 22), arm (n = 8), leg (n = 7), ribs (n = 6), hip (n = 4), spine (n = 3), fingers (n = 3), pelvis (n = 2), and wrist (n = 1), although spine X-rays were not performed in all [102]. In an observational study of cardiac transplantation recipients, rapid bone loss occurred in the initial 6 months (lumbar spine) or 1 year (femoral neck) after transplant [5]. During the second and third years, however, a significant loss of radial bone mass occurred (2.1% and 2.9%, respectively) [5]. In a small study of adult survivors of adolescent cardiac transplantation, the forearm was the site with the greatest bone loss [71]. In a study of renal transplant patients (n = 69), although the main sites of bone loss were at the hip or lumbar spine, 22% had osteoporosis and 35% had osteopenia at the wrist [68]. In summary, evidence exists both for and against a role for PTH in the later phases of bone loss after transplantation.

VI. TRANSPLANT-INDUCED OSTEOPOROSIS AND PTH: HISTOMORPHOMETRIC EVIDENCE

Direct histomorphometric analyses of bone biopsies in transplant patients are scant, and those that are available probably reflect early changes associated with glucocorticoid use, at which stage PTH does not have an important role. The histomorphometric changes of GIO, and, by extrapolation, those in early transplant, are not consistent with the histomorphometric changes associated with chronic excess PTH. In pure GIO, there is a decrease in wall thickness of trabecular packets, in trabecular thickness, and in cancellous bone volume (see Figure 3) [17, 103]. One histomorphometric study in renal transplant patients, performed when glucocorticoid doses were high, showed changes which are similar to those of GIO, namely a decrease in osteoid surface [104]. Histomorphometric analysis of 6 cardiac transplant survivors who were transplanted within the previous 10 years

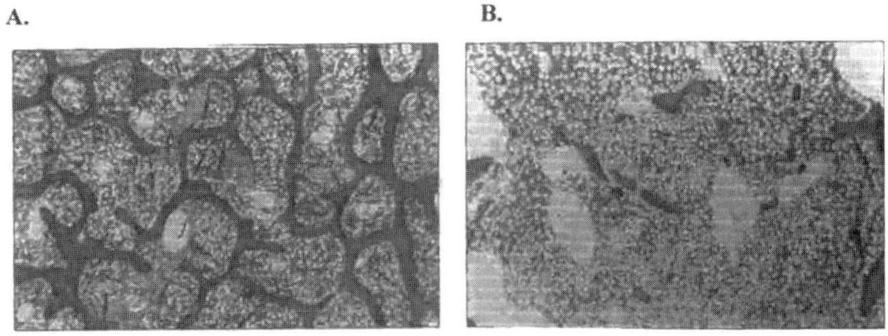

FIGURE 3 **A:** Normal trabecular bone from a 30-year-old patient. Note the thick, serpiginous trabecular plates with excellent connectivity. Arrows indicate areas of osteoid, consistent with bone formation. **B:** Severe osteoporosis in a 30-year-old patient receiving long-term glucocorticoid therapy. Multiple isolated bone islands are present, and little evidence of bone formation is noted. Histomorphometrically, dynamic measures of bone formation are profoundly reduced, indicating that remodeling has been uncoupled. Reproduced with permission from Fitzpatrick et al. [113].

showed an absence of hyperparathyroid bone disease, although the results were quite varied between patients [3]. In primary hyperparathyroidism, the predominant picture is different, namely cortical thinning [105] with maintenance of cancellous bone volume (see Figure 4)

Furthermore, trabecular connectivity is relatively well maintained in primary hyperparathyroidism [106], whereas in GIO and likely in early transplant bone loss, trabecular microarchitecture is typically disrupted with a reduction in connectivity [17, 103, 107]. Dynamic histomorphometric indices provide further contrasts between PTH and GIO-associated bone loss. The early phase of glucocorticoid use is associated with increased osteoclast activity and is similar in this respect to the accelerated bone resorption of primary hyperparathyroidism. Chronic glucocorticoid use decreases the bone formation rate and shortens the lifespan of the active osteoblastic population [17]. The mineralization rate and adjusted apposition rate fall, consistent with a decrease in bone turnover [108]. Osteoid seam thickness is normal or reduced [17, 18].

Similarly, in renal transplant patients, a decrease in osteoid and osteoblast surfaces, adjusted bone formation rate, and prolonged mineralization lag time was found [104]. Although bone disease in kidney transplant patients can be complicated by other factors such as osteomalacia and adynamic bone disease, impaired osteoblastogenesis and early osteoblast apoptosis were seen in this study [104]. Evidence for osteoblast apoptosis in the proximity of osteoid seams or in the medullary space was observed in the majority of the patients [104]. PTH, in contrast, increases bone formation by enhancing the number and activity of osteoblasts [109, 110]. Mineralization rate and adjusted apposition rate rise in primary hyperparathyroidism, along with a widening of the osteoid seams [110]. A summary of these comparisons is presented in Table 2. It is important to realize, however, that the histomorphometric effects of PTH,

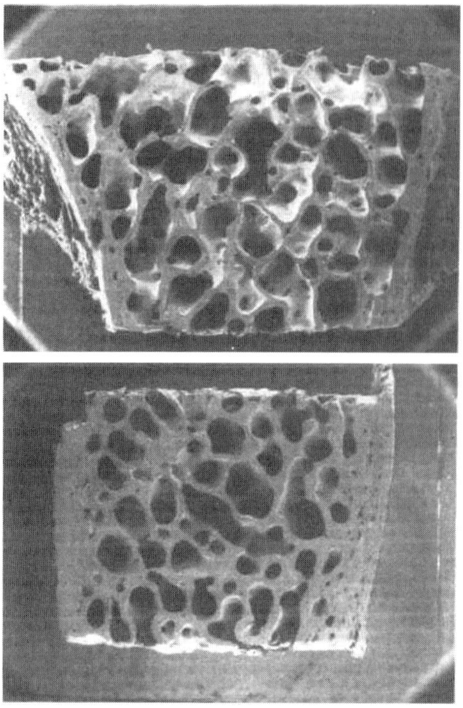

FIGURE 4 Scanning electron micrographs of iliac crest biopsies of a patient with primary hyperparathyroidism (top) and an age- and sex-matched control subject (bottom). Note the thinning of cortices in the patient with primary hyperparathyroidism as well as the maintenance of cancellous bone and trabecular connectivity. Reprinted with permission from Parisien et al. [105].

glucocorticoids, and calcineurin inhibitors could, when considered together, be different from their individual effects.

VII. BONE FORMATION RECOVERY: IS THERE A ROLE FOR PTH?

Bone formation recovers as glucocorticoid doses are lowered after transplantation. It could be speculated that PTH might actually be protective, rather than detrimental, after transplantation. This observation is consistent with the recoupling that occurs in the second phase of bone loss after transplantation, albeit at a higher rate of bone turnover. One could infer that the elevated PTH allows bone formation rates to recover, and thus serves a restorative function, allowing bone mass to stabilize. Further support for a protective effect of PTH after transplant can be found in a study of 47 men followed for 1 year after cardiac transplant, in whom intact PTH levels

TABLE 2 Comparison of Histomorphometric Parameters in Glucocorticoid-Induced Osteoporosis and Primary Hyperparathyroidism

Parameter	GIO (chronic, steady state changes)	Primary hyperparathyroidism
Osteoblast activity	Decreased	Increased
Osteoclast activity	Decreased	Increased
Bone formation rate	Decreased	Increased
Mineralization rate	Decreased	Increased
Adjusted apposition rate	Decreased	Increased
Osteoid seams	No change or decreased	Widened
Trabecular connectivity	Decreased	Maintained or increased
Cancellous bone volume	Decreased	Maintained or increased

tended to be higher in men who did not experience fracture (37 ± 15 versus 69 ± 46 pg/mL; $P < 0.06$) [85]. Support for this hypothesis can be found in the improvement in lumbar spine density that occurs with time, although it is accompanied by decreases at the radial site [5].

On a cellular level, there is some evidence to suggest that elevated PTH in the post-transplant setting might have a beneficial effect on osteoblasts. In a histomorphometric study of 20 patients who had undergone renal transplant [104], impaired osteoblastogenesis and early osteoblast apoptosis were found. Importantly, the osteoblast surface correlated positively with pre- and post-transplant PTH levels, suggesting that PTH might have a protective effect by preserving osteoblast survival. Moreover, post-transplant apoptosis was rare in patients with pre-transplant secondary hyperparathyroidism. If PTH was indeed preserving osteoblasts, this would be consistent with the known effects of intermittent PTH treatment to increase bone formation by preventing osteoblast apoptosis [111].

VIII. CONCLUSION

The weight of the dynamic, densitometric, and histomorphometric evidence reviewed in this chapter indicates that PTH does not play an important role in organ transplant–associated bone loss, particularly in the early phase. The predominant mechanism for the early, rapid bone loss is most likely to be the effects of glucocorticoids. In the later period after transplantation, there is evidence to suggest that elevated PTH levels, likely caused by calcineurin inhibitor-associated renal insufficiency, may play a contributory role to ongoing bone loss, although clear histomorphometric evidence is lacking, and other evidence has provided conflicting results. Whether intermittent PTH therapy might have a beneficial effect in transplantation osteoporosis, as it does in GIO [112], remains to be seen.

REFERENCES

1. Cohen, A. and E. Shane. (2003). Osteoporosis after solid organ and bone marrow transplantation. *Osteoporos Int.* 14(8):617–630.
2. Guo, C.Y., A. Johnson, T.J. Locke, and R. Eastell. (1998). Mechanisms of bone loss after cardiac transplantation. *Bone.* 22(3):267–271.
3. Glendenning, P., G.N. Kent, B.D. Adler, L. Matz, I. Watson, G.J. O'Driscoll, and D.M. Hurley. (1999). High prevalence of osteoporosis in cardiac transplant recipients and discordance between biochemical turnover markers and bone histomorphometry. *Clin Endocrinol (Oxf).* 50(3):347–355.
4. Thiebaud, D., M.A. Krieg, D. Gillard-Berguer, A.F. Jacquet, J.J. Goy, and P. Burckhardt. (1996). Cyclosporine induces high bone turnover and may contribute to bone loss after heart transplantation. *Eur J Clin Invest.* 26(7):549–555.
5. Shane, E., M. Rivas, D.J. McMahon, R.B. Staron, S.J. Silverberg, M.J. Seibel, D. Mancini, R.E. Michler, K. Aaronson, V. Addesso, and S.H. Lo. (1997). Bone loss and turnover after cardiac transplantation. *J Clin Endocrinol Metab.* 82(5):1497–1506.
6. Epstein, S. (1995). Post-transplantation bone disease: the role of immunosuppressive agents and the skeleton. *J Bone Miner Res.* 11(1):1–7.
7. Abdelhadi, M., S.A. Eriksson, S. Ljusk Eriksson, B.G. Ericzon, and J. Nordenstrom. (1995). Bone mineral status in end-stage liver disease and the effect of liver transplantation. *Scand J Gastroenterol.* 30(12):1210–1215.
8. Shane, E., M.C. Rivas, S.J. Silverberg, T.S. Kim, R.B. Staron, and J.P. Bilezikian. (1993). Osteoporosis after cardiac transplantation. *Am J Med.* 94(3):257–264.
9. Rodino, M.A. and E. Shane. (1998). Osteoporosis after organ transplantation. *Am J Med.* 104(5):459–469.
10. Weinstein, R.S., R.L. Jilka, A.M. Parfitt, and S.C. Manolagas. (1998). Inhibition of osteoblastogenesis and promotion of apoptosis of osteoblasts and osteocytes by glucocorticoids. Potential mechanisms of their deleterious effects on bone. *J Clin Invest.* 102(2):274–282.
11. Canalis, E. and A. Giustina. (2001). Glucocorticoid-induced osteoporosis: summary of a workshop. *J Clin Endocrinol Metab.* 86(12):5681–5685.
12. Plotkin, L.I., R.S. Weinstein, A.M. Parfitt, P.K. Roberson, S.C. Manolagas, and T. Bellido. (1999). Prevention of osteocyte and osteoblast apoptosis by bisphosphonates and calcitonin. *J Clin Invest.* 104(10):1363–1374.
13. O'Brien, C.A., D. Jia, L.I. Plotkin, T. Bellido, C.C. Powers, S.A. Stewart, S.C. Manolagas, and R.S. Weinstein. (2004). Glucocorticoids act directly on osteoblasts and osteocytes to induce their apoptosis and reduce bone formation and strength. *Endocrinology.* 145(4):1835–1841.
14. Weinstein, R.S., J.R. Chen, C.C. Powers, S.A. Stewart, R.D. Landes, T. Bellido, R.L. Jilka, A.M. Parfitt, and S.C. Manolagas. (2002). Promotion of osteoclast survival and antagonism of bisphosphonate-induced osteoclast apoptosis by glucocorticoids. *J Clin Invest.* 109(8):1041–1048.
15. Canalis, E. (1996). Clinical review 83: Mechanisms of glucocorticoid action in bone: implications to glucocorticoid-induced osteoporosis. *J Clin Endocrinol Metab.* 81(10):3441–3447.
16. Canalis, E. and A.M. Delany. (2002). Mechanisms of glucocorticoid action in bone. *Ann NY Acad Sci.* 966:73–81.
17. Dempster, D.W., M.A. Arlot, and P.J. Meunier. (1983). Mean wall thickness and formation periods of trabecular bone packets in corticosteroid-induced osteoporosis. *Calcif Tissue Int.* 35(4-5):410–417.
18. Dempster, D.W. (1989). Bone histomorphometry in glucocorticoid-induced osteoporosis. *J Bone Miner Res.* 4(2):137–141.
19. Lane, N.E. and B. Lukert. (1998). The science and therapy of glucocorticoid-induced bone loss. *Endocrinol Metab Clin North Am.* 27(2):465–483.

20. Lukert, B.P. and L.G. Raisz. (1990). Glucocorticoid-induced osteoporosis: pathogenesis and management. *Ann Intern Med*. 112(5):352–364.
21. Lukert, B.P. and L.G. Raisz. (1994). Glucocorticoid-induced osteoporosis. *Rheum Dis Clin North Am*. 20(3):629–650.
22. Feldman, D. and A.V. Krishnan. Glucocorticoid effects on calcium metabolism and bone in the development of osteopenia, in Osteoporosis, C. Christiansen, J.S. Johansen, and B.J. Riis, eds., p. 1106, 1987. Copenhagen: Osteopress.
23. Rickers, H., A. Deding, C. Christiansen, P. Rodbro, and J. Naestoft. (1982). Corticosteroid-induced osteopenia and vitamin D metabolism. Effect of vitamin D2, calcium phosphate and sodium fluoride administration. *Clin Endocrinol (Oxf)*. 16(4): 409–415.
24. Kimberg, D.V., R.D. Baerg, E. Gershon, and R.T. Graudusius. (1971). Effect of cortisone treatment on the active transport of calcium by the small intestine. *J Clin Invest*. 50(6):1309–1321.
25. Lund, B., T.L. Storm, F. Melsen, L. Mosekilde, R.B. Andersen, C. Egmose, and O.H. Sorensen. (1983). Bone mineral loss, bone histomorphometry and vitamin D metabolism in patients with rheumatoid arthritis on long-term glucocorticoid treatment. *Clin Rheumatol*. 4(2):143–149.
26. Suzuki, Y., Y. Ichikawa, E. Saito, and M. Homma. (1983). Importance of increased urinary calcium excretion in the development of secondary hyperparathyroidism of patients under glucocorticoid therapy. *Metabolism*. 32(2):151–156.
27. Hahn, T.J., L.R. Halstead, S.L. Teitelbaum, and B.H. Hahn. (1979). Altered mineral metabolism in glucocorticoid-induced osteopenia. Effect of 25-hydroxyvitamin D administration. *J Clin Invest*. 64(2):655–665.
28. Gennari, C., B. Imbimbo, M. Montagnani, M. Bernini, P. Nardi, and L.V. Avioli. (1984). Effects of prednisone and deflazacort on mineral metabolism and parathyroid hormone activity in humans. *Calcif Tissue Int*. 36(3):245–252.
29. Lukert, B.P. and J.S. Adams. (1976). Calcium and phosphorus homeostasis in man. Effect of corticosteroids. *Arch Intern Med*. 136(11):1249–1253.
30. Guo, C.Y., H. Weiler, and S.A. Atkinson. (2001). Elevated intact parathyroid hormone is associated with reduced biochemical markers of bone formation and resorption measured in blood in infant piglets receiving oral dexamethasone for 15 days. *Biol Neonate*. 80(4):295–299.
31. Fucik, R.F., S.C. Kukreja, G.K. Hargis, E.N. Bowser, W.J. Henderson, and G.A. Williams. (1975). Effect of glucocorticoids on function of the parathyroid glands in man. *J Clin Endocrinol Metab*. 40(1):152–155.
32. Au, W. (1976). Cortisol stimulation of parathyroid hormone secretion by rat parathyroid glands in organ culture. *Science* (193):1015–1017.
33. Sugimoto, T., A.J. Brown, C. Ritter, J. Morrissey, E. Slatopolsky, and K.J. Martin. (1989). Combined effects of dexamethasone and 1,25-dihydroxyvitamin D3 on parathyroid hormone secretion in cultured bovine parathyroid cells. *Endocrinology*. 125(2):638–641.
34. Peraldi, M.N., E. Rondeau, V. Jousset, A. el M'Selmi, R. Lacave, F. Delarue, J.M. Garel, and J.D. Sraer. (1990). Dexamethasone increases preproparathyroid hormone messenger RNA in human hyperplastic parathyroid cells in vitro. *Eur J Clin Invest*. 20(4):392–397.
35. Van Staa, T.P., R. Eastell, I.P. Barton, R. Rizzoli, M.K. Javaid, and C. Cooper. (2003). The value of bone turnover markers in the prediction of vertebral fracture in patients using oral glucocorticoids. *J Bone Miner Res*. 18(suppl 2):F097.
36. Titus, L., E. Jackson, M.S. Nanes, J.E. Rubin, and B.D. Catherwood. (1991). 1,25-dihydroxyvitamin D reduces parathyroid hormone receptor number in ROS 17/2.8 cells and prevents the glucocorticoid-induced increase in these receptors: relationship to adenylate cyclase activation. *J Bone Miner Res*. 6(6):631–637.
37. Ziegler, R. and C. Kasperk. (1998). Glucocorticoid-induced osteoporosis: prevention and treatment. *Steroids*. 63(5-6):344–348.

38. Urena, P., A. Iida-Klein, X.F. Kong, H. Juppner, H.M. Kronenberg, A.B. Abou-Samra, and G.V. Segre. (1994). Regulation of parathyroid hormone (PTH)/PTH-related peptide receptor messenger ribonucleic acid by glucocorticoids and PTH in ROS 17/2.8 and OK cells. *Endocrinology*. 134(1):451–456.
39. Yamamoto, I., J.T. Potts, Jr., and G.V. Segre. (1988). Glucocorticoids increase parathyroid hormone receptors in rat osteoblastic osteosarcoma cells (ROS 17/2). *J Bone Miner Res*. 3(6):707–712.
40. Rodan, S.B., M.K. Fischer, J.J. Egan, P.M. Epstein, and G.A. Rodan. (1984). The effect of dexamethasone on parathyroid hormone stimulation of adenylate cyclase in ROS 17/2.8 cells. *Endocrinology*. 115(3):951–958.
41. Wong, G.L. (1979). Basal activities and hormone responsiveness of osteoclast-like and osteoblast-like bone cells are regulated by glucocorticoids. *J Biol Chem*. 254(14): 6337–6340.
42. Kaji, H., T. Sugimoto, M. Kanatani, K. Nishiyama, and K. Chihara. (1997). Dexamethasone stimulates osteoclast-like cell formation by directly acting on hemopoietic blast cells and enhances osteoclast-like cell formation stimulated by parathyroid hormone and prostaglandin E2. *J Bone Miner Res*. 12(5):734–741.
43. Conaway, H.H., D. Grigorie, and U.H. Lerner. (1997). Differential effects of glucocorticoids on bone resorption in neonatal mouse calvariae stimulated by peptide and steroid-like hormones. *J Endocrinol*. 155(3):513–521.
44. Cosman, F., J. Nieves, J. Herbert, V. Shen, and R. Lindsay. (1994). High-dose glucocorticoids in multiple sclerosis patients exert direct effects on the kidney and skeleton. *J Bone Miner Res*. 9(7):1097–1105.
45. Lane, N.E., S. Goldring, J. Stewart, and S. Morris. (2003). Biochemical markers of bone turnover in glucocorticoid-treated patients are altered by calcium supplementation: preliminary results from ACTIVATE trial. *J Bone Miner Res*. 18(suppl 2):SA324.
46. Gram, J., P. Junker, H.K. Nielsen, and J. Bollerslev. (1998). Effects of short-term treatment with prednisolone and calcitriol on bone and mineral metabolism in normal men. *Bone*. 23(3):297–302.
47. Hahn, T.J., L.R. Halstead, and D.T. Baran. (1981). Effects off short term glucocorticoid administration on intestinal calcium absorption and circulating vitamin D metabolite concentrations in man. *J Clin Endocrinol Metab*. 52(1):111–115.
48. Slovik, D.M., R.M. Neer, J.L. Ohman, F.C. Lowell, M.B. Clark, G.V. Segre, and J.T. Potts, Jr. (1980). Parathyroid hormone and 25-hydroxyvitamin D levels in glucocorticoid-treated patients. *Clin Endocrinol (Oxf)*. 12(3):243–248.
49. Seeman, E., R. Kumar, G.G. Hunder, M. Scott, H. Heath, 3rd, and B.L. Riggs. (1980). Production, degradation, and circulating levels of 1,25-dihydroxyvitamin D in health and in chronic glucocorticoid excess. *J Clin Invest*. 66(4):664–669.
50. Leboff, M.S., J.P. Wade, S. Mackowiak, G. el-Hajj Fuleihan, M. Zangari, and M.H. Liang. (1991). Low dose prednisone does not affect calcium homeostasis or bone density in postmenopausal women with rheumatoid arthritis. *J Rheumatol*. 18(3):339–344.
51. Paz-Pacheco, E., G.E. Fuleihan, and M.S. LeBoff. (1995). Intact parathyroid hormone levels are not elevated in glucocorticoid-treated subjects. *J Bone Miner Res*. 10(11):1713–1718.
52. Hattersley, A.T., K. Meeran, J. Burrin, P. Hill, R. Shiner, and H.K. Ibbertson. (1994). The effect of long- and short-term corticosteroids on plasma calcitonin and parathyroid hormone levels. *Calcif Tissue Int*. 54(3):198–202.
53. Dovio, A., L. Perazzolo, G. Osella, M. Ventura, A. Termine, E. Milano, and A. Bertolotto. (2003). and A. Angeli. Immediate fall of serum osteocalcin and transient increase of bone resorption markers in the course of high-dose, short-term glucocorticoid therapy in young patients with multiple sclerosis, in 3rd International Congress on Glucocorticoid-Induced Osteoporosis. Turin, Italy.
54. Nielsen, H.K., K. Thomsen, E.F. Eriksen, P. Charles, T. Storm, and L. Mosekilde. (1988). The effects of high-dose glucocorticoid administration on serum bone gamma

carboxyglutamic acid-containing protein, serum alkaline phosphatase and vitamin D metabolites in normal subjects. *Bone Miner.* 4(1):105–113.

55. Pearce, G., D.A. Tabensky, P.D. Delmas, H.W. Baker, and E. Seeman. (1998). Corticosteroid-induced bone loss in men. *J Clin Endocrinol Metab.* 83(3):801–806.
56. Manelli, F., S. Bossoni, G. Bugari, R. Carpinteri, D. Godi, E. Agabiti Rosei, J.D. Veldhuis, and A. Giustina. (2001). Chronic glucocorticoid treatment alters the spontaneous pulsatile parathyroid hormone (PTH) secretory pattern in humans (abstract). 83rd Annual Meeting of the Endocrine Society:OR 42-46.
57. Rich, G.M., G.H. Mudge, G.L. Laffel, and M.S. LeBoff. (1992). Cyclosporine A and prednisone-associated osteoporosis in heart transplant recipients. *J Heart Lung Transplant.* 11(5):950–958.
58. Wilmink, J.M., J. Bras, S. Surachno, J.L. van Heyst, and J.M. van der Horst. (1989). Bone repair in cyclosporin treated renal transplant patients. *Transplant Proc.* 21(1 Pt 2): 1492–1494.
59. Movsowitz, C., S. Epstein, F. Ismail, M. Fallon, and S. Thomas. (1989). Cyclosporin A in the oophorectomized rat: unexpected severe bone resorption. *J Bone Miner Res.* 4(3):393–398.
60. Epstein, S., I.R. Dissanayake, G.R. Goodman, A.R. Bowman, H. Zhou, Y. Ma, and W.S. Jee. (2001). Effect of the interaction of parathyroid hormone and cyclosporine a on bone mineral metabolism in the rat. *Calcif Tissue Int.* 68(4):240–247.
61. Sambrook, P.N., P.J. Kelly, D. Fontana, T. Nguyen, A. Keogh, P. Macdonald, P. Spratt, J. Freund, and J.A. Eisman. (1994). Mechanisms of rapid bone loss following cardiac transplantation. *Osteoporos Int.* 4(5):273–276.
62. Valimaki, M.J., K. Kinnunen, R. Tahtela, E. Loyttyniemi, K. Laitinen, P. Makela, P. Keto, and M. Nieminen. (1999). A prospective study of bone loss and turnover after cardiac transplantation: effect of calcium supplementation with or without calcitonin. *Osteoporos Int.* 10(2):128–136.
63. Lems, W.F., M.I. Gerrits, J.W. Jacobs, R.M. van Vugt, H.J. van Rijn, and J.W. Bijlsma. (1996). Changes in (markers of) bone metabolism during high dose corticosteroid pulse treatment in patients with rheumatoid arthritis. *Ann Rheum Dis.* 55(5):288–293.
64. Stein, B., B.P. Halloran, T. Reinhardt, G.W. Engstrom, C.W. Bales, M.K. Drezner, K.L. Currie, M. Takizawa, J.S. Adams, and S. Epstein. (1991). Cyclosporin-A increases synthesis of 1,25-dihydroxyvitamin D3 in the rat and mouse. *Endocrinology.* 128(3):1369–1673.
65. Cvetkovic, M., G.N. Mann, D.F. Romero, X.G. Liang, Y. Ma, W.S. Jee, and S. Epstein. (1994). The deleterious effects of long-term cyclosporine A, cyclosporine G, and FK506 on bone mineral metabolism in vivo. *Transplantation.* 57(8):1231–1237.
66. Aringer, M., H.P. Kiener, M.D. Koeller, O. Artemiou, A. Zuckermann, G. Wieselthaler, W. Klepetko, G. Seidl, F. Kainberger, P. Bernecker, J.S. Smolen, and P. Pietschmann. (1998). High turnover bone disease following lung transplantation. *Bone.* 23(5):485–488.
67. Monegal, A., M. Navasa, N. Guanabens, P. Peris, F. Pons, M.J. Martinez de Osaba, J. Ordi, A. Rimola, J. Rodes, and J. Munoz-Gomez. (2001). Bone disease after liver transplantation: a long-term prospective study of bone mass changes, hormonal status and histomorphometric characteristics. *Osteoporos Int.* 12(6):484–492.
68. Cayco, A.V., J. Wysolmerski, C. Simpson, M.A. Mitnick, C. Gundberg, A. Kliger, M. Lorber, D. Silver, G. Basadonna, A. Friedman, K. Insogna, D. Cruz, and M. Bia. (2000). Posttransplant bone disease: evidence for a high bone resorption state. *Transplantation.* 70(12):1722–1728.
69. Shane, E., D. Mancini, K. Aaronson, S.J. Silverberg, M.J. Seibel, V. Addesso, and D.J. McMahon. (1997). Bone mass, vitamin D deficiency, and hyperparathyroidism in congestive heart failure. *Am J Med.* 103(3):197–207.
70. Boncimino, K., D.J. McMahon, V. Addesso, J.P. Bilezikian, and E. Shane. (1999). Magnesium deficiency and bone loss after cardiac transplantation. *J Bone Miner Res.* 14(2):295–303.

71. Cohen, A., L.J. Addonizio, J.M. Lamour, V. Addesso, R.B. Staron, P. Gao, and E. Shane. (2004). Osteoporosis in adult survivors of adolescent cardiac transplantation may be related to hyperparathyroidism, mild renal insufficiency and increased bone turnover. *J Heart Lung Transplant.* (In press.)
72. Shane, E., V. Addesso, P.B. Namerow, D.J. McMahon, S.H. Lo, R.B. Staron, M. Zucker, S. Pardi, S. Maybaum, and D. Mancini. (2004). Alendronate versus calcitriol for the prevention of bone loss after cardiac transplantation. *N Engl J Med.* 350(8):767–776.
73. Cruz, D.N., H.M. Brickel, J.J. Wysolmerski, C.G. Gundberg, C.A. Simpson, A.S. Kliger, M.I. Lorber, G.P. Basadonna, A.L. Friedman, K.L. Insogna, and M.J. Bia. (2002). Treatment of osteoporosis and osteopenia in long-term renal transplant patients with alendronate. *Am J Transplant.* 2(1):62–67.
74. Floreani, A., A. Mega, L. Tizian, P. Burra, P. Boccagni, V. Baldo, S. Fagiuoli, R. Naccarato, and G. Luisetto. (2001). Bone metabolism and gonad function in male patients undergoing liver transplantation: a two-year longitudinal study. *Osteoporos Int.* 12(9):749–754.
75. Monegal, A., M. Navasa, N. Guanabens, P. Peris, F. Pons, M.J. Martinez de Osaba, A. Rimola, J. Rodes, and J. Munoz-Gomez. (2001). Bone mass and mineral metabolism in liver transplant patients treated with FK506 or cyclosporine A. *Calcif Tissue Int.* 68(2):83–86.
76. Compston, J.E., S. Greer, S.J. Skingle, D.M. Stirling, C. Price, P.J. Friend, and G. Alexander. (1996). Early increase in plasma parathyroid hormone levels following liver transplantation. *J Hepatol.* 25(5):715–718.
77. Segal, E., Y. Baruch, R. Kramsky, B. Raz, A. Tamir, and S. Ish-Shalom. (2003). Predominant factors associated with bone loss in liver transplant patients—after prolonged post-transplantation period. *Clin Transplant.* 17(1):13–19.
78. Lee, A.H., R.L. Mull, G.F. Keenan, P.E. Callegari, M.K. Dalinka, H.J. Eisen, D.M. Mancini, V.J. DiSesa, and M.F. Attie. (1994). Osteoporosis and bone morbidity in cardiac transplant recipients. *Am J Med.* 96(1):35–41.
79. Van Cleemput, J., W. Daenen, P. Geusens, P. Dequeker, F. Van De Werf, and J. VanHaecke. (1996). Prevention of bone loss in cardiac transplant recipients. A comparison of biphosphonates and vitamin D. *Transplantation.* 61(10):1495–1499.
80. Meys, E., F. Terreaux-Duvert, T. Beaume-Six, G. Dureau, and P.J. Meunier. (1993). Bone loss after cardiac transplantation: effects of calcium, calcidiol and monofluorophosphate. *Osteoporos Int.* 3(6):322–329.
81. Cueto-Manzano, A.M., S. Konel, A.J. Freemont, J.E. Adams, B. Mawer, R. Gokal, and A.J. Hutchison. (2000). Effect of 1,25-dihydroxyvitamin D3 and calcium carbonate on bone loss associated with long-term renal transplantation. *Am J Kidney Dis.* 35(2):227–236.
82. Valero, M.A., C. Loinaz, L. Larrodera, M. Leon, E. Moreno, and F. Hawkins. (1995). Calcitonin and bisphosphonates treatment in bone loss after liver transplantation. *Calcif Tissue Int.* 57(1):15–19.
83. Hawkins, F.G., M. Leon, M.B. Lopez, M.A. Valero, L. Larrodera, I. Garcia-Garcia, C. Loinaz, and E. Moreno Gonzalez. (1994). Bone loss and turnover in patients with liver transplantation. *Hepatogastroenterology.* 41(2):158–161.
84. Gandhi, M.K., S. Lekamwasam, I. Inman, S. Kaptoge, L. Sizer, S. Love, P.W. Bearcroft, T.P. Milligan, C.P. Price, R.E. Marcus, and J.E. Compston. (2003). Significant and persistent loss of bone mineral density in the femoral neck after haematopoietic stem cell transplantation: long-term follow-up of a prospective study. *Br J Haematol.* 121(3):462–468.
85. Shane, E., M. Rivas, R.B. Staron, S.J. Silverberg, M.J. Seibel, J. Kuiper, D. Mancini, V. Addesso, R.E. Michler, and P. Factor-Litvak. (1996). Fracture after cardiac transplantation: a prospective longitudinal study. *J Clin Endocrinol Metab.* 81(5):1740–1746.
86. Leidig-Bruckner, G., S. Hosch, P. Dodidou, D. Ritschel, C. Conradt, C. Klose, G. Otto, R. Lange, L. Theilmann, R. Zimmerman, M. Pritsch, and R. Ziegler. (2001). Frequency and predictors of osteoporotic fractures after cardiac or liver transplantation: a follow-up study. *Lancet.* 357(9253):342–347.

87. Eastell, R., E.R. Dickson, S.F. Hodgson, R.H. Wiesner, M.K. Porayko, H.W. Wahner, S.L. Cedel, B.L. Riggs, and R.A. Krom. (1991). Rates of vertebral bone loss before and after liver transplantation in women with primary biliary cirrhosis. *Hepatology*. 14(2):296–300.
88. Haagsma, E.B., C.J. Thijn, J.G. Post, M.J. Slooff, and C.H. Gips. (1988). Bone disease after orthotopic liver transplantation. *J Hepatol*. 6(1):94–100.
89. Schlosberg, M., C. Movsowitz, S. Epstein, F. Ismail, M.D. Fallon, and S. Thomas. (1989). The effect of cyclosporin A administration and its withdrawal on bone mineral metabolism in the rat. *Endocrinology*. 124(5):2179–84.
90. Movsowitz, C., S. Epstein, M. Fallon, F. Ismail, and S. Thomas. (1988). Cyclosporin-A in vivo produces severe osteopenia in the rat: effect of dose and duration of administration. *Endocrinology*. 123(5):2571–2577.
91. Sambrook, P., J. Birmingham, S. Kempler, P. Kelly, S. Eberl, N. Pocock, M. Yeates, and J. Eisman. (1990). Corticosteroid effects on proximal femur bone loss. *J Bone Miner Res*. 5(12):1211–1216.
92. Laan, R.F., W.C. Buijs, L.J. van Erning, J.A. Lemmens, F.H. Corstens, S.H. Ruijs, L.B. van de Putte, and P.L. van Riel. (1993). Differential effects of glucocorticoids on cortical appendicular and cortical vertebral bone mineral content. *Calcif Tissue Int*. 52(1):5–9.
93. Reid, I.R. and S.W. Heap. (1990). Determinants of vertebral mineral density in patients receiving long-term glucocorticoid therapy. *Arch Intern Med*. 150(12):2545–2548.
94. Reid, I.R., M.C. Evans, and J. Stapleton. (1992). Lateral spine densitometry is a more sensitive indicator of glucocorticoid-induced bone loss. *J Bone Miner Res*. 7(10):1221–1225.
95. Lo Cascio, V., E. Bonucci, B. Imbimbo, P. Ballanti, D. Tartarotti, G. Galvanini, L. Fuccella, and S. Adami. (1984). Bone loss after glucocorticoid therapy. *Calcif Tissue Int*. 36(4):435–438.
96. Bilezikian, J.P., S.J. Silverberg, E. Shane, M. Parisien, and D.W. Dempster. (1991). Characterization and evaluation of asymptomatic primary hyperparathyroidism. *J Bone Miner Res*. 6 Suppl 2:S85–S89; discussion S121–S124.
97. Silverberg, S.J., E. Shane, L. de la Cruz, D.W. Dempster, F. Feldman, D. Seldin, T.P. Jacobs, E.S. Siris, M. Cafferty, M.V. Parisien, and et al. (1989). Skeletal disease in primary hyperparathyroidism. *J Bone Miner Res*. 4(3):283–291.
98. Dempster, D.W., F. Cosman, M. Parisien, V. Shen, and R. Lindsay. (1993). Anabolic actions of parathyroid hormone on bone. *Endocr Rev*. 14(6):690–709.
99. Khosla, S., L.J. Melton, 3rd, R.A. Wermers, C.S. Crowson, W. O'Fallon, and B. Riggs. (1999). Primary hyperparathyroidism and the risk of fracture: a population-based study. *J Bone Miner Res*. 14(10):1700–1707.
100. Kenny, A.M., D.C. MacGillivray, C.C. Pilbeam, H.D. Crombie, and L.G. Raisz. (1995). Fracture incidence in postmenopausal women with primary hyperparathyroidism. *Surgery*. 118(1):109–114.
101. Van Staa, T.P., H.G. Leufkens, L. Abenhaim, B. Zhang, and C. Cooper. (2000). Use of oral corticosteroids and risk of fractures. *J Bone Miner Res*. 15(6):993–1000.
102. Ramsey-Goldman, R., J.E. Dunn, D.D. Dunlop, F.P. Stuart, M.M. Abecassis, D.B. Kaufman, C.B. Langman, M.H. Salinger, and S.M. Sprague. (1999). Increased risk of fracture in patients receiving solid organ transplants. *J Bone Miner Res*. 14(3):456–463.
103. Chappard, D., E. Legrand, M.F. Basle, P. Fromont, J.L. Racineux, A. Rebel, and M. Audran. (1996). Altered trabecular architecture induced by corticosteroids: a bone histomorphometric study. *J Bone Miner Res*. 11(5):676–685.
104. Rojas, E., R.G. Carlini, P. Clesca, A. Arminio, O. Suniaga, K. De Elguezabal, J.R. Weisinger, K.A. Hruska, and E. Bellorin-Font. (2003). The pathogenesis of osteodystrophy after renal transplantation as detected by early alterations in bone remodeling. *Kidney Int*. 63(5):1915–1923.

105. Parisien, M., S.J. Silverberg, E. Shane, L. de la Cruz, R. Lindsay, J.P. Bilezikian, and D.W. Dempster. (1990). The histomorphometry of bone in primary hyperparathyroidism: preservation of cancellous bone structure. *J Clin Endocrinol Metab*. 70(4):930–938.
106. Parisien, M., R.W. Mellish, S.J. Silverberg, E. Shane, R. Lindsay, J.P. Bilezikian, and D.W. Dempster. (1992). Maintenance of cancellous bone connectivity in primary hyperparathyroidism: trabecular strut analysis. *J Bone Miner Res*. 7(8):913–919.
107. Dalle Carbonare, L., M.E. Arlot, P.M. Chavassieux, J.P. Roux, N.R. Portero, and P.J. Meunier. (2001). Comparison of trabecular bone microarchitecture and remodeling in glucocorticoid-induced and postmenopausal osteoporosis. *J Bone Miner Res*. 16(1):97–103.
108. Chavassieux, P., P. Pastoureau, M.C. Chapuy, P.D. Delmas, and P.J. Meunier. (1993). Glucocorticoid-induced inhibition of osteoblastic bone formation in ewes: a biochemical and histomorphometric study. *Osteoporos Int*. 3(2):97–102.
109. MacDonald, B.R., J.A. Gallagher, and R.G. Russell. (1986). Parathyroid hormone stimulates the proliferation of cells derived from human bone. *Endocrinology*. 118(6):2445–2449.
110. Dempster, D.W., M. Parisien, S.J. Silverberg, X.G. Liang, M. Schnitzer, V. Shen, E. Shane, D.B. Kimmel, R. Recker, R. Lindsay, and J.P. Bilezikian. (1999). On the mechanism of cancellous bone preservation in postmenopausal women with mild primary hyperparathyroidism. *J Clin Endocrinol Metab*. 84(5):1562–1566.
111. Jilka, R.L., R.S. Weinstein, T. Bellido, P. Roberson, A.M. Parfitt, and S.C. Manolagas. (1999). Increased bone formation by prevention of osteoblast apoptosis with parathyroid hormone. *J Clin Invest*. 104(4):439–446.
112. Lane, N.E., S. Sanchez, G.W. Modin, H.K. Genant, E. Pierini, and C.D. Arnaud. (1998). Parathyroid hormone treatment can reverse corticosteroid-induced osteoporosis. Results of a randomized controlled clinical trial. *J Clin Invest*. 102(8):1627–1633.
113. Fitzpatrick, L., Glucocorticoid-induced osteoporosis, in Atlas of Osteoporosis, 2nd edition, E.S. Orwoll, ed., p. 138, 2003. Philadelphia: Current Medicine.

CHAPTER 10

The Role of Hypogonadism in the Evolution of Bone Loss before and after Cardiac Transplantation

Hans-Ulrich Stempfle, MD, PhD
Department of Cardiology, Medizinische Poliklinik–Innenstadt,
Ludwig–Maximilians–University, Munich, Germany

I. INTRODUCTION

Osteoporosis is a well-known complication after cardiac transplantation, attributed to the side effects of immunosuppressive agents [1, 2]. Hypogonadism may play an important role in the multifactorial pathogenesis of the immunosuppressive-induced bone loss. This chapter will review the skeletal effects of sex-steroid deficiency and its therapy before and after cardiac transplantation.

Hypogonadism is a clinical condition characterized by low serum levels of gonadal hormones in association with specific symptoms, including diminished libido, erectile dysfunction in men, anemia, impaired vitality, and reduced muscle and bone mass. The loss of gonadal function in either sex stimulates the production of osteoblasts and osteoclasts, resulting in an increase in bone turnover with an imbalance between bone formation and resorption. These changes are mediated by up-regulating the production and action of cytokines including interleukin-6 (IL-6) as well as the expression of two subunits of the IL-6 receptor, IL-6Rα and gp130 [3, 4, 5, 6, 7]. The loss of gonadal function furthermore may increase the sensitivity of mechanisms regulating osteoclast function and activity to IL-6 and IL-1[8]. Sex-steroid deficiency also causes osteoblast apoptosis and, in addition, anti-apoptotic effects on osteoclasts, resulting in a shortening of the working lifespan of the osteoblast and an extension of the working lifespan of the osteoclast [9, 10, 11]. The latter is likely to be responsible for the deeper resorption cavities and hence the trabecular perforation seen in states of estrogen deficiency.

II. THE ROLE OF CALCINEURIN-PHOSPHATASE INHIBITORS IN REGULATION OF GONADAL HORMONES

A. Cyclosporine

Cyclosporine A (CsA) is widely used to prevent acute rejection after organ transplantation. Studies within the last two decades have delineated several negative skeletal effects of CsA [12]. The role of CsA on gonadal function is, however, not well understood.

In vitro and animal studies have demonstrated that CsA inhibits testosterone biosynthesis in isolated, interstitial cells from rat Leydig cells [13]. The results indicated that CsA acts in multiple ways that include an inhibition of luteinizing hormone (LH)-stimulated and cAMP-stimulated intracellular cholesterol transport into the Leydig cells and a decrease in testosterone production by testicular inhibition of steroidogenic enzymes. In particular, CsA inhibits the activity of 17α-hydroxylase, a cytochrome P-450-dependent enzyme, in an uncompetitive manner and of 17β-hydroxysteroid dehydrogenase (3ß-HSD), a cytochrome P-450-independent enzyme, in a competitive manner. The activity of 3ß-HSD was also inhibited in prepubertal rats after administration of relatively low doses of CsA (1–2 mg/kg/d), resulting in a decrease in serum testosterone and the number of spermatids and spermatozoa [14]. Furthermore, the motility and the fertilizing abililty of spermatozoa were reduced. Although testicular weight remained unchanged in this study, much higher doses of CsA (20-40 mg/kg/d) caused it to decrease in a previous study performed in adult rats [15].

It is still unclear whether CsA induces hypogonadism as a direct effect on the gonads or via centrally mediated mechanisms that inhibit the hypothalamic–pituitary axis, or by both means. Sikka et al. demonstrated that the CsA-induced decrease in testosterone was mainly mediated through the hypothalamic–pituitary axis by suppressed serum LH levels [16, 17, 18]. The site of CsA action was probably the hypothalamus, since the normal LH stimulatory response to gonadotropin-releasing hormone (GnRH) was normal. Although central nervous system toxicity of CsA is well documented, it is unclear whether CsA crosses the blood–brain barrier [19, 20, 21, 22]. In contrast, Seethalakshmi et al. found a direct inhibitory effect of CsA on testosterone biosynthesis in the rat testis, associated with a significant, dose-dependent elevation of serum LH and follicle-stimulating hormone (FSH) levels [14]. Despite the known nephrotoxicity of CsA, most animal studies have excluded renal insufficiency as a mechanism for both hypo- and hypergonadotrophic hypogonadism. In five of six nephrectomized rats with serum creatinine twice the normal value, testicular function and fertility were relatively maintained [23]. Other ways in which CsA causes testicular dysfunction might be in a reduction of the number of LH receptors and a suppression of the heme formation, thus compromising the hemoprotein-dependent steroidogenic enzyme activities [24].

Different results concerning gonadal hormones were found by Erben et al., who demonstrated a highturnover osteopenia in the axial skeleton of aged male rats after administration of lowdose cyclosporine for 4 weeks, without any changes in serum testosterone levels [25]. The control group also had low testosterone levels, however, indicating that hypogonadism was common in this aged rat population. This may explain why CsA administration did not significantly reduce testosterone. In a similar model, very high doses of oral CsA, with trough levels of CsA between 800 and 1250 ng/ml, lowered serum total and free testosterone in male rats [26]. Testosterone replacement with slow-release pellets increased serum testosterone levels but was unable to prevent CsA-induced bone loss. These results were surprising because androgens inhibit osteoclastogenesis [27] and *in vivo* evidence suggests that testosterone has antiresorptive properties [28, 29]. The authors concluded that hypoandrogenemia is only a minor factor in CsA-induced bone loss and that the antiresorptive potency of testosterone is low. Animal studies have demonstrated that the negative effects of CsA on gonads and the hypothalamic–pituitary axis are reversed after withdrawal of CsA [30].

B. Tacrolimus

The macrolide lactone tacrolimus (FK506) is a newer immunosuppressive drug in organ transplantation that has been demonstrated to be more potent and effective than CsA [31]. After forming a complex with the immunophilin FKBP (FK506-binding protein), the complex acts in a similar fashion to the cyclosporine-immunophilin complex, resulting in inhibition of calmodulin followed by inhibition of interleukin-2 gene transcription and proliferation of cytotoxic T-lymphocytes. In experimental models, tacrolimus leads to significant loss of trabecular bone volume that is even more pronounced than that observed with CsA [32]. There are limited data on the role of tacrolimus on gonadal function. Although tacrolimus acts in a similar way to CsA at a molecular level after binding to the immunophilin FKBP, Tai et al. found both *in vivo* and *in vitro* that short-term tacrolimus treatment caused no adverse effects on the function and morphology of rat Leydig cells or on serum testosterone and LH levels [33]. These results were confirmed in an animal model demonstrating that even long-term tacrolimus treatment does not lower serum free and total testosterone [26]. On the other hand, tacrolimus dose-dependently decreased sperm counts and motility through a direct action on the sperm in the epididymis without change in the testicular production of sperm [34]. So far the reason for the discrepancies between

CsA and tacrolimus with regards to their gonadal effects remains to be established.

III. THE EFFECTS OF GLUCOCORTICOIDS ON GONADAL HORMONES

There are wellknown glucocorticoid-induced effects on the production of sex hormones [35, 36, 37, 38]. Animal studies have shown that dexamethasone decreased the synthesis and release of LH at the pituitary level in female rats [39]. Glucocorticoids also blunt FSH-induced estrogen production in cultured rat granulosa cells [40]. Longterm treatment with glucocorticoids inhibits LH secretion in response to luteinizing hormone–releasing hormone in women and, to a lesser degree, in men [41]. In contrast, McAdams et al. demonstrated a normal LH and FSH secretory response after GnRH was administered, indicating that glucocorticoid therapy suppresses the secretion of GnRH by the hypothalamus [42]. A 24-hour administration of cortisol suppressed plasma testosterone by abolishing or flattening the nocturnal rise without effects on testosterone during the day. In this study LH and FSH showed a significant increase during the second part of the night [35] with normal values during the day. The data indicated that the cortisol-induced suppression of testosterone is not mediated by LH. Furthermore glucocorticoids reduce adrenal production of androstenedione due to suppression of ACTH, which can result in adrenal atrophy [43]. Longterm glucocorticoid excess has been thought to cause increased bone resorption and activation of bone remodeling due to deficiency in gonadal hormones [44]. Recently Weinstein et al. demonstrated that in mice the adverse skeletal effects of glucocorticoids override those of sex-steroid deficiency [45]. The authors found that BMD, vertebral strength, and histomorphometric indices were similar in intact and orchidectomized animals receiving prednisolone, suggesting that the adverse skeletal effects of hypogonadism and glucocorticoid excess are not additive.

The role of reduced secretion of gonadal hormones in the pathogenesis of the deleterious skeletal effects of glucocorticoids has not been fully elucidated. Studies are often based on observations in small groups of patients receiving longterm glucocorticoid treatment for severe diseases [44, 46, 47, 48], which themselves could cause hypogonadism rather than its being a consequence of a glucocorticoid therapy [47]. Evidence for the latter is supported by a recent study showing a 4.6% decrease in spinal BMD in men after 6 months of treatment with 50 mg/d of prednisolone, despite maintenance of a normal testosterone/sex hormone binding globulin ratio [49]. Similarly, Weinstein et al. demonstrated that serum unbound testosterone concentration and seminal vesicle weight in mice were not diminished when prednisolone was administered alone [45].

IV. THE EFFECT OF ANTIPROLIFERATIVE AGENTS ON GONADAL HORMONES

A. Azathioprine and Mycophenolate Mofetil

Azathioprine and mycophenolate mofetil are frequently used in combination with calcineurin-phosphatase inhibitors and glucocorticoids after transplantation. Nieszporek et al. found suppressed serum testosterone levels in combination with a blunted LH response to gonadotropin-releasing hormone after renal transplantation in patients receiving azathioprine in combination with prednisone [50]. Other investigators reported normal testosterone levels in patients receiving glucocorticoids and azathioprine after kidney transplantation [51]. Animal studies do not suggest any significant testicular toxicity as a result of azathioprine or mycophenolate mofetil treatment. Furthermore, short-term studies in rats showed no effect of either azathioprine or mycophenolate mofetil on bone volume when administered as single agents [52, 53].

B. Sirolimus (Rapamycin)

Sirolimus is a highly potent immunosuppressive agent that has recently become available for organ transplantation [54]. It is structurally related to tacrolimus, but its mechanism of immunosuppression differs. Whereas tacrolimus, like CsA, interferes with early events of T-cell activation by blocking calcineurin activity, sirolimus prevents progression from the G1 to the S phase in T cells by blocking downstream IL-2R signaling [55]. Furthermore sirolimus inhibits T-cell responses to cytokines and blocks lymphocytic proliferation at a point further upstream than occurs with the antiproliferative agents discussed above. Hence sirolimus should act synergistically with antiproliferative agents and calcineurin inhibitors. Data on the effect of sirolimus on gonadal hormones are limited. Kaczmarek et al. recently demonstrated decreased serum testosterone levels associated with a significant increase in gonadotrophic hormones in patients receiving sirolimus after heart transplantation [56]. An immunosuppressive regimen that included CsA, prednisone, and sirolimus also caused dramatic reductions in sperm count, percentage of normally shaped sperm heads, and sperm motility in a single young male kidney transplant recipient [57]. Cessation of sirolimus treatment was followed by complete normalization of the sperm parameters. The following mechanism might be responsible for these findings. The development of the male germ cells in the seminiferous tubule consists of spermatogonial proliferation and meiosis. The stem cell factor/c-kit system regulates germ cell proliferation, meiosis, and apoptosis using a rapamycin-sensitive PI3 kinase/AKT/p70S6k/cyclin D3 pathway. Disruption of PI3 kinase-binding to cKit *in vivo* will therefore result in male sterility because of inhibition of the early stages of spermatogenesis [58].

V. CLINICAL FEATURES OF HYPOGONADISM AFTER CARDIAC TRANSPLANTATION

There are limited clinical data concerning the role of single immunosuppressive agents on sex-hormone deficiency and bone loss after organ transplantation. Handelsman et al. evaluated testicular function in male renal transplants who were receiving either CsA alone or a combination of azathioprine and prednisone as immunosuppressive therapy [59]. There were no differences in clinical or hormonal indices of testicular function including serum testosterone, LH, FSH, estradiol, and prolactin. A similar immunosuppressive regimen was used in a comparable study evaluating the role of gonadal hormones on bone metabolism in renal transplant patients [60]. Serum testosterone in men was normal and did not predict bone loss, while serum estradiol in women was an independent predictor of bone status in multivariate analysis. Discrepant results were reported using CsA within a combination immunosuppressive regimen [61, 62, 63]. Low serum testosterone with normal LH and FSH levels was found in a small group of cardiac and renal transplant recipients, indicating hypogonadotropic hypogonadism [64]. A recent study demonstrated low serum testosterone levels in 70% of male patients after renal transplantation, which were negatively influenced by the use of calcineurin-phosphatase inhibitors [61].

After heart transplantation, patients usually receive a combination immunosuppressive therapy, which includes calcineurin-phosphatase inhibitors, glucocorticoids, and antiproliferative drugs. This situation makes it more difficult to address the effect of a single immunosuppressive agent on gonadal hormones. Furthermore, doses of calcineurin-phosphatase inhibitors are usually higher after cardiac transplantation, possibly explaining the increased hormonal and skeletal side effects when compared with renal transplants. Shane et al. detected a significant relationship between low levels of serum testosterone and rates of femoral neck bone loss during the first 6 months after cardiac transplantation [65]. In most studies, testosterone levels return to normal by 6–12 months after transplantation [65, 66]. Hypogonadism is quite common early after cardiac transplantation, occurring in up to 50% of men [67, 68]. The role of low androgen levels in the evolution of bone loss after cardiac transplantation is, however, less clear. Guo et al. [69], who also reported decreased serum testosterone and dehydroepiandrosterone levels in heart transplant recipients, found only a positive correlation to the time after transplantation, without any correlation with BMD or markers of bone and mineral metabolism. In contrast, low serum total testosterone levels and free testosterone index were still seen in

20% of male patients 3 years after heart transplantation in those patients treated with cyclosporine and 2.5–5 mg/day of prednisone [70]. Hypogonadism was associated with a significant decrease in bone mineral density (BMD) [71] (see Figure 1). Furthermore, all hypogonadal patients showed low serum gonadotropins that increased after stimulation with gonadotropin-releasing hormone, indicating hypothalamic hypogonadism.

Tacrolimus, a newer immunosuppressive agent is replacing CsA with increasing frequency in immunosuppressive regimens. Clinical data on the influence of tacrolimus-based immunosuppression on the skeleton and gonadal hormones are limited. A recent prospective, longitudinal study revealed low serum total testosterone and free testosterone index in 30% of male transplant recipients [72]. Hypogonadal patients also showed low gonadotropin levels with a normal increase after stimulation with GnRH, indicating that tacrolimus-based immunosuppression is associated with hypothalamic hypogonadism. In contrast to evidence from animal and *in vitro* studies, CsA and tacrolimus combined with glucocorticoids and antiproliferative agents cause a comparable prevalence of sex-hormone deficiency and similar rates of bone loss in clinical studies [73].

The impairment of renal function associated with calcineurin-phosphatase inhibitors may have some longterm influence on gonadal hormones after heart transplantation. Thus far, however, no correlation between mild renal insufficiency and the prevalence of hypogonadism in the early phase after cardiac transplantation has been documented. The threshold of nephrotoxicity that is necessary to alter androgen metabolism remains unclear.

Aging also effects serum total and free testosterone levels in healthy men. Harman et al. documented a prevalence of hypogonadism, defined by low levels of serum total testosterone, in 12%, 19%, 28%, and 49% in men in their 50s, 60s, 70s, and 80s, respectively [74]. The effect of age should therefore be taken in account when assessing the prevalence of

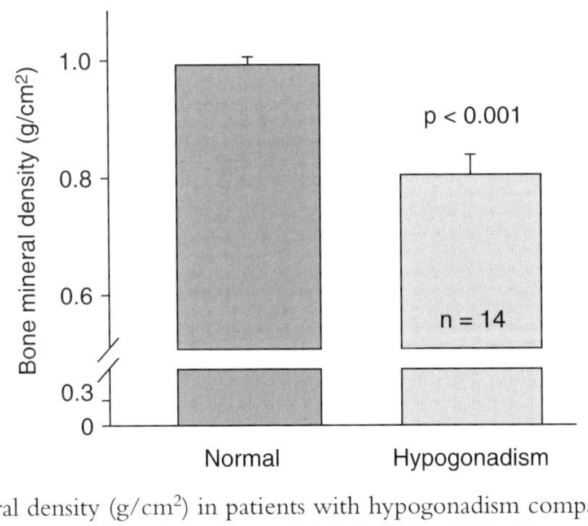

FIGURE 1 Bone mineral density (g/cm^2) in patients with hypogonadism compared to patients with normal testosterone after heart transplantation. (From Stief, J. Sohn, H.Y., Stempfle, H.U. (2004) Role of immunosuppression induced hypogonadism on bone loss after cardiac transplantation. Dtsch Med Wochenschrift. 129:1674–1678.)

immunosuppressive-induced hypogonadism. On the other hand, a recent study showed that low serum total testosterone and a low free testosterone index were also quite common in younger patients (see Figure 2) after heart transplantation, supporting the negative role of immunosuppressive therapy on gonadal hormones [75, 76].

VI. CLINICAL FEATURES OF HYPOGONADISM BEFORE CARDIAC TRANSPLANTATION

Data on gonadal function in congestive heart failure are limited. Two studies in male patients with congestive heart failure (CHF) found that serum dehydroepiandrosterone (DHEA) levels were significantly lower than in healthy controls [77, 78]. Diminished cardiac output and digoxin therapy appear to have opposing effects on testosterone, estradiol, and luteinizing hormone concentrations [79]. Depression of the levels of these hormones was significantly correlated with a decrease in cardiac index while elevation was associated with digoxin therapy of long duration. The effect of cardiac output is most marked on serum testosterone and that of digoxin on serum estradiol. In 5 men with severe left ventricular dysfunction and markedly reduced plasma testosterone, gonadal hormones normalized within 2 months after implantation of a ventricular assist device [80]. In an animal model of heart failure, Syrian hamsters with cardiomyopathy were found to have very low testosterone levels and testicular weights along with depressed reproductive function [81]. Low levels of testosterone are quite common in male patients with congestive heart failure, most likely attributable to chronic illness and increased oxidative stress [78, 82]. Approximately 30% of men evaluated before transplantation have biochemical evidence of hypogonadism [83]. Stief et al. recently investigated the relative

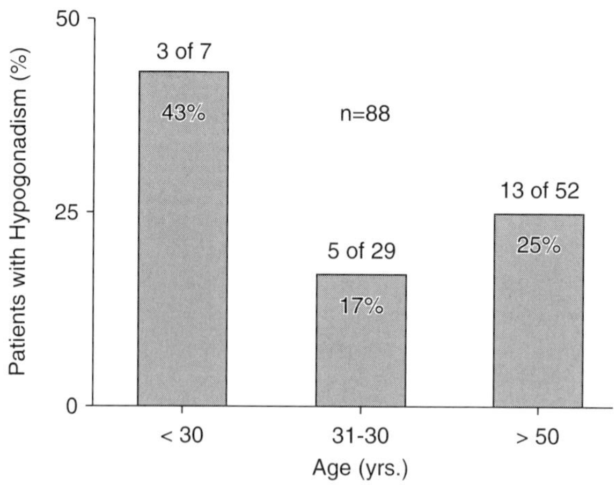

FIGURE 2 Age distribution of hypogonadal patients under a cyclosporine A-based immunosuppressive therapy. (From Stief, J., Sohn, H.Y., Stempfle, H.U. (2004). Role of immunosuppression induced hypogonadism on bone loss after cardiac transplantation. Dtsch Med Wochenschrift. 129:1674–1678.)

roles of previous congestive heart failure and immunosuppressive therapy in post-transplantation hypogonadism [84]. In 20 male patients with previous congestive heart failure, the mean testosterone level decreased significantly after transplantation (433ng/dl versus 314ng/dl; $p = 0.024$) (see Figure 3). Six of the 20 (30%) patients with CHF had low serum testosterone levels, indicating hypogonadotrophic hypogonadism. Six months after heart transplantation, all 6 patients remained hypogonadal. Additionally, 3 more transplant patients (15%) developed hypogonadism within the study period. In a second small study, 80% of heart failure patients showed a decrease in serum testosterone levels after starting tacrolimus-based immunosuppression for cardiac transplantation [85].

The role of sex hormone deficiency on the evolution of bone loss in patients with congestive heart failure is, however, not clear. Other factors such as high-dose glucocorticoid therapy, renal insufficiency, hyperparathyroidism, vitamin D deficiency, immobilization, and a history of exposure to heparin or loop diuretics may also reduce BMD. Furthermore there are no data on the effects of sexhormone replacement therapy on BMD in patients with congestive heart failure. If treatment is required, transdermal testosterone preparations are preferred to injectable administration because of the frequent use of warfarin in these patient groups.

VII. PREVENTION AND MANAGEMENT OF HYPOGONADISM

Studies on the role of testosterone replacement therapy in men are limited, and no studies have been done on hormone replacement in women after

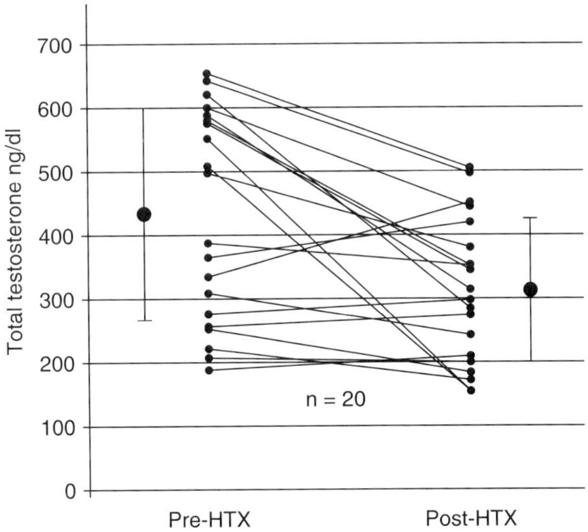

FIGURE 3 Serum total testosterone before (pre) and after (post) heart transplantation (HTx) (normal range 350-900 ng/dl). (From Stief, J., and Stempfle, H-U. (2004). Post-transplantation hypogonadism: A reflection of sex steroids deficiency due to previous congestive heart failure or an immunosuppressive side effect? *J Bone Miner Res.* 19: Suppl 1, abstract)

cardiac transplantation. Most transplantation centers consider hormone replacement therapy in postmenopausal and premenopausal amenorrheic women and truly hypogonadal men who do not have contraindications.

A recent study evaluated the effect of testosterone replacement therapy on bone loss in hypogonadal cardiac transplant patients [75, 76]. Osteoporosis prevention therapy also included calcium and vitamin D. Hypogonadal patients showed no significant additional increase in BMD over a two year study period compared with a control group with normal gonadal function, despite testosterone replacement therapy that resulted in normalization of hormone levels (see Figure 4). Clinical symptoms such as vitality, sexual dysfunction, and mood improved in most patients, however.

Furthermore, evidence suggests that estrogen derived from peripheral aromatization of androgens is critical for the maintenance of bone mass in men as well as in women [86, 87]. Szulc et al. found, in a cross-sectional cohort analysis of men, that low serum levels of bioavailable 17ß-estradiol are associated with high bone turnover and low BMD [88].

Because of the lack of clinical data, the rationale for hormone replacement therapy in female transplant recipients is based on animal studies that show that estrogen prevents CsA-induced bone loss [89] and on clinical studies in which estrogens improved BMD in women treated with glucocorticoids [90].

Several transplantation-related factors must be considered, however, before initiating hormone replacement therapy. First, since estrogen enhances hepatic metabolism of CsA, daily dosing of estrogen and progesterone is preferred over cyclic administration to avoid fluctuating CsA levels after transplantation. Moreover, dose adjustments of CsA may be necessary. Second, animal data suggest that immunoreactivity against transplantation antigens can be influenced by sex steroid hormones.

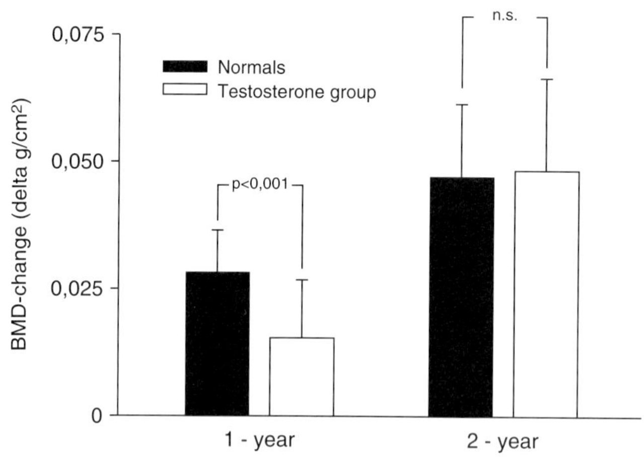

FIGURE 4 Increase of bone mineral density (g/cm^2) after one and two years in normogonadal vs. testosterone substituted patients after heart transplantation. (From Stief, J., Sohn, H.Y., Stempfle, H.U. 2004). Role of immunosuppression induced hypogonadism on bone loss after cardiac transplantation. Dtsch Med Wochenschrift. 129:1674–1678.)

Hirasawa et al. showed that estradiol antagonizes the immunosuppressive activity of CsA [91, 92]. In contrast, testosterone in combination with CsA prolonged graft survival time significantly. Because clinical data are lacking, careful monitoring to detect transplant rejection after estrogen replacement seems appropriate. Third, anecdotal reports suggest that estrogen replacement therapy alone is not sufficient to prevent bone loss during the first year after transplantation in postmenopausal women. Finally, potential risks of testosterone therapy include acceleration of hyperlipidemia in patients already prone to atherosclerosis from immunosuppressive agents, hypertension, and diabetes. Furthermore, the risk of prostatic cancer may be higher in an immunosuppressed patient.

In summary, hypogonadism is frequently found both before and after cardiac transplantation and may play a role in the multifactorial pathogenesis of immunosuppression-induced bone loss. Data on the influence of hormone replacement therapy on the rate of bone loss after organ transplantation are limited and mostly negative. If hormone replacement therapy is given after transplantation, recommendations for monitoring should be strictly followed [93].

REFERENCES

1. Epstein, S. (1996). Post-transplantation bone disease: the role of immunosuppressive agents and the skeleton. *J Bone Miner Res.* 11:1–7.
2. Rodino, M.A., and Shane, E. (1998). Osteoporosis after organ transplantation. *Am J Med.* 104:459–469.
3. Manolagas, S.C. (1998). The role of IL-6 type cytokines and their receptors in bone. *Ann NY Acad Sci.* 840:194–204.
4. Lin, S. C., Yamate, T., Taguchi, Y., Borba, V.Z., Girasole, G., O'Brien, C.A., Bellido, T., Abe, E., Manolagas, S.C. (1997). Regulation of the gp80 and gp130 subunits of the IL-6 receptor by sex steroids in the murine bone marrow. *J Clin Invest.* 100:1980–1990.
5. Bellido, T., Girasole, G., Jilka, R.L., Crabb, D., and Manolagas, S.C. (1993). Demonstration of androgen receptors in bone marrow stromal cells and their role in the regulation of transcription from the human interleukin-6 (IL-6) gene promoter. *J Bone Miner Res.* 8 Suppl 1, S.131 abstract
6. Jilka, R.L., Hangoc, G., Girasole, G., Passeri, G., Williams, D.C., Abrams, J.S., Boyce, B., Broxmeyer, H., and Manolagas, S.C. (1992). Increased osteoclast development after estrogen loss: Mediation by interleukin-6. *Science.* 257:88–91.
7. Passeri, G., Girasole, G., Jilka, R.L., and Manolagas, S.C. (1993). Increased interleukin-6 production by murine bone marrow and bone cells after estrogen withdrawal. *Endocrinology.* 133:822–828.
8. Manolagas, S.C., and Jilka, R.L. (1995). Bone marrow, cytokines and bone remodeling. *N Engl J Med.* 332:305–311.
9. Weinstein, R.S., Jilka, R.L., Parfitt, A.M., and Manolagas, S.C. (1997). The effects of androgen deficiency on murine bone remodelling and bone mineral density are mediated via cells of the osteoblastic lineage. *Endocrinology.* 138:4013–4021.
10. Kousteni S., Chen, J.R., Bellido, T.M., Han, L.L., Ali, A.A., O'Brien C.A., Plotkin, L., Fu, Q., Mancino A.T., Wen, Y., Vertino, A.M., Powers, C., Steward, S.A., Ebert, R.H., Parfitt A.M., Weinstein, R.S., Jilka, R.L., and Manolagas, S.C. (2002). Reversal of bone loss in mice by nongenotrophic signalling of sex steroids. *Science.* 298:843–846.

11. Manolagas, S.C. (2000). Birth and death of bone cells: basic regulatory mechanisms and implications for the pathogenesis and treatment of osteoporosis. *Endocrine Reviews*. 21:115–137.
12. Shane, E., and Epstein, S. (1994). Immunosuppresive therapy and the skeleton. *Trends Endocrinol Metab*. 5:169–175.
13. Seethalakshmi, L., Flores, C., Malhotra, R.K., Pallias, J.D., Tharakan, D., Khauli, R.B., and Menon, M. (1992). The mechanism of cyclosporine's action in the inhibition of testosterone biosynthesis by rat leydig cells in vitro. *Transplantation*. 53:190–195.
14. Seethalakshmi, L., Flores, C., Carboni, A., Bala, R., Diamond, D.A., and Menon, M. (1990). Cyclosporine: Its effects on testicular function and fertility in the prepubertal rat. *J Androl*. 11:17–24.
15. Seethalakshmi, L., Menon, M., Malhotra, R.K., and Diamond, D.A. (1987). Effect of cyclosporine A on male reproduction in rats. *J Urol*. Part 2 138:991–995.
16. Sikka, S.C., Bhasin, S., Coy, D.C., Koyle, M.A., Swerdloff, R.S., and Rajfer, J. (1988). Effects of cyclosporine on the hypothalamic-pituitary-gonadal axis in the male rat: Mechanism of action. *Endocrinology*. 123:1069–1074.
17. Sikka, S.C., Coy, D.C., Lemmi, C.A.E., and Rajfer, J. (1988). Effect of cyclosporine on steroidogenesis in rat leydig cells. *Transplantation*. 46:886–889.
18. Rajfer, J., Sikka, S.C., Lemmi, C., and Koyle, M.A. (1987). Cyclosporine inhibits testosterone biosynthesis in the rat testis. *Endocrinology*. 121:586–589.
19. Nooter, K., Meershoek B., Spans, W., Sonneveld, P., Oostrum, R., and Deurloo, J. (1984). Blood and tissue distribution of cyclosporine A after a single oral dose in the rat. *Experientia*. 40:559.
20. Kochi, S., Takanaga, H., Matsuo, H., Naito, M., Tsuruo, T., and Sawada, Y. (1999). Effect of cyclosporine A or tacrolimus on the function of blood-brain barrier cells. *Eur J Parmacol*. 372:287–295.
21. Ried, M., Gibbons, S., Kwik, D., VanBuren, C.T., Flechner, S., and Kahan, B.D. (1983). Cyclosporine levels in human tissues of patients treated for one week to one year. *Transplant Proc*. (Suppl. 1) 15:2434.
22. Atkinson, K., Boland, J., Britton, K., and Biggs, J. (1983). Blood and tissue distribution of cyclosporine in humans and mice. *Transplant Proc*. 15:2430.
23. Seethalakshmi, L., Diamond, D.A., Malhotra, R.K., Mazanitis, S.C., Kumar, S., and Menon, M. (1988). Cyclosporin-induced testicular dysfunction: a separation of the nephrotoxic component and an assessment of a 60-day recovery period. *Transplant Proc*. 20:1005–1010.
24. Krueger, B.A., Trakshel, G.M., Sluss, P.M., and Maines, M.D. (1991). Cyclosporin-mediated depression of luteinizing hormone receptors and heme biosynthesis in rat tests: a possible mechanism for decrease in serum testosterone. *Endocrinology*. 129:2647–2654
25. Erben, R.G., Stangassinger, M., and Gärtner, R. (1998). Skeletal effects of low-dose cyclosporin A in aged male rats: Lack of relationship to serum testosterone levels. *J Bone Miner Res*. 13:79–87.
26. Bowman, A.R., Sass, D.A., Dissanayake, I.R., Ma, Y.F., Liang, H., Yuan, Z., Jee, W.S.S., and Epstein, S. (1997). The role of testosterone in cyclosporine-induced osteopenia. *J Bone Miner Res*. 12:607–615.
27. Bellido, T., Jilka, R.L., Boyce, B.F., Girasole, G., Broxmeyer, H., Dalrymple, S.A., Murray, R., and Manolagas S.C. (1995). Regulation of interleukin-6, osteoclastogenesis, and bone mass by androgens. *J Clin Invest*. 95:2886–2895.
28. Vanderschueren, D., Van Herck, E., Suiker A.M.H., Visser, W.J., Schot, L.P.C., and Buillon, R. (1992). Bone and mineral metabolism in aged male rats: Short and long term effects of androgen deficiency. *Endocrinology*. 130:2906–2916.
29. Wakley, G.K., Schutte, H.D.J., Hannon, K.S., and Turner, R.T. (1991). Androgen treatment prevents loss of cancellous bone in the orchidectomized rat. *J Bone Miner Res*. 6:325–330.

30. Sikka, S.C., Koyle, M.A., Swerdloff, R.S., Rajfer, J. (1988). Reversibility of cyclosporine-induced hypoandrogenism in rats. *Transplantation*. 45(4), 784–787.
31. Rinaldi, M., Pellegrini, C., Martinelli, L., et al. (1997). FK506 effectiveness in reducing acute rejection after heart transplantation: a prospective randomized study. *J Heart Lung Transplant*. 16:1001.
32. Cvetkovic, M., Mann, G.N., Romero, D.F., Liang, X.G., Ma, Y., Jee, W.S., and Epstein, S. (1994). The deleterious effects of long-term cyclosporine A, cyclosporine G, and FK506 on bone mineral metabolism in vivo. *Transplantation*. 57:1231–1237.
33. Tai, J., Tze, W.T., Murase, N., and Starzl, T.E. (1994). Effect of FK506 on rat leydig cell function—in vivo and in vitro study. *Metabolism*. 43:533–537.
34. Hisatomi, A., Fujihira, S., Fujimoto, Y., Fujii, T., Mine, Y., and Ohara, K. (1995). Effect of Prograf (FK506) on spermatogenesis in rats. *Toxicology*. 109:75–83.
35. Doerr, P., and Pirke, K.M. (1976). Cortisol induced suppression of plasma testosterone in normal adult males. *J Clin Endocrinol Metab*. 43:622–629.
36. Heersche JN, Jez DH, Aubin J, Sodek J(1981). Regulation of hormone responsiveness of bone in vitro by corticosteroids, PTH, PGE2 and calcitonin, in hormonal control of kalzium metabolism, Talmage, R.V., ed., 1981, pp. 157–162. Amsterdam.
37. Lukert, B.P., and Raisz, L.G. (1990). Glucocorticoid-induced osteoporosis: pathogenesis and management. *Annals of Intern Med*. 112:352–364.
38. Canalis, E. (1996). Mechanisms of glucocorticoid action in bone: implications to glucocorticoid-induced osteoporosis. *J Clin Endocrinol Metab*. 81(10):3441–3447. Review. No abstract available.
39. Baldwin, D.M., and Sawyer, C.H. (1974). Effects of dexamethasone on LH release and ovulation in the cyclic rat. *Endocrinology*. 94:1397.
40. Hsueh A.J., Erickson, G.F. (1978). Glucocorticoid inhibition of FSH induced estrogen production in cultured rat granulosa cells. *Steroids*. 32:639–648.
41. Sakakura, M., Takebe, K., and Nakagawa, S. (1975). Inhibition of luteinizing hormone secretion induced by synthetic LRH by long-term treatment with glucocorticoids in human subjects. *J Clin Endocrinol Metab*. 40:774–779.
42. MacAdams, M.R., White, R.H., and Chipps, B.E. (1986). Reduction of serum testosterone levels during chronic glucocorticoid therapy. *Annals of Internal Medicine*. 104:648–651.
43. Crilly, R.G., Cawood, M., Marshall, D.H., and Nordin, B.E. (1978). Hormonal status in normal, osteoporotic and corticosteroid-treated postmenopausal women. *J R Soc Med*. 71:733–736.
44. Kream, B.E., and Lukert, B.P. (2002). Clinical and basic aspects of glucocorticoid action in bone. In Principles of Bone Biology, Bilezikian, J.P., Raisz, L.G., Rodan, G.A., eds., 2002, pp. 723–740. San Diego: Academic Press.
45. Weinstein, R.S., Jia, D., Powers, C.C., Steward, S.A., Jilka, R.L., Parfitt, A.M., and Manolagas, S.C. (2004). The skeletal effects of glucocorticoid excess override those of orchidectomy in mice. *Endocrinology*. 145:1980–1987.
46. MacAdams, M.R., White, R.H., and Chipps, B.E. (1986). Reduction of serum testosterone levels during chronic glucocorticoid therapy. *Ann Intern Med*. 104:648–651.
47. Montecucco, C., Caporali, R., Caprotti, P., Caprotti, M., and Notario, A. (1992). Sex hormones and bone metabolism in postmenopausal rheumatoid arthritis treated with two different glucocorticoids: a potential contributory factor in steroid-induced osteoporosis. *Metabolism*. 51:1458–1462.
48. Hampson, G., Bhargava, N., Cheung, J., Vaja, S., Seed, PT., Fogelman, I. (2002). Low circulating estradiol and adrenal androgens concentrations in men on glucocorticoids: a potential contributory factor in steroid-induced osteoporosis. *Metabolism*. 51:1458–1462.
49. Pearce, G., Tabensky, D.A., Delmas, P.D., Baker, H.W.D., and Seeman, E. (1998). Corticosteroid-induced bone loss in men. *J Clin Endocrinol Metab*. 83:801–806.

50. Nieszporek, T., Grzeszczak, W., Kokot, F., Zukowska-Szczechowska, E., Kusmierski, S., and Szkodny, A. (1989). Influence of type of immunosuppressive therapy on secretion of somatotropin and function of the pituitary-adrenal and pituitary-gonadal axis in patients with a kidney transplant. *Nephron*. 53:65–69.
51. Handelsman, D.J., Ralec, V.L., Tiller, D.J., Horvath, J.S., and Turtle, J.R. (1981). Testicular function after renal transplantation. *Clin Endocrinol*. 14:527–538.
52. Bryer, H.P., Isserow, J.A., Armstrong, E.C., Mann, G.N., Rucinski, B., Buchinsky, F.J., Romero, D.F., and Epstein, S. (1995). Azathioprine alone is bone sparing and does not alter cyclosporin A-induced osteopenia in the rat. *J Bone Miner Res*. 10(1):132–138.
53. Dissanayake, I.R., Goodman, G.R., Bowman, A.R., Ma, Y., Pun, S., Jee, W.S., and Epstein, S. (1998). Mycophenolate mofetil: a promising new immunosuppressant that does not cause bone loss in the rat. *Transplantation*. 65(2), 275–278.
54. Rapamune US Study Group, and Kahan, B.D. (2000). Efficiacy of sirolimus compared with azathioprine for reduction of acute renal allograft rejection: a randomized multicenter study. *Lancet*. 356:194–202.
55. Kelly, P., Gruber, S., Behbod, F., and Kahan, B. (1997). Sirolimus, a new potent immunosuppressive agent. *Pharmacotherapy*. 17:1148–1156.
56. Kaczmarek, I., Groetzner, J., Adamidis, I., Landwehr, P., Mueller, M., Vogeser, M., Gerstorfer, M., Überfuhr, P., Meiser, B., and Reichard, B. (2003). Sirolimus impairs gonadal function in heart transplant recipients. *American J Transplant*, Online Issue
57. Bererhi, L., Flamant, M., Martinez, F., Karras, A., Thervet, E., and Legendre C. (2002). Rapamycin-induced oligospermia. *Transplantation*. 76:885–886.
58. Blume-Jensen, P., Jiang, G., Hyman, R, et al. (2000). Kit/stem cell factor receptor-induced activation of phosphatidylinositol 3'-kinase is essential for male fertility. *Nat Genet*. 24:157.
59. Handelsman, D.J., McDowell, I.F.W., Caterson, I.D., Tiller, D.J., Hall, B.M., and Turtle J.R. (1984). Testicular function after renal transplantation: comparison of Cyclosporin A with azathioprine and prednisone combination regimes. *Clinical Nephrology*. 22:144–148.
60. Cueto-Manzano, A.M., Freemont A.J., Adams, J.E., Mawer, B., Gokal, R., and Hutchison A.J. (2001). Association of sex hormone status with the bone loss of renal transplant patients. *Nephrol Dial Transplant*. 16:1245–1250.
61. Tauchmanovà, L., Carrano, C., Sabbatini, M., De Rosa, M., Orio, F., Palomba, S., Cascella, T., Lombardi, G., Federico, S., and Colao, A. (2004). Hypothalamic-pituitary-gonadal axis function after successful kidney transplantation in men and women. *Human Reproduction*. 19:867–873.
62. Peces, R., de la Torre, M., and Urra, J.M. (1994). Pituitary-testicular function in cyclosporin-treated renal transplant patients. *Nephrology Dialysis Transplantation*. 9(10):1453–1455
63. Saha, M.T., Saha, M.H.T., Niskanen, L.K., Salmela, K.T., and Pasternack, A.I. (2002). Time course of serum prolactin and sex hormones following successful renal transplantation. *Nephron*. 92:735–737.
64. Ramirez, G., Narvarte, J., Bittle, P.A., Ayers-Chastain, C., and Dean, S.E. (1991). Cyclosporine-induced alterations in the hypothalamic hypophyseal gonadal axis in transplant patients. *Nephron*. 58:27–32.
65. Shane, E., Rivas, M., McMahon, D.J., Staron, R.B., Silverberg, S.J., Seibel, M.J., Mancini, D., Michler, R.E., Aaronson, K., Addesso, V., and Lo, S.H. (1997). Bone loss and turnover after cardiac transplantation. *J Clin Endocrinol Metab*. 82:1497–1506.
66. Sambrook, P.N., Kelly, P.J., Keogh, A.M., Macdonald, P., Spratt, P., Freund, J., and Eisman, J.A. (1994). Bone loss after heart transplantation: A prospective study. *J Heart Lung Transplant*. 13:116–121.
67. Muchmore, J.S., Cooper, D.K.C., Ye, Y., Schlegel, V.T., and Zuhdi, N. (1991). Loss of vertebral bone density in heart transplant patients. *Transplantation Proceedings*. 23:1184–1185.

68. Muchmore, J.S., Cooper, K.C., Ye, Y., Schlegel, V., Pribil, A., and Zuhdi, N. (1992). Prevention of loss of vertebral bone density in heart transplant patients. *J Heart Lung Transplant*. 11:959–964.
69. Guo, C-Y., Johnson, A., Locke, T.J., and Eastell, R. (1998). Mechanisms of bone loss after cardiac transplantation. *Bone*. 22:267–271.
70. Stempfle, H.U., Werner, C., Echtler, S., Wehr, U., Rambeck, W.A., Siebert, U., Überfuhr, P., Angermann, C.E., Theisen, K., and Gärtner, R. (1999). Prevention of osteoporosis after cardiac transplantation. A prospective, randomized, double-blind trial with calcitriol. *Transplantation*. 68:523–530.
71. Stempfle, H.U., Werner, C., Siebert, U., Assum, T., Wehr, U., Rambeck, W.A., Meiser, B., Theisen, K., and Gartner, R. (2002). The role of tacrolimus (FK506)-Based immunosuppression on bone mineral density and bone turnover after cardiac transplantation: a prospective, longitudinal, randomized, double-blind trial with calcitriol. *Transplantation*. 73:547–552.
72. Werner, C., Assum, T., Angermann, C.E., Gärtner, R., Meiser, B., and Stempfle, H.U. (1999). Vergleich der Auswirkungen von FK506 und Cyclosporin A auf den Knochenstoffwechsel – Prävention der Osteoporose nach Herztransplantation durch Calcitriol. *Z Kardiol*. 88(1):127
73. Harman, S.M., Metter, E.J., Tobin, J.D., Pearson, J., and Blackman, M.R. (2001). Longitudinal effects of aging on serum total and free testosterone levels in healthy men. *J Clin Endocrinol Metab*. 86:724–731.
74. Stief, J., Sohn, H.Y., Alt, A., Überfuhr, P., Theisen, K., and Stempfle, H.U. (2004). Role of immunosuppression-induced hypogonadism on bone loss after cardiac transplantation. *Dtsch Med Wochenschrift*. 129:1674–1678.
75. Stief, J., Sohn, H.Y., Alt, A., Überfuhr, P., Theisen, K., and Stempfle, H.U. (2004). Role of immunosuppression induced hypogonadism on bone loss after cardiac transplantation. DMW (in press).
76. Anker S.D., Chua, T.P., Ponikowski, P., Harrington D., Swan, J.W., Kox, W.J, Poole-Wilson, P.A., and Coats A.J.S. (1997). Hormonal changes and catabolic/anabolic imbalance in chronic heart failure and their importance for cardiac cachexia. *Circulation* 96:526–534.
77. Moriyama, Y., Yasue, H., Yoshimura, M., Mizuno, Y., Nishiyama, K., Tsunoda, R., Kawano, H., Kugiyama, K., Ogawa, H., Saito, Y., and Nakao, K. (2000). The plasma levels of dehydroepiandrosterone sulfate are decreased in patients with chronic heart failure in proportion to the severity. *J Clin Endocrinol Metab* 85:1834–40.
78. Tappler, B., and Katz, M. (1979). Pituitary-gonadal dysfunction in low-output cardiac failure. *Clin Endocrinol* 10:219–226.
79. Noirhomme, P., Jaquet, L., Underwood, M., El Khoury, G., Goenen, M., and Dion, R. (1999). The effect of chronic mechanical circulatory support on neuroendocrine activation in patients with end-stage heart failure. *Eur J Cardiothorac Surg* 16:63–67.
80. Ottenweller, J.E., Tapp, W.N., Creighton, D., and Natelson, B.H. (1988). Aging, stress and chronic disease interact to suppress plasma testosterone in syrian hamsters. *J Gerontol* 43:175–180.
81. Kontoleon, P.E., Anastasiou-Nana, M., Papapetrou, P.D., Alexopoulos, G., Ktenas, V., Rapti, A.C., Tsagalou, E.P., and Nanas, J.N. (2003). Hormonal profile in patients with congestive heart failure. *International Journal of Cardiology* 87:179–183.
82. Stempfle, H.U., Frost, R., Sonne, C., Theisen, K., and Gärtner, R. (2002). Bone loss and prevention of osteoporosis in congestive heart failure. *J Heart Transplant* 21(1), 158.
83. Stief, J., Gaertner, R., Überfuhr, P., Theisen, K., Stempfle, H.-U. (2004). Post-transplantation hypogonadism: A reflection of sex steroids deficiency due to previous congestive heart failure or an immunosuppressive side effect? *J Bone Miner Res* 19: Suppl 1, abstract.
84. Stempfle, H.U., Werner, C., Echtler, S., Assum, T., Meiser, B., Angermann, C.E., Theisen, K., and Gärtner, R. (1998). Rapid trabecular bone loss after cardiac transplantation using FK506 (Tacrolimus) based immunosuppression. *Transplant Proceedings* 30:1132–1133.
85. Riggs, B.L., Khosla, S., and Melton L.J. 3rd (1998). A unitary model for involutional osteoporosis: estrogen deficienca causes both type I and type II osteoporosis in

postmenopausal women and contributes to bone loss is aging men. *J Bone Miner Res* 13(5), 763–773.
86. Khosla, S., Melton L.J. 3rd, Atkinson, E.J., O'Fallon, W.M., Klee, G.G., and Riggs, B.L. (1998). Relationship of serum sex steroid levels and bone turnover markers with bone mineral density in men and women: a key role for bioavailable estrogen. *J Clin Endocrinol Metab* 83:2266–2274.
87. Szulc, P., Munoz, F., Claustrat, B., Garnero, P., Marchand, F., Duboeuf, F., and Delmas, P.D. (2001). Bioavailible estradiol may be an important determinant of osteoporosis in men: The MINOS Study. *J Clin Endocrinol Metab* 86:192–199.
88. Joffe I, Katz I, Jacobs T, Epstein S (1992). 17a-Estradiol prevents osteopenia in the oophorectomized rat treated with cyclosporin-A. *Endocrinology* 130:1578–1586.
89. McIlwain, H.H. (2003). Glucocorticoid-Induced osteoporosis: pathogenesis, diagnosis, and management. *Preventive Medicine* 36:243–249.
90. Hirasawa, K., and Kamada, N. (1992). Female sex hormone, estradiol, antagonizes the immunosuppressive activity of cyclosporine in rat organ transplantation. *Transplant Proc* (1), 408–409.
91. Hirasawa, K., and Enosawa, S. (1991). Sex-associated differences in organ transplantation: different effects of steroid hormones, testosterone, estradiol, progesterone, and prednisolone on the survival time of allogeneic skin graft in rats treated with cyclosporin A. *Transplant Proc* 23(1 Pt 1), 714–715.
92. Rhoden, E.L., and Morgentaler A. (2004). Risks of testosterone-replacement therapy and recommendations for monitoring. *N Engl J Med* 350:482–492.

CHAPTER 11

Pathogenesis of Transplantation Bone Disease: A Unifying Hypothesis

Richard Eastell, MD, FRCP, FRCPath, FmedSci
Kim E. Naylor, PhD, BSc
Annie M. Cooper, MD, FRCP
Bone Metabolism Group, Division of Clinical Sciences (North), University of Sheffield, Sheffield, England

I. INTRODUCTION

This chapter addresses the pathophysiology of bone loss after cardiac transplantation. There are three reasons for considering just one type of transplantation. Firstly, there have been many publications in this field. Secondly, cardiac transplantation is performed mainly in men and so avoids the profound changes that result from estrogen deficiency associated with menopause in women. Thirdly, there may be some bone loss prior to cardiac transplantation, but the severe osteodystrophy found in patients awaiting transplantation of organs such as the kidney is not seen.

Low bone mass prior to transplantation is likely to contribute to the increased risk of fracture after transplantation. Other contributing factors include immobility and the use of glucocorticoids, heparin, and loop diuretics such as furosemide. The evidence that bone loss and fracture risk are greater in the first year after transplantation is considered elsewhere in this book.

II. A PROPOSED MODEL

Guo et al. proposed a model [1] in which bone loss after cardiac transplantation results from an increase in the rate of bone turnover in association with remodeling imbalance (Figure 1). This imbalance is in part a consequence of the inhibition of bone formation by glucocorticoids. It is likely that this inhibition is a result of an increase in the rate of osteoblast apoptosis [2]. The increase in bone turnover may result from a number of factors, including hypogonadism (low

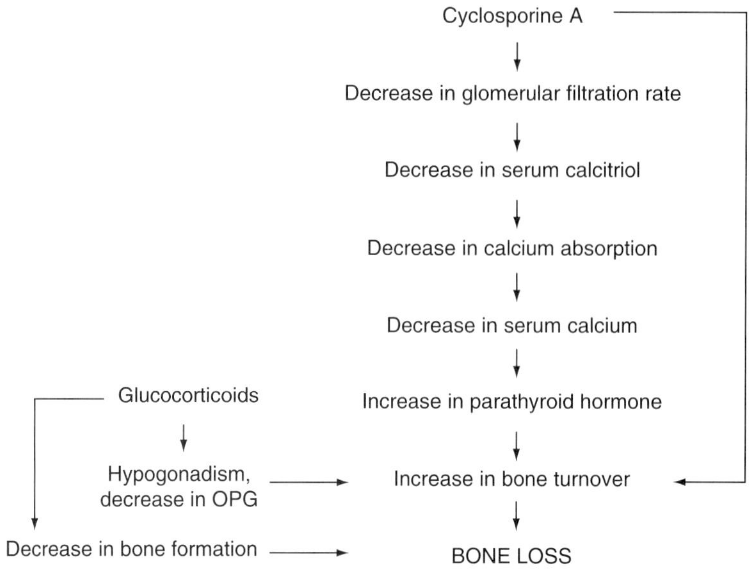

FIGURE 1 A model for explaining biochemical changes after cardiac transplantation. Cyclosporine A increases bone turnover directly and by increasing PTH. Paradoxically, the hypomagnesemia that results from cyclosporine A therapy inhibits bone turnover. The effects of glucocorticoids are most marked in the first year after the transplant. Modified from Guo et al. (1998), *Bone*. 22:267–271.

testosterone in men), immunosuppressants such as cyclosporine A, and increased parathyroid hormone (PTH) secretion. Hypogonadism is most likely caused by high doses of glucocorticoids. The increase in PTH is multifactorial and may be related in part to the inhibition of intestinal calcium absorption secondary to high-dose glucocorticoids and a decline in synthesis of calcitriol that is associated with renal impairment. Cyclosporine A [3] and tacrolimus [4] are well known to cause renal impairment.

This model applies to the early post-transplantation period. As pointed out by Cohen and Shane [5], the later phase of transplantation-related bone loss does not include the effects of glucocorticoids, as doses of these are usually sharply reduced after the first six months and may be stopped one to two years after surgery.

III. EVIDENCE FOR THE PROPOSED MODEL

A. Evidence for an Increased Rate of Bone Turnover

Bone turnover can be assessed by bone histomorphometry (see Chapter 8) or by biochemical markers of bone turnover. Bone turnover markers may reflect osteoblastic activity (osteocalcin, bone alkaline phosphatase, type I procollagen propeptides from the C- and N-terminal) or osteoclastic activity (deoxypyridinoline, type I collagen telopeptides from the C- and N-terminal). Markers of osteoclast activity reflect the rate of bone resorption, and the ones most studied are deoxypyrinoline (DPD) and the C- and N-telopeptide of type I collagen (CTX and NTX). These markers are increased in patients after cardiac transplantation, especially during the first year [1, 6]. Markers of osteoblastic activity reflect the rate of bone formation (in the absence of any defect in mineralization) and osteocalcin (OC) has been most commonly studied. Conflicting results have been reported in studies of the changes occurring after transplantation. Increased OC has been observed throughout the post-transplantation period in some studies [1], whereas in others, suppression in the first months after transplantation is followed by increased levels [6]. The differences between studies may be due to differences in the doses of glucocorticoid administered and in the fragments of OC captured in the assay. Bone alkaline phosphatase has also been reported to be elevated in patients after cardiac transplantation [1].

There are three reasons why bone turnover remains elevated late after transplantation (and after glucocorticoid administration has stopped). First, a decrease in glomerular filtration rate alone will result in an increase in OC [7]. Second, immunosuppressive agents such as cyclosporine A may have a direct effect on the rate of bone turnover. Finally, fractures may result in an increase in bone turnover markers, reflecting fracture repair.

It is likely that glucocorticoids are an important determinant of the changes in osteocalcin. Thus the early reduction in osteocalcin levels [6] follows the same time course as the dosing with glucocorticoids in that the lowest OC levels are observed during the period when the highest doses are given. Further, serum OC correlates with the daily dose of prednisolone [1]. This effect of glucocorticoids on OC is well described in other disease states [8].

The effect of glucocorticoids on bone resorption markers has also been studied. A recent study measured serum C terminal telopeptide of type I collagen (CTX) in cardiac transplant patients and found that levels were significantly lower in patients receiving glucocorticoid-free treatment compared to those taking glucocorticoids [9].

It has been suggested that increased bone resorption after transplantation may be related to the effect of glucocorticoids and other immunosuppressive agents on the synthesis of osteoprotegerin by osteoblasts [10]. Osteoprotegerin (OPG) is a decoy receptor for RANK ligand (RANKL) and is produced by several cell types including osteoblasts and arterial cells. OPG blocks the RANK–RANKL signalling pathway, inhibiting osteoclastogenesis and osteoclast function and resulting in a decrease in bone turnover. Hofbauer et al. [11] assessed the effects of glucocorticoids on OPG and RANKL expression in human osteoblastic lineage cells. They found that dexamethasone inhibited OPG and stimulated RANKL production by osteoblastic lineage cells, indicating a potential mechanism for glucocorticoid-induced bone loss. There is further evidence that OPG has a role in the development of post-transplantation osteoporosis. Fahrleitner et al. measured serum OPG in cardiac transplant patients both cross-sectionally and in a separate 6-month prospective study [10]. In the cross-sectional cohort, serum OPG was correlated with bone density of the femoral neck. In the prospective cohort, OPG had decreased by 41% 3 months following cardiac transplant. In a study of renal transplant patients, Sato et al. [12] found that serum OPG levels decreased significantly 14 and 28 days after renal transplant compared to pretransplant levels.

Serum magnesium changes profoundly after cardiac transplantation. The decrease in serum magnesium that is commonly found is likely to be a consequence of cyclosporine A therapy. Boncimino et al. [13] have reported that low serum magnesium is associated with a smaller increase in bone turnover markers and lower rates of bone loss. A low serum magnesium results in resistance to the action of PTH, and very low levels of serum magnesium can result in functional hypoparathyroidism. Thus, the low serum magnesium levels found in patients after cardiac transplantation may protect the skeleton by making it more resistant to the effects of PTH.

B. Evidence for an Increase in PTH

This topic is considered in detail in Chapter 9. Elevated PTH after transplantation has been reported in some but not all studies [14–20]. Guo et al. reported a correlation between serum PTH and OC, suggesting that PTH may contribute to increased bone turnover. This increase in PTH was related to the decrease in serum calcium and increase in serum creatinine [1]. One week of alphacalcidol therapy suppressed PTH and NTX for one to four weeks, suggesting that the increase in PTH was driving the increase in NTX (see Figure 2).

This suppression of PTH and NTX has recently been shown to be even greater after 12 months of calcitriol therapy [21].

C. Evidence for Changes in Serum Calcium and Calcium Absorption

Boncimino et al. [13] measured serum calcium prior to and three months after cardiac transplantation and found no change. Our observations were similar, but we found a transient decrease in serum calcium within the first months of surgery that is a consequence of the transient decrease in serum albumin. Surgery often causes a decrease in serum albumin, and this is considered an "acute phase reactant."

D. Evidence for a Decrease in Serum Calcitriol

1-alpha hydroxylation of vitamin D takes place in the proximal renal tubule and is regulated by serum phosphate, calcium, PTH, and calcitriol itself.

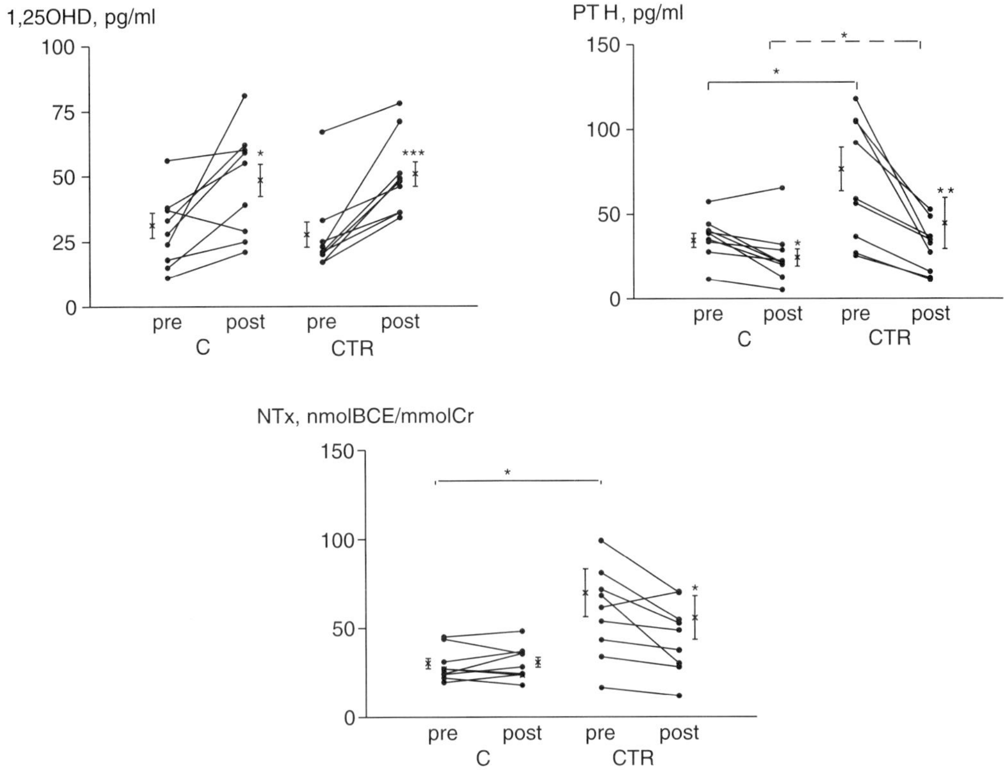

FIGURE 2 We administered alphacalcidol (2 micrograms/day) to 9 male cardiac transplant recipients and 9 age-matched controls. Following 7 days of treatment, there were significant increases in urinary calcium, serum phosphate, and strontium absorption. The graph shows the significant increase in serum calcitriol ($p<0.001$, ***) and the significant suppression in serum PTH ($p<0.01$, **) and urinary NTX excretion ($p<0.05$, *) in the men after cardiac transplantation (CTR). The levels of PTH and NTX decreased towards those found at baseline in the control (C) group.

Serum phosphate is elevated in patients after cardiac transplantation as a result of renal impairment [1], and this presumably predominates over other regulatory influences and results in decreased calcitriol production. Serum calcitriol correlates with serum creatinine levels [1].

The effect of alphacalcidol administration is to increase serum calcitriol levels (see Figure 2) and hence to reverse the increase in PTH and NTX, suggesting a central role for calcitriol in the pathogenesis of transplant bone disease. This human study is supported by a study in rats showing that calcitriol prevents cyclosporine A–induced bone loss [22].

E. Evidence for Decrease in Glomerular Filtration Rate

There is ample evidence for a decrease in glomerular filtration rate, as assessed by creatinine clearance, after cardiac transplantation. It is likely that this results from the administration of immunosuppressive drugs such as cyclosporine A and tacrolimus [23–25].

F. Evidence for Hypogonadism

Hypogonadism is most marked in men during the first few months after transplantation [26]. This time course would be consistent with an effect of glucocorticoids, which suppress testosterone by a direct effect on the testis and by inhibiting the secretion of gonadotrophins. However, there is some evidence for residual hypogonadism even later [1, 27]. There is also a decrease in the production of adrenal androgens, as shown by a decrease in dehydroepiandrosterone sulfate (DHEA-S), resulting from adrenal suppression by glucocorticoids [1].

The effect of testosterone on bone is a topic of recent debate. Testosterone has direct effects on bone formation and resorption [28, 29], but more importantly, it acts as a substrate for the production of estrogen (by aromatase) and hence inhibits bone resorption. Thus, low levels of testosterone (and DHEA-S) might be expected to increase bone turnover [30] and cause a relative reduction in bone formation.

Fahrleitner et al. [31] found that male hypogonadal cardiac transplant patients treated with ibandronate had a better bone density response if also treated with testosterone. However, a recent study of tacrolimus-based immunosuppression in cardiac transplant patients demonstrated a significant reduction in bone density despite calcium and hormone supplementation in hypogonadal patients [4].

IV. IMPLICATIONS OF THE MODEL FOR TREATMENT

An understanding of the pathogenesis of a disorder may provide the foundation for guiding treatment approaches. Thus, the lower the dose of glucocorticoids, the less the bone loss. Similarly, the increase in bone turnover induced by cyclosporine A should respond to antiresorptive therapy such as bisphosphonates. It would be unwise, however, to proceed with bisphosphonates alone as this might cause a further increase in PTH. It is logical to give at least high-dose calcium supplements, and possibly an active form of vitamin D such as calcitriol or alphacalcidol as well; calcitriol given for two years appears more effective in preventing bone loss than calcium alone [32]. This might explain why alendronate was no more effective than calcitriol on preventing bone loss after cardiac transplantation [21]. It would also seem logical to replace testosterone in men who are deficient. This may have adverse effects on lipids, however, and if the original cardiovascular disease was a consequence of hyperlipidemia, this form of therapy may not be desirable. Until there have been further randomized controlled trials of testosterone, this form of treatment should be used with caution and only in truly hypogonadal patients who are monitored carefully.

V. SUMMARY

Drugs that are used to prevent rejection appear to have an important role to play in bone loss after cardiac transplantation. Indeed, this is also true for other forms of organ transplantation [5]. The most convincing biochemical change is the increase in serum parathyroid hormone in the later post-transplant period, along with the decrease in serum magnesium, which may be the cause of the increase in bone resorption. It is less clear whether bone formation increases early after transplantation, or shows an early decrease followed by an increase. This uncertainty may relate to the dose of glucocorticoid administered to prevent rejection. It is likely that cyclosporine A and other immunosuppressives are important determinants of the increased bone turnover, through effects on renal function and hence on calcitriol levels and calcium absorption; the importance of any direct effect on bone is unclear in humans. Glucocorticoid therapy [34] is a potential contributor to the fracture syndrome. The latter may be countered by bisphosphonates such as alendronate [35]; the decrease in calcium absorption may be countered by the administration of calcitriol, or of calcium and vitamin D.

REFERENCES

1. Guo, C.Y., Johnson, A., Locke, T.J., Eastell, R. (1998). Mechanisms of bone loss after cardiac transplantation. *Bone*. 22:267–271.
2. Weinstein, R.S., Jilka, R.L., Parfitt, A.M., Manolagas, S.C. (1998). Inhibition of osteoblastogenesis and promotion of apoptosis of osteoblasts and osteocytes by glucocorticoids. Potential mechanisms of their deleterious effects on bone. *J Clin Invest*. 102:274–282.
3. Kahan, B.D. (1989). Cyclosporine [see comments]. *N Engl J* Med. 321:1725–1738.
4. Stempfle, H.U., Werner, C., Siebert, U., Assum, T., Wehr, U., Rambeck, W.A., Meiser, B., Theisen, K., Gartner, R. (2002). The role of tacrolimus (FK506)-based immunosuppression on bone mineral density and bone turnover after cardiac transplantation: a prospective, longitudinal, randomized, double-blind trial with calcitriol. *Transplantation*. 73:547–552.
5. Cohen, A., Shane, E. (2003). Osteoporosis after solid organ and bone marrow transplantation. *Osteoporos Int*. 14:617–630.
6. Shane, E., Rivas, M., McMahon, D.J., Staron, R.B., Silverberg, S.J., Seibel, M.J., Mancini, D., Michler, R.E., Aaronson, K., Addesso, V., Lo, S.H. (1997). Bone loss and turnover after cardiac transplantation. *J Clin Endocrinol Metab*. 82:1497–1506.
7. Delmas, P.D., Wilson, D.M., Mann, K.G., Riggs, B.L. (1983). Effect of renal function on plasma levels of bone gla-protein. *J Clin Endocrinol Metab*. 57:1028–1030.
8. Prummel, M.F., Wiersinga, W.M., Lips, P., Sanders, G.T.B., Sauerwein, H.P. (1991). The course of biochemical parameters of bone turnover during treatment with corticosteriods. *J Clin Endocrinol Metab*. 72:382–386.

9. Hofle, G., Holzmuller, H., Gouya, G., Hergan, K., Hubmann, M., Langer, P., Drexel, H. (2003). Lower serum beta-CrossLaps in male cardiac transplant recipients treated without prednisolone. *Transpl Int.* 16:523–528.
10. Fahrleitner, A., Prenner, G., Leb, G., Tscheliessnigg, K.H., Piswanger-Solkner, C., Obermayer-Pietsch, B., Portugaller, H.R., Berghold, A., Dobnig, H. (2003). Serum osteoprotegerin is a major determinant of bone density development and prevalent vertebral fracture status following cardiac transplantation. *Bone.* 32:96–106.
11. Hofbauer, L.C., Gori, F., Riggs, B.L., Lacey, D.L., Dunstan, C.R., Spelsberg, T.C., Khosla, S. (1999). Stimulation of osteoprotegerin ligand and inhibition of osteoprotegerin production by glucocorticoids in human osteoblastic lineage cells: potential paracrine mechanisms of glucocorticoid-induced osteoporosis. *Endocrinol.* 140:4382–4389.
12. Sato, T., Tominaga, Y., Iwasaki, Y., Kazama, J.J., Shigematsu, T., Inagaki, H., Watanabe, I., Katayama, A., Haba, T., Uchida, K., Fukagawa, M. (2001). Osteoprotegerin levels before and after renal transplantation. *Am J Kidney Dis.* 38:S175-S177.
13. Boncimino, K., McMahon, D., Addesso, V., Bilezikian, J.P., Shane, E. (1999). Magnesium deficiency and bone loss after cardiac transplantation. *J Bone Miner Res.* 14:295–303.
14. Rich, G.M., Mudge, G.H., Laffel, G.L., LeBoff, M.S. (1992). Cyclosporine A and prednisone-associated osteoporosis in heart transplant recipients. *J Heart Lung Transplant.* 11:950–958.
15. Shane, E., Rivas, M., Staron, R.B., Silverberg, S.J., Seibel, M.J., Kuiper, J., Mancini, D., Addesso, V., Michler, R.E., Factor-Litvak, P. (1996). Fracture after cardiac transplantation: a prospective longitudinal study. *J Clin Endocrinol Metab.* 81:1740–1746.
16. Lee, A.H., Mull, R.L., Keenan, G.F., Callegari, P.E., Dalinka, M.K., Eisen, H.J., Mancini, D.M., Disesa, V.J., Attie, M.F. (1994). Osteoporosis and bone morbidity in cardiac transplant recipients. *Am J Med.* 96:35–41.
17. Compston, J.E., Greer, S., Skingle, S.J., Stirling, D.M., Price, C., Friend, P.J., Alexander, G. (1996). Early increase in plasma parathyroid hormone levels following liver transplantation. *J Hepatol.* 25:715–718.
18. Brandenberger, G., Schnedecker, B., Spiegel, K., Mettauer, B., Geny, B., Sacrez, J., Lampert, E., Lonsdorfer, J. (1995). Parathyroid function in cardiac transplant patients: evaluation during physical exercise. *Eur J Appl Physiol.* 70:401–406.
19. Glendenning, P., Kent, G.N., Adler, B.D., Matz, L., Watson, I., O'Driscoll, G.J., Hurley, D.M. (1999). High prevalence of osteoporosis in cardiac transplant recipients and discordance between biochemical turnover markers and bone histomorphometry. *Clin Endocrinol (Oxf).* 50:347–355.
20. Thiebaud, D., Krieg, M.A., Gillard-Berguer, D., Jacquet, A.F., Goy, J.J., Burckhardt, P. (1996). Cyclosporine induces high bone turnover and may contribute to bone loss after heart transplantation. *Eur J Clin Invest.* 26:549–555.
21. Shane, E., Addesso, V., Namerow, P.B., McMahon, D.J., Lo, S.H., Staron, R.B., Zucker, M., Pardi, S., Maybaum, S., Mancini, D. (2004). Alendronate versus calcitriol for the prevention of bone loss after cardiac transplantation. *N Engl J Med.* 350:767–776.
22. Epstein, S., Schlosberg, M., Fallon, M., Thomas, S., Movsowitz, C., Ismail, F. (1990). 1,25 dihydroxyvitamin d3 modifies cyclosporine-induced bone loss. *Calcif Tissue Int.* 47:152–157.
23. Myers, B.D., Sibley, R., Newton, L., Tomlanovich, S.J., Boshkos, C., Stinson, E., Luetscher, J.A., Whitney, D.J., Krasny, D., Coplon, N.S. (1988). The long-term course of cyclosporine-associated chronic nephropathy. *Kidney Int.* 33:590–600.
24. Bertani, T., Ferrazzi, P., Schieppati, A., Ruggenenti, P., Gamba, A., Parenzan, L., Mecca, G., Perico, N., Imberti, O., Remuzzi, A.,. (1991). Nature and extent of glomerular injury induced by cyclosporine in heart transplant patients. *Kidney Int.* 40:243–250.
25. Burke, J.F., Jr., Pirsch, J.D., Ramos, E.L., Salomon, D.R., Stablein, D.M., Van Buren, D.H., West, J.C. (1994). Long-term efficacy and safety of cyclosporine in renal-transplant recipients. *N Engl J Med.* 331:358–363.

26. Sambrook, P.N., Kelly, P.J., Fontana, D., Nguyen, T., Keogh, A., Macdonald, P., Spratt, P., Freund, J., Eisman, J.A. (1994). Mechanisms of rapid bone loss following cardiac transplantation. *Osteoporos Int.* 4:273–276.
27. Stempfle, H.U., Werner, C., Echtler, S., Wehr, U., Rambeck, W.A., Siebert, U., Uberfuhr, P., Angermann, C.E., Theisen, K., Gartner, R. (1999). Prevention of osteoporosis after cardiac transplantation: a prospective, longitudinal, randomized, double-blind trial with calcitriol. *Transplantation.* 68:523–530.
28. Falahati-Nini, A., Riggs, B.L., Atkinson, E.J., O'Fallon, W.M., Eastell, R., Khosla, S. (2000). Relative contributions of testosterone and estrogen in regulating bone resorption and formation in normal elderly men. *J Clin Invest.* 106:1553–1560.
29. Leder, B.Z., LeBlanc, K.M., Schoenfeld, D.A., Eastell, R., Finkelstein, J.S. (2003). Differential effects of androgens and estrogens on bone turnover in normal men. *J Clin Endocrinol Metab.* 88:204–210.
30. Guo, C.Y., Jones, T.H., Eastell, R. (1997). Treatment of isolated hypogonadotropic hypogonadism and its effect on bone mineral density and bone turnover. *J Clin Endocrinol Metab.* 82:658–665.
31. Fahrleitner, A., Prenner, G., Tscheliessnigg, K.H. (2002). Testosterone supplementation has additional benefits on one metabolism in cardiac transplant recipients receiving intravenous bisphosphonate treatment: a prospective study, 17 ed., p. S388.
32. Sambrook, P., Henderson, N.K., Keogh, A., Macdonald, P., Glanville, A., Spratt, P., Bergin, P., Ebeling, P., Eisman, J. (2000). Effect of calcitriol on bone loss after cardiac or lung transplantation. *J Bone Miner Res.* 15:1818–1824.
33. Henderson, K., Eisman, J., Keogh, A., Macdonald, P., Glanville, A., Spratt, P., Sambrook, P. (2001). Protective effect of short-term calcitriol or cyclical etidronate on bone loss after cardiac or lung transplantation. *J Bone Miner Res.* 16:565–571.
34. Weinstein, R.S., Jilka, R.L., Parfitt, A.M., Manolagas, S.C. (1998). Inhibition of osteoblastogenesis and promotion of apoptosis of osteoblasts and osteocytes by glucocorticoids. Potential mechanisms of their deleterious effects on bone. *J Clin Invest.* 102:274–282.
35. Weinstein, R.S., Manolagas, S.C. (2000). Apoptosis and osteoporosis. *Am J Med.* 108:153–164.

PART III

Clinical Features of Transplantation Bone Disease

CHAPTER 12

Bone Disease after Kidney Transplantation

S.L-S. Fan, MRCP
Department of Nephrology and Transplantation, The Royal London Hospital, London, England

John Cunningham, DM, FRCP
Department of Nephrology, University College London Hospitals,
The Middlesex Hospital, London, England

I. INTRODUCTION

The recipient of a successful kidney transplant is catapulted from the often limited existence on dialysis into a world with better quality of life, freedom from dialysis, and many other advantages. As counterpoint to this, the transition can also be seen as one that moves the patient from an environment laden with restrictions, comorbidities, and high mortality to a new environment that, while less burdened with restrictions, remains hazardous in the contexts of comorbidity and high mortality. The median life span of a kidney transplant is of the order of 10 to 12 years with an annual graft loss rate of approximately 5% [1]. Kidney function usually deteriorates with the passage of time, with the result that the transplant population as a whole can be described as a population suffering from chronic renal insufficiency (chronic kidney disease, or CKD), which is often progressive and of variable severity. On top of this somewhat unhappy scenario, the kidney transplant recipient is further burdened with the need for a regimen of immunosuppressive agents, which, although they have been progressively refined over the years, still bring considerable toxicity to the picture.

II. TERMINOLOGY

The lack of cohesion between the basic science and practice that has developed in the field of osteoporosis and that developed in renal osteodystrophy has led to confusion as to appropriate terminology [2]. Descriptive terms applied to osteoporosis are not applicable to renal osteodystrophy, and vice versa.

It is important to recognize that the low bone mineral density (BMD) frequently encountered in dialysed and transplanted patients does not necessarily constitute a diagnosis of osteoporosis, and, conversely, a "normal" bone density does not necessarily translate to a healthy skeleton in the CKD patient. Strictly speaking, osteoporosis should be diagnosed only according to the WHO criteria (bone mineral density T score −1 to −2.5 defining osteopenia and below −2.5 defining osteoporosis), which were developed in a female Caucasian postmenopausal population. The patient groups under consideration here differ conspicuously from the WHO database: they are of both genders, diverse ethnicity, and variable age; in addition, they may suffer from conditions that can cause secondary osteoporosis, including hyperparathyroidism, adynamic bone disease, and hypogonadism, as a result of their underlying disease and/or therapy.

A recent consensus statement from the National Institutes of Health (NIH) is of greater relevance to the CKD and transplanted population. As defined by the NIH, osteoporosis is "a skeletal disorder characterized by compromised bone strength predisposing to an increased risk of fracture Bone strength reflects the integration of two main features—bone density and bone quality" [3]. An important implication of this definition is that bone strength and fracture risk (by far the most important clinical endpoints of this type of bone disease) are determined by a combination of bone density, architecture, turnover, damage accumulation, and efficiency of repair. Of these variables, only bone mineral density is easy to measure in the clinical setting, which frequently leads to inappropriate emphasis being placed on this parameter in the absence of sufficient information on the other important determinants of bone strength.

Thus the term osteoporosis is potentially quite misleading in the CKD population and also in transplant recipients, implying as it does a diagnosis when only one of several determinants of bone strength, namely BMD, has been measured. Equally, the finding of "normal" BMD in patients after renal transplantation does not exclude the possibility of substantially increased fracture risk, as there may be important abnormalities of bone microarchitecture and turnover.

Similar notes of caution are appropriate in regard to quantitative computed tomographic (qCT) measurements of bone density and also in the use of biochemical bone markers. qCT may well have other advantages over dual energy X-ray absorptiometry (DXA, or DEXA), however, in that defined areas of interest can be examined with less contamination from extraneous artifacts such as localized sclerosis, degenerative change, and soft tissue calcification [4, 5]. In the case of biochemical markers, most of the available information has been obtained in patients without renal disease, and the utility of these markers in the assessment of fracture risk in CKD and transplantation is extremely limited. They may, however, have an increasingly important role in the assessment of bone turnover rate. At present, parathyroid hormone (PTH) is the most frequently used biochemical surrogate for this, but measurement of biochemical markers of bone formation and resorption (bone-specific alkaline phosphatase and c-telopeptide are the most studied to date [6–8]) may allow more precise assessment of bone turnover rate, although their value in renal failure still needs to be confirmed [9–11]. At present these indirect measures fall somewhat short of the ideal, and the only truly reliable measure of bone turnover is bone biopsy following double tetracycline labelling *in vivo* [12, 13].

III. SUBSTRATE: THE CKD PATIENT AT THE TIME OF TRANSPLANTATION

The dialysed CKD population comes to transplantation with a degree of skeletal degradation that is variable but frequently severe. These patients manifest a spectrum of bone diseases collectively falling under the umbrella of renal osteodystrophy [14]. These diseases range from, at one extreme, severe hyperparathyroid bone disease with greatly accelerated bone turnover and extensive woven bone, to a pathologically low level of bone turnover (the adynamic bone disorder/adynamic bone disease/aplastic bone disease) at the other extreme. In the latter instance, parameters of bone formation and bone resorption are both depressed, and PTH concentration is either frankly low, or relatively so in the context of the uraemic environment [15]. At both these extremes there are important functional ramifications, the most important of which are reduction of BMD and greatly increased fracture risk [16, 17], although the correlation between BMD and fracture risk is not good in CKD and transplanted populations. This has obvious implications for clinical trials that have focused mainly on BMD as a surrogate of fracture risk. Patients with extremely low bone turnover also appear to suffer from the effects of an impaired ability to dispose of calcium loads (loss of skeletal buffering), with the result that episodes of hypercalcemia are frequent, as is the development of soft tissue calcification [18].

Current therapies for advanced CKD are dominated by control of hyperphosphatemia (using a combination of dialysis, diet, and phosphate binders) and judicious use of active metabolites of vitamin D (alfacalcidol, calcitriol, paricalcitol, doxercalciferol, and 22-oxacalcitriol) as replacement therapy for deficient endogenous calcitriol. These therapies, while often highly effective, have many imperfections, with the result that some patients continue to manifest excessively high or low serum parathyroid hormone levels, associated with undesirably high or low bone turnover rates. Current therapeutic strategies for the regulation of PTH, calcium, and phosphorus are designed to give the best possible chance of achieving normal bone turnover rates while minimizing the risk of soft tissue calcification [19]. In most patients these targets are not met, reflecting the inadequacies of the available therapies.

In addition to the negative skeletal impact of chronic uremia, a number of other factors may injure the skeleton in this patient population. Lack of mobility, tobacco consumption, diabetes (type 1 and type 2), and hypogonadism (affecting both men and women) are likely to be important contributors to adversity these patients face. It is not surprising, therefore, that reduction of BMD and an increase of fracture rate are prominent in the CKD setting and persist into the post-transplant period [20–22].

IV. POST-TRANSPLANT BONE DISEASES

A high proportion of recipients of solid-organ transplants are likely to manifest metabolic bone disease, with or without mechanical deterioration of the skeleton, and the condition is both severe and unusually complex in the kidney transplant recipient. The majority of kidney transplants take place after a considerable period of advanced and usually end-stage kidney disease treated by dialysis. Most of these patients have one of the several forms of renal osteodystrophy. After a renal transplant, some of them continue to manifest widely differing forms of osteodystrophy and, as is discussed in the chapter by Faugere and Malluche, different forms of osteodystrophy may coexist in the same patient [23].

For obvious reasons, in subjects with normal kidney (and hepatic, pulmonary, and cardiac) function, the emphasis has been on the progressive bone loss that occurs with aging and which predicts increased fracture rates [24, 25], morbidity, and mortality. Considerable progress has been made in identifying and refining effective treatments for this very large osteoporotic population. While these treatments remain far from perfect, a number of strategies now have a powerful evidence base [26] and the field remains in a state of evolution [27–29].

In contrast, patients with reduced levels of kidney function, whose metabolic bone disease has historically been termed renal osteodystrophy, have been the subject of intense study focused particularly on the florid disturbances to their mineral metabolism and calcium regulating hormones [30]. That these patients develop severe bone disease has been recognized for many decades, but until recently there has been surprisingly little focus on the issues of bone density, mechanical integrity, and the clinical sequelae thereof. In addition, there has been little integration between the focus on renal osteodystrophy in CKD and post–renal transplant populations, and that on low bone density and osteoporosis in the more general sense.

While osteoporotic fractures are very common and cause significant morbidity, occurring predominantly at the vertebrae or ribs (areas of predominant cancellous bone) [20, 31, 32], avascular necrosis is an extremely debilitating condition that affects the weight-bearing long bones. This latter disease, considered in depth in Chapter 19, is characterised by aseptic ischaemic death of osteoblasts and chondrocytes [33]. The subsequent resorption of necrotic tissue reduces bone strength and leads to the characteristic radiological changes (crescent-shaped subchondral lucency, bony collapse, and patchy areas of sclerosis) [34]. Joint space is initially preserved. The pathogenesis of this condition in transplant patients is related to glucocorticoids [35, 36] and possibly hyperparathyroidism [37]. Now that modern immunosuppressive regimens use lower doses of steroids than previously, the incidence has decreased [38]. The reader is referred to Chapter 19 for a more detailed discussion of the subject.

Calcineurin inhibitors are also associated with a particular painful bone syndrome. In this uncommon condition, periarticular pain is associated with soft-tissue swelling, no joint effusion, and vasomotor skin changes in affected areas. There are many aspects of this condition that are similar to Sudek's osteodystrophy or reflex sympathetic dystrophy (now termed "complex regional pain syndrome") [39, 40]. This condition is dose-dependent, however, and can often respond dramatically to reduction in calcineurin inhibitor dose [41]. Other therapies that have been shown to be effective (albeit in small studies) are calcium channel blockers [42], calcitonin, and bisphosphonates. Isotopic radionucleotide scanning and MRI can aid diagnosis of this condition. The pathogenesis is unknown, but intraosseous hypertension leading to bone infarction and osteonecrosis has been implicated by some authors [43].

A. Evolution of Skeletal Abnormalities Following Transplantation

Successful renal transplantation is the most effective treatment available for the uremic syndrome. Bone and mineral metabolism is dramatically improved in a number of ways. Phosphate excretory capacity is restored, which greatly reduces the overall level of stimulatory input to the parathyroid glands. The newly transplanted kidney synthesizes calcitriol promptly after transplantation, although often inadequately, particularly if the achievement level of kidney function is suboptimal (see Table 1). This provision of endogenous calcitriol contributes further to the reduction in parathyroid activity. Observational studies have shown that there is almost invariably a dramatic reduction in the serum PTH concentration following transplantation, but it is important to note that this is rarely complete [44].

TABLE 1 Effect of renal function

Uremia	Good graft	Poor graft/recurrent CKD
↓ Ca	↑ Ca	↓ Ca
↑ Pi	↓ Pi	↑ Pi
↓ calcitriol	↑ calcitriol	↓ calcitriol
↓ VDR	↑ VDR	↓ VDR
↓ Ca receptor	↑ Ca receptor	↓ Ca receptor
↑ PTH	↓ PTH	↑ PTH

VDR—vitamin D receptor; PTH—parathyroid hormone; Pi—inorganic phosphate

Thus even in cases where the allograft function is outstandingly good, PTH frequently remains slightly elevated [45]. In some patients, this persistent hyperparathyroidism is sufficient to generate overt hypercalcemia and probably results from increased parathyroid gland mass as a result of previous hyperplasia, complicated by the presence of unsuppressable areas of nodular hyperplasia [46]. In these areas, the abnormal parathyroid cells lack the machinery to respond appropriately to suppressive inputs from calcium and calcitriol as a result of under-expression of the extracellular calcium sensing receptor (CaR) and of the nuclear vitamin D receptor (VDR) [47]. Moreover, polymorphisms of the VDR may also contribute to persistence of hyperparathyroidism after renal transplant [44]. While the provision of adequate calcitriol by the transplanted kidney is likely to up-regulate both the VDR and the CaR, and the removal of uraemic toxins by the new kidney probably improves VDR function further, apoptosis in hyperplastic parathyroid glands is an extremely slow process. Reduction of parathyroid cell hypertrophy probably occurs promptly after successful transplantation; apoptotic reversal of the hyperplastic process is likely to be limited and of little or no clinical significance.

Despite the improvement of many factors driving renal osteodystrophy, fracture rates are substantially increased following kidney transplantation. The transplant procedure has the effect of taking a population of patients in whom fracture rates are already high and rendering them higher still. For example, women aged 25 to 44 who have undergone kidney transplantation suffer from fracture rates 18 times higher than in comparable individuals from the normal population [48]. In patients aged 45 to 64, the fracture rate is 34 times higher than in the normal population [48]. Other studies attest to the increase in fracture rate that occurs following renal transplantation [21, 22]. Meanwhile, a survey of lung transplant patients confirmed that chronic pain was more common in those with low bone mineral density and accompanied by significantly impaired quality of life [49].

Although data linking the causality of increased fracture risk to post-transplant bone loss are limited, a considerable number of observational studies have demonstrated rapid reduction of BMD during the first 3 to 12 months after transplantation [50] with partial and in some cases near complete stabilization thereafter [51]. The reduction of BMD during the early rapid phase of bone loss is sometimes spectacularly high, with evidence that diabetic recipients of kidney/pancreas transplants may fare even worse than non-diabetic transplant recipients [53]. Loss rates during the first 3 months as high as 20% per annum have been documented in some of the studies reported [52], although most reports have documented mean bone loss during the first year following transplantation at 5 to 10% [50, 54].

Of great importance is the observation that bone loss is nearly universal and that it is poorly predicted by pretransplant BMD [52]. Thus, measurement of bone mineral density at the time of transplantation is at best an imperfect predictor of the need for effective prophylaxis, and an argument can be made for the implementation of preventative strategies in all patients irrespective of baseline BMD, subject to safety and efficacy considerations.

Post–renal transplant hypophosphatemia is a long-recognized, common condition that, when severe, can have important implications for the skeleton [55]. Persistent hyperparathyroidism, relative vitamin D deficiency, and use of glucocorticoids and cyclosporine have all been implicated as possible causes. The identification of circulating phosphatonins in tumor-induced osteomalacia [56, 57], autosomal dominant hypophosphataemic rickets [58], and X-linked hypophosphatemia (via mutations to the PHEX gene) [59] raises the possibility that abnormalities of the regulatory system of renal phosphate proximal tubular transporters may also exist in some post-transplant patients. Certainly it has been shown that there is a PTH-independent humoral mediator in some post-transplant patients with hypophosphataemia [60]. The clinical consequence of hypophosphatemia is that patients are at further risk of osteomalacia and osteoporosis.

B. Pathogenesis of Post-Transplant Osteoporosis: The Role of Immunosuppressive Drugs

This topic is described in detail in other chapters. The combination of pre-existing osteodystrophy, persisting hyperparathyroidism, and hypophosphataemia after transplantation, and the posttransplant drug regimens that are used, leads to an unfortunate combination of decreased bone formation and increased bone resorption.

After transplantation, the effect of glucocorticoids on bone dominates the picture [61]. These drugs are powerful skeletal toxins even without pre-existing metabolic bone disease. Doses of prednisolone as low as 7.5mg daily are associated with significant reduction of bone density and increase of fracture rate [62]. At the cellular level, glucocorticoids reduce bone formation in transplanted patients by a number of direct mechanisms associated with increased apoptosis of osteoblasts, impaired osteoblastogenesis, and reduction of osteoblast number [63]. Several osteoblast gene products are down-regulated, including type 1 collagen, osteocalcin, bone morphogenetic proteins, and transforming growth factor β (TGF-β). Glucocorticoid-treated patients experience a decrease in osteoprotegerin (OPG) and an increase in receptor activated ligand for NFκβ (RANKL) production [64]. This leads to accelerated osteoclastogenesis. Glucocorticoid-treated patients also experience varying degrees of hypogonadatrophic hypogonadism, which adds additional impetus to the switch from bone formation to bone resorption. Finally, glucocorticoids may be associated with the development or augmentation of secondary hyperparathyroidism via a reduction in intestinal calcium absorption and an increase in calciuria.

The calcineurin inhibitors, cyclosporine [65] and tacrolimus [66], exhibit very powerful skeletal effects in some animal models, although in the clinical arena it has been harder to demonstrate clear-cut consequences of these agents. In part this almost certainly reflects the dominant role of glucocorticoids and the extremely complex metabolic environment that exists following kidney transplantation. Nevertheless, *in vivo* studies in rats have consistently shown the development of a severe high turnover osteopenia in cyclosporine- and tacrolimus-treated animals. Serum levels of osteocalcin and calcitriol were increased in these animals. Of note is that several antiresorptive therapies, in particular bisphosphonates, raloxifene, and estrogen, demonstrably attenuate the bone loss in this rat model [67, 68].

Of course, any negative impact of cyclosporine or tacrolimus must be seen in the context of the indirect skeletal benefits that result from these treatments. Calcineurin inhibitors have led to a dramatic reduction in the cumulative glucocorticoid exposure of transplant recipients. At present, the weight of evidence suggests that cyclosporin and tacrolimus probably differ little in their skeletal impact in recipients of kidney transplants. Furthermore, the negative impact of these agents, at least in renal transplant recipients, is probably relatively minor when compared to that of glucocorticoids. Nevertheless, the possibility remains that, by accelerating resorption in a group of patients with coexisting glucocorticoid-induced reduction of bone formation, calcineurin inhibitors may significantly exacerbate unwanted glucocorticoid effects.

Despite extensive use over several decades, there is no evidence that azathioprine has significant skeletal toxicity, and the same applies to mycophenolate mofetil. In both cases, however, it should be emphasized that their invariable deployment as part of a combination regimen could easily mask minor unwanted effects. Of note is that sirolimus, unlike the calcineurin inhibitors, has no adverse effect in the *in vivo* rat model [69, 70]. Human clinical data are lacking.

Finally, no convincing data have emerged to implicate the biological induction agents directly in the natural history of post-transplant bone disease. Indirectly, however, they may well be protective if their use results in reduced glucocorticoid exposure.

An important issue relating both to pathogenesis and to the development of clinical strategies is the heterogeneity of bone lesions seen in transplant recipients. Studies in which bone histology was examined have tended to make matters more complex rather than less. These issues are discussed at length in Chapter 13, but suffice to say that the bone lesions that develop in kidney transplant recipients are difficult to predict, either on the basis of the pretransplant bone disease or by means of indirect measures such as bone mineral density, PTH, direct biochemical markers of bone metabolism, or drug exposure [23]. A further problem is that strikingly different lesions may on occasion coexist in the same patient. These observations point to the great difficulty in devising appropriate treatment regimens, and the near certainty that protective strategies will have to be individualized and implemented with a much higher degree of sophistication than is presently the case.

V. MANAGEMENT

Prevention and treatment of the abnormalities of mineral and bone metabolism after renal transplantation must be considered in the knowledge that these patients almost invariably have chronic kidney disease with at least some reduction of renal function (see Table 2). Thus, the recommendations set out by many national bodies, such as the Kidney Disease Quality Outcomes Initiative (K/DOQI) clinical practice guidelines, for nontransplanted patients with CKD stages 3 and 4 that relate to the evaluation and treatment of disorders of calcium, phosphorus, and PTH metabolism may be equally relevant, albeit frequently forgotten, in transplanted patients [19]. Although not formally studied, it is our impression that basic management of uremic hyperparathyroidism, hyperphosphatemia, and acidosis is not a sufficiently high priority during routine follow-up after kidney transplantation.

Nonetheless, the kidney transplant patient faces particular problems that should be directly addressed. Early severe hypophosphatemia is common and can persist in some patients even 1 year after transplantation [71]. Phosphorus supplementation may be required to maintain a minimum serum phosphate concentration greater than 0.48 mmol/l in the short term and greater than 0.81 mmol/l in the long term. However, phosphorus supplementation leads to hyperparathyroidism when used to treat other hypophosphatemic states and could potentiate or delay the resolution of the increased PTH secretion that is commonly observed after kidney transplantation. It would therefore be sensible to titrate the dose of such supplements such that only the lowest necessary is prescribed. While hyperparathyroidism often improves after transplantation, despite normalization of serum creatinine concentration, it has been reported that PTH concentrations can remain high in approximately 50% of patients [45]. Thus, patients may also need supplementation with calcium and vitamin D analogs to suppress hyperparathyroidism and thereby lessen

TABLE 2 Drug therapies for post-transplant bone loss

Antiresorptives	Formation stimulators
Vitamin D	Fluoride
Calcium	PTH
Oestrogen	Growth hormone
Bisphosphonates	Anabolic steroids
Calcitonin	Calcimimetics (if PTH low)
SERMS	Calcilytics (via PTH)
Calcimimetics (if PTH high)[a]	
Osteoprotegerin	

[a] The effect of calcimimetics would depend on the initial PTH concentration. Elevated PTH would be reduced whereas PTH cycling might be induced if initial PTH was low.

phosphaturia. Parathyroid surgery may be required in a minority of cases despite successful renal transplantation.

A pragmatic approach to the issues just described would be to monitor serum calcium, phosphorous, and bicarbonate concentrations at a minimum of fortnightly intervals for the initial 3 months after transplantation and monthly thereafter until 1 year after transplant. PTH concentrations can be monitored less frequently; monthly for the first 3 months and quarterly until 1 year after transplant is reasonable. One year after transplantation, the intensity of monitoring can be titrated according to the level of kidney function, the severity of hyperparathyroidism, and the timing and type of therapeutic interventions.

Because of the important differences between the general osteoporosis population and the renal osteodystrophy population, the implications of a low BMD measurement in the transplant recipient, and in turn the appropriate clinical response to that measurement, are likely to be uncertain. It is generally accepted that minimizing exposure to glucocorticoids can reduce bone loss and osteonecrosis. Even so, the use of established agents of proven benefit in the treatment of postmenopausal women with osteoporosis is currently highly speculative with a remarkably weak evidence base, at least in terms of important clinical outcomes in transplant recipients. As indicated previously, identification of the patient most at risk of fracture requires an ability to measure the quality and strength of bone much more precisely than is presently the case. BMD measurement appears to be a much less robust surrogate for fracture in the CKD and transplant populations than it is in the osteoporosis population at large. Clinical decisions based solely on BMD measurement are, therefore, quite likely to be inappropriate. So also may be conclusions drawn from studies of preventative strategies in which BMD is used as the primary endpoint. The therapy may be quite effective at preventing the loss of BMD following transplantation, but this does not necessarily translate to a parallel reduction in fracture risk.

During the early phase of rapid bone loss, histological studies have generally shown that bone resorption rates are increased relative to bone formation [61, 63]. Despite the cautionary provisos given above, this suggests that antiresorptive agents would be a reasonable therapy, although perhaps not in all patients. Some precedent for this view comes from the extensive evidence showing that bisphosphonates effectively retard loss of bone density in glucocorticoid-treated patients without renal disease [72, 73], and from some studies showing a reduction of fracture risk as well [74]. Bisphosphonate use in the post-transplant setting has been reported in a number of studies and is now quite widely utilized in clinical practice, albeit on the basis of fairly weak evidence. The bisphosphonate studies have generally examined the protective effect of these agents given at the time of transplantation. Fan et al. [52] used a small dose of intravenous pamidronate in male renal transplant recipients. This was a fairly small, randomized, controlled study in which the untreated patients lost bone at a rate similar to that reported in previous observational studies. Pamidronate-treated patients experienced no significant reduction of bone mineral density during the one year study period (see Figure 1). The study was too small to assess clinical outcomes such as fracture risk. In a later report, Fan et al. [75] restudied the same patients 4 years after transplantation. No further bisphosphonate treatment had been given, and thus it was not wholly unexpected that patients who had received pamidronate 4 years earlier appeared to have lost less bone than controls (see Figure 2).

Other studies have looked at ibandronate and zoledronate. Intravenous ibandronate was given by Grotz et al. [76] in a randomized study of 80 patients. Bone mineral density decreased substantially in the untreated patients but not in those who received ibandronate. There was evidence of a reduction in vertebral fracture rate in ibandroante-treated patients as judged by vertebral morphometry in this study. Further, an entirely unexpected observation was an apparent decrease in the number of rejection episodes and enhanced graft survival in the ibandronate-treated patients. This observation remains unexplained and has not been reported in other studies. Zoledronate, a highly potent third-generation bisphosphonate, when given at the time of renal transplantation also slowed bone loss during the early post-transplant period, but these effects were not sustained over 3 years [77]. No adverse effects were reported in relation to pamidronate, ibandronate, or zoledronate in these studies, although bisphosphonates have been implicated rarely as a cause of acute renal failure (through acute tubular necrosis and collapsing focal segmental sclerosis) [65, 78].

Oral alendronate has been evaluated in the context of a controlled study in which 2 groups of patients received 2 grams of calcium daily and a small

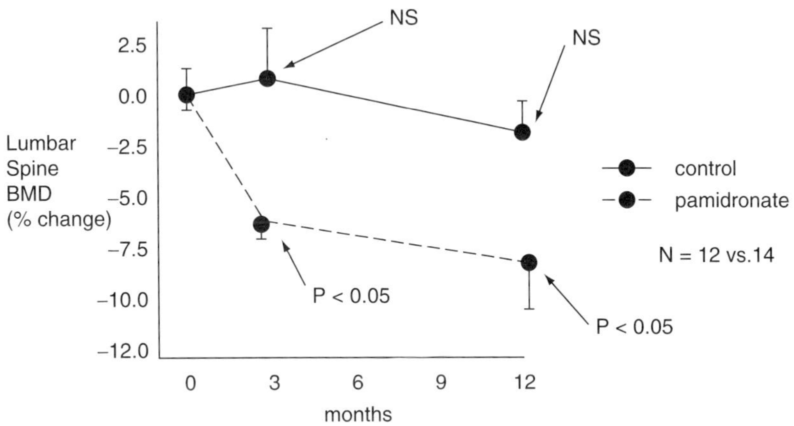

FIGURE 1 Loss of BMD following transplantation and protection using pamidronate given at 0.5 mg/kg BW at the time of transplantation and repeated 4 weeks later. Males only. Redrawn from Fan et al. (2000). Pamidronate therapy as prevention of bone loss following renal transplantation. *Kidney Int.* 57:684–690. Used with permission.

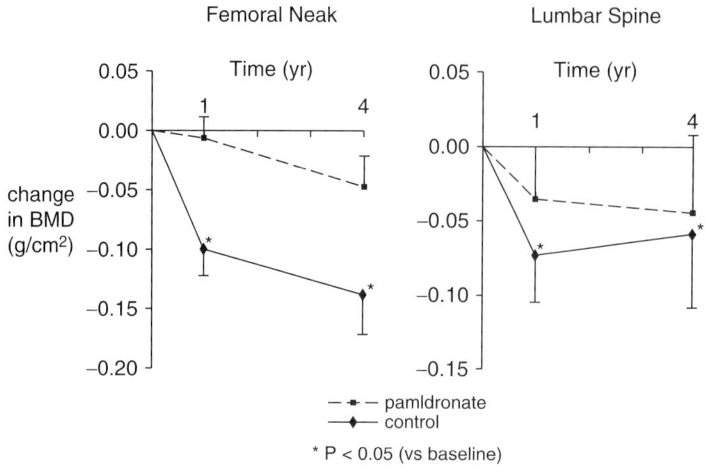

FIGURE 2 Long-term effects of early pamidronate (0.5 mg/kg BW) given at transplantation and repeated at 4 weeks. Redrawn from Fan et al. (2003). Long-term effects on bone mineral density of pamidronate given at the time of renal transplantation. *Kidney Int.* 63:2275–2279. Used with permission.

dose of calcitriol for 6 months after kidney transplantation. One of the groups additionally received alendronate. In this study, a striking disparity in BMD as an outcome measure was observed. Patients receiving alendronate with calcium and calcitriol experienced an increase in lumbar spine BMD of 6.3%, whereas those receiving just calcium and calcitriol experienced a reduction of 5.8% [79].

Antiresorptive therapy with calcitonin has yielded results less impressive than those obtained with bisphosphonates, with little or no convincing protection demonstrated [80]. Calcitonin is also expensive, and the need for parenteral administration is also a drawback in countries where the intranasal formulation is not available.

Studies using vitamin D and calcium, a regimen recommended by many national bodies and expert groups for patients receiving glucocorticoid treatment [81], appear to be ineffective in the setting of kidney transplantation. The use of calcitriol, however, appears to hold more promise [82], although the picture is mixed and far from convincing. On theoretical grounds at least, it would be expected that the utility of calcitriol in this setting could depend quite heavily on the level of graft function and thus on the adequacy or otherwise of endogenous calcitriol production. Studies of calcitriol may have suffered from this heterogeneity, and it is possible that calcitriol has a more important role in the subgroup of patients with demonstrably low endogenous calcitriol production rates. A further problem with calcitriol and other active vitamin D metabolites is their relatively narrow therapeutic window. It is extremely easy to induce hypercalcemia or hypercalciuria, both of which are highly undesirable in patients in whom the transplanted organ already faces a number of other threats from immunological and drug toxicity.

Estrogen and selective estrogen receptor modulators (SERMs) have not been evaluated as thoroughly as bisphosphonates. Results of studies using raloxifene in postmenopausal osteoporotic women are encouraging [83], but there are few data in renal transplant patients, and, particularly in light of increasing concern regarding safety of estrogen [84], it is difficult to recommend their use with the specific aim of improving skeletal health in transplant recipients. These patients are already at exceptionally high risk of cardiovascular disease, and the level of risk introduced by estrogen therapy in this context remains unclear.

A. Augmentation of Bone Formation

It would appear logical to use antiresorptive therapy as primary prevention against future fracture in transplant patients or as therapy for patients with evidence of osteoporosis and high bone turnover. However, many patients suffer atraumatic fractures despite "non-osteoporotic" BMD. Although unproven, therapy directed at correcting abnormalities of bone turnover irrespective of BMD might enhance bone quality and prevent future fractures. For patients with low bone turnover, therapies that might be appropriate are sodium fluoride and PTH, both powerful skeletal anabolic agents. Sodium fluoride has been shown in a number of studies to increase BMD substantially [85] and, at least when used judiciously in the context of its narrow therapeutic window, to reduce vertebral fracture rates [86]. Over-dosage is, however, a major concern, the consequences of which are evident in areas of endemic fluorosis, as well as in some of the earlier studies utilizing larger doses of sodium fluoride as treatment for osteoporosis. No studies examining the use of fluoride in renal transplant recipients have been published, although in a study of 203 cardiac transplant recipients given background therapy with calcium 1 g and calcidiol 25 micrograms daily, the addition of disodium monofluorophosphate led to significant increases in BMD [87]. Despite its potential, however, sodium fluoride treatment would be difficult and quite possibly hazardous in renal transplant patients, in whom multiple other drug therapies coupled with variable kidney function could profoundly affect fluoride clearance rates.

PTH has anabolic effects on the skeleton [88, 89]. Early studies in osteoporotic patients demonstrated clear increases in BMD [90, 91]. Following the development of synthetic human PTH 1-84 and the 1-34 N-terminal fragment in pharmaceutical form, a surge of additional evidence has attested to its efficacy in patients with documented osteoporosis [88, 92, 93]. Considerable increases in BMD have been reported, along with reduction of fracture rate. The applicability of this treatment in kidney transplant recipients is unclear. Many of these patients will have already suffered from the effects of excess PTH, and it is clear that when used therapeutically, PTH dose is important. Relatively small intermittent doses have a net anabolic effect on the skeleton, whereas prolonged high levels of PTH, as seen in uremia, are clearly net catabolic. Theoretically, PTH treatment seems most likely to be appropriate in renal transplant recipients in whom low PTH, together with other pointers, suggest the likelihood of low bone turnover. This would include previously parathyroidectomized patients. PTH injections might well increase bone turnover in these patients with useful consequences for both BMD and bone strength.

New oral therapies may allow this approach to be exploited indirectly. Calcimimetic agents, which increase the sensitivity of the extracellular calcium receptor (CaR) to ambient calcium concentration, thereby lowering both PTH and calcium simultaneously, are being evaluated in the CKD populations and appear to be highly effective treatments for hyperparathyroidism [94]. If their half-life is short, compounds of this type could be used to induce PTH cycling in a way that might augment bone formation. Likely candidates for this approach would be patients in whom unperturbed PTH remains modestly elevated; in these patients, intermittent dosing with a short-acting calcimimetic agent could be used to cycle PTH in a manner similar to the profile achieved with daily subcutaneous injections.

Calcilytic agents also act on the CaR, but in reverse fashion. Thus calcilytics decrease the sensitivity of the CaR to calcium, resulting in an increase in the secretion of PTH. These agents, used either alone or in combination with calcimimetics, might be capable of generating PTH cycling of greater amplitude than the calcimimetics alone. Anabolic effects on rat bone have been demonstrated [95]. The relevance to transplanted patients of therapies directly or indirectly involving PTH is highly speculative at this stage but merits further study.

Osteoprotegerin (OPG), the decoy receptor for RANKL, forms part of the final common path for the regulation of osteoclastogenesis. It has a central role in the maintenance of normal bone turnover, and abnormalities of RANKL-OPG balance have been implicated in many bone disease states including post-transplant osteoporosis. Thus, directly manipulating this effector pathway might prove to be a powerful tool for the manipulation of bone turnover. Single doses of recombinant OPG have been shown to have a sustained half-life and potent antiresorptive effects in rats [96].

Growth hormone is clearly of benefit in growth hormone–deficient adults, in the context of both their body composition and bone mineral density [97]. It is not clear at the moment whether these benefits can be achieved in patients with partial growth-hormone deficiency or in growth hormone–sufficient individuals. Further work will be needed to evaluate the role of growth hormone in this patient group.

B. Who Should Be Treated and How?

In this population, bone loss and fracture rate following transplantation are both so high that all patients must be considered at high risk. BMD measurement at the time of transplantation, while appearing to be a sensible precaution, in fact has little objective justification. This is mainly because of the poor correlation between BMD and fracture rate among transplant recipients, and also the lack of ability of baseline BMD to predict the magnitude of subsequent bone loss following transplantation. It is, therefore, hard to see how measurement of BMD would inform a decision as to which patients should receive prophylaxis. Because virtually all patients lose bone substantially in the early phase, neither is it logical to defer assessment to 6 or 12 months following transplantation and base therapeutic intervention on the magnitude of bone loss that has occurred. This is tantamount to shutting the stable door after the horse has bolted. It is clear from the available evidence that the decision as to whether or not to treat, and how to treat, should be made at the time of transplantation or very soon afterwards.

Based on currently available evidence, choice of therapy favors bisphosphonates on the grounds that the database justifying their use is greater than for any other intervention. They also have established benefit in preventing the reduction of BMD following transplantation, albeit with the proviso that there may or may not be a beneficial effect on fracture risk as well. The gains, therefore, are uncertain, and the decision to treat should be heavily weighted by the perceived level of toxicity and risk of treatment. Here the bisphosphonate experience is generally reassuring in the context of adverse clinical outcomes, since very little evidence exists of important skeletal or other toxicity of clinical importance. Against this must be set the undoubted concern that bisphosphonates remain in the skeleton for extended periods (many years) and that skeletal toxicity may, therefore, arise very late. Furthermore, with such a broad range of bone turnover in patients at the time of transplantation, the effect of a powerful antiresorptive agent given to, for example, a patient with adynamic bone disorder, needs to be considered very carefully. Histological evidence obtained in transplanted patients who have received bisphosphonate points to a considerable increase in the likelihood of low turnover lesions [98].

A reasonable compromise position, taking account both of the possible clinical benefit and the concern driven by histological studies, would be to give bisphosphonates only to those patients who have at least indirect evidence of normal or raised bone turnover at the time of transplantation. Ideally this would be based on bone histology at the time of transplantation, although this would be unrealistic in most cases. Practically speaking, this would be based on surrogates such as the degree of hyperparathyroidism as judged by serum PTH. (In one ongoing study conducted by the authors, patients with intact PTH of less than 150 pg/ml are excluded from treatment with bisphosphonates.) As discussed earlier, however, such a "one size fits all" approach to a condition as heterogeneous as post-transplant bone disease is illogical. Individualizing therapy according to risk stratification (including clinical predictors, bone mass, turnover, microarchitecture, and microfracture) will require a greater degree of sophistication than is currently achievable.

Most of the focus to date has been on the early period of rapid bone loss following transplantation. While it is certainly the case that this period probably offers the best opportunity for useful intervention, there remains a large body of established transplant recipients who collectively experience an extremely high fracture rate. Among renal transplant patients, a majority manifest varying degrees of CKD, and it is likely that many of these patients receive inadequate attention to what is, in effect, recurrence of uraemic renal osteodystrophy. Although robust evidence is lacking, conventional treatment using phosphate binders and vitamin D analogues to maintain plasma concentrations of calcium, phosphorus, and PTH within their respective target ranges is logical and probably has beneficial effects on bone turnover [99]. The best form of additional intervention in this group remains unclear, although certainly the combination of calcium, calcitriol, and alendronate has been found exceedingly effective in a single study to date [100]. Whether these patients should receive additional therapies, and upon what measures such therapy should be based, remains uncertain.

Hypogonadism, which is frequently present in transplanted patients, is almost certainly underinvestigated and undertreated. Judicious use of testosterone in hypogonadal males, especially those with low bone mineral density and a history of fracture, is likely to be reasonably safe and is certainly logical, albeit without a robust evidence base at this stage. Similar arguments can probably be advanced for hypogonadal women, although safety is a significant concern in such a high-risk population. It is difficult to recommend SERMs at this stage, there being no convincing evidence as to their efficacy in regard to either direct clinical or surrogate outcomes. Nevertheless, on theoretical grounds at least, raloxifene may have a role, and it should, along with estrogen and testosterone therapies in appropriate subpopulations, be evaluated in properly controlled studies.

Although much used in the pre-erythropoietin era, anabolic steroids in the CKD population are now used infrequently. Recently, however, a number of studies have attested to the benefits of anabolic steroid use in regard to hemoglobin, body composition, and general well-being [101]. In these studies, nandrolone was used and appeared well tolerated at doses of 100 mg per month. This approach has not been tested in the transplant population, but because these patients have a high prevalence of fragility fractures and nutritional deficiency and/or poor body composition, anabolic steroids certainly merit careful evaluation in selected subgroups.

C. Development of New Immune-Suppressive Regimens

There is little doubt that the principal villain of the piece to date has been the glucocorticoid component of immunosuppressive regimens. The effect of glucocorticoids on the skeleton sits very uncomfortably alongside the substrate of a skeleton damaged by longstanding CKD. The scenario may be further exacerbated by the concomitant use of calcineurin inhibitors. A major effort has been building over the past few years to develop immunosuppressive regimens that are at least as effective as current standard therapies, while engendering less toxicity. These regimens have frequently involved minimal and in some cases zero glucocorticoid exposure. It is likely that an important outcome of these developments will be less severe bone disease following transplantation. Sadly, however, the extensive industry-funded trials that have been conducted to evaluate new immunosuppressive agents have rarely included a skeletal dimension. Thus a great opportunity to evaluate the natural history of bone disease following transplantation in large numbers of patients, and at the same time develop a large and robust database, has been missed. It is to be hoped that those designing immunosuppressive protocols in the future will be cognizant of the importance of skeletal morbidity following transplantation and the potential benefits of new immunosuppressive agents and protocols in the avoidance of this often intractable problem.

REFERENCES

1. Cecka, J.M. (2002). The UNOS Renal Transplant Registry. *Clin Transpl.* 1-20.
2. Cunningham, J., Sprague, S.M., Cannata-Andia, J., Coco, M., Cohen-Solal, M., Fitzpatrick, L., et al. (2004). Osteoporosis in chronic kidney disease. *Am J Kidney Dis.* 43:566–571.
3. Anonymous. (2000). Osteoporosis prevention, diagnosis, and therapy. *NIH Consens Statement.* 17:1–45.
4. Karantanas, A.H., Kalef-Ezra, J.A., Sferopoulos, G., Siamopoulos, K.C. (1996). Quantitative computed tomography for spinal bone mineral measurements in chronic renal failure. *Br J Radiol.* 69:132–136.
5. Lechleitner, P., Krimbacher, E., Genser, N., Fridrich, L., Zur, N.D., Helweg, G., et al. (1994). Bone mineral densitometry in dialyzed patients: quantitative computed tomography versus dual photon absorptiometry. *Bone.* 15:387–391.
6. Takahashi, M., Naitou, K., Ohishi, T., Nagano, A. (2003). Comparison of biochemical markers of bone turnover and bone mineral density between hip fracture and vertebral fracture. *J Clin Densitom.* 6:211–218.
7. Delmas, P.D., Hardy, P., Garnero, P., Dain, M. (2000). Monitoring individual response to hormone replacement therapy with bone markers. *Bone.* 26:553–560.
8. Bollen, A.M., Kiyak, H.A., Eyre, D.R. (1997). Longitudinal evaluation of a bone resorption marker in elderly subjects. *Osteoporos Int.* 7:544–549.
9. Ferreira, M.A. (2000). Diagnosis of renal osteodystrophy: when and how to use biochemical markers and non-invasive methods; when bone biopsy is needed. *Nephrol Dial Transplant.* 15 Suppl 5:8–14.
10. Siggelkow, H., Eidner, T., Lehmann, G., Viereck, V., Raddatz, D., Munzel, U., et al. (2003). Cytokines, osteoprotegerin, and RANKL in vitro and histomorphometric indices of bone turnover in patients with different bone diseases. *J Bone Miner Res.* 18:529–538.
11. Urena, P., Hruby, M., Ferreira, A., Ang, K.S., De Vernejoul, M.C. (1996). Plasma total versus bone alkaline phosphatase as markers of bone turnover in hemodialysis patients. *J Am Soc Nephrol.* 7:506–512.

12. Martin, K.J., Olgaard, K., Coburn, J.W., Coen, G.M., Fukagawa, M., Langman, C., et al. (2004). Diagnosis, assessment, and treatment of bone turnover abnormalities in renal osteodystrophy. *Am J Kidney Dis*. 43:558–565.
13. Trueba, D., Sawaya, B.P., Mawad, H., Malluche, H.H. (2003). Bone biopsy: indications, techniques, and complications. *Semin Dial*. 16:341–345.
14. Hruska, K.A., Teitelbaum, S.L. (1995). Renal osteodystrophy. *N Engl J Med*. 333:166–174.
15. Hruska, K.A. (1997). Renal osteodystrophy. *Baillieres Clin Endocrinol Metab*. 11:165–194.
16. Coco, M., Rush, H. (2000). Increased incidence of hip fractures in dialysis patients with low serum parathyroid hormone. *Am J Kidney Dis*. 36:1115–1121.
17. Lindberg, J.S., Moe, S.M. (1999). Osteoporosis in end-state renal disease. *Semin Nephrol*. 19:115–122.
18. Parfitt, A.M. (2003). Renal bone disease: a new conceptual framework for the interpretation of bone histomorphometry. *Curr Opin Nephrol Hypertens*. 12:387–403.
19. Renal Association Standards Subcommittee. Treatment of adult patients with renal failure: recommended standards and audit measures, 3rd ed. London: Royal College of Physicians, 2 A.D.
20. Durieux, S., Mercadal, L., Orcel, P., Dao, H., Rioux, C., Bernard, M., et al. (2002). Bone mineral density and fracture prevalence in long-term kidney graft recipients. *Transplantation*. 74:496–500.
21. Grotz, W.H., Mundinginger, F.A., Gugel, B., Exner, V., Kirste, G., Schollmeyer, P. (1994). Bone fracture and osteodensitometry with dual energy X-ray absorpiometry in kidney transplant recipients. *Transplantation*. 58:912–915.
22. Nisbeth, U., Lindh, E., Ljunghall, S., Backman, U., Fellstrom, B. (1999). Increased fracture rate in diabetes mellitus and females after renal transplantation. *Transplantation*. 67:1218–1222.
23. Monier-Faugere, M.C., Mawad, H., Qi, Q., Friedler, R.M., Malluche, H.H. (2000). High prevalence of low bone turnover and occurrence of osteomalacia after kidney transplantation. *J Am Soc Nephrol*. 11:1093–1099.
24. Cummings, S.R., Black, D.M., Nevitt, M.C., Browner, W., Cauley, J., Ensrud, K., et al. (1993). Bone density at various sites for prediction of hip fracture. *Lancet*. 341:72–75.
25. Marshall, D., Johnell, O., Wedel, H. (1996). Meta-analysis of how well measures of bone mineral density predict occurrence of osteoporotic fractures. *BMJ*. 312:1254–1259.
26. Eastell, R. (1998). Treatment of postmenopausal osteoporosis. *N Engl J Med*. 338:736–746.
27. Cuddihy, M.T., Gabriel, S.E., Crowson, C.S., Atkinson, E.J., Tabini, C., O'Fallon, W.M., et al. (2002). Osteoporosis intervention following distal forearm fractures: a missed opportunity. *Arch Intern Med*. 162:421–426.
28. Heaney, R.P. (2003). Is the paradigm shifting. *Bone*. 33:457–465.
29. Robert, P., Heaney, R.P. (2003). Remodeling and skeletal fragility. *Osteoporos Int*. 14:12–15.
30. Torres, A., Lorenzo, V., Salido, E. (2002). Calcium metabolism and skeletal problems after transplantation. *J Am Soc Nephrol*. 13:551–558.
31. Collier, J. (2002). Commentary on: Bone mineral density and fracture prevalence in long-term kidney graft recipients. *Transplantation*. 74:438–439.
32. Patel, S., Kwan, J.T., McCloskey, E., McGee, G., Thomas, G., Johnson, D., et al. (2001). Prevalence and causes of low bone density and fractures in kidney transplant patients. *J Bone Miner Res*. 16:1863–1870.
33. Metselaar, H.J., van Steenberge, E.J., Bijnen, A.B., Jeekel, J.J., van Linge, B., Weimar, W. (1985). Incidence of osteonecrosis after renal transplantation. *Acta Orthop Scand*. 56:413–415.
34. Zizic, T.M. (1991). Osteonecrosis. *Curr Opin Rheumatol*. 3:481–489.

35. Mankin, H.J. (1992). Nontraumatic necrosis of bone (osteonecrosis). *N Engl J Med.* 326:1473–1479.
36. Chang, C.C., Greenspan, A., Gershwin, M.E. (1993). Osteonecrosis: current perspectives on pathogenesis and treatment. *Semin Arthritis Rheum.* 23:47–69.
37. Nehme, D., Rondeau, E., Paillard, F., Moreau, J.F., Nussaume, O., Kanfer, A., et al. (1989). Aseptic necrosis of bone following renal transplantation: relation with hyperparathyroidism. *Nephrol Dial Transplant.* 4:123–128.
38. Parfrey, P.S., Farge, D., Parfrey, N.A., Hanley, J.A., Guttman, R.D. (1986). The decreased incidence of aseptic necrosis in renal transplant recipients—a case control study. *Transplantation.* 41:182–187.
39. Munoz-Gomez, J., Collado, A., Gratacos, J., Campistol, J.M., Lomena, F., Llena, J., et al. (1991). Reflex sympathetic dystrophy syndrome of the lower limbs in renal transplant patients treated with cyclosporin A. *Arthritis Rheum.* 34:625–630.
40. Torregrosa, J.V., Campistol, J.M. (1999). Reflex sympathetic dystrophy syndrome in renal transplant patients: a mysterious and misdiagnosed entity. *Nephrol Dial Transplant.* 14:1364–1365.
41. Ybarra, J., Crespo, M., Torregrosa, J.V., Fuster, D., Campistol, J.M., Oppenheimer, F. (2003). Reflex sympathetic dystrophy syndrome in renal transplanted patients under immunosuppression with tacrolimus. *Transplant Proc.* 35:2937–2939.
42. Gauthier, V.J., Barbosa, L.M. (1994). Bone pain in transplant recipients responsive to calcium channel blockers. *Ann Intern Med.* 121:863–865.
43. Zizic, T.M. (1990). Avascular necrosis of bone. *Curr Opin Rheumatol.* 2:26–37.
44. Messa, P., Sindici, C., Cannella, G., Miotti, V., Risaliti, A., Gropuzzo, M., et al. (1998). Persistent secondary hyperparathyroidism after renal transplantation. *Kidney Int.* 54:1704–1713.
45. Pietschmann, P., Vychytil, A., Woloszczuk, W., Kovarik, J. (1991). Bone metabolism in patients with functioning kidney grafts: increased serum levels of osteocalcin and parathyroid hormone despite normalisation of kidney function. *Nephron.* 59:533–536.
46. Parfitt, A.M. (1982). Hypercalcemic hyperparathyroidism following renal transplantation: differential diagnosis, management, and implications for cell population control in the parathyroid gland. *Miner Electrolyte Metab.* 8:92–112.
47. Slatopolsky, E., Brown, A., Dusso, A. (1999). Pathogenesis of secondary hyperparathyroidism. *Kidney Int.* Suppl 73:S14-S19.
48. Ramsey-Goldman, R., Dunn, J.E., Dunlop, D.D., Stuart, F.P., Abecassis, M.M., Kaufman, D.B., et al. (1999). Increased risk of fracture in patients receiving solid organ transplants. *J Bone Miner Res.* 14:456–463.
49. Dodd, V.A., Staron, R.B., Papadopoulos, A., Evans, L., Schulman, L.L., Jorgensen, B., et al. (1999). Bone densitometry should be included in the evaluation of candidates for lung transplantation. *J Transpl Coord.* 9:119–123.
50. Almond, M.K., Kwan, J.T., Evans, K., Cunningham, J. (1994). Loss of regional bone mineral density in the first 12 months following renal transplantation. *Nephron.* 66:52–57.
51. Grotz, W.H., Mundinger, F.A., Gugel, B., Exner, V.M., Kirste, G., Schollmeyer, P.J. (1995). Bone mineral density after kidney transplantation: a cross-sectional study in 190 graft recipients up to 20 years after transplantation. *Transplantation.* 59:982–986.
52. Fan, S.L.-S., Almond, M.K., Ball, E., Evans, K., Cunningham, J. (2000). Pamidronate therapy as prevention of bone loss folowing renal transplantation. *Kidney Int.* 57:684–690.
53. Chiu, M.Y., Sprague, S.M., Bruce, D.S., Woodle, E.S., Thistlethwaite J.R.J., Josephson, M.A. (1998). Analysis of fracture prevalence in kidney-pancreas allograft recipients. *J Am Soc Nephrol.* 9:677–683.
54. Dalen, N., Alvestrand, A. (1973). Bone mineral content in chronic renal failure and after renal transplantation. *Clin Nephrol.* 1:338–346.

55. Moorhead, J.F., Wills, M.R., Ahmed, K.Y., Baillod, R.A., Varghese, Z., Tatler, G.L. (1974). Hypophosphataemic osteomalacia after cadaveric renal transplantation. *Lancet*. 1:694–697.
56. Strewler, G.J. (2001). FGF23, hypophosphatemia, and rickets: has phosphatonin been found. *Proc Natl Acad Sci U S A*. 98:5945–5946.
57. Fukumoto, S., Yamashita, T. (2002). Fibroblast growth factor-23 is the phosphaturic factor in tumor-induced osteomalacia and may be phosphatonin. *Curr Opin Nephrol Hypertens*. 11:385–389.
58. White, K.E., Jonsson, K.B., Carn, G., Hampson, G., Spector, T.D., Mannstadt, M., et al. (2001). The autosomal dominant hypophosphatemic rickets (ADHR) gene is a secreted polypeptide overexpressed by tumors that cause phosphate wasting. *J Clin Endocrinol Metab*. 86:497–500.
59. Drezner, M.K. (2000). PHEX gene and hypophosphatemia. *Kidney Int*. 57:9–18.
60. Green, J., Debby, H., Lederer, E., Levi, M., Zajicek, H.K., Bick, T. (2001). Evidence for a PTH-independent humoral mechanism in post-transplant hypophosphatemia and phosphaturia. *Kidney Int*. 60:1182–1196.
61. Julian, B.A., Laskow, D.A., Dubovsky, J., Dubovsky, E.V., Curtis, J.J., Quarles, L.D. (1991). Rapid loss of verebral mineral density after renal transplantation. *N Eng J Med*. 325:544–50.
62. Van Staa, T.P., Leufkens, H.G., Abenhaim, L., Zhang, B., Cooper, C. (2000). Use of oral corticosteroids and risk of fractures. *J Bone Miner Res*. 15:993–1000.
63. Rojas, E., Carlini, R.G., Clesca, P., Arminio, A., Suniaga, O., De Elguezabal, K., et al. (2003). The pathogenesis of osteodystrophy after renal transplantation as detected by early alterations in bone remodeling. *Kidney Int*. 63:1915–1923.
64. Sasaki, N., Kusano, E., Ando, Y., Yano, K., Tsuda, E., Asano, Y. (2001). Glucocorticoid decreases circulating osteoprotegerin (OPG): possible mechanism for glucocorticoid induced osteoporosis. *Nephrol Dial Transplant*. 16:479–482.
65. Movsowitz, C., Epstein, S., Fallon, M., Ismail, F., Thomas, S. (1988). Cyclosporin A in vivo produces severe osteopenia in the rat. Effect of dose and duration of administration. *Endocrinology*. 123:2571–2577.
66. Cvetkovic, M., Mann, G.N., Romero, D.F., Liang, X.G., Ma, Y., Jee, W.S., et al. (1994). The deleterious effects of long-term cyclosporine A, cyclosporine G, and FK506 on bone mineral metabolism in vivo. *Transplantation*. 57:1231–1237.
67. Bowman, A.R., Sass, D.A., Marshall, I., Ma, Y.F., Liang, H., Jee, W.S., et al. (1996). Raloxifene analog (LY117018 HCL) ameliorates cyclosporin A-induced osteopenia in oophorectomized rats. *J Bone Miner Res*. 11:1191–1198.
68. Sass, D.A., Bowman, A.R., Yuan, Z., Ma, Y., Jee, W.S., Epstein, S. (1997). Alendronate prevents cyclosporin A-induced osteopenia in the rat. *Bone*. 21:65–70.
69. Romero, D.F., Buchinsky, F.J., Rucinski, B., Cvetkovic, M., Bryer, H.P., Liang, X.G., et al. (1995). Rapamycin: a bone sparing immunosuppressant. *J Bone Miner Res*. 10:760–768.
70. Joffe, I., Katz, I., Sehgal, S., Bex, F., Kharode, Y., Tamasi, J., et al. (1993). Lack of change of cancellous bone volume with short-term use of the new immunosuppressant rapamycin in rats. *Calcif Tissue Int*. 53:45–52.
71. Felsenfeld, A.J., Gutman, R.A., Drezner, M., Llach, F. (1986). Hypophosphatemia in long-term renal transplant recipients: effects on bone histology and 1,25-dihydroxy-cholecalciferol. *Miner Electrolyte Metab*. 12:333–341.
72. Cohen, S., Levy, R.M., Keller, M., Boling, E., Emkey, R.D., Greenwald, M., et al. (1999). Risedronate therapy prevents corticosteroid-induced bone loss: a twelve-month, multicenter, randomized, double-blind, placebo-controlled, parallel-group study. *Arthritis Rheum*. 42:2309–2318.
73. Sambrook, P.N., Kotowicz, M., Nash, P., Styles, C.B., Naganathan, V., Henderson-Briffa, K.N., et al. (2003). Prevention and treatment of glucocorticoid-induced osteoporosis: a comparison of calcitriol, vitamin D plus calcium, and alendronate plus calcium. *J Bone Miner Res*. 18:919–924.

74. Miller, P.D. (2001). Bisphosphonates for the prevention and treatment of corticosteroid-induced osteoporosis. *Osteoporos Int.* 12 Suppl 3:S3-10.
75. Fan, S.L., Kumar, S., Cunningham, J. (2003). Long-term effects on bone mineral density of pamidronate given at the time of renal transplantation. *Kidney Int.* 63:2275–2279.
76. Grotz, W., Nagel, C., Poeschel, D., Cybulla, M., Petersen, K.G., Uhl, M., et al. (2001). Effect of ibandronate on bone loss and renal function after kidney transplantation. *J Am Soc Nephrol.* 12:1530–1537.
77. Schwarz, C., Mitterbauer, C., Heinze, G., Woloszczuk, W., Haas, M., Oberbauer, R. (2004). Nonsustained effect of short-term bisphosphonate therapy on bone turnover three years after renal transplantation. *Kidney Int.* 65:304–309.
78. Rodd, C. (1904). Bisphosphonates in dialysis and transplantation patients: efficacy and safety issues. *Perit Dial Int.* 21 Suppl 3:S256-S260.
79. Kovac, D., Lindic, J., Kandus, A., Bren, A.F. (2001). Prevention of bone loss in kidney graft recipients. *Transplant Proc.* 33:1144–1145.
80. Grotz, W.H., Rump, L.C., Niessen, A., Schmidt-Gayk, H., Reichelt, A., Kirste, G., et al. (1998). Treatment of osteopenia and osteoporosis after kidney transplantation. *Transplantation.* 66:1004–1008.
81. Eastell, R., Reid, D.M., Compston, J., Cooper, C., Fogelman, I., Francis, R.M., et al. (1998). A UK Consensus Group on management of glucocorticoid-induced osteoporosis: an update. *J Intern Med.* 244:271–292.
82. De Sevaux, R.G., Hoitsma, A.J., Corstens, F.H., Wetzels, J.F. (2002). Treatment with vitamin D and calcium reduces bone loss after renal transplantation: a randomized study. *J Am Soc Nephrol.* 13:1608–1614.
83. Kanis, J.A., Johnell, O., Black, D.M., Downs RWJ, Sarkar, S., Fuerst, T., et al. (2003). Effect of raloxifene on the risk of new vertebral fracture in postmenopausal women with osteopenia or osteoporosis: a reanalysis of the Multiple Outcomes of Raloxifene Evaluation trial. *Bone.* 33:293–300.
84. Anonymous. (2002). Risks and benefits of estrogen plus progestin in healthy postmenopausal women: principal results From the Women's Health Initiative randomized controlled trial. *JAMA.* 288:321–333.
85. Morabito, N., Gaudio, A., Lasco, A., Vergara, C., Tallarida, F., Crisafulli, G., et al. (2003). Three-year effectiveness of intravenous pamidronate versus pamidronate plus slow-release sodium fluoride for postmenopausal osteoporosis. *Osteoporos Int.* 14:500–506.
86. Ringe, J.D., Setnikar, I. (2002). Monofluorophosphate combined with hormone replacement therapy in postmenopausal osteoporosis: an open-label pilot efficacy and safety study. *Rheumatol Int.* 22:27–32.
87. Meys, E., Terreaux-Duvert, F., Beaume-Six, T., Dureau, G., Meunier, P.J. (1993). Bone loss after cardiac transplantation: effects of calcium, calcidiol and monofluorophosphate. *Osteoporos Int.* 3:322–329.
88. Hodsman, A.B., Hanley, D.A., Ettinger, M.P., Bolognese, M.A., Fox, J., Metcalfe, A.J., et al. (2003). Efficacy and safety of human parathyroid hormone-(1-84) in increasing bone mineral density in postmenopausal osteoporosis. *J Clin Endocrinol Metab.* 88:5212–5220.
89. Frolik, C.A., Black, E.C., Cain, R.L., Satterwhite, J.H., Brown-Augsburger, P.L., Sato, M., et al. (2003). Anabolic and catabolic bone effects of human parathyroid hormone (1-34) are predicted by duration of hormone exposure. *Bone.* 33:372–379.
90. Mitlak, B.H., Williams, D.C., Bryant, H.U., Paul, D.C., Neer, R.M. (1992). Intermittent administration of bovine PTH-(1-34) increases serum 1,25-dihydroxyvitamin D concentrations and spinal bone density in senile (23 month) rats. *J Bone Miner Res.* 7:479–484.
91. Slovik, D.M., Rosenthal, D.I., Doppelt, S.H., Potts J.T.J., Daly, M.A., Campbell, J.A., et al. (1986). Restoration of spinal bone in osteoporotic men by treatment with human parathyroid hormone (1-34) and 1,25-dihydroxyvitamin D. *J Bone Miner Res.* 1:377–381.

92. Cappuzzo, K.A., Delafuente, J.C. (2004). Teriparatide for severe osteoporosis. *Ann Pharmacother.* 38:294–302.
93. Neer, R.M., Arnaud, C.D., Zanchetta, J.R., Prince, R., Gaich, G.A., Reginster, J.Y., et al. (2001). Effect of parathyroid hormone (1-34) on fractures and bone mineral density in postmenopausal women with osteoporosis. *N Engl J Med.* 344:1434–1441.
94. Block, G.A., Martin, K.J., de Francisco, A.L., Turner, S.A., Avram, M.M., Suranyi, M.G., et al. (2004). Cinacalcet for secondary hyperparathyroidism in patients receiving hemodialysis. *N Engl J Med.* 350:1516–1525.
95. Gowen, M., Stroup, G.B., Dodds, R.A., James, I.E., Votta, B.J., Smith, B.R., et al. (2000). Antagonizing the parathyroid calcium receptor stimulates parathyroid hormone secretion and bone formation in osteopenic rats. *J Clin Invest.* 105:1595–1604.
96. Capparelli, C., Morony, S., Warmington, K., Adamu, S., Lacey, D., Dunstan, C.R., et al. (2003). Sustained antiresorptive effects after a single treatment with human recombinant osteoprotegerin (OPG): a pharmacodynamic and pharmacokinetic analysis in rats. *J Bone Miner Res.* 18:852–858.
97. Weaver, J.U., Monson, J.P., Noonan, K., John, W.G., Edwards, A., Evans, K.A., et al. (1995). The effect of low dose recombinant human growth hormone replacement on regional fat distribution, insulin sensitivity, and cardiovascular risk factors in hypopituitary adults. *J Clin Endocrinol Metab.* 80:153–159.
98. Coco, M., Glicklich, D., Faugere, M.C., Burris, L., Bognar, I., Durkin, P., et al. (2003). Prevention of bone loss in renal transplant recipients: a prospective, randomized trial of intravenous pamidronate. *J Am Soc Nephrol.* 14:2669–2676.
99. Cueto-Manzano, A.M., Konel, S., Freemont, A.J., Adams, J.E., Mawer, B., Gokal, R., et al. (2000). Effect of 1,25-dihydroxyvitamin D3 and calcium carbonate on bone loss associated with long-term renal transplantation. *Am J Kidney Dis.* 35:227–236.
100. Giannini, S., Dangel, A., Carraro, G., Nobile, M., Rigotti, P., Bonfante, L., et al. (2001). Alendronate prevents further bone loss in renal transplant recipients. *J Bone Miner Res.* 16:2111–2117.
101. Navarro, J.F., Mora, C., Macia, M., Garcia, J. (2002). Randomized prospective comparison between erythropoietin and androgens in CAPD patients. *Kidney Int.* 61:1537–1544.

CHAPTER 13

Histologic Abnormalities of Bone before and after Kidney Transplantation

Marie-Claude Monier-Faugere,
Hartmut H. Malluche, MD
Division of Nephrology, University of Kentucky Medical Center,
Lexington, KY

The bone diseases that develop after solid-organ transplantation have generated a great deal of interest because of (1) the severity of their complications, especially osteoporosis, which leads to increased risk of bone pain and fractures, (2) the increasing number of transplanted patients, (3) the prolonged survival rate, (4) the addition of new immunosuppressive drugs that may lessen the need for glucocorticoids, and (5) the availability of new FDA-approved therapeutic agents that could prevent or treat the transplant-related osteoporosis.

All solid-organ transplantations share the deleterious impact of immunotherapy, in particular glucocorticoids, on calcium and bone metabolism. However, bone disease after kidney transplantation is unique. At the time of transplantation, kidney transplant recipients already suffer from various forms of renal osteodystrophy, that is, abnormalities in bone volume, bone turnover, and bone mineralization [1–3] that might affect post-transplant bone disease. Also, even though renal function improves after kidney transplantation, patients may still show various degrees of renal insufficiency, which may worsen over time and may impact bone. Moreover, the number of diabetic patients on chronic dialysis undergoing kidney transplantation has increased [4]. Types I and II diabetic patients have been shown to be at increased risk for fractures, especially hip fractures [5], and to have low bone turnover [6, 7].

Due to the complexity of the factors involved in post-transplant bone disease, it is useful to describe bone status at time of transplantation and the changes that occur thereafter.

I. PRETRANSPLANT BONE DISEASE

A. Renal Osteodystrophy

Despite a mostly common initial pathogenic pathway, renal osteodystrophy is not a uniform bone disease. The forms of renal osteodystrophy comprise: (1) predominant hyperparathyroid bone disease, (2) low-turnover bone disease including osteomalacia and adynamic bone disease, and (3) mixed uremic osteodystrophy. Transformation from one form to another can occur [8].

1. Predominant Hyperparathyroid Bone Disease

Predominant hyperparathyroid bone disease (PHBD) is characterized by a marked increase in bone turnover. Irregularly-shaped trabeculae display numerous abnormal remodeling sites, and an unusually high number of bone cells that are irregular in arrangement and shape.

Deep, irregular resorption cavities often dissect or tunnel through the trabeculae. Numerous enlarged osteoclasts contain multiple nuclei with prominent nucleoli. Osteoblast shape changes from cuboidal to polygonal or spindle-shaped. The usual palisade-like monolayer of osteoblasts can be replaced by atypical multilayered arrangements of cells with variable orientation toward the bone surface. Osteoid surface and volume increase, and osteoid seams can thicken because of collagen overproduction. The resulting osteoid is primarily of the woven, irregular type. Because collagen fibers accumulate toward the bone surfaces and are deposited between osteoblasts and toward the bone marrow, peritrabecular and bone marrow fibrosis result. In advanced cases, fibrosis replaces the bone marrow entirely. Numerous irregular osteocytic lacunae within woven osteoid and mineralized bone result from the increased number of osteoblasts entrapped in bone, and the mineral apposition rate and the extent and number of mineralizing sites are notably increased. Calcium deposition in woven osteoid proceeds diffusely, irregularly, and incompletely.

A marked increase in bone turnover often leads to cancellization of the cortical bone. This causes a net decrease in cortical bone volume most evident in the appendicular skeleton. PHBD is usually associated with high bone volume, but malnutrition, immobilization, or other factors can markedly reduce bone volume. Also, areas of high bone mass may be adjacent to pseudocysts consisting primarily of hyperplastic or fibrotic bone marrow. In any case, bone strength cannot be equated with high bone volume in PHBD patients because the irregular trabeculae may lose their proper three-dimensional architecture and connectivity. Also, the poorly mineralized trabeculae consist mainly of mechanically deficient woven bone, resulting in a propensity to fracture. This disease creates particularly fragile, fracture-prone bone; thus, the use of the term "osteosclerosis" is inappropriate.

2. *Low-Turnover Bone Diseases*

Representing the other end of the spectrum from PHBD, low-turnover renal osteodystrophy is marked by a profound decrease in active remodeling sites. There are two separate entities, low-turnover osteomalacia (LTOM) and adynamic bone disease (ABD).

LTOM is characterized by an accumulation of unmineralized matrix in which a diminution in mineralization precedes or is more pronounced than the inhibition of collagen deposition. Although bone volume/tissue volume may vary, mineralized bone volume is always low. The increased lamellar osteoid volume results from the presence of wide osteoid seams that cover much of the trabecular surface. Most of the trabecular surfaces are covered by lining cells. The occasional presence of woven bone buried within the trabeculae indicates past high bone turnover. Osteoclasts, when present, are usually seen within trabecular bone or at the small fraction of trabecular surface left without osteoid covering.

With ABD, bone volume is frequently reduced. Reduced mineralization is coupled with a parallel decrease in bone formation. ABD is characterized by few osteoid seams and few osteoblasts. Osteoclast number may be low normal or elevated.

3. *Mixed Uremic Osteodystrophy*

Mixed uremic osteodystrophy (MUO) is caused primarily by defective mineralization with or without increased bone formation and by increased parathyroid hormone activity on bone, features that may coexist to varying degrees in different patients. Bone volume is extremely variable and depends on the dominant pathogenic cause. Other features include increased numbers of remodeling sites and usually an increase in osteoclasts. Active foci with numerous cells, peritrabecular fibrosis, and woven osteoid seams coexist with adjacent lamellar sites with a lower cellular activity. Therefore, greater production of lamellar or woven osteoid causes the accumulation of osteoid with normal or increased thickness of osteoid seams. Although active mineralizing surfaces are often present in woven bone with higher mineralization rate and diffuse labeling, mineralization surfaces may be low in lamellar bone with a low mineral apposition rate.

4. *Evolution of Renal Osteodystrophy*

In the past, diversity in bone lesions was partly attributed to the accumulation of aluminum in bone with resulting aluminum toxicity. The major sources of aluminum contamination in ESRD patients are aluminum-containing phosphate binders and high aluminum content of water and dialysate. High morbidity and mortality accompany severe aluminum intoxication.

Today, aluminum dialysate content is under better control, and aluminum-containing phosphate binders have largely been replaced with calcium salts or other phosphate binders. To overcome parathyroid gland overactivity, therapeutic regimens ensuring better control of serum calcium and phosphorus levels and correction of calcitriol deficiency are also widely used.

In a study in which the changing pattern of renal osteodystrophy was analyzed in 2,248 patients over 13 years, distribution of the four histological forms varied [9]. MUO was initially found in the majority of patients, but a decrease has occurred in recent years. LTOM is now seen in few patients. Bone abnormalities are now polarized in patients on dialysis. Most patients present with either variable degrees of hyperparathyroidism or adynamic bone disease. The number of patients with ABD, which was first described in 1984, has increased markedly and now affects 30–50% of the dialysis population, depending on the center. Patients with this abnormality have abnormal calcium homeostasis [10], higher incidence of fractures, more bone pain, delayed fracture healing, and higher morbidity and mortality than those exhibiting other histological abnormalities [11].

II. POST–KIDNEY TRANSPLANT BONE DISEASE

A. Histological Aspects of Post–Kidney Transplant Bone Disease

1. Bone Loss

Bone loss after kidney transplantation is a well-established phenomenon. Rapid bone loss can be demonstrated as soon as 6 months to 1 year after grafting [12–14], with lower rates of bone loss thereafter (up to 10 years) [15–17]. Glucocorticoid therapy has been shown to be one of the main factors responsible for post-transplant bone loss (*vide infra*). An indirect corroboration to this statement is provided by the results of a study by Briner et al. [18]. In this study, efforts were made to keep doses of glucocorticoids, as well as duration of glucocorticoid treatment, to a minimum. On average, there was no decrease in bone volume. Those patients who lost bone had high bone volume at the time of transplantion and reached normal values one year after grafting. Those patients with low bone volume at transplantation increased into the normal range by the end of the study [18].

2. Alterations in Bone Turnover

The few studies that address the histological alterations in bone turnover are somewhat conflicting. There are several potential explanations for some of these discrepancies. The early studies were conducted at a time when bone aluminum accumulation was highly prevalent in patients on chronic dialysis [18–20], and other trace elements such as iron were found to accumulate in bone [21]. In the more recent reports, aluminum accumulation in bone has virtually disappeared. Moreover, inclusion of patients in most studies was highly selective. Patients were often treated with the same immunosuppressive therapy regimens, and bone biopsies were performed at a standardized time from 6 months to up to 10 years. Most investigations reported homogeneity of histologic changes in the populations they studied. Heterogeneity of histological abnormalities was noted in only a few reports [17, 19, 22].

Some studies noted high prevalence of high bone turnover associated with persistence of secondary hyperparathyroidism [15, 18, 23–25]. Normal bone turnover was observed in pediatric patients [22] and in 75% of adult patients with GFR >70 mL/min [26]. The majority of studies, however, found low bone turnover characterized by delayed mineralization (mineralization lag time >50 days) without osteoid accumulation and with or without increased number of osteoclasts, a histologic picture that resembled adynamic bone disease [12, 15–17, 21, 27, 28].

3. *Alterations in Mineralization*

As stated previously, numerous studies showed that mineralization lag time was increased to more than 50 days. However, the definition of focal or generalized osteomalacia encompasses not only an increase in mineralization lag time but also focal or generalized increases in osteoid thickness (>20 μm). Before 1990, there were few reports of osteomalacia developing after kidney transplantation [19, 29, 30], and these cases were mainly due to uncorrected hypophosphatemia. In a more recent cross-sectional study of 57 kidney transplant recipients who had stable renal function and normal serum phosphate concentrations, and who were not receiving treatment for osteoporosis, it was found that 15.8% had generalized osteomalacia, and 21.1% had focal osteomalacia [17]. A high prevalence of mineralization defects was also observed, however, associated with signs of secondary hyperparathyroidism (mixed renal osteodystrophy) [16] or normal bone turnover [26].

B. Factors Influencing Post-Transplant Bone Disease

1. *Bone Loss*

Post-transplant bone loss is a result of an imbalance between bone formation and resorption. Although the etiology is multifactorial, evidence is overwhelming that glucocorticoids play a major role. There is an inverse relationship between cumulative and mean doses of prednisone and bone volume [12, 17]. The effects of glucocorticoids in transplant recipients resemble those observed in glucocorticoid-induced osteoporosis [31, 32]. Time after transplantation is inversely related to bone volume [17]. The impact of cyclosporine on bone loss is controversial. *In vitro* data, animal experiments, and some human studies point to a negative effect of cyclosporine on bone mass when administered [23, 33, 34] on its own, but another human study did not find any histologic differences in bone between patients treated only with cyclosporine and those treated only with prednisone and azathioprine [35]. It is conceivable that the profound effects of high-dose glucocorticoids may mask the effects of cyclosporine on bone in the majority of post–kidney transplant patients.

Most kidney transplant recipients lose bone, but not all suffer from fractures. The fracture rate is as high as 10% during the first 2 years after grafting [36, 37] and the cumulative fracture rate is 40% in patients transplanted for more than 5 years [38]. These data point to the importance of bone status at time of transplantation. If bone volume is low at time of transplantation, the chance that the bone loss reaches levels below the fracture threshold (bone volume <14%) is greater than when bone volume is normal or elevated at time of transplantation. Also, patients with diabetes and adynamic bone disease have a higher risk of developing fracture even when on dialysis and more so after transplantation [5, 39].

2. *Bone Turnover*

Among kidney transplant recipients, there is a subset of patients who present with high bone turnover (approximately 25%) [17]. In the case of patients who have severe hyperparathyroid bone disease at time of transplantation that does not improve after grafting, there may have been prior development of nodular hyperplasia of the parathyroid glands, which appears unresponsive to the improvement in kidney function. In other instances, the mild to moderate increase in bone turnover could be a result of deterioration in kidney function and/or to glucocorticoid-sparing regimens, which did not drastically alter the bone disease present at time of grafting [18].

The majority of kidney transplant recipients, however, present with low bone turnover or adynamic bone disease, characterized by decreased bone formation and delayed mineralization with normal or increased osteoclast number. In a cross-sectional study of kidney transplant recipients, bone turnover, as assessed by activation frequency, was inversely correlated with the cumulative dose of glucocorticoids [17]. It is well documented that glucocorticoids depress osteoblastogenesis and promote osteoblast and osteocyte apoptosis [40]. In a recent study, patients underwent bone biopsies at the time of kidney transplantation and 22 to 160 days later [41]. There was a decline in osteoid and osteoblast surfaces and in bone formation, and mineralization was delayed. None of the baseline biopsies revealed apoptotic osteoblasts, as assessed by cell DNA fragmentation measured by the method of transferase-mediated uridine triphosphate nick end labeling (TUNEL). In approximately half the patients, the post-transplant biopsies showed apoptotic osteoblasts and in some cases apoptotic osteocytes. Patients with apoptotic osteoblasts had a smaller number of osteoblasts and lower circulating serum phosphate concentrations than those without apoptotic osteoblasts. Serum phosphate levels correlated positively with osteoblast number and negatively with apoptotic osteoblast number. Moreover, osteoblast surface correlated negatively with the cumulative dose of glucocorticoids and positively with parathyroid hormone (PTH) levels, reflecting the known effect of PTH to prevent osteoblast apoptosis [40].

3. Mineralization

In early reports, osteomalacia after kidney transplantation was attributed to hypophosphatemia [19, 29, 30]. However, more recent studies, in which phosphate supplementation is frequent and serum phosphate levels are maintained in the normal range, suggest that other factors may be important. In a cross-sectional study, both general and focal osteomalacia was observed in a rather large number of patients despite normal circulating calcitriol concentrations; however, no relationship could be detected with hypophosphatemia or bone aluminum accumulation and the observed mineralization defect [17, 26]. There is no current evidence that glucocorticoids impair mineralization. As the mineralization defect occurred despite normal calcitriol levels, it is possible that osteoblasts may have been resistant to vitamin D, either because of an abnormal vitamin D receptor or a post-receptor defect. Larger studies may be needed to unravel the determining factors leading to post-transplantation mineralization defects. Potential causes include subtle changes in phosphate homeostasis with mild deficiencies not detectable *in vivo* by current methods, low serum levels of 25-OH vitamin D, possibly due to preexisting nephrotic syndrome or malnutrition; or effects of other immosuppressive drugs, such as tacrolimus, sirolimus, mycophenolic acid, etc.

C. Prevention and Treatment of Post-Transplant Bone Disease

Overall, there is a lack of information regarding the effects on bone histology of the various treatments that have been used to prevent or treat post-transplant bone disease. However, inferences can be drawn from data obtained on the effects of the different agents in osteoporotic patients, in moderate renal failure, or in normal conditions in experimental animals.

Because bone status at time of transplantation may impact the development of bone abnormalities during the post-transplant period, it is advisable to monitor bone mass in patients on dialysis, especially those awaiting kidney transplantation. Also, avoidance of adynamic bone disease should be attempted by limiting overzealous treatment with calcitriol or its analogs and/or calcium salts, especially in diabetic patients.

After transplantation, glucocorticoid-sparing regimens have been shown to have a positive effect on bone volume and bone turnover [18]. However, such regimens are not always practicable. Alternative approaches have been tested to prevent or treat bone loss.

In patients with severe persistent hyperparathyroidism six months after transplantation that is associated with hypercalcemia, parathyroidectomy is often inevitable. However, the risk of developing adynamic bone disease is increased if the majority of the parathyroid gland mass is removed [42].

Several treatment modalities have been tested to prevent bone loss after transplantation; these include calcium supplementation, active vitamin D or its analogs, and antiresorptive agents such as bisphosphonates and calcitonin.

Vitamin D or its analogs, with or without calcium supplementation, has been shown to prevent bone loss after transplantation in some studies [43–45], though others did not find a beneficial effect [46]. Vitamin D therapy might be useful for those patients with mild increase in bone turnover or in patients with a mineralization defect. It should be kept in mind, however, that prolonged treatment may result in excessive lowering of bone turnover [47].

Various bisphosphonates (e.g., etidronate, alendronate, clodronate, ibandronate, pamidronate, and zoledronic acid) have been used in kidney transplant patients in an attempt to prevent or treat bone loss after grafting [48–62]. Overall, they prevent bone loss. However, in one placebo controlled study, histologic examination showed that at time of transplantation, 50% of patients presented with adynamic bone disease, while by 6 months after transplantation, all patients receiving pamidronate had adynamic bone disease and 50% of the placebo patients had decreased bone turnover [61]. Whether or not improved bone mineral density with adynamic bone histology is beneficial and maintains long-term bone health in renal transplant recipients requires further study.

Calcitonin is an antiresorptive agent, which has been shown to prevent bone loss after grafting and alleviate bone pain [55, 56]. However, it was also shown that a mineralization defect develops in ovariectomized and normal experimental animals treated with calcitonin. The mineralization defect was assessed by three independent methods including bone histology, bone biomechanics, and ultrastructural mineral characteristics of iliac crest bone determined by gravimetry and Fourier transform infrared spectroscopy [63, 64].

All these agents may have beneficial effects on bone mass, but they have some unwanted potential effects on bone turnover and mineralization. New therapeutic agents such as teriparatide (rhPTH-(1-34)) might be efficient in preventing bone loss due to its anabolic effects [65, 66], especially in patients with low bone turnover.

In conclusion, despite great interest in the bone disease developing after kidney transplantation, more studies are needed to address the effects of the available therapeutic agents on bone turnover and bone mineralization.

REFERENCES

1. Malluche, H., and Faugere, M.C. (1990). Renal bone disease 1990: an unmet challenge for the nephrologist. *Kidney Int*. 38(2):193–211.

2. Sherrard, D. J., Hercz, G., Pei, Y., Maloney, N.A., Greenwood, C., Manuel, A., Saiphoo, C., Fenton, S.S., and Segre, G.V. (1993). The spectrum of bone disease in end-stage renal failure—an evolving disorder. *Kidney Int.* 43(2):436–442.
3. Hruska, K.A., and Teitelbaum, S.L. (1995). Renal osteodystrophy. *N Engl J Med.* 33:166–174.
4. U.S. Renal Data System, USRDS 2002 Annual Report: Atlas of End-Stage Renal Disease in the United States, NIH and NIDDK, Bethesda, MD, 2002.
5. Nicodemus, K.K., and Folsom, A.R. (2001). Type 1 and type 2 diabetes and incident hip fractures in postmenopausal women. *Diabetes Care.* 24(7):1192–1197.
6. Aubia, J., Serrano, S., Marinoso, L., Hojman, L., Diez, A., Lloveras, J., and Masramon, J. (1988). Osteodystrophy of diabetics in chronic dialysis: a histomorphometric study. *Calcif Tissue Int.* 42(5):297–301.
7. Malluche, H.H., and Monier-Faugere, M.C. (1992). Risk of adynamic bone disease in dialyzed patients. *Kidney Int Suppl.* 38:S62–67.
8. Malluche, H.H., and Faugere, M.C. (1986). *Atlas of Mineralized Bone Histology.* New York: Karger.
9. Monier-Faugere, M.C., and Malluche, H.H. (1996). Trends in renal osteodystrophy: a survey from 1983 to 1995 in a total of 2248 patients. *Nephrol Dial Transplant.* 11(Suppl 3):111–120.
10. Kurz, P., Monier-Faugere, M.C., Bognar, B., Werner, E., Roth, P., Vlachojannis, J., and Malluche, H.H. (1994). Evidence for abnormal calcium homeostasis in patients with adynamic bone disease. *Kidney Int.* 46(3):855–861.
11. Coco, M., and Rush, H. (2000). Increased incidence of hip fractures in dialysis patients with low serum parathyroid hormone. *Am J Kidney Dis.* 36(6):1115–1121.
12. Julian, B.A., Laskow, D.A., Dubovsky, J., Dubovsky, E.V., Curtis, J.J., and Quarles, L.D. (1991). Rapid loss of vertebral mineral density after renal transplantation. *N Engl J Med.* 325(8):544–550.
13. Almond, M.K., Kwan, J.T., Evans, K., and Cunningham, J. (1994). Loss of regional bone mineral density in the first 12 months following renal transplantation. *Nephron.* 66(1):52–57.
14. Horber, F.F., Casez, J.P., Steiger, U., Czerniak, A., Montandon, A., and Jaeger, P. (1994). Changes in bone mass early after kidney transplantation. *J Bone Miner Res.* 9(1):1–9.
15. Carlini, R.G., Rojas, E., Arminio, A., Weisinger, J.R., and Bellorin-Font, E. (1998). What are the bone lesions in patients with more than four years of a functioning renal transplant? *Nephrol Dial Transplant.* 13 Suppl 3:103–104.
16. Carlini, R.G., Rojas, E., Weisinger, J.R., Lopez, M., Martinis, R., Arminio, A., and Bellorin-Font, E. (2000). Bone disease in patients with long-term renal transplantation and normal renal function. *Am J Kidney Dis.* 36(1):160–166.
17. Monier-Faugere, M.C., Mawad, H., Qi, Q., Friedler, R.M., and Malluche, H.H. (2000). High prevalence of low bone turnover and occurrence of osteomalacia after kidney transplantation. *J Am Soc Nephrol.* 11(6):1093–1099.
18. Briner, V.A., Thiel, G., Monier-Faugere, M.C., Bognar, B., Landmann, J., Kamber, V., and Malluche, H.H. (1995). Prevention of cancellous bone loss but persistence of renal bone disease despite normal 1,25 vitamin D levels two years after kidney transplantation. *Transplantation.* 59(10):1393–1400.
19. Bonomini, V., Feletti, C., Di Felice, A., and Buscaroli, A. (1984). Bone remodelling after renal transplantation (RT). *Adv Exp Med Biol.* 178:207–216.
20. Martins, L., Queiros, J., Ferreira, A., Henriques, A.C., Sarmento, A.M., Pereira, M.C., and Guimaraes, S. (2000). Renal osteodystrophy: histologic evaluation after renal transplantation. *Transplant Proc.* 32(8):2599–2601.
21. Velasquez-Forero, F., Mondragon, A., Herrero, B., and Pena, J.C. (1996). Adynamic bone lesion in renal transplant recipients with normal renal function. *Nephrol Dial Transplant.* 11 Suppl 3:58–64.

22. Sanchez, C.P., Salusky, I.B., Kuizon, B.D., Ramirez, J.A., Gales, B., Ettenger, R.B., and Goodman, W.G. (1998). Bone disease in children and adolescents undergoing successful renal transplantation. *Kidney Int.* 53(5):1358–1364.
23. Aubia, J., Masramon, J., Serrano, S., Llovelas, J., and Marinoso, L. (1988). Bone histology in renal transplantation patients receiving cyclosporin [letter]. *Lancet.* 1:1048.
24. Torres, A., Rodriguez, A.P., Concepcion, M.T., Garcia, S., Rufino, M., Martin, B., Perez, L., Machado, M., de Bonis, E., Losada, M., Hernandez, D., and Lorenzo, V. (1998). Parathyroid function in long-term renal transplant patients: importance of pre-transplant PTH concentrations. *Nephrol Dial Transplant.* 13 Suppl 3:94–97.
25. Parfitt, A.M. (1982). Hypercalcemic hyperparathyroidism following renal transplantation: differential diagnosis, management, and implications for cell population control in the parathyroid gland. *Miner Electrolyte Metab.* 8(2):92–112.
26. Montalban, C., de Francisco, A.L., Marinoso, M.L., Zubimendi, J.A., Garcia Unzueta, M., Amado, J.A., and Arias, M. (2003). Bone disease in long-term adult kidney transplant patients with normal renal function. *Kidney Int Suppl* (85):S129–132.
27. Cueto-Manzano, A.M., Konel, S., Hutchison, A.J., Crowley, V., France, M.W., Freemont, A.J., Adams, J.E., Mawer, B., and Gokal, R. (1999). Bone loss in long-term renal transplantation: histopathology and densitometry analysis. *Kidney Int.* 55(5):2021–2029.
28. Parker, C.R., Freemont, A.J., Blackwell, P.J., Grainge, M.J., and Hosking, D.J. (1999). Cross-sectional analysis of renal transplantation osteoporosis. *J Bone Miner Res.* 14(11):1943–1951.
29. Moorhead, J.F., Wills, M.R., Ahmed, K.Y., Baillod, R.A., Varghese, Z., and Tatler, G.L. (1974). Hypophosphataemic osteomalacia after cadaveric renal transplantation. *Lancet.* 1(7860):694–697.
30. Felsenfeld, A.J., Gutman, R.A., Drezner, M., and Llach, F. (1986). Hypophosphatemia in long-term renal transplant recipients: effects on bone histology and 1,25-dihydroxycholecalciferol. *Miner Electrolyte Metab.* 12(5–6):333–341.
31. Meunier, P.J., Dempster, D.W., Edouard, C., Chapuy, M.C., Arlot, M., and Charhon, S. (1984). Bone histomorphometry in corticosteroid-induced osteoporosis and Cushing's syndrome. *Adv Exp Med Biol.* 171:191–200.
32. Dempster, D.W., Arlot, M.A., and Meunier, P.J. (1983). Mean wall thickness and formation periods of trabecular bone packets in corticosteroid-induced osteoporosis. *Calcif Tissue Int.* 35(4–5):410–417.
33. Nacher, M., Aubia, J., Serrano, S., Marinoso, M.L., Hernandez, J., Bosch, J., Diez, A., Puig, J.M., and Lloveras, J. (1994). Effect of cyclosporine A on normal human osteoblasts in vitro. *Bone Miner.* 26(3):231–243.
34. Movsowitz, C., Epstein, S., Fallon, M., Ismail, F., and Thomas, S. (1988). Cyclosporin-A in vivo produces severe osteopenia in the rat: effect of dose and duration of administration. *Endocrinology.* 123:2571–2577.
35. Cueto-Manzano, A.M., Konel, S., Crowley, V., France, M.W., Freemont, A.J., Adams, J.E., Mawer, B., Gokal, R., and Hutchison, A. J. (2003). Bone histopathology and densitometry comparison between cyclosporine a monotherapy and prednisolone plus azathioprine dual immunosuppression in renal transplant patients. *Transplantation.* 75(12):2053–2058.
36. Nisbet, N.W., and Menage, J. (1981). The fate of allogeneic grafts of intact bone marrow in immunologically tolerant recipients and after abrogation of the tolerance. *Br J Exp Pathol.* 62(3):215–221.
37. Ramsey-Goldman, R., Dunn, J.E., Dunlop, D.D., Stuart, F.P., Abecassis, M.M., Kaufman, D.B., Langman, C.B., Salinger, M.H., and Sprague, S.M. (1999). Increased risk of fracture in patients receiving solid organ transplants. *J Bone Miner Res.* 14(3):456–463.
38. Durieux, S., Mercadal, L., Orcel, P., Dao, H., Rioux, C., Bernard, M., Rozenberg, S., Barrou, B., Bourgeois, P., Deray, G., and Bagnis, C.I. (2002). Bone mineral density and fracture prevalence in long-term kidney graft recipients. *Transplantation.* 74(4):496–500.
39. Coco, M., and Rush, H. (2000). Increased incidence of hip fractures in dialysis patients with low serum parathyroid hormone. *Am J Kidney Dis.* 36(6):1115–1121.

40. Weinstein, R.S., Jilka, R.L., Parfitt, A.M., and Manolagas, S.C. (1998). Inhibition of osteoblastogenesis and promotion of apoptosis of osteoblasts and osteocytes by glucocorticoids. Potential mechanisms of their deleterious effects on bone. *J Clin Invest.* 102(2):274–282.
41. Rojas, E., Carlini, R.G., Clesca, P., Arminio, A., Suniaga, O., De Elguezabal, K., Weisinger, J.R., Hruska, K.A., and Bellorin-Font, E. (2003). The pathogenesis of osteodystrophy after renal transplantation as detected by early alterations in bone remodeling. *Kidney Int.* 63(5):1915–1923.
42. Charhon, S.A., Berland,Y.F., Olmer, M.J., Delawari, E., Traeger, J., and Meunier, P.J. (1985). Effects of parathyroidectomy on bone formation and mineralization in hemodialyzed patients. *Kidney Int.* 27(2):426–435.
43. Lobo, P.I., Cortez, M.S., Stevenson, W., and Pruett, T.L. (1995). Normocalcemic hyperparathyroidism associated with relatively low 1:25 vitamin D levels post-renal transplant can be successfully treated with oral calcitriol. *Clin Transplant.* 9(4):277–281.
44. Jeffery, J.R., Leslie, W.D., Karpinski, M.E., Nickerson, P.W., and Rush, D.N. (2003). Prevalence and treatment of decreased bone density in renal transplant recipients: a randomized prospective trial of calcitriol versus alendronate. *Transplantation.* 76(10): 1498–1502.
45. El-Agroudy, A.E., El-Husseini, A.A., El-Sayed, M., and Ghoneim, M.A. (2003). Preventing bone loss in renal transplant recipients with vitamin D. *J Am Soc Nephrol.* 14(11):2975–2979.
46. Cueto-Manzano, A.M., Konel, S., Freemont, A.J., Adams, J.E., Mawer, B., Gokal, R., and Hutchison, A. J. (2000). Effect of 1,25-dihydroxyvitamin D3 and calcium carbonate on bone loss associated with long-term renal transplantation. *Am J Kidney Dis.* 35(2): 227–236.
47. Baker, L.R., Abrams, L., Roe, C.J., Faugere, M.C., Fanti, P., Subayti, Y., and Malluche, H. H. (1989). 1,25(OH)2D3 administration in moderate renal failure: a prospective double-blind trial. *Kidney Int.* 35(2):661–669.
48. Arlen, D.J., Lambert, K., Ioannidis, G., and Adachi, J.D. (2001). Treatment of established bone loss after renal transplantation with etidronate. *Transplantation.* 71(5):669–673.
49. Kovac, D., Lindic, J., Kandus, A., and Bren, A. F. (2000). Prevention of bone loss with alendronate in kidney transplant recipients. *Transplantation.* 70(10):1542–1543.
50. Torregrosa, J.V., Moreno, A., Gutierrez, A., Vidal, S., and Oppenheimer, F. (2003). Alendronate for treatment of renal transplant patients with osteoporosis. *Transplant Proc.* 35(4):1393–1395.
51. Koc, M., Tuglular, S., Arikan, H., Ozener, C., and Akoglu, E. (2002). Alendronate increases bone mineral density in long-term renal transplant recipients. *Transplant Proc.* 34(6):2111–2113.
52. Cruz, D.N., Brickel, H.M., Wysolmerski, J.J., Gundberg, C.G., Simpson, C.A., Kliger, A.S., Lorber, M.I., Basadonna, G. P., Friedman, A.L., Insogna, K.L., and Bia, M.J. (2002). Treatment of osteoporosis and osteopenia in long-term renal transplant patients with alendronate. *Am J Transplant.* 2(1):62–67.
53. Giannini, S., Dangel, A., Carraro, G., Nobile, M., Rigotti, P., Bonfante, L., Marchini, F., Zaninotto, M., Dalle Carbonare, L., Sartori, L., and Crepaldi, G. (2001). Alendronate prevents further bone loss in renal transplant recipients. *J Bone Miner Res.* 16(11):2111–2117.
54. Kovac, D., Lindic, J., Kandus, A., and Bren, A.F. (2001). Prevention of bone loss in kidney graft recipients. *Transplant Proc.* 33(1–2):1144–1145.
55. Grotz, W.H., Rump, L.C., Niessen, A., Schmidt-Gayk, H., Reichelt, A., Kirste, G., Olschewski, M., and Schollmeyer, P. J. (1998). Treatment of osteopenia and osteoporosis after kidney transplantation. *Transplantation.* 66(8):1004–1008.
56. Grotz, W., Rump, J.A., Niessen, A., Schmidt-Gayk, H., and Schollmeyer, P. (1998). Treatment of bone pain after kidney transplantation. *Transplant Proc.* 30(5):2114–2116.
57. Sellers, E., Sharma, A., and Rodd, C. (1998). The use of pamidronate in three children with renal disease. *Pediatr Nephrol.* 12(9):778–781.

58. Fan, S. L., Almond, M.K., Ball, E., Evans, K., and Cunningham, J. (2000). Pamidronate therapy as prevention of bone loss following renal transplantation1. *Kidney Int.* 57(2):684–690.
59. Nam, J.H., Moon, J.I., Chung, S. S., Kim, S.I., Park, K.I., Song, Y.D., Kim, K.R., Lee, H. C., Huh, K., and Lim, S.K. (2000). Pamidronate and calcitriol trial for the prevention of early bone loss after renal transplantation. *Transplant Proc.* 32(7):1876.
60. Grotz, W., Nagel, C., Poeschel, D., Cybulla, M., Petersen, K. G., Uhl, M., Strey, C., Kirste, G., Olschewski, M., Reichelt, A., and Rump, L.C. (2001). Effect of ibandronate on bone loss and renal function after kidney transplantation. *J Am Soc Nephrol.* 12(7):1530–1537.
61. Coco, M., Glicklich, D., Faugere, M.C., Burris, L., Bognar, I., Durkin, P., Tellis, V., Greenstein, S., Schechner, R., Figueroa, K., McDonough, P., Wang, G., and Malluche, H. (2003). Prevention of bone loss in renal transplant recipients: a prospective, randomized trial of intravenous pamidronate. *J Am Soc Nephrol.* 14(10):2669–2676.
62. Schwarz, C., Mitterbauer, C., Heinze, G., Woloszczuk, W., Haas, M., and Oberbauer, R. (2004). Nonsustained effect of short-term bisphosphonate therapy on bone turnover three years after renal transplantation. *Kidney Int.* 65(1):304–309.
63. Monier-Faugere, M.C., Geng, Z., Qi, Q., Arnala, I., and Malluche, H.H. (1996). Calcitonin prevents bone loss but decreases osteoblastic activity in ovariohysterectomized beagle dogs. *J Bone Miner Res.* 11(4):446–455.
64. Pienkowski, D., Doers, T.M., Monier-Faugere, M.C., Geng, Z., Camacho, N.P., Boskey, A.L., and Malluche, H.H. (1997). Calcitonin alters bone quality in beagle dogs. *J Bone Miner Res.* 12(11):1936–1943.
65. Slovik, D.M., Rosenthal, D.I., Doppelt, S. H., Potts, J.T., Jr., Daly, M.A., Campbell, J.A., and Neer, R. M. (1986). Restoration of spinal bone in osteoporotic men by treatment with human parathyroid hormone (1-34) and 1,25-dihydroxyvitamin D. *J Bone Miner Res.* 1(4):377–381.
66. Neer, R.M., Arnaud, C.D., Zanchetta, J.R., Prince, R., Gaich, G.A., Reginster, J.Y., Hodsman, A.B., Eriksen, E.F., Ish-Shalom, S., Genant, H.K., Wang, O., and Mitlak, B.H. (2001). Effect of parathyroid hormone (1-34) on fractures and bone mineral density in postmenopausal women with osteoporosis. *N Engl J Med.* 344(19):1434–1441.

CHAPTER 14

Bone Disease Following Kidney–Pancreas and Pancreas Transplantation

Stuart M. Sprague, DO
Division of Nephrology and Hypertension, Evanston Northwestern Healthcare,
Northwestern University Feinberg School of Medicine, Evanston, IL

I. INTRODUCTION

Organ transplantation is the optimal form of therapy for those with diabetes and/or kidney disease. Improvement in immunosuppressive therapy has increased allograft survival; however, this enhanced survival has led to the emergence of and appreciation of transplant complications such as bone disease. Bone and mineral disorders are common in patients with diabetes and a universal complication in those with chronic kidney disease prior to transplantation. Several different pathogenetic mechanisms may be involved and may ultimately lead to one or more types of bone disease, including osteitis fibrosa cystica as a result of secondary hyperparathyroidism, some form of low-turnover bone disease (osteomalacia, adynamic bone disease, and aluminum bone disease), osteoporosis, osteosclerosis, and β_2-microglobulin amyloidosis. Low-turnover bone disease is especially prevalent in diabetic patients. In addition, hypogonadism, metabolic acidosis, and certain medications (loop diuretics, heparin, glucocorticoids, antiepileptics, and calcineurin inhibitors) may also affect bone health. Superimposed on these underlying bone diseases are disorders of mineral metabolism, which occur following successful transplantation and include the effects of medications, persistence of underlying metabolic disorders, development of hyperphosphaturia, and the recurrence of varying degrees of renal insufficiency. These disorders of mineral metabolism and the associated bone disease lead to the development of fractures following transplantation.

Pancreas transplantation rarely occurs in the absence of severe underlying kidney disease and simultaneous kidney transplantation. Furthermore, there are very limited data on bone disease following pancreas transplantation. Thus, the following discussion on the role of pancreas transplantation and diabetes on transplant bone disease will consider the data obtained from kidney transplantation.

II. FRACTURES FOLLOWING TRANSPLANTATION

Patients with chronic kidney disease prior to transplantation are at increased risk of fracture with vertebral fracture prevalence as high as 21% and the relative risk of hip fracture increased by 2- to 14 fold. Fracture risk is increased with older age, female gender, Caucasian race [1], duration of dialysis [2], diabetic nephropathy [3], peripheral vascular disease [1], low spine bone mineral density (BMD), and lower parathyroid hormone (PTH) levels. Following successful kidney transplantation, studies report fracture rates between 5% and 44% [4–14]. The causes of this wide range of reported fracture rates are many, including whether the fracture data were obtained by questionnaire or patient encounter. The variation likely also reflects differences in post-transplant timing of the studies, as the more time has passed since transplantation, the higher the reported fracture rate [4–14]. More importantly, the spread may also be attributed to the fraction of transplant recipients with diabetes mellitus in the various studies. Patients with diabetes receiving a kidney–pancreas transplant have fracture rates as high as 40% and 49% post-transplantation [15, 16]. As shown in Table 1, transplant recipients have a markedly higher risk of fracture compared to the general population with those undergoing a simultaneous kidney–pancreas being at significantly greater risk [6]. The magnitude of the increased fracture risk faced by the transplant recipient can also be appreciated when comparing hospitalizations for fracture. Abbott et al. found that in 33,479 transplant recipients, 3 years or less post-transplant, the relative risk of being hospitalized for a fracture was 4.59 compared with the general population [17]. Fractures occur both peripherally and centrally (see Figure 1), whereas 6 studies have documented a higher fracture rate at peripheral sites

TABLE 1 Age- and gender-specific initial fracture estimated relative risk compared to general population in kidney and kidney–pancreas transplant recipients surviving at least 30 days. Adapted from Ramsey-Goldman et al. (1999). Increased risk of fracture in patients receiving solid organ transplants. *J Bone Miner Res.* 14:456–463.

Age (in years)	Kidney	Kidney–Pancreas
Female		
25-44	18.51	38.63
45-64	34.03	54.91
Male		
25-44	4.74	13.19
45-64	4.88	80.73

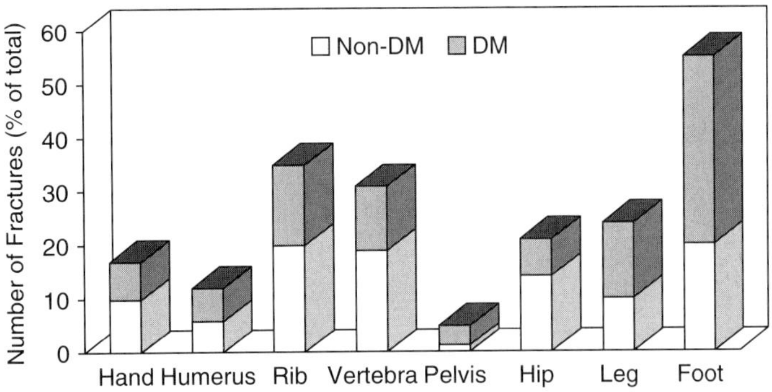

FIGURE 1 Distribution of post-transplant fractures in diabetic and nondiabetic kidney and kidney–pancreas transplant recipients. Number of fractures expressed as the percentage of total fractures. Fractures occur both peripherally (feet and ankles) and centrally (in the ribs, hip, or vertebrae), with the diabetic patients being at particular risk for peripheral fractures. [Adapted from references 6, 15, and 16.]

[4, 7–10, 16]. Patients with a history of diabetes mellitus are at particular risk for peripheral fractures [16].

Risk factors identified for fracture include duration of hemodialysis prior to transplant [12], time since transplant [12], female gender (particularly if post-menopausal) [10, 12], BMD scores below the normal range [10], kidney failure from diabetes [10], history of fracture prior to transplant [10], and age greater than 45 [4]. By contrast, obesity was associated with a decreased risk of fracture [10]. In addition, although having a low BMD puts a recipient at increased risk for fracture, many patients with low BMDs do not experience a fracture, so BMD does not discriminate between those who will and will not fracture [10].

III. BONE MINERAL DENSITY

Patients with chronic kidney disease have an increased prevalence of low BMD at the spine, hip, and distal radius. Risk factors for a low BMD include female gender, Caucasian race, amenorrhea, lower weight or body mass index (BMI), elevated PTH, duration of hemodialysis, and previous kidney transplantation. Recipients of kidney or combined kidney–pancreas allografts rapidly lose bone after transplantation [18–35]. Decreases in BMD, measured by dual x-ray absorptiometry scans (DXA), have been observed as early as 3 to 6 months following transplant. Almond et al. found a 3.93% drop in femoral neck BMD in male transplant recipients at 3 months [33]. Julian et al. observed a lumbar spine BMD decline of 6.8% at 6 months [31]. Investigators who have obtained serial BMD scans at both the lumbar spine (mainly trabecular bone) and femoral neck (predominately cortical bone) have found bone loss at both sites [18, 25, 27, 28, 32–35]. In contrast to these findings, a few investigators have not documented BMD loss following transplantation and have attributed their results to differing effects of immunosuppression (cyclosporine had a beneficial effect compared with azathioprine [20], deflazacort was associated with less bone loss than prednisone [23, 24], and tacrolimus-treated patients gained bone, while cyclosporine-treated patients lost bone [30]) or the influence of the vitamin D receptor genotype bb [21]. Risk factors for post-transplant bone loss have been identified, but not all studies implicate the same ones. These risks include total glucocorticoid exposure [12, 20, 22, 36, 37], dialysis duration prior to transplantation [38], and time since transplantation [12, 36, 39].

Some investigators have identified increasing time since transplantation as a risk, yet others examining BMD trends 2 or more years after transplant have not demonstrated continued bone loss. In 12 such studies several years after transplant, 3 did not demonstrate a significant drop [22, 35, 40], 6 noted improvements in BMD [19, 27, 37, 41–43], 1 showed a slight improvement in the lumbar spine accompanied by a small decline at the femoral neck [44], and 2 found that while some patients improve, some worsen [45, 46]. The authors of one of these last two studies found that allograft recipients with declining bone density scores differed from those with stable bone densities. The former had biomarkers indicating a high-turnover bone state while the latter did not [45]. However, despite the improvements in BMD that some studies have shown following the first year after transplantation, most studies demonstrate that BMDs measured up to 12 years after transplantation remain low [11, 29, 35, 39, 43, 45–56].

IV. BONE BIOMARKERS

Data evaluating bone markers following transplantation are limited and not specific for pancreas or kidney–pancreas transplantation. The majority of studies evaluating post-transplant PTH trends demonstrate that PTH levels decrease following transplantation [22, 24, 30, 34, 40, 42, 54, 57–62]. Of these 13 studies, 8 note that despite the decline, levels remain elevated [22, 34, 40, 54, 57–59, 62]. At least one study found that an increased PTH concentration was associated with declining bone density, though this has not been uniformly observed [50, 63].

Alkaline phosphatase levels have an unpredictable trend after transplantation [22, 24, 30, 34, 40, 43, 57, 60, 64–68]. Of six cross-sectional studies, two noted that levels were higher than normal post-transplant [51, 69], while four found no difference from control [50, 53, 70, 71]. Glucocorticoid use has been associated with an alkaline phosphatase decrease [13, 65]. Whether alkaline phosphatase helps predict the risk of bone loss is unclear. One study found no correlation between alkaline phosphatase levels and bone loss at the lumbar spine [42], but another found that elevated alkaline phosphatase levels correlated with low femoral neck BMD [13].

At least five studies have shown that osteocalcin declines with time post-transplantation [34, 57, 62, 64, 67]. Several studies have found an association between trends in osteocalcin and PTH [53, 58, 72–74]. Most cross-sectional studies note that osteocalcin is elevated after transplant [24, 51, 53,

70, 71, 73], while one found it to be normal [46]. At least one study noted an association between osteocalcin and dropping BMD scores [63], though another did not [46].

Urinary collagen cross links have been found to either decrease or remain unchanged following transplantation [24, 34, 40, 60, 64]. Two cross-sectional studies found the levels to be elevated [51, 53], while one noted levels within the normal range [70]. In one study the urinary collagen cross links trends correlated with PTH as well as with alkaline phosphatase [60]. Cruz et al. found that elevated levels of urinary collagen cross links and serum osteocalcin were associated with decreases in BMD [45].

V. BONE HISTOLOGY

Performing bone biopsies following transplantation is rare in day-to-day clinical practice. Unfortunately, there are no studies evaluating bone histology in recipients of pancreatic transplants. Studies in kidney transplant recipients have revealed that bone histomorphometry results could not have been predicted from other, less invasive clinical tests. The bone biopsy results of at least 373 kidney transplant recipients, on no specific therapy for bone loss [21, 31, 43, 48, 50, 75-81], reveal that the lesions found in transplant patients vary widely. Sanchez et al. performed biopsies on children and adolescents and found 66% to have normal bone histology post-transplant [78]; in most series, however, only a minority of patients have normal bone histology following transplantation [11, 43, 77]. Although many patients have low bone turnover on biopsy [31, 43, 48, 75, 76, 80, 81], many others display high turnover [11, 77–79, 81]. There is no clear-cut pattern even when accounting for time post-transplantation. Cueto-Manzano et al. obtained baseline bone biopsies at a mean of 133±75 months post transplant and repeated them 12 months later [43]. Without specific treatment directed at bone disease, 71% of patients undergoing biopsies had different histological findings on the second biopsy compared with the first.

Julian et al. found that declines in PTH correlated with decreases in bone turnover indices [31] in patients undergoing bone biopsy at baseline and again at six months. In contrast to these findings, several other studies were unable to demonstrate an association between PTH or alkaline phosphatase and biopsy findings [50, 76, 78–81]. Cueto-Manzano et al. found no significant association between transformation to adynamic bone and PTH reduction [43].

VI. PATHOPHYSIOLOGY

A. Pretransplant Bone Disease

Patients awaiting transplantation frequently manifest significant and often severe metabolic bone disease as a consequence of progressive dysfunction of their failing organ. Patients maintained on dialysis for end-stage kidney disease invariably manifest severe derangements of mineral and skeletal metabolism and the calcium-regulating hormones. Standard therapies aim to minimize the impact of these disorders, but are successful only to a degree [82]. Direct assessment of skeletal health is relatively difficult to assess *in vivo* (in contrast to, for example, parathyroid function, vitamin D metabolism, and other easily measured metabolic parameters), and it is not unusual for patients receiving kidney transplants to do so at a time when renal osteodystrophy is protracted and/or severe. In contrast to patients without diabetes, diabetic patients are much more likely to have relatively low PTH levels and a much higher prevalence of low turnover or adynamic bone disease [83]. *In vitro* studies have demonstrated that exposure to elevated glucose concentrations may stimulate cellular proliferation while inhibiting calcium uptake, resulting in bone that is structurally impaired [84]. Clinically, these patients are likely to experience reduction of bone mineral density [85]. Thus, the skeletal starting point at the time of organ transplantation is far from ideal.

B. Skeletal Effects of Immunosuppressive Drugs

1. *Glucocorticoids*

Glucocorticoids in high doses (e.g., ≥ 50 mg/day of prednisone or prednisolone) are commonly prescribed immediately following transplantation, with subsequent dose reduction over several weeks and transient increases during rejection episodes. Exposure varies with the number and management of rejection episodes and with the practice of transplantation programs. The introduction of cyclosporine A (CsA), tacrolimus, and more recently rapamycin and daclizumab have reduced glucocorticoid requirements. However, in most transplant programs there is still sufficient exposure, particularly during the first few months after transplantation, to cause substantial bone loss. Glucocorticoids reduce BMD predominantly at trabecular sites, and even relatively small doses are associated with markedly increased fracture risk. Glucocorticoids cause direct and profound reductions in bone formation by decreasing osteoblast replication, differentiation, and lifespan, and by inhibiting genes for type I collagen, osteocalcin, insulin-like growth factors, bone morphogenetic proteins and other bone matrix proteins, transforming growth factor β (TGF-β), and receptor activator for NFκB-ligand (RANK-L). Direct effects of glucocorticoids on bone resorption are minor relative to effects on formation. However, steroids may increase bone resorption indirectly, by inhibiting osteoprotegerin, resulting in increased osteoclast formation, inhibiting synthesis of gonadal steroids, and inducing hyperparathyroidism secondary to reduced intestinal and renal calcium absorption [86]. These clinical consequences are particularly severe in the presence of preexisting and/or continuing hyperparathyroidism, calcium deficiency, vitamin D deficiency, malnutrition, or relative immobility, many of which may coexist in the transplant recipient.

2. *Calcineurin Inhibitors: Cyclosporine A and Tacrolimus*

The introduction of CsA to transplantation regimens was associated with a marked reduction in rejection episodes and an improvement in survival. CsA inhibits calcineurin, a T-cell phosphatase, and reduces T-cell function via suppression of regulatory genes expressing products such as IL-2, interleukin receptors, and the proto-oncogenes, H-ras and c-myc [87]. Although *in vitro* studies demonstrated that CsA inhibits bone resorption in cultured bone [88, 89], *in vivo* rodent studies suggest that CsA has independent adverse effects on bone and mineral metabolism that could contribute to bone loss after organ transplantation [87]. In the rat, CsA administration caused severe bone loss, particularly in trabecular bone, that was associated with marked increases in both bone resorption and formation and increased levels of osteocalcin and 1,25-vitamin D [87]. The CsA-mediated bone loss was associated with testosterone deficiency [90], independent of renal function [87] and attenuated by parathyroidectomy [91]. Anti-resorptive agents such as estrogen, raloxifene, calcitonin, and alendronate prevented CsA-induced bone loss [87]. CsA may cause bone loss by direct effects on calcineurin genes expressed in osteoclasts [92] or indirectly via alterations in T-cell function [93]. These animal studies suggest that CsA could be responsible for the high-turnover aspects of post-transplantation bone disease. However, the effects of CsA on the human skeleton are still unclear, particularly in view of reports that kidney transplant patients receiving CsA in a steroid-free regimen [20, 94, 95] do not appear to lose bone.

Tacrolimus (FK506), another calcineurin inhibitor, inhibits cytokine gene expression, T-cell activation, and T-cell proliferation, and also causes trabecular bone loss in the rat [87]. Fewer studies have evaluated the skeletal effects of FK506 in humans; it has been associated with post-transplantation bone loss, however, although it is not always possible to distinguish clearly between the effects of the calcineurin inhibitor and those of glucocorticoids. Whether tacrolimus differs importantly from CsA in this respect is unknown.

3. *Other Immunosuppressive Agents*

Limited information is available regarding the effects of other immunosuppressive drugs on BMD and bone metabolism. Azathioprine, sirolimus (rapamycin), and mycophenolate mofetil do not cause bone loss in the rat model. The skeletal effects of newer agents, such as daclizumab, have not been studied. However, by reducing glucocorticoid requirements, they may be relatively beneficial to the skeleton.

VII. EVALUATION FOR POST-TRANSPLANT BONE DISEASE

Given that transplant recipients lose bone and are at ongoing increased risk for fracture, long-term monitoring of their "bone risk" is warranted. Specific evaluation protocols have not been tested, and various approaches are likely useful. The National Kidney Foundation's recent Kidney Disease Outcome Quality Initiative (K/DOQI) recommends the following in the evaluation of transplant recipients: Serum levels of calcium, phosphorus, total CO_2, and plasma intact parathyroid hormone should be monitored following kidney transplantation, and bone mineral density should be measured at time of transplant and at 1 year and 2 years post-transplant [96]. These recommendations are opinion-based, and Table 2 summarizes our approach for long-term monitoring.

VIII. MANAGEMENT OF BONE DISEASE

Virtually all studies have shown that bone loss is most rapid immediately following transplantation. Fractures may occur very early and affect patients with both low and normal BMD. Most patients (even those with normal BMD) should therefore have preventive therapy instituted immediately following transplantation. In addition, the population of patients who received transplants months or years ago is growing, and many of these patients have never been evaluated or treated for bone disease.

Therapeutic studies in patients undergoing kidney transplantation are limited in number, and there are no studies specific to kidney–pancreas recipients. The majority of therapeutic trials are in patients undergoing other solid-organ transplantation. These studies have focused on the use of

TABLE 2 Recommendations for evaluation of the transplant recipient

1. Monitor BMD by DXA at the lumbar spine and femoral neck within one month pre- or post-transplantation.
2. Obtain a baseline PTH.
3. Follow serum calcium, albumin, phosphorous. and total CO_2 concentrations.
4. Within 6–12 months of transplant, repeat the BMD measurement.
5. If BMD shows a decline (>5% decrease or half of a standard deviation), recheck the PTH and vitamin D level and intake, and evaluate gonadal status (LH, FSH, estradiol, total testosterone, and prolactin in the setting of impotence, amenorrhea, oligomenorrhea, or complete cessation of menses).
6. If bone mineral density is decreasing as just described in 5, recheck BMD yearly.
7. If bone mineral density is stable (less than 5% decline yearly), recheck every 2 years.
8. If the PTH was initially elevated, monitor at least yearly.
9. Perform a bone biopsy if bone loss continues as measured by BMD and if the etiology of the bone disease is not clear.

vitamin D metabolites and antiresorptive drugs, particularly the bisphosphonates.

Vitamin D metabolites may reduce post-transplantation bone loss by reversing glucocorticoid-induced decreases in intestinal calcium absorption and by mitigating secondary hyperparathyroidism [97]. Theoretically, they could reduce glucocorticoid exposure by virtue of their immunomodulatory effects. There have been no studies evaluating the use of the parent form of vitamin D and only one prospective study utilizing calcidiol (25-hydroxyvitamin D_3) in the prevention or treatment of post–kidney transplant bone disease. The use of 500 mg calcium and 50 μg calcidiol increased neither proximal femur nor lumbar BMD in 6 patients treated for 1 year after transplantation [98]. There are also very few studies with calcitriol (1, 25-dihydroxyvitamin D_3) for the prevention or treatment of bone disease after kidney transplantation. The results of these studies are not conclusive. Cueto-Manzano et al. were unable to demonstrate protection from ongoing bone loss with calcitriol and calcium when started in patients a mean of 119 months following transplantation [43]. In a preliminary report, however, we were able to demonstrate an increase in BMD of the femoral neck, lumbar spine, and radius following 12 months of calcitriol and calcium treatment compared to double placebo [99] when used to prevent early post-transplantation bone loss. Similar protection in BMD was observed in both diabetic and nondiabetic subjects.

Several studies [7, 28, 34, 100-102] suggest that bisphosphonates may be useful in either preventing or treating bone loss following renal transplantation. Administration of intravenous pamidronate at time of transplantation and 1 month later was shown to prevent lumbar spine and proximal femoral bone loss at 1 year [28]. The use of the more potent biphosphonate, ibandronate, administered at time of transplantation and 3, 6, and 9 months after transplantation also resulted in a significant protective effect on BMD in the lumbar spine and proximal femur at 1 year [34]. A small study ($n = 20$) compared the use of oral alendronate with calcitriol. A regimen that included alendronate (10 mg/day), calcium carbonate (2 g/day), and calcitriol (0.25 μg/day) was associated with a 6.3% increase in lumbar spine BMD in the first 6 months after transplantation, compared to a decrease of 5.8% with calcium and calcitriol alone [101]. Another trial compared therapy for 1 year with either alendronate, calcitriol, and calcium, or calcitriol and calcium treatment alone in 40 kidney transplant recipients in whom therapy was begun an average of 5 years after transplantation. This study reported an increase of 5% at the lumbar spine and 4.5% at the femoral neck in the alendronate-treated group [100]. BMD remained stable in the patients treated with calcitriol and calcium. Finally, Haas et al. evaluated bone biopsies in 6 patients given placebo and 7 patients who received zoledronic acid and found similar resolution of the high-turnover lesions in both groups; those receiving zoledronic acid, however, had significant improvement in trabecular calcification [102]. Thus, bisphosphonates may be promising for the management of post-transplant bone loss. This may be especially true immediately following transplantation and in those patients with high-turnover bone lesions. Controversies remain regarding the optimal administration of bisphosphonates, however: whether continuous or intermittent therapy should be used, the duration of therapy, the level of renal impairment at which bisphosphonates should be avoided, whether they are safe in kidney transplant recipients with low-turnover bone disease and their utility following pediatric transplantation. Finally, one must be cautious in the use of bisphosphonates as there are reports of development of sclerosing focal segmental glomerulonephritis following the use of pamidronate.

There are essentially no data on the use of calcitonin or hormone replacement therapy following transplantation. Hypogonadism is a common sequela in patients with chronic kidney disease and may persist following transplantation, thus an evaluation of gonadal status would be appropriate. The potential benefits of either estrogen replacement or testosterone therapy have to be weighed against the potential risks in the individual patient.

Diabetics with kidney failure tend not to have severe hyperparathyroidism, but the condition may persist following successful kidney–pancreas transplantation. This usually resolves within 1 to 2 years of transplantation, and thus these patients generally require periodic monitoring. Mild elevations of parathyroid hormone, in the range of 1–2 times the upper limit of normal, may not be a problem. If the parathyroid hormone is persistently elevated (>500–600 by intact assay) and there is associated hypercalcemia and/or hypophosphatemia that does not respond to or is worsened by oral Vitamin D analogues, parathyroidectomy should be considered.

IX. SUMMARY AND CONCLUSIONS

Information concerning bone disease following pancreas or kidney–pancreas transplantation is very limited. Thus, our understanding must be extrapolated from the data available from the kidney transplant population. Pretransplantation bone disease and post-transplantation immunosuppressive regimens combining high doses of glucocorticoids and calcineurin inhibitors interact to produce a variety of bone and mineral disorders, which result in rapid bone loss and increased fracture rates. Patients undergoing kidney–pancreas transplantation as well as diabetics receiving kidney transplants have greater fracture rates compared to nondiabetic kidney recipients. Bone biopsy information reveals that bone disease in kidney transplant recipients is not a single entity; studies demonstrate uncoupling of bone turnover, with many biopsies exhibiting features of increased bone resorption and decreased bone formation. Unfortunately, bone biomarkers have not been shown to be useful probes to distinguish the underlying process. Although BMD is used as a surrogate for bone disease, BMD does not predict fractures in the kidney–pancreas transplant population. Management of these patients should combine assessment and treatment of pretransplantation bone disease with preventive therapy in the immediate post-transplantation period, since most bone loss occurs in the first months following successful grafting. In addition, bone mass measurement and therapy of bone loss in the long-term organ transplant recipient should be addressed. There are no pretransplantation variables that reliably predict post-transplantation bone loss and fracture risk in the individual patient. Therefore, all transplant recipients should be considered at risk for post-transplantation bone loss and fractures. Although recent observations suggest that rates of bone loss and fracture may be lower in patients treated with the newer immunosuppressive regimens, morbidity from transplantation bone loss remains unacceptably high. Therapeutic trials have shown promise to decrease bone loss, but no trial has demonstrated an effect on preventing fractures.

REFERENCES

1. Stehman-Breen, C.O., Sherrard, D.J., Alem, A.M., Gillen, D.L., Heckbert, S.R., Wong, C.S., Ball, A., Weiss, N.S. (2000). Risk factors for hip fracture among patients with end-stage renal disease. *Kidney Int.* 58:2200–2205.
2. Alem, A.M., Sherrard, D.J., Gillen, D.L., Weiss, N.S., Beresford, S.A., Heckbert, S.R., Wong, C., Stehman-Breen, C. (2000). Increased risk of hip fracture among patients with end-stage renal disease. *Kidney Int.* 58:396–399.
3. Ball, A.M., Gillen, D.L., Sherrard, D., Weiss, N.S., Emerson, S.S., Seliger, S.L., Kestenbaum, B.R., Stehman-Breen, C. (2002). Risk of hip fracture among dialysis and renal transplant recipients. *JAMA.* 288:3014–3018.
4. Elmstedt, E., Svahn, T. (1981). Skeletal complications following renal transplantation. *Acta Orthop Scand.* 52:279–286.
5. Davidson, J.K., Tsakiris, D., Briggs, J.D., Junor, B.J. R. (1985). Osteonecrosis and fractures following renal transplantation. *Clinical Radiol.* 36:27–35.
6. Ramsey-Goldman, R.R., Dunn, J.E., Dunlop, D.D., Stuart, F.P., Abecassis, M.M., Kaufman, D.B., Langman, C.B., Salinger, M.H., Sprague, S.M. (1999). Increased risk of fracture in patients receiving solid organ transplants. *J Bone Miner Res.* 14:456–463.
7. Arlen, D.J., Lambert, K., Ioannidis, G., Adachi, J. (2001). Treatment of established bone loss after renal transplantation with etidronate. *Transplantation.* 71:669–673.
8. O'Shaughnessy, E.A., Dahl, D.C., Smith, C.L., Kasiske, B.L. (2002). Risk factors for fractures in kidney transplantation. *Transplantation.* 74:362–366.
9. Durieux, S., Mercadal, L., Orcel, P., Dao, H., Rioux, C., Bernard, M., Rozenberg, S., Barrou, B., Bourgeous, P., Deray, G., Bagnis, C.I. (2002). Bone mineral density and fracture prevalence in long-term kidney graft recipients. 74:496–500.
10. Grotz, W.H., Mundinger, F.A., Gugel, B., Exner, V., Kirste, G., Schollmeyer, P.J. (1994). Bone fracture and osteodensitometry with dual energy x-ray absorptiometry in kidney transplant recipients. *Transplantation.* 58:912–915.
11. Parker, C.R., Freemont, A.J., Blackwell, P.J., Grainge, M.J., Hosking, D.J. (1999). Cross-sectional analysis of renal tranpslantation osteoporosis. *J Bone Miner Res.* 14:1943–1951.
12. Patel, S., Kwan, J.T. C., McCloskey, E., McGee, G., Thomas, G., Johnson, D., Wills, R., Ogunremi, L., Barron, J. (2001). Prevalence and causes of low bone density and fractures in kidney transplant patients. *J Bone Miner Res.* 16:1863–1870.

13. D'Angelo, A., Calo, L., Giannini, S., Carraro, G., Bonfante, L., Favaro, S., Zaninotto, M., Perin, N., Di Landro, D., Rigotti, P., Antonello, A. (2000). Parathyroid hormone and bone metabolism in kidney-transplanted patients. *Clin Nephrol.* 53:19–22.
14. Nam, J.H., Moon, J.I., Chung, S.S., Kim, S.I., Park, K.I., Song, Y.D., Kim, K.R., Lee, H.C., Huh, K., Lim, S.K. (2000). Prevalence and risk factors for vertebral fractures in renal transplants. *Transplant Proc.* 32:1877.
15. Chiu, M.Y., Sprague, S.M., Bruce, D.S., Woodle, E.S., Thistlethwaite, J.R., Josephson, M.A. (1998). Analysis of fracture prevalence in kidney-pancreas allograft recipients. *J Am Soc Nephrol.* 9:677–683.
16. Nisbeth, U., Lindh, E., Ljunghall, S., Backman, U., Feller, B. (1999). Increased fracture rate in diabetes mellitus and females after renal transplantation. *Transplantation.* 67:1218–1222.
17. Abbott, K.C., Oglesby, R.J., Hypolite, I.O., Kirk, A.D., Ko, C.W., Welch, P.G., Agodoa, L.Y., Duncan, W.E. (2001). Hospitalizations for fractures after renal transplantation in the United States. *Annals of Epidemiology.* 11:450–457.
18. Kwan, J.T., Almond, M.K., Evans, K., Cunningham, J. (1992). Changes in total body bone mineral content and regional bone mineral density in renal patients following renal transplantation. *Mineral and Electrolyte Metabolism.* 18:166–168.
19. Feber, J., Cochat, P., Braillon, P., Castelo, F., Martin, X., Glastre, C., Chapuis, F., David, L., Meunier, P.J. (1994). Bone mineral density after renal transplantation in children. *Journal of Pediatrics.* 6:870–875.
20. McIntyre, H.D., Menzies, B., Rigby, R., Perry-Kenne, D.A., Hawley, C.M., Hardie, I.R. (1995). Long-term bone loss after renal transplantation: comparison of immunosuppressive regimens. *Clinical Transplantation.* 9:20–24.
21. Torres, A., Machado, M., Concepcion, M.T., Martin, N., Lorenzo, V., Hernadez, D., Rodriguez, A.P., Rodriguez, A., de Bonis, E., Gonzalez-Posada, J.M., Hernandez, A., Salido, E. (1996). Influence of vitamin D receptor genotype on bone mass changes after renal transplantation. *Kidney Int.* 50:1726–1733.
22. Yun, Y.S., Kim, B.J., Hong, S.P., Lee, T.W., Lim, C.G., Kim, M.J. (1996). Changes of bone metabolism indices in patients receiving immunosuppressive therapy including low doses of steroids after renal transplantation. *Transplantation Proceedings.* 28:1561–1564.
23. Kim, M.S., Kim, Y.S., Lim, S.K., Kim, S.I., Moon, J.I., Park, K. (1998). Effect of deflazacort on bone mineral density in renal transplant recipients. *Transplantation Proceedings.* 30:3041–3042.
24. Lippuner, K., Casez, J.-P, Horber, F.F., Jaeger, P. (1998). Effects of deflazacort versus prednisone on bone mass, body composition and lipid profile: a randomized double blind study in kidney transplant patients. *J Clin Endocrinol Metab.* 83:3795–3802.
25. Smets, Y.F. C., van der Pijl, J.W., Ringers, J., de Fijter, J.W., Lemkes, H.H. P., Hamdy, N.A.T. (1998). Pattern of bone loss after simultaneous pancreas-kidney transplantation: a prospective study. *Transplantation Proceedings.* 30:326.
26. Isiklar, I., Akin, O., Demirag, A., Niron, E.A. (1998). Changes in bone mineral density after renal transplantation. *Transplantation Proceedings.* 30:814–185.
27. Moreno, A., Torregrosa, J.V., Pons, F., Campistol, J.M., Martinez de Osaba, M.J., Oppenheimer, F. (1999). Bone mineral density after renal transplantation. *Transplantation Proceedings.* 31:2322–2323.
28. Fan, S.L. S., Almond, M.K., Ball, E., Evans, K., Cunningham, J. (2000). Pamidronate therapy as prevention of bone loss following renal transplantation. *Kidney Int.* 57:684–690.
29. Kokado, Y., Takahara, S., Ichimaru, N., Toki, K., Kyo, M., Permpongkosol, S., Kojima, Y., Inoue, T., Wang, J.D., Okuyama, A. (2000). Factors influencing vertebral bone density after renal transplantation. *Transpl Int.* 13:S431-S435.
30. Goffin, E., Devogelaer, J.-P, Lalaoui, A., Depresseux, G., De Naeyer, P., Squifflet, J.-P, Pirson, Y., van Ypersele de Strihou, C. (2002). Tacrolimus and low-dose steroid

immunosuppression preserves bone mass after renal transplantation. *Transpl Int.* 15:73–80.

31. Julian, B.A., Laskow, D.A., Dubovsky, J., Dubovsky, E.V., Curtis, J.J., Quarles, L.D. (1991). Rapid loss of vertebral mineral density after renal transplantation. *N Engl J Med.* 325:544–550.
32. Horber, F.F., Casez, J.P., Steiger, U., Czerniak, A., Montandon, A., Jaeger, P. (1994). Changes in bone mass early after kidney transplantation. *J Bone Miner Res.* 9:1–9.
33. Almond, M.K., Kwan, J.T., Evans, K., Cunningham, J. (1994). Loss of regional bone mineral density in the first 12 months following renal transplantation. *Nephron.* 66:52–57.
34. Grotz, W., Nagel, C., Poeschel, D., Cybulla, M., Petersen, K.G., Uhl, M., Strey, C., Kirste, G., Olschewski, M., Reichelt, A., Rump, L.C. (2001). Effect of ibandronate on bone loss and renal function after kidney transplantation. *J Am Soc Nephrol.* 12:1530–1537.
35. Grotz, W.H., Mundinger, F.A., Gugel, B., Exner, V.M., Kirste, G., Schollmeyer, P.J. (1995). Bone mineral density after kidney transplantation. A cross-sectional study in 190 graft recipients up to 20 years after transplantation. *Transplantation.* 59:982–986.
36. Ugur, A., Guvener, N., Isiklar, I., Turan, M., Erdal, R., Haberal, M. (2001). Osteoporosis after renal transplantation: single center experience. *Transplantation.* 71:645–649.
37. Nowacka-Cieciura, E., Durlik, M., Cieciura, T., Lewandowska, D., Baczkowska, T., Kukla, K., Lao, M., Szmidt, J., Rowinski, W. (2002). Steroid withdrawal after renal transplantation-risks and benefits. *Transplantation Proceedings.* 34:560–563.
38. Aroldi, A., Tarantino, A., Montagnino, G., Cesana, B., Cocucci, C., Ponticelli, C. (1997). Effects of three immunosuppressive regimens on vertebral bone density in renal transplant recipients: a prospective study. *Transplantation.* 63:380–386.
39. Bagni, B., Gilli, P., Cavallini, A., Bagni, I., Marzola, M.C., Orzincolo, C., Wahner, H.W. (1994). Continuing loss of vertebral mineral density in renal transplant recipients. *European Journal of Nuclear Medicine.* 21:108–112.
40. Hurst, G., Alloway, R., Hathaway, D., Somerville, D., Hughes, T., Gaber, A. (1998). Stabilization of bone mass after renal transplant with preemptive care. *Transplantation Proceedings.* 30:1327–1328.
41. Yazawa, K., Ishikawa, T., Ichikawa, Y., Shin, J., Usui, Y., Hanafusa, T., Fukunishi, T., Sakai, R., Nagano, S., Fujita, N., Mizuno, K. (1998). Positive effects of kidney transplantation on bone mass. *Transplantation Proceedings.* 30:3031–3033.
42. Kim, H., Chang, K., Lee, T., Kwon, J., Park, S. (1998). Bone mineral density after renal transplantation. *Transplantation Proceedings.* 30:3029–3030.
43. Cueto-Manzano, A.M., Konel, S., Freemont, A.J., Adams, J.E., Mawer, B., Gokal, R., Hutchinson, A.J. (2000). Effect of 1,25-dihydroxyvitamin D3 and calcium carbonate on bone loss associated with long-term renal transplantation. *American Journal of Kidney Diseases.* 35:227–236.
44. Grotz, W.H., Rump, L.C., Niessen, A., Schmidt-Gayk, H., Reichelt, A., Kirste, G., Olschewski, M., Schollmeyer, P.J. (1998). Treatment of osteopenia and osteoporosis after kidney transplantation. *Transplantation.* 66:1004–1008.
45. Cruz, D., Wysolmerski, J.J., Brickel, H., Gundberg, C.G., Simpson, C.A., Mitnick, M.A. E., Kliger, A.S., Lorber, M.I., Basadonna, G.P., Friedman, A.L., Insogna, K.L., Bia, M.J. (2001). Parameters of high bone-turnover predict bone loss in renal transplant patients: a longitudinal study. *Transplantation.* 72:83–88.
46. Brandenburg, V.M., Ketteler, M., Fassbender, W.J., Heussen, N., Freuding, T., Floege, J., Ittel, T.H. (2002). Development of lumbar bone mineral density in the late course after kidney transplantation. *Am J Kidney Dis.* 40:1066–1074.
47. Smets, Y.F., van der Pilj, J.W., de Fijter, J.W., Ringers, J., Lemkes, H.H., Hamdy, N.A. (1998). Low bone mass and high incidence of fractures after successful simultaneous pancreas-kidney transplantation. *Nephrology Dialysis Transplantation.* 13:1250–1255.
48. Velasquez-Forero, F., Mondragon, A., Herrero, B., Pena, J.C. (1996). Adynamic bone lesion in renal transplant recipients with normal renal function. *Nephrology Dialysis Transplantation.* 11 Suppl. 3:58–64.

49. Braun, W.E., Richmond, B.J., Protiva, D.A., Gifford, R.W., Straffon, R.A. (1999). The incidence and management of osteoporosis, gout, and avascular necrosis in recipients of renal allografts functioning more than 20 years (level 5A) treated with prednisone and azathioprine. *Transplantation Proceedings*. 31:1366–1369.
50. Carlini, R.G., Rojas, E., Weisinger, J.R., Lopez, M., Martinis, R., Arminio, A., Bellorin-Font, E. (2000). Bone disease in patients with long-term renal transplantation and normal renal function. *American Journal of Kidney Diseases*. 36:160–166.
51. Heaf, J., Tvedgaard, E., Kanstrup, I.-L, Fogh-Andersen, N. (2000). Bone loss after renal transplantation: role of hyperparathyroidism, acidosis, cyclosporine and systemic disease. *Clin Transplantation*. 14:457–463.
52. Ellis, E.N., Floyd-Gimon, D.M., Berry, P.L., Wells, T.G., Seibert, J., Belsha, C. (2000). Risk factors for bone mineral density loss in pediatric renal transplant patients. *Pediatr Transplantation*. 4:146–150.
53. Cayco, A.V., Wysolmerski, J., Simpson, C., Mitnick, M.A., Gundberg, C., Kliger, A., Lorber, M., Silver, D., Basadonna, G., Friedman, A., Insogna, K., Cruz, D., Bia, M. (2000). Posttransplant bone disease: evidence for a high bone resorption state. *Transplantation*. 70:1722–1728.
54. Kovac, D., Lindic, J., Kandus, A., Bren, A.F. (2001). Bone mineral density in kidney transplant recipients. *Transplantation Proceedings*. 33:3668–3669.
55. Pichette, V., Bonnardeaux, A., Prudhomme, L., Gagne, M., Cardinal, J., Ouimet, D. (1996). Long-term bone loss in kidney transplant recipients: a cross-sectional and longitudinal study. *Am J Kidney Dis*. 28:105–114.
56. Wolpaw, T., Deal, C.L., Fleming-Brooks, S., Bartucci, M.R., Schulak, J.A., Hricik, D.E. (1994). Factors influencing vertebral bone density after renal transplantation. *Transplantation*. 58:1186–1189.
57. Boiskin, I., Epstein, S., Ismail, F., Thomas, S.B., Raja, R. (1989). Serum osteocalcin and bone mineral metabolism following successful renal transplantation. *Clin Nephrol*. 31:316–322.
58. Schmidt, H., Stracke, H., Schatz, H., Scheuermann, E.H., Fassbinder, W., Schoeppe, W. (1989). Osteocalcin serum levels in patients following renal transplantation. *Klin Wochenschr*. 67:297–303.
59. Saha, H.H., Salmela, K.T., Ahonen, P.J., Pietila, K.O., Morsky, P.J., Mustonen, J.T., Lalla, M.L., Pasternack, A.I. (1994). Sequential changes in vitamin D and calcium metabolism after successful renal transplantation. *Scand J Urol Nephrol*. 28:21–27.
60. Withold, W., Degenhardt, S., Heins, M., Grabensee, B., Reinauer, H. (1995). Monitoring of bone resorption after renal transplantation by measuring the urinary excretion of pyridinium cross-links. *Eur J Clin Chem Clin Biochem*. 33:15–21.
61. Bonnin, M.R., Gonzalez, M.T., Grino, J.M., Cruzado, J.M., Bover, J., Martinez, J.M., Navarro, M.A. (1997). Changes in serum osteocalcin levels in the follow-up of kidney transplantation. *Ann Clin Biochem*. 34:651–655.
62. Barbarykin, D., Adamsone, I., Amerika, D., Folkmane, I., Rozental, R. (1999). Disorders of calcium metabolism at various times after renal transplantation. *Annals of Transplantation*. 4:46–53.
63. Kusec, V., Smalcelj, R., Cvijetic, S., Rozman, B., Skreb, F. (2000). Determinants of reduced bone mineral density and increased bone turnover after kidney transplantation: cross-sectional study. *Croat Med* J.41:396–400.
64. Westeel, F.P., Mazouz, H., Ezaitouni, F., Hottelart, C., Ivan, C., Fardellone, P., Brazier, M., El Elsper, I., Petit, J., Achard, J.M., Pruna, A., Fournier, A. (2000). Cyclosporine bone remodeling effect prevents steroid osteopenia after kidney transplantation. *Kidney Int*. 58:1788–1796.
65. Cundy, T., Kanis, J.A. (1987). Rapid suppression of plasma alkaline phosphatase activity after renal transplantation in patients with osteodystrophy. *Clin Chim Acta*. 164:285–291.
66. van Straalen, J.P., Sanders, E., Prummel, M.F., Sanders, G.T. (1991). Bone-alkaline phosphatase as indicator of bone formation. *Clin Chim Acta*. 201:27–33.

67. Withold, W., Friedrich, W., Degenhardt, S. (1997). Serum bone alkaline phosphatase is superior to plasma levels of bone matrix proteins for assessment of bone metabolism in patients receiving renal transplants. *Clin Chim Acta.* 261:105–115.
68. Withold, W., Degenhardt, S., Grabensee, B., Reinauer, H. (1995). Comparison between serum levels of bone alkaline phosphatase and the carboxy-terminal propeptide of type I procollagen as markers of bone formation in patients following renal transplantation. *Clin Chim Acta.* 239:143–151.
69. Epstein, S., Traberg, H., Raja, R., Poser, J. (1985). Serum and dialysate osteocalcin levels in hemodialysis and peritoneal dialysis patients and after renal transplantation. *J Clin Endocrinol Metab.* 60:1253–1256.
70. Reusz, G.S., Szabo, A.J., Peter, F., Kenesei, E., Sallay, P., Latta, K., Szabo, A., Szabo, A., Tulassay, T. (2000). Bone metabolism and mineral density following renal transplantation. *Arch Dis Child.* 83:146–151.
71. Pietschmann, P., Vychytil, A., Woloszczuk, W., Kovarik, J. (1991). Bone metabolism in patients with functioning kidney grafts: increased serum levels of osteocalcin and parathyroid hormone despite normalisation of kidney function. *Nephron.* 59:533–536.
72. Amado, J.A., Riancho, J.A., De Francisco, A.L., Cotorruelo, J.G., Feijanes, J., Arias, M., Napal, J., Gonzalez-Macias, J. (1989). Hyperparathyroidism is responsible for the increased levels of osteocalcin in patients with normally functioning kidney grafts. *Nephron.* 52:209–215.
73. Dumoulin, G., Hory, B., Nguyen, N.U., Bresson, C., Fournier, V., Bouhaddi, M., Chalopin, J.M., Saint-Hillier, Y., Regnard, J. (1997). No trend toward a spontaneous improvement of hyperparathyroidism and high bone turnover in normocalcemic long-term renal transplant recipients. *Am J Kidney Dis.* 29:746–753.
74. Giannini, S., D'Angelo, A., Carraro, G., Antonello, A., Di Landro, D., Marchini, F., Plebani, M., Zaninotto, M., Rigotti, P., Sartori, L., Crepaldi, G. (2001). Persistently increased bone turnover and low bone density in long-term survivors to kidney transplantation. *Clinical Nephrology.* 56:353–363.
75. Briner, V.A., Thiel, G., Monier-Faugere, M.C., Bognar, B., Landmann, J., Kamber, V., Malluche, H.H. (1995). Prevention of cancellous bone loss but persistence of renal bone disease despite normal 1,25 vitamin D levels two years after kidney transplantation. *Transplantation.* 59:1393–1400.
76. Carlini, R.G., Rojas, E., Arminio, A., Weisinger, J.R., Bellorin-Font, E. (1998). What are the bone lesions in patients with more than four years of a functioning renal transplant. *Nephrol Dial Transplant* 13 Suppl. 3:103–104.
77. Cueto-Manzano, A.M., Konel, S., Hutchison, A.J., Crowley, V., France, M.W., Freemont, A.J., Adams, J.E., Mawer, B., Gokal, R. (1999). Bone loss in long-term renal transplantation: histopathology and densitometry analysis. *Kidney Int.* 55:2021–2029.
78. Sanchez, C.P., Salusky, I.B., Kuizon, B.D., Ramirez, J.A., Gales, B., Ettenger, R.B., Goodman, W.G. (1998). Bone disease in children and adolescents undergoing successful renal transplantation. *Kidney Int.* 53:1358–1364.
79. Weisinger, J.R., Carlini, R.G., Rojas, E., Bellorin-Font, E. (1999). Bone disease after renal transplantation. *Transplant Proc.* 31:3033–3034.
80. Monier-Faugere, M.C., Mawad, H., Qi, Q., Friedler, R.M., Malluche, H.H. (2000). High prevalence of low bone turnover and occurrence of osteomalacia after kidney transplantation. *J Am Soc Nephrol.* 11:1093–1099.
81. Parker, C.R., Blackwell, P.J., Freemont, A.J., Hosking, D.J. (2002). Biochemical measurements in the prediction of histologic subtype of renal transplant bone disease in women. *Am J Kidney Dis.* 40:385–396.
82. Hruska, K.A., Teitelbaum, S.L. (1995). Renal osteodystrophy. *N Engl J Med.* 333:166.
83. Ho, L.T., Sprague, S.M. (2002). Renal osteodystrophy in chronic renal failure. *Seminars in Nephrology.* 22:488–493.
84. Balint, E., Szabo, P., Marshall, C.F., Sprague, S.M. (2001). Glucose-induced inhibition of in vitro bone mineralization. *Bone.* 28:21–28.

85. Schober, H.C., Han, Z.H., Foldes, A.J., Shih,, M.S., Rao, D.S., Balena, R., Parfitt, A.M. (1998). Mineralized bone loss at different sites in dialysis patients: implications for prevention. *J Am Soc Nephrol.* 9:1225-1233.
86. Rubin, M.R., Bilezikian, J.P. (2002). Clinical review 151: The role of parathyroid hormone in the pathogenesis of glucocorticoid-induced osteoporosis: a re-examination of the evidence. *J Clin Endocrinol Metab.* 87:4033–4041.
87. Epstein, S. (1996). Post-transplantation bone disease: the role of immunosuppressive agents and the skeleton. *J Bone Miner Res.* 11:1–7.
88. Stewart, P.J., Stern, P.H. (1989). Cyclosporines: correlation of immunosuppressive activity and inhibition of bone resorption. *Calcif Tissue Int.* 45:222–226.
89. Stewart, P.J., Stern, P.H. (1989). Interaction of cyclosporine A and calcitonin on bone resorption in vitro. *Horm Metab Res.* 21:194–197.
90. Bowman, A.R., Sass, D.A., Dissanayake, I.R., Ma, Y.F., Liang, H., Yuan, Z., Jee, W.S., Epstein, S. (1997). The role of testosterone in cyclosporine-induced osteopenia. *J Bone Miner Res.* 12:607–615.
91. Epstein, S., Dissanayake, I.R., Goodman, G.R., Bowman, A.R., Zhou, H., Ma, Y., Jee, W.S. (2001). Effect of the interaction of parathyroid hormone and cyclosporine a on bone mineral metabolism in the rat. *Calcif Tissue Int.* 68:240–247.
92. Awumey, E.M., Moonga, B.S., Sodam, B.R., Koval, A.P., Adebanjo, O.A., Kumegawa, M., Zaidi, M., Epstein, S. (1999). Molecular and functional evidence for calcineurin-A alpha and beta isoforms in the osteoclast: novel insights into cyclosporin A action on bone resorption. *Biochem Biophys Res Commun.* 254:248–252.
93. Buchinsky, F.J., Ma, Y., Mann, G.N., Rucinski, B., Bryer, H.P., Romero, D.F., Jee, W.S., Epstein, S. (1996). T lymphocytes play a critical role in the development of cyclosporin A-induced osteopenia. *Endocrinology.* 137:2278–2285.
94. Ponticelli, C., Aroldi, A. (2001). Osteoporosis after organ transplantation. *Lancet.* 357:1623.
95. Grotz, W., Mundinger, A., Gugel, B., Exner, V., Reichelt, A., Schollmeyer, P. (1994). Missing impact of cyclosporine on osteoporosis in renal transplant recipients. *Transplant Proc.* 26:2652–2653.
96. National Kidney Foundation. (1999). K/DOQI Clinical Practice Guidelines for Bone Metabolism and Disease in Chronic Kidney Disease. Am J Kidney Dis 42:(suppl 3)S1-S202.
97. Sambrook, P. (1999). Alfacalcidol and calcitriol in the prevention of bone loss after organ transplantation. *Calcif Tissue Int.* 65:341–343.
98. Lippuner, K., Haller, B., Casez, J.P., Montandon, A., Jaeger, P. (1996). Effect of disodium monofluorophosphate, calcium and vitamin D supplementation on bone mineral density in patients chronically treated with glucocorticosteroids: a prospective, randomized, double-blind study. *Miner Electrolyte Metab.* 22:207–213.
99. Josephson, M.A., Schumm, L.P., Chiu, M.Y., Marshall, C., Sprague, S.M. (2000). Calcium and calcitriol prophylaxis against post-transplant bone loss. (abstract) *J Am Soc Nephrol.* 11:720A.
100. Giannini, S., D'Angelo, A., Carraro, G., Nobile, M., Rigotti, P., Bonfante, L., Marchini, F., Zaninotto, M., Carbonare, L.D., Sartori, L., Crepaldi, G. (2001). Alendronate prevents further bone loss in renal transplant recipients. *J Bone Miner Res.* 16:2111–2117.
101. Kovac, D., Lindic, J., Kandus, A., Bren, A.F. (2001). Prevention of bone loss in kidney graft recipients. *Transplant Proc.* 33:1144–1145.
102. Haas, M., Leko-Mohr, Z., Roschger, P., Kletzmayr, J., Schwarz, C., Mitterbauer, C., Steininger, R., Grampp, S., Klaushofer, K., Delling, G., Oberbauer, R. (2003). Zoledronic acid to prevent bone loss in the first 6 months after renal transplantation. *Kidney Int.* 63:1130-1136.

CHAPTER 15

Bone Disease after Liver Transplantation

Nuria Guañabens, MD
Ana Monegal, MD
Metabolic Bone Diseases Unit, Department of Rheumatology, Hospital Clínic, Barcelona, Spain

I. INTRODUCTION

Liver transplantation is now a well-established treatment for end-stage liver failure, but the survivors' quality of life may be reduced by the development of fractures, which is one of the main complications. This is a problem, particularly since the number of liver transplant recipients has been increasing in the last few years. In Spain, the number of patients undergoing liver transplantation increased from 495 in 1993 to 1033 in 2002, and liver transplantation at present represents up to 28% of the total solid-organ transplant procedures (see Figure 1) [1].

In the development of bone loss and fractures after liver transplantation, pretransplant bone disease and post-transplant factors such as the use of immunosuppressive agents, including glucocorticoids, cyclosporine A, and tacrolimus (FK506), play an important role. In recent years, however, it has been suggested that rates of bone loss and fracture may be lower than previously reported, mainly because of the newer immunosuppressive regimens that are less reliant on glucocorticoids.

This chapter is focused on the frequency, risk factors, and pathogenesis of bone loss and osteoporotic fractures after liver transplantation, and on the therapeutic approaches to this bone disease.

II. POST-TRANSPLANTATION BONE LOSS

Rates of bone loss increase during the first few months after liver transplantation. Thus, lumbar BMD decreases by roughly 6% at 3 months after

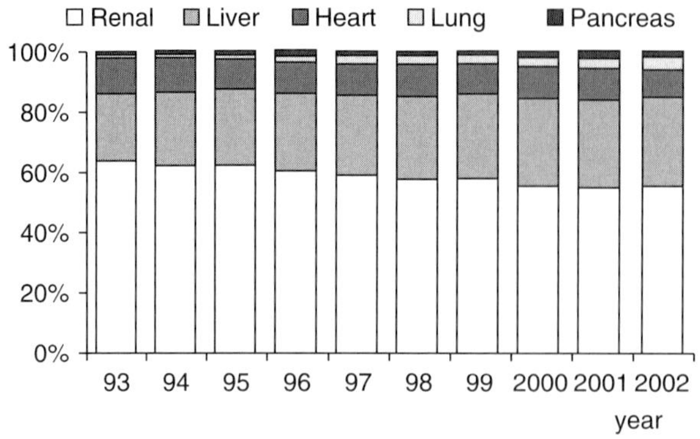

FIGURE 1 Percentage of different types of solid-organ transplant procedures in Spain over the last decade.

liver transplantation, with a progressive and significant increase after 1 year of follow-up. Moreover, lumbar BMD reaches baseline values 2 years after transplantation (see Figure 2) [2]. Most of the longitudinal studies show similar rates of bone loss in the lumbar spine during the first 12 months, when BMD declines from 3.5 to 5.7%, with subsequent spontaneous recovery [3, 4]. However, earlier studies, as well as some later ones, reported greater or zero bone loss, respectively. Thus, in the 1990s a marked decline in lumbar BMD shortly after liver transplantation was reported in series

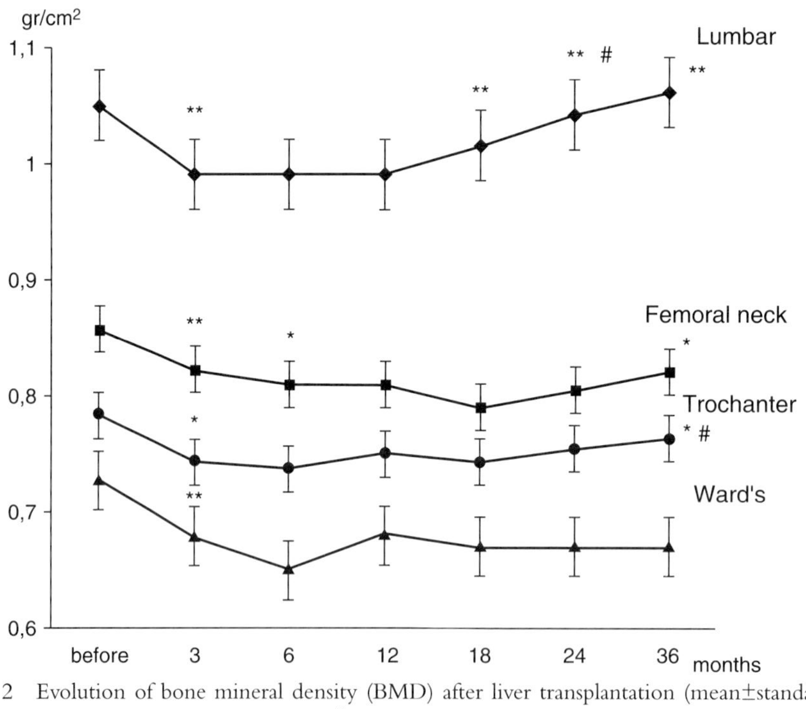

FIGURE 2 Evolution of bone mineral density (BMD) after liver transplantation (mean±standard error). *P <0.05 Manova repeated measures analysis. **P <0.000 Manova repeated measures analysis; # no differences to base-line values [2]. Reproduced from *Osteoporos Int.* 12:485–492 with permission of Springer-Verlag London Ltd.

including mostly patients with end-stage cholestatic liver disease treated with immunosuppressive regimens using high doses of glucocorticoids [5, 6]. In contrast, some recent studies have reported no significant changes in lumbar BMD or even small increases at short-term follow-up [7, 8]. Few longitudinal studies have assessed lumbar BMD changes at more than 2 years of follow-up. After this point, when BMD is similar to or slightly higher than that before transplantation [2, 5, 9], there are no significant changes during a long-term follow-up [10].

Femoral BMD has a different pattern of evolution following liver transplantation. After a marked decrease of up to 4% in femoral neck BMD during the first 3–6 months, there is a delayed and incomplete improvement at 3 years, since differences still persist in relation to baseline values (see Figure 2) [2]. Other studies have also observed a sustained reduction in femoral neck BMD at 18–24 months after liver transplantation [9]. Thereafter, BMD remained stable in a 15-year follow-up study [10].

III. FRACTURES AFTER LIVER TRANSPLANTATION

A high proportion of patients develop fractures during the first 6–12 months after liver transplantation. Available data indicate that fracture incidence ranges from 22 to 65% [5, 11], although most series have shown an incidence of vertebral fractures around 30% (see Table 1) [2, 12, 13]. Similarly, we have reported vertebral fractures in 33% of patients during the first year after transplantation [2]. The differences observed among the various studies may be partially related both to the severity and etiology of the liver disease and to the immunosuppressive regimens. Thus, the higher rates were reported in the earliest studies involving patients with cholestatic diseases with immunosuppressive approaches that were highly reliant on glucocorticoids [5]. By contrast, the lowest rates of fracture were described in studies with only symptomatic fractures taken into account [9] and in recent studies performed in patients with better bone health prior to transplantation together with the use of lower doses and shorter duration of glucocorticoid therapy [7]. Most studies have assessed vertebral fracture rates during short-term follow-up. Interestingly, a long-term follow-up study showed that few patients have their first fracture in the third and fourth year after liver transplantation [13].

A low rate of nonvertebral fractures has been reported, ranging from 7 to 9%, with discrepancy in fracture sites among studies. Thus, while the most common site affected in one study was the hip [9], others have reported different sites of fracture including ribs, sacrum, arms, and legs [5, 13–15].

IV. BIOCHEMICAL AND HORMONAL PARAMETERS

Before liver transplantation, patients may show a decrease in total serum calcium, but serum concentrations of albumin-corrected calcium, as well as serum ionized calcium concentrations, are usually normal [2, 16, 17]. Moreover, patients with end-stage liver disease normally show low or normal circulating concentrations of parathyroid hormone (PTH), despite low or in some cases normal 25-hydroxyvitamin D concentrations [2, 16–18]. Thus, serum 25-hydroxyvitamin D has been found to be significantly lower in cirrhotic patients than in healthy controls. In fact, serum 25-hydroxyvitamin D levels were below normal in 64% of patients before liver transplantation [19]. In the same study, 25 of 58 (43%) cirrhotic patients had decreased serum concentrations of PTH. In addition, abnormalities in gonadal hormones have been reported. In male patients, testosterone values are normal or below normal, with higher sex hormone binding globulin, estradiol, and estrone levels compared to control subjects; testosterone levels are related to liver failure, since the most severely affected patients have the lowest testosterone values [2, 17, 20]. Gonadotropin levels (follicle-stimulating and luteinizing hormones) are normal or low, suggesting a combined failure of the hypothalamic–pituitary system and gonads [2, 20].

After liver transplantation, along with normalization of liver function and the consequences of the immunossuppresive regimens, marked changes occur in hormonal status. A significant increase in serum PTH levels is frequently described after liver transplantation [2, 18, 21, 22, 23]. After an early increase in the first month after transplantation, by 3 months the levels decline [21] or, more frequently, remain elevated during long-term follow-up. In some cases PTH levels are normal, though higher than pretransplant values [18, 24]. Moreover, serum creatinine values increase over the same period [2, 8, 23, 25], and both parameters display a positive correlation after liver transplantation. The low pretransplant serum 25-hydroxyvitamin D levels [2, 8, 16] show a highly significant increase within 3 months of transplantation [2, 18, 21, 26], and levels continue to increase over the first year. In men, there is a rapid decrease in sex hormone binding globulin following liver transplantation associated with an increase in total testosterone levels, resulting in a significant

TABLE 1 Incidence of bone fractures after liver transplantation

Author	Cases (n)	Fractures (%)	Follow-up (months)
Haagsma, 1988	26	38	24
Porayko, 1991	146	22	24
Eastell, 1991[a]	20	65	36
Arnold, 1992	48	31	15
Park, 1996	25	24	12
Ninkovic, 2000	37	27	3
Hay, 2001[a]	34	47	12
Leidig-Bruckner, 2001	130	33	48
Monegal, 2001	45	33	12

[a] Only cholestatic patients.

increase in the free testosterone index. High estrone and estradiol levels tend to decrease at 6 months after transplantation [2, 20].

Analysis of changes in biochemical markers of bone turnover prior to transplantation shows an increase in most bone resorption markers including hydroxyproline, free pyridinoline, and deoxypyridinoline crosslinks [2, 18, 19]. Nevertheless, when assessing biochemical markers of bone formation, cirrhotic patients display low [2, 17] or normal serum levels of osteocalcin, with normal or high values of bone-specific alkaline phosphatase and procollagen type I C propeptide. It should be pointed out, however, that collagen-related markers of bone turnover may be elevated as a consequence of liver fibrosis, reflecting liver collagen metabolism in addition to bone remodeling [27].

In accordance with histomorphometric data, biochemical markers of bone turnover increase early after liver transplantation, suggesting a high bone-turnover status. Moreover, liver transplant patients show a significant rise in bone resorption markers immediately after transplantation, as well as a slower increase in bone formation marker levels, which may suggest an imbalance between bone formation and resorption in the first months after liver transplantation [2, 19]. Thereafter, the few available data suggest that bone resorption markers remain elevated at 1 year after liver transplantation, as do bone formation markers such as osteocalcin, with increased mean levels at 1, 2, and 3 years [2, 8, 19].

V. HISTOMORPHOMETRIC DATA

Studies using histomorphometric analysis of bone in liver transplant patients are scarce [2, 26, 28, 29]. In patients with end-stage liver disease, bone biopsies before transplantation reveal a low bone turnover when compared with healthy controls [26, 28]. Nevertheless, differences in resorptive indices are seen between patients with prevalent vertebral fractures before transplantation and those without, with higher values in the former [2].

After liver transplantation, a significant increase in bone turnover has been observed. Thus, all histomorphometric studies of bone biopsies at three or six months after liver transplantation showed a significant increase in bone formation parameters such as osteoid volume and osteoid and osteoblast surface indices, as well as bone formation rate [2, 28], when compared with pretransplant data [2, 26, 28]; no significant differences in structural parameters were observed. Moreover, some results suggest that indices of resorption also tend to increase in the earlier post-transplant period, since a trend toward an increase in the resorption cavity size has been reported by Vedi et al. [28]. No evidence of osteomalacia in patients after liver transplantation has been found.

Limited histomorphometric data have been obtained concerning specific characteristics of patients who develop bone loss and fractures after liver transplantation, probably because of the small number of biopsies. In three patients with a continuous decrease in bone mineral density one year after liver transplantation, persistant low bone formation has been described [26]. In addition, bone biopsies obtained six months after liver transplantation suggest that patients who developed fractures in the first year after transplantation have significant differences in structural indices (lower bone surface density and trabecular number, as well as a higher trabecular separation) than nonfractured patients [2]. However, there are no baseline histomorphometric data that predict fracture risk in the post-transplant period.

VI. RISK FACTORS FOR FRACTURES AND BONE LOSS

Assessment of risk factors for developing fractures after liver transplantation demonstrates that no pretransplant indicator reliably predicts the risk of fracture in a given patient. Some conditions have been identified as major risk factors for fractures, however; these include low BMD and vertebral fractures before transplantation, as well as older age, the type of liver disease, and retransplantation. In addition, the immunosuppressive regimens used in liver transplantation play a key role in the development of bone loss and fractures (see Table 2).

Bone disease is common in patients with end-stage liver disease. Thus, osteoporosis by densitometric criteria (T-score ≤ -2.5 or Z-score ≤ -2) has been found in 24 to 37% of patients, depending on the series [2, 19, 30]. Most studies have reported that osteoporosis or osteopenia in the lumbar spine was present in a greater proportion of patients than osteoporosis or osteopenia in the proximal femur [19], although one study in a large cohort of patients showed lower femoral neck BMD measurements [30]. When considering the severity of the hepatic damage as a risk factor for developing pretransplant bone disease, most studies found no differences in the frequency of osteoporosis according to the severity of the liver disease classified using the Child-Pugh score [30]. Patients with more advanced liver disease (Child-Pugh C), however, have been found to have lower femoral Z-scores than Child-Pugh B patients [19]. In addition, it has been reported that severity and duration of liver disease are major risk factors for osteoporosis in women with primary biliary cirrhosis [31]. Few studies have assessed the rate of vertebral fractures in patients with severe chronic liver

TABLE 2 Risk factors for bone loss and fractures after liver transplantation

Pretransplantation	-Low bone mass (osteoporosis)[a]
	-Vertebral fractures[a]
	-Etiology of the liver disease[a]
Post-transplantation	-Immunosuppressive agents[a]
	-Immobilization
Other	-Advanced age
	-Variable individual susceptibility
	-Re-transplantation

[a] Main risk factors.

diseases prior to transplantation, but the average reported prevalence is close to 20–30% [19, 32].

Both features—pretransplant low BMD and fractures—are the major predictors of osteoporotic fractures after liver transplantation. Thus, Leidig-Bruckner et al. found in a long-term follow-up study that only vertebral fractures before transplantation were independent predictors for incident fractures following liver transplantation [13]. Also, a short-term prospective study showed that 46% of patients with 1 prevalent fracture and 62% of those with 2 or more prevalent fractures had a new vertebral fracture in the first 3 months [32]. Another prospective study identified osteoporosis, diagnosed according to densitometric criteria, as an independent risk factor for developing fractures during the first year after liver transplantation (odds ratio 5.6, 95% CI 1.31–24.53) [2].

Another relevant risk factor for fractures is the underlying liver disease. Patients with cholestatic liver disease, such as primary biliary cirrhosis and primary sclerosing cholangitis, seem to be more at risk than patients with other liver diseases for developing fractures after transplantation [11, 13, 33]. In some series, this has been observed together with a higher rate of pretransplant fractures [11] or low BMD [3, 11]. In addition, greater age was associated with an increased risk of fracture in some series, since patients with fracture were older than those withou [2], although in another study age did not contribute to vertebral fracture risk [13]. Other identified contributing factors for fractures include retransplantation [33] and postmenopausal status [3].

In addition to identified risk factors for developing fractures after liver transplantation, several conditions related to bone loss during this period may indirectly contribute to risk of fracture. Post-transplantation bone loss in the first 3 months has been associated with the number of postoperative inpatient days [26], an excess of bone resorption relative to bone formation [18], and an individual susceptibility determined by a specific polymorphism of the vitamin D receptor gene [34].

Immunosuppressive therapy also contributes to the development of bone loss and fractures. Glucocorticoids seem to play a key role. The initial rapid bone loss and the highest rate of fractures following liver transplantation occur with the highest doses, their withdrawal accelerates the recovery of lumbar BMD [35], and the use of low doses for a short time may be involved in a lower rate of fractures and less bone loss [7]. However, most studies have failed to demonstrate differences in the cumulative dose of glucocorticoids between patients with fractures and those without [2, 13] or a correlation between cumulative dose and BMD evolution [2, 8, 35]. In addition to glucocorticoids, other immunosuppressive agents such as cyclosporine (CsA) and FK506 frequently used in liver transplantation may influence bone disease. Both drugs induce high bone turnover and bone loss in rats [36], but their independent effects in transplant patients are not well established. Giannini et al. found that at one year after liver transplantation, femoral BMD was negatively associated with serum CsA

47. Reeves, H.L., Francis, R.M., Manas, D.M., Hudson, M., Day, C.P. (1998). Intravenous bisphosphonate prevents symptomatic osteoporotic vertebral collapse in patients after liver trasplantation. *Liver Transpl Surg*. 4:404–409.
48. Dodidou, P., Bruckner, T., Hosch, S., Haas, M., Klar, E., Sauer, P. et al. (2003). Better late than never? Experience with intravenous pamidronate treatment in patients with low bone mass or fractures following cardiac or liver transplantation. *Osteoporos Int*. 14:82–89.

CHAPTER 16

Bone Disease in Patients before and after Cardiac Transplantation

Adi Cohen, MD
Department of Medicine,
Durham: Veterans Affairs Medical Center, Durham, NC

Elizabeth Shane, MD
Department of Medicine, Columbia University
College of Physicians and Surgeons, New York, NY

I. INTRODUCTION

Cardiac transplantation has become an established therapy for end-stage heart disease, and recent years have seen a marked improvement in short- and long-term survival. One-year survival in patients transplanted after 1992 approximates 85%, and 5-year survival is 68% [1]. Advances in immunosuppressive therapies have contributed to these improved survival rates, and many patients are currently treated with regimens that combine glucocorticoids with calcineurin inhibitors (cyclosporine or tacrolimus), azathioprine, rapamycin, or mycophenolate mofetil. Unfortunately, both glucocorticoids and calcineurin inhibitors have specific adverse effects on the skeleton. It is thought that the independent and interrelated skeletal effects of glucocorticoids and calcineurin inhibitors lead to a form of bone disease characterized by rapid bone loss and high rates of fracture. These skeletal complications can significantly affect the quality of life of cardiac transplant recipients and represent a therapeutic challenge in the management of these patients.

In this chapter, we will discuss the clinical features of osteoporosis in cardiac transplant recipients as well as the mechanisms of bone loss that may occur both before and after transplantation. Additionally, we will address treatment strategies that may benefit patients with this unique type of bone disease.

II. BONE DISEASE PRIOR TO CARDIAC TRANSPLANTATION

Unlike renal and liver failure, congestive heart failure (CHF) is not associated with a specific type of bone disease. However, patients approaching cardiac transplant can experience bone insults related to drugs such as heparin, or loop diuretics (which cause prerenal azotemia), immobility, and vitamin D deficiency. Thus, evaluations of bone mineral density (BMD) in such populations have shown that osteoporosis and osteopenia are common in patients with severe CHF. In a study of 91 patients with severe CHF (New York Heart Association functional class III or IV) [2], osteopenia (defined as bone mineral density T score between −1.0 and −2.5) was present in 43% at the lumbar spine, 47% at the total hip, and 42% at the femoral neck. Osteoporosis (defined as BMD T score ≤ −2.5) was present in 7% at the lumbar spine, 6% at the total hip, and 19% at the femoral neck. In a second study evaluating femoral neck BMD, similar prevalence rates of osteoporosis and osteopenia were observed in 36 candidates for cardiac transplantation [3]. In addition, prospective studies that have evaluated patients prior to transplantation have documented lumbar spine osteoporosis (T score ≤ −2.5 or Z score < −2.0) in 12–40% of patients [4–7]. Another study of 58 patients found that vertebral bone density measured by single-energy CT scan before transplantation was approximately 20% lower than age-matched controls [8]. Measurement of biochemical markers of bone turnover in this population suggests the presence of increased bone resorption [2, 3]. Markers of bone formation have been both higher [9] and lower [10, 11] than healthy controls.

Patients with CHF may have abnormal bone and mineral homeostasis related to both the pathophysiology and the therapy of their cardiac disease. Patients with end-stage cardiac disease may have risk factors for osteoporosis such as older age, postmenopausal status, physical inactivity, and excessive use of tobacco and alcohol. Therapy with anticoagulants, such as heparin and warfarin, could contribute to bone loss [12]. Long-term use of heparin has been associated with bone mineral density losses [13, 14] and vertebral fractures [15] in observational studies of pregnant women, and there is biochemical evidence of decreased bone formation and increased bone resorption in an animal model exposed to heparin [16]. The consequences of multiple short courses of heparin therapy are not clear. Warfarin, which is more likely to be used chronically in patients with heart failure, blocks vitamin K–dependent gamma-carboxylation of osteocalcin and thus affects its binding to calcium [12]. A large retrospective cohort study found increased fracture risk associated with warfarin use [17], while a prospective observational study with 3.5 years of follow-up did not find increased fracture risk [18]. Therapy with loop diuretics increases urinary calcium losses [11] and has been associated with increased fracture risk [19, 20]. Impaired renal function, associated with CHF or its therapy, may lead to secondary hyperparathyroidism, abnormal vitamin D metabolism, and abnormal mineral homeostasis [2, 9].

Vitamin D deficiency may contribute to abnormalities in bone metabolism in this patient population. Lower serum 25-hydroxyvitamin D (25OHD) and 1,25 dihydroxyvitamin D [1,25$(OH)_2$D] levels were found in a study comparing CHF patients to healthy controls [10], and a study evaluating 101 patients with CHF has documented very low levels of 25OHD (≤ 9 ng/mL) and $1,25(OH)_2D$ (≤ 15 pg/mL) in 17 and 26%, respectively [2]. Physical inactivity may lead to inadequate sunlight exposure and in turn to low serum 25OHD levels. Severe right ventricular failure may be associated with passive intestinal congestion that impairs vitamin D absorption and liver congestion that could cause decreased hepatic synthesis of 25OHD. Renal insufficiency may be related to decreased 1-alpha hydroxylase activity and reduced synthesis of $1,25(OH)_2D$. Alterations in vitamin D action may also affect calcium metabolism in patients with heart failure. In a study of 75 postmenopausal Japanese women with CHF, the FF genotype of the vitamin D receptor was associated with increased urinary calcium losses and higher rates of bone loss at the spine [11].

III. BONE DISEASE AFTER CARDIAC TRANSPLANTATION

Factors that affect bone health before transplantation, such as older age, secondary hyperparathyroidism, and abnormal vitamin D metabolism, may persist or worsen after transplantation. In addition, cardiac transplant recipients are exposed to immunosuppressive medications that are thought to have specific negative effects upon bone metabolism and skeletal health. Most patients receive glucocorticoids, which are associated with profound suppression of bone formation (Chapter 3). In addition, glucocorticoid administration is associated with an early period of increased bone resorption followed by decreased bone resorption. Patients are usually also treated with calcineurin inhibitors (cyclosporine and tacrolimus), which have been associated with rapid bone loss in animal models [21]. Other immunosuppressive agents used after cardiac transplantation, such as azathioprine, rapamycin, and mycophenolate mofetil, have not been associated with a specific bone disease.

A. BMD after Cardiac Transplantation

Cross-sectional studies evaluating cardiac transplant recipients an average of 2–4 years after transplantation have documented lumbar spine and femoral neck osteoporosis in a substantial percentage of patients. In a study of 40 transplant recipients who had been treated with 1000 mg/day of calcium and 50,000 IU/week of vitamin D, Z scores ≤ −2 were found in 28% at the lumbar spine and 20% at the femoral neck [22]. In a study of 32 patients who were not receiving calcium or vitamin D, osteoporosis (T score < −2.5) at one or both of these sites was found in 41% of patients [23]. In a recent study comparing 9 patients receiving cyclosporine in a glucocorticoid-free regimen to 12 patients treated with both cyclosporine and glucocorticoids, osteoporosis (T score ≤ −2.5 at the lumbar spine or femoral neck) was documented in approximately 30% in both groups [24]. Some cross-sectional studies have found correlations between BMD and time since transplantation [25, 26], while others have not [22, 27].

Cross-sectional studies have also documented low bone density in pediatric recipients of cardiac transplants, who are exposed to drugs that affect the skeleton during a period of growth and bone mineral accrual. In 19 adolescents evaluated an average of 19 months after cardiac transplantation, BMD was 12% lower at the lumbar spine and 13% lower at the femoral neck than published norms matched for gender and age [28]. In another study of nine adult survivors of cardiac transplantation, osteoporosis (Z score adolescent ≤ −2.0) was present in 56% at the lumbar spine, 33% at the femoral neck, and 100% at the one-third site of the radius [29]. It is not clear whether adolescent transplant recipients have low BMD due to failure of bone mass acquisition or due to an actual period of bone mineral loss.

Several investigators have prospectively measured BMD in observational studies of adult transplant recipients, and they have found that the most rapid rate of BMD decline occurs in the first 6 to 12 months after transplantation. Lumbar spine BMD falls 3 to 9% over the first post-transplant year [5, 30–33], generally stabilizes after the first 6 to 12 months [30, 32], and may increase by the third post-transplant year [30] (see Figure 1a). Femoral neck BMD declines 9 to 11% over the first post-transplant year [5, 30–32] and stabilizes thereafter [30] (see Figure 1b). At the distal radius, continuing bone loss has been documented over 3 years of follow-up [30]. Another study, observing patients after cardiac transplantation performed in 1999, 2000, and 2001, found smaller declines in BMD, possibly due to the reduction of post-transplant glucocorticoid doses in recent years [34] (see Figure 1). Some studies have found associations between the rate of bone loss and glucocorticoid dose [30] as well as older age at transplant [8], while others have not found these relationships [32, 35].

B. Fractures after Cardiac Transplantation

Cross-sectional studies surveying spinal radiographs in populations of transplant recipients have documented prevalent vertebral fractures in 22–42% [9, 22–24, 36]. Studies of patients referred for evaluation of bone health have documented prevalent vertebral fractures in up to 56% [25, 26]. Prospective observational studies have found an incidence of fractures ranging from 15 to 36% [4, 31, 37] in the first year. In a study by Shane et al. (n=47), fractures occurred in 36% of patients during the first post-transplant year. The majority involved the spine, and 85% of patients who sustained fractures did so within the first 6 months [37]. Similarly Leidig-Bruckner et al. observed that nearly one-third of 105 patients had

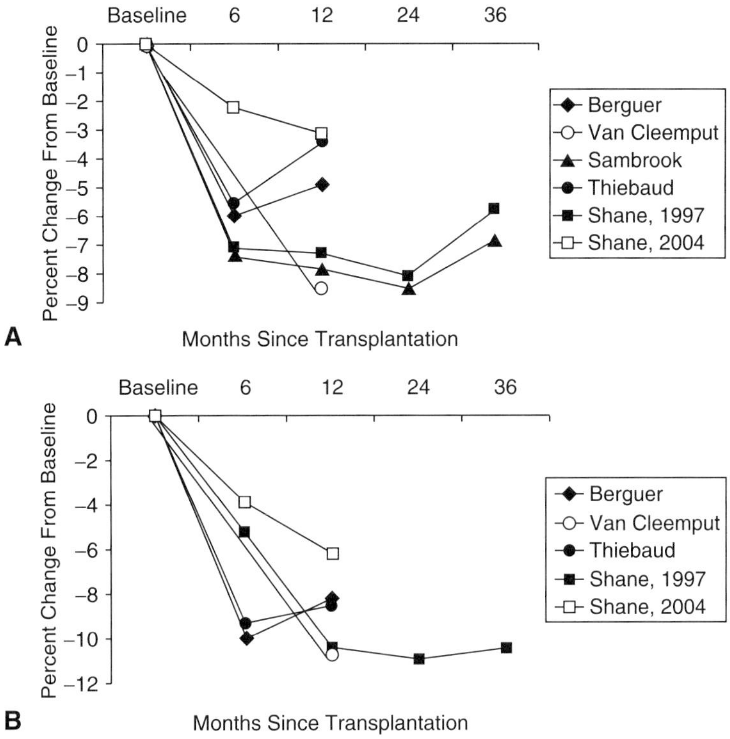

FIGURE 1 Early post-transplantation bone loss at the lumbar spine (A) and hip (B) is generally followed by stabilization after 6 to 12 months, and increases in lumbar spine BMD have been observed in the third year after transplantation.

sustained a vertebral fracture by the end of the third year after heart transplantation [4].

Glucocorticoid [4, 37] and cyclosporine [37] exposure has not been related to fracture risk, probably because most patients receive high and relatively consistent doses. Other factors may have relevance as clinical predictors, however. In a cross-sectional study of 51 males (11–120 months after cardiac transplantation) utilizing high spatial resolution magnetic resonance imaging of the calcaneus, certain aspects of bone structure, such as increased trabecular separation and decreased trabecular number, correlated with increased prevalence of vertebral fractures [36]. Leidig-Bruckner et al. found that a lumbar spine BMD T score < -1 (hazard ratio 3.1; 95% CI: 1.2 to 7.9) and older age (hazard ratio for each 5 year increase, 1.34; 95% CI: 1.03 to 1.75) conferred a greater risk of vertebral fracture over a mean follow-up time of 3.7 years [4] (see Figure 2). Shane et al. found relationships between fracture incidence and both pretransplantation femoral neck BMD and age, but only for women [37]. In male patients, those who fractured sustained significantly more bone loss at the femoral neck during the first 6 months [37].

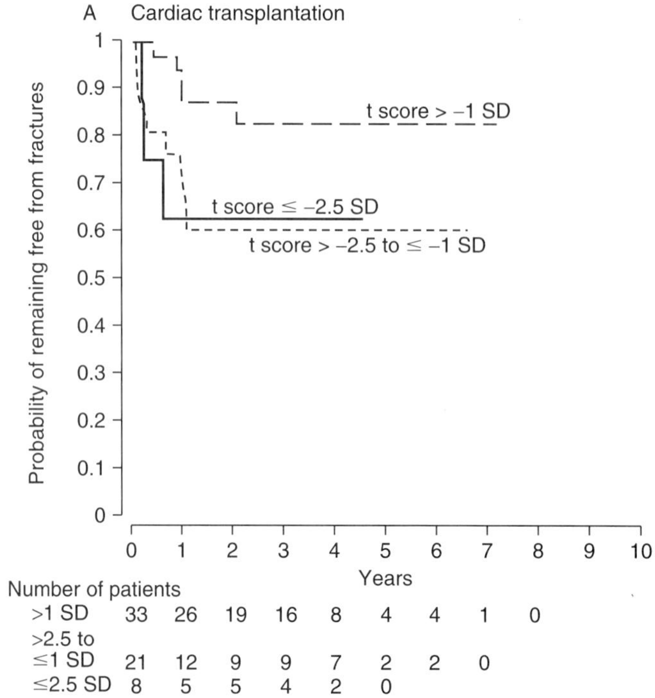

FIGURE 2 Effect of pretransplant lumbar spine BMD on risk of vertebral fracture after cardiac transplantation: Kaplan-Meier analysis. **t* scores. From Leidig-Bruckner et al. (2001). Frequency and predictors of osteoporotic fractures after cardiac or liver transplantation: a follow-up study. *The Lancet*. 357:342–347. Reprinted with permission from Elsevier.

C. Bone Turnover Markers and the Mechanism of Bone Loss after Cardiac Transplantation

In studies evaluating recipients of cardiac transplants, there is biochemical evidence of two distinct phases of abnormal bone turnover. An early period of rapid bone loss occurs in the first six months, during which there is evidence of uncoupling of bone turnover with decreased bone formation and increased bone resorption (see Figure 3). These changes occur in the context of high glucocorticoid doses used in the early post-transplant period and are consistent with the changes generally observed in patients using glucocorticoids alone, though the increase in bone resorption markers may be more pronounced. As glucocorticoid doses are tapered, bone formation recovers with recoupling of bone formation and resorption, albeit at the expense of higher bone turnover. During this second phase, rates of bone loss and fracture are considerably slower.

In prospective studies observing patients from the time of transplantation, there are transient increases in markers of bone resorption and decreases in markers of bone formation (osteocalcin) soon after transplantation [30, 33]. As glucocorticoid doses are tapered after the first 6 months, there are further changes in bone turnover. While some

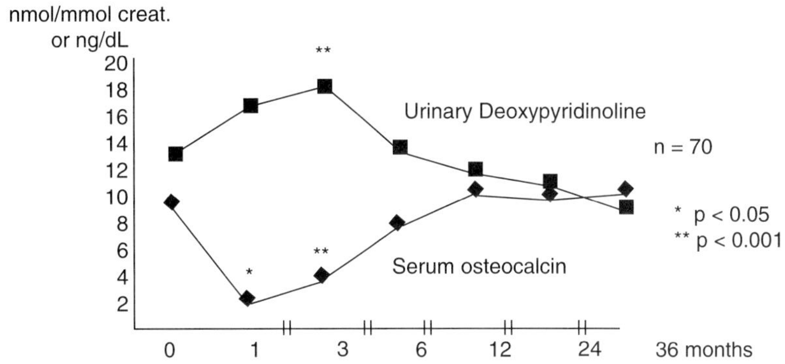

FIGURE 3 Serum osteocalcin concentration and urinary excretion of deoxypyridinoline after cardiac transplantation. The biochemical pattern seen in the early post-transplant period provides evidence for increased bone resorption (deoxypyridinoline) and decreased bone formation (osteocalcin), and thus suggests uncoupling of bone remodeling. Adapted from Shane et al. (1997). Bone loss and turnover after cardiac transplantation. *J Clin Endocrinol Metab.* 82(5):1497–1506. Copyright 1997, The Endocrine Society.

studies find a return of bone turnover markers towards the upper end of the normal range by 6–12 months after transplantation [30, 33], others document frankly elevated markers of resorption and formation at 18 months after transplantation [32].

The majority of cross-sectional studies, evaluating patients at a variety of time points after transplantation, have documented increased osteocalcin, a marker of bone formation [9, 22, 23, 25, 27]. Additionally, some cross-sectional studies have found elevations in markers of bone resorption [23, 27]. Serum osteocalcin levels may be difficult to interpret as osteocalcin is excreted by the kidney and may accumulate when creatinine clearance falls below 30mL/min [38]. Since most patients evaluated after cardiac transplantation have only mild renal insufficiency, it is likely that the elevations in osteocalcin seen in this population represent an actual increase in bone turnover. These increases in bone formation contrast with the low-turnover state and decreased osteocalcin levels found in patients on long-term glucocorticoids alone [39, 40], and suggest that factors other than glucocorticoid exposure contribute to the bone disease seen after transplantation.

D. Hormonal Factors

Heart transplantation may lead to secondary hyperparathyroidism, which could contribute to the high bone turnover state consistently observed in long-term heart transplant recipients. Elevated parathyroid hormone (PTH) levels have been observed in 21–72% of post-transplant patients evaluated in 3 cross-sectional studies [22, 23, 27]. In a fourth cross-sectional study, evaluating adult survivors of adolescent cardiac transplantation, elevated PTH levels were observed in 75% of patients [29]. In this patient population, a role for PTH in the pathogenesis of bone loss was also suggested by the high prevalence of osteoporosis at the one-third radius (100%) [29], a site sensitive to the catabolic effects of sustained PTH action.

The well-known nephrotoxic effects of cyclosporine and tacrolimus may lead to decreased synthesis of 1,25(OH)$_2$D and resultant hyperparathyroidism. In 70 patients followed for 3 years after cardiac transplantation, decreases in 1,25(OH)$_2$D were observed throughout the first year, and the decline in 1,25(OH)$_2$D concentrations, as well as elevated PTH levels, correlated with deteriorating renal function [30]. Decreased calcium absorption in the setting of glucocorticoid therapy may also contribute to secondary hyperparathyroidism. In the study [22] with the lowest prevalence of hyperparathyroidism (21%), all patients had received treatment with calcium (1000 mg/day) and vitamin D (50,000 IU/week), which could have suppressed PTH secretion. Interestingly, in 60 post-transplant patients evaluated by Boncimino et al. [41], those with lower magnesium levels had significantly lower PTH concentrations and lower rates of femoral neck bone loss, suggesting that magnesium deficiency may be protective in this regard.

In addition, hypogonadism may occur in the post-transplant period. In male cardiac transplant recipients, testosterone has been shown to fall immediately after transplantation and normalize after 6–12 months [30, 33]. The fall may be related to suppression of the hypothalamic–pituitary–gonadal axis during recovery from the surgery, as well as the high doses of glucocorticoids used in the immediate post-transplant period. Decreased gonadal hormones may thus be a factor in the post-transplantation bone loss observed in both men and women.

IV. MANAGEMENT OF OSTEOPOROSIS IN RECIPIENTS OF CARDIAC TRANSPLANTATION

Since increased bone turnover, deficiency of active vitamin D, and low testosterone have all been implicated in the pathophysiology of osteoporosis after cardiac transplantation, most therapies have been aimed at correcting these conditions. The majority of therapeutic trials have focused on the use of vitamin D metabolites and antiresorptive agents. As an extensive discussion of the management of post-transplantation osteoporosis is provided in Chapters 23 and 24, this section will provide only a brief summary of prevention and treatment strategies relating to osteoporosis after cardiac transplantation.

A. Vitamin D Metabolites

Treatment with parent vitamin D, in doses of 400–1000 IU/day, has not been sufficient to prevent bone loss after cardiac transplantation [30, 32, 42].

Benefits have been found, however, with the use of vitamin D metabolites, such as calcidiol and calcitriol. In a study by Garcia-Delgado et al., patients treated with 32,000 IU/week of oral calcidiol for 18 months had improvements in lumbar spine BMD after transplantation, while patients treated with oral etidronate or nasal calcitonin exhibited decreases in BMD [6]. In contrast, Van Cleemput et al. found that 0.25 to 1 μg/day of oral alfacalcidol therapy attenuated but did not eliminate bone loss in a comparison made to a group receiving oral etidronate [43].

In a study by Stempfle et al., a low dose of calcitriol (0.25 μg/day) did not provide a statistically significant benefit compared to placebo in patients who began therapy several months after transplantation [44] (see Figure 4). However, 6 months of therapy with a higher dose of calcitriol (0.5 μg/day), given immediately after cardiac or lung transplantation, was associated with attenuation of lumbar spine bone loss compared to an untreated reference group in a study by Henderson et al. [45]. The benefit of this short-term therapy waned, and bone loss resumed after calcitriol was discontinued. The same group evaluated longer-term use of calcitriol (0.5–0.75 μg/day) in 65 heart and lung transplant recipients in a recent 2-year, double-blind study [46]. All subjects received calcium and were randomized to receive placebo, 12 months of calcitriol, or 24 months of calcitriol. Lumbar spine bone loss was similar among all three groups. There was, however, significantly less femoral bone loss after 12 months in the groups that received calcitriol (3.9% and 1.2% versus 6.6% in controls; $p < 0.05$). As with the prior study, the benefits of calcitriol waned after its cessation, and by 24 months, femoral neck bone loss in the group that had stopped therapy after 12 months was

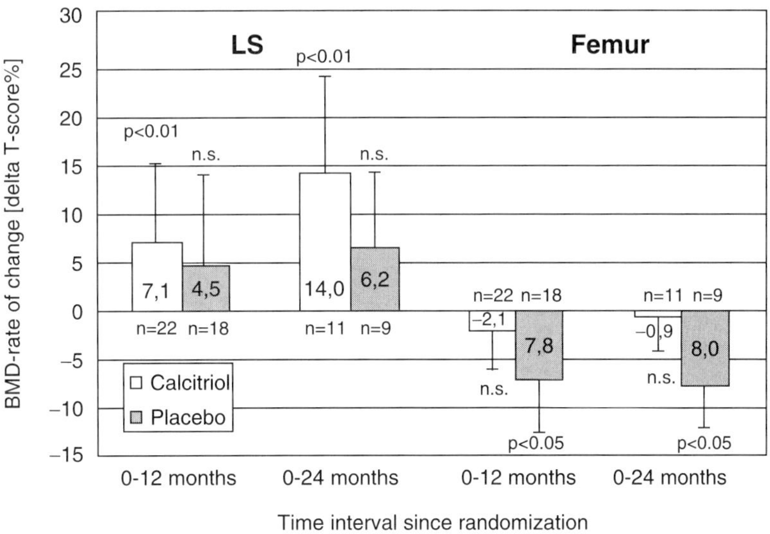

FIGURE 4 Changes in BMD during the two-year study period in calcitriol-treated versus placebo-treated patients. Randomization took place several months after transplantation and after the most rapid phase of bone loss. From: Stempfle et al. (2002). The role of tacrolimus (FK506)-based immunosuppression on bone mineral density and bone turnover after cardiac transplantation: a prospective, longitudinal, randomized, double-blind trial with calcitriol. *Transplantation*. 73(4):547–552.

similar to that of controls (7.4% versus 8.2%). Additionally, hypercalcemia and hypercalcuria were common in this study, occurring in 18% and 59% of calcitriol-treated subjects, respectively.

Two studies [7, 34] that compared calcitriol to potent bisphosphonates (alendronate and pamidronate) are discussed in the next section.

B. Bisphosphonates

Etidronate has been evaluated in several studies but has not been effective in preventing or treating bone loss in recipients of heart transplants [6, 43]. Several investigators have studied intravenous pamidronate for the prevention of bone loss in the early transplant period [7, 34, 42, 47]. In a 1-year, open-label study using the two bisphosphonates sequentially, a single intravenous dose of pamidronate (60 mg), followed by cyclic etidronate (400 mg for 2 weeks every 3 months) and daily oral calcitriol (0.25 μg/day), prevented lumbar spine and femoral neck bone loss and reduced fracture rates in heart transplant recipients compared to historical controls [47]. In another nonrandomized trial, 11 cardiac transplant recipients with osteoporosis prior to transplantation (BMD T score < –2.5) were treated with calcium (1 g/day), vitamin D (1000 IU/day), and intravenous pamidronate (60 mg every 3 months) for 3 years [42]. Although pamidronate was started an average of 6 months after the graft, lumbar spine BMD increased 14.3% compared to baseline, and femoral neck BMD, which decreased 3.4% in the first year, recovered totally after 3 years of treatment.

Bisphosphonates have been compared to calcitriol in two randomized trials. Bianda et al. reported lumbar spine and femoral neck bone loss of only 1.9% and 1.4%, respectively, at 12 months after transplantation, in patients (n = 14) who received calcium (1 g/day) and a small dose of pamidronate (0.5 mg/kg every 3 months). In patients (n = 12) randomized to a combination of calcium (1 g/day), nasal calcitonin (200 IU/day), and calcitriol (0.25–0.5 μg/day) given only for the first 3 months, lumbar spine BMD fell by 7.4% and femoral neck BMD by 6.3% [7]. A second trial compared patients randomized to treatment with either oral alendronate (10 mg/day; n = 74) or oral calcitriol (0.5 μg/day; n = 75) for 1 year [34]. They were compared to each other and, in a secondary analysis, to a nonrandomized untreated reference group (n = 27). All participants received calcium (945 mg/day elemental calcium) and vitamin D (1000 IU/day). The intention-to-treat analysis found no significant differences in bone loss or fracture incidence between the alendronate- and calcitriol-treated groups. Reference subjects lost significantly more bone mass at the spine and femoral neck, however (see Figure 5). Additionally, more reference subjects sustained fractures (13.6% versus 3.6–6.8%), although the difference was not statistically significant. As expected, hypercalcemia and hypercalciuria occurred frequently (8% and 27%, respectively) in the calcitriol-treated patients [34]. In a follow-up study conducted over a

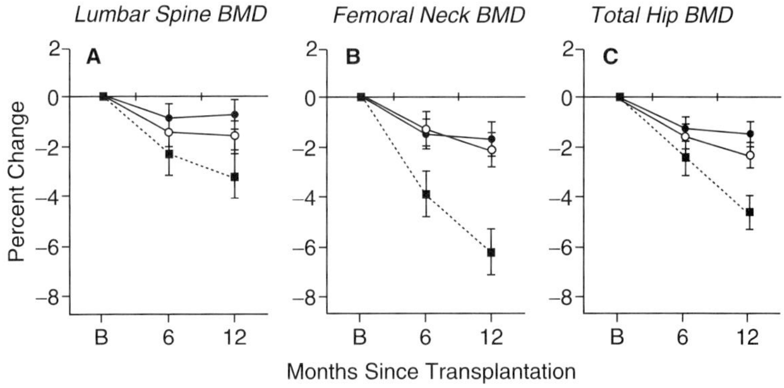

FIGURE 5 Intention to treat analysis of mean percentage change in BMD from baseline (B) in alendronate (closed circle) and calcitriol (open circle) arms. The nonrandomized reference group is shown in the closed squares. Data are ± SEM. From Shane et al. (2004). Alendronate versus calcitriol for the prevention of bone loss after cardiac transplantation. *N Engl J Med.* 350:767-776. Copyright © 2004 Massachusetts Medical Society.

second year, patients evaluated 12 months after the cessation of calcitriol had a rise in markers of bone turnover that did not occur in those who had been treated with alendronate [48]. Despite the increase in bone turnover, BMD remained stable in both groups during 12 months of observation after cessation of alendronate and calcitriol therapy [48].

These two studies [7, 34] initiated treatment in the immediate post-transplant period, at a mean of two to three weeks after the graft. In patients treated several months after transplantation, both oral clodronate and intravenous pamidronate have been beneficial for the treatment of established bone loss [49, 50].

C. Other Therapies

Since mechanical loading is an osteogenic stimulus, exercise training after transplantation may be beneficial to bone. In a small, randomized study by Braith et al., 8 cardiac transplant recipients enrolled in a resistance exercise training program and treated with alendronate (10 mg/day) beginning 2 months after transplantation had greater improvements in lumbar spine and femoral neck BMD during the ensuing 6 months when compared to a group receiving alendronate without exercise training [51].

Gonadal hormone replacement therapy may also be beneficial. Fahrleitner et al. evaluated male cardiac transplant recipients treated with intravenous ibandronate and found that hypogonadal men who received testosterone supplementation had an improved BMD response at one year compared to hypogonadal men who did not receive testosterone [52]. Hormone replacement therapy has been shown to protect the skeleton in women receiving glucocorticoids [39], but it has not been studied in female recipients of cardiac transplantation. Gonadal hormone replacement therapy may have risks in both male and female cardiac transplant recipients. Testosterone replacement therapy may cause prostatic hypertrophy, hyperlipidemia, and abnormal liver enzymes, and it should be reserved for men with true hypogonadism. Recent data suggest increased rates of coronary events and stroke in postmenopausal women treated with estrogen and progesterone [53]. Thus the risk of therapy could outweigh the benefits in most female cardiac transplant recipients.

Calcitonin has also been studied in recipients of cardiac transplants, but it has been found to be relatively ineffective in preventing or treating bone loss [6, 54, 55].

V. CONCLUSIONS

In recipients of cardiac transplants, the actions of several medications and clinical factors interact to produce cumulative deleterious effects on the skeleton, leading to rapid bone loss and increased incidence of fractures. Early rapid bone loss has been observed after transplantation, and the majority of fractures occur in the first six months. Although more recent studies [34] suggest that rates of bone loss and fracture may be lower than those found in studies conducted in the early 1990s, it is still prudent to initiate aggressive measures to prevent transplantation osteoporosis. Management of these patients should combine assessment and treatment of pretransplantation bone disease with preventive therapy in the immediate post-transplantation period. Treatment of established osteoporosis after cardiac transplantation is also beneficial. Most therapeutic trials have focused on the use of vitamin D metabolites and antiresorptive agents. Calcitriol, due to its narrow therapeutic window, is not recommended as a first-line agent for post-transplantation osteoporosis. Data from clinical trials suggest that bisphosphonates are safe and effective for the prevention and treatment of osteoporosis after cardiac transplantation, and should be considered in all cardiac transplant recipients.

REFERENCES

1. Hosenpud, J.D., Bennett, L.E., Keck, B.M., Boucek, M.M., Novick, R.J. (2001). The registry of the International Society for Heart and Lung Transplantation: sixteenth official report. *J Heart Lung Transplant.* 20:805–815.
2. Shane, E., Mancini, D., Aaronson, K., et al. (1997). Bone mass, vitamin D deficiency, and hyperparathyroidism in congestive heart failure. *Am J Med.* 103:197–207.
3. Kerschan-Schindl, K., Strametz-Juranek, J., Heinze, G., et al. (2003). Pathogenesis of bone loss in heart transplant candidates and recipients. *J Heart Lung Transplant.* 22:843–850.
4. Leidig-Bruckner, G., Hosch, S., Dodidou, P., et al. (2001). Frequency and predictors of osteoporotic fractures after cardiac or liver transplantation: a follow-up study. *Lancet.* 357:342–347.
5. Berguer, D.G., Krieg, M.A., Thiebaud, D., et al. (1994). Osteoporosis in heart transplant recipients: a longitudinal study. *Transplant Proc.* 26:2649–2651.

6. Garcia-Delgado, I., Prieto, S., Gil-Fraguas, L., Robles, E., Rufilanchas, J.J., Hawkins, F. (1997). Calcitonin, etidronate, and calcidiol treatment in bone loss after cardiac transplantation. *Calcif Tissue Int.* 60:155–159.
7. Bianda, T., Linka, A., Junga, G., et al. (2000). Prevention of osteoporosis in heart transplant recipients: a comparison of calcitriol with calcitonin and pamidronate. *Calcif Tissue Int.* 67:116–121.
8. Muchmore, J.S., Cooper, D.K., Ye, Y., Schlegel, V.T., Zuhdi, N. (1991). Loss of vertebral bone density in heart transplant patients. *Transplant Proc.* 23:1184–1185.
9. Lee, A.H., Mull, R.L., Keenan, G.F., et al. (1994). Osteoporosis and bone morbidity in cardiac transplant recipients. *Am J Med.* 96:35–41.
10. Schleithoff, S.S., Zittermann, A., Stuttgen, B., et al. (2003). Low serum levels of intact osteocalcin in patients with congestive heart failure. *J Bone Miner Metab.* 21:247–252.
11. Nishio, K., Mukae, S., Aoki, S., et al. (2003). Congestive heart failure is associated with the rate of bone loss. *J Intern Med.* 253:439–446.
12. Rosen, H.N. Drugs that affect bone metabolism, in UpToDate, Rose, B.D., ed. 2003, . Wellesley, MA: UpToDate.
13. Dahlman, T.C., Sjoberg, H.E., Ringertz, H. (1994). Bone mineral density during long-term prophylaxis with heparin in pregnancy. *Am J Obstet Gynecol.* 170:1315–1320.
14. Barbour, L.A., Kick, S.D., Steiner, J.F., et al. (1994). A prospective study of heparin-induced osteoporosis in pregnancy using bone densitometry. *Am J Obstet Gynecol.* 170:862–869.
15. Dahlman, T.C. (1993). Osteoporotic fractures and the recurrence of thromboembolism during pregnancy and the puerperium in 184 women undergoing thromboprophylaxis with heparin. *Am J Obstet Gynecol.* 168:1265–1270.
16. Muir, J.M., Andrew, M., Hirsh, J., et al. (1996). Histomorphometric analysis of the effects of standard heparin on trabecular bone in vivo. *Blood.* 88:1314–1320.
17. Caraballo, P.J., Heit, J.A., Atkinson, E.J., et al. (1999). Long-term use of oral anticoagulants and the risk of fracture. *Arch Intern Med.* 159:1750–1756.
18. Jamal, S.A., Browner, W.S., Bauer, D.C., Cummings, S.R. (1998). Warfarin use and risk for osteoporosis in elderly women. Study of Osteoporotic Fractures Research Group. *Ann Intern Med.* 128:829–832.
19. Tromp, A.M., Ooms, M.E., Popp-Snijders, C., Roos, J.C., Lips, P. (2000). Predictors of fractures in elderly women. *Osteoporos Int.* 11:134–140.
20. Heidrich, F.E., Stergachis, A., Gross, K.M. (1991). Diuretic drug use and the risk for hip fracture. *Ann Intern Med.* 115:1–6.
21. Epstein, S. (1996). Post-transplantation bone disease: the role of immunosuppressive agents and the skeleton. *J Bone Miner Res.* 11:1–7.
22. Shane, E., Rivas, M.C., Silverberg, S.J., Kim, T.S., Staron, R.B., Bilezikian, J.P. (1993). Osteoporosis after cardiac transplantation. *Am J Med.* 94:257–264.
23. Glendenning, P., Kent, G.N., Adler, B.D., et al. (1999). High prevalence of osteoporosis in cardiac transplant recipients and discordance between biochemical turnover markers and bone histomorphometry. *Clin Endocrinol (Oxf).* 50:347–355.
24. Hofle, G., Holzmuller, H., Gouya, G., et al. (2003). Lower serum beta-CrossLaps in male cardiac transplant recipients treated without prednisolone. *Transpl Int.* 16:523–528.
25. Rich, G.M., Mudge, G.H., Laffel, G.L., LeBoff, M.S. (1992). Cyclosporine A and prednisone-associated osteoporosis in heart transplant recipients. *J Heart Lung Transplant.* 11:950–958.
26. Fahrleitner, A., Prenner, G., Leb, G., et al. (2003). Serum osteoprotegerin is a major determinant of bone density development and prevalent vertebral fracture status following cardiac transplantation. *Bone.* 32:96–106.
27. Guo, C.Y., Johnson, A., Locke, T.J., Eastell, R. (1998). Mechanisms of bone loss after cardiac transplantation. *Bone.* 22:267–271.
28. Braith, R.W., Howard, C., Fricker, F.J., Mitchell, M., Edwards, D.G. (2000). Glucocorticoid-induced osteopenia in adolescent heart transplant recipients. *J Heart Lung Transplant.* 19:840–845.

29. Cohen, A., Addonizio, L.J., Lamour, J.M., et al. (2004). Osteoporosis in adult survivors of adolscent cardiac transplantation may be related to hyperparathyroidism, mild renal insufficiency and increased bone turnover. *J Heart Lung Transplant.* In Review.
30. Shane, E., Rivas, M., McMahon, D.J., et al. (1997). Bone loss and turnover after cardiac transplantation. *J Clin Endocrinol Metab.* 82:1497–1506.
31. Van Cleemput, J., Daenen, W., Nijs, J., Geusens, P., Dequeker, J., Vanhaecke, J. (1995). Timing and quantification of bone loss in cardiac transplant recipients. *Transpl Int.* 8:196–200.
32. Thiebaud, D., Krieg, M.A., Gillard-Berguer, D., Jacquet, A.F., Goy, J.J., Burckhardt, P. (1996). Cyclosporine induces high bone turnover and may contribute to bone loss after heart transplantation. *Eur J Clin Invest.* 26:549–555.
33. Sambrook, P.N., Kelly, P.J., Fontana, D., et al. (1994). Mechanisms of rapid bone loss following cardiac transplantation. *Osteoporos Int.* 4:273–276.
34. Shane, E., Addesso, V., Namerow, P.B., et al. (2004). Alendronate versus calcitriol for the prevention of bone loss after cardiac transplantation. *N Engl J Med.* 350(8):767–776.
35. Sambrook, P.N., Kelly, P.J., Keogh, A.M., et al. (1994). Bone loss after heart transplantation: a prospective study. *J Heart Lung Transplant.* 13:116–120; discussion 121.
36. Link, T.M., Lotter, A., Beyer, F., et al. (2000). Changes in calcaneal trabecular bone structure after heart transplantation: an MR imaging study. *Radiology.* 217:855–862.
37. Shane, E., Rivas, M., Staron, R.B., et al. (1996). Fracture after cardiac transplantation: a prospective longitudinal study. *J Clin Endocrinol Metab.* 81:1740–1746.
38. Delmas, P.D., Wilson, D.M., Mann, K.G., Riggs, B.L. (1983). Effect of renal function on plasma levels of bone Gla-protein. *J Clin Endocrinol Metab.* 57:1028–1030.
39. Lane, N.E., Lukert, B. (1998). The science and therapy of glucocorticoid-induced bone loss. *Endocrinol Metab Clin North Am.* 27:465–483.
40. Dempster, D.W. (1989). Bone histomorphometry in glucocorticoid-induced osteoporosis. *J Bone Miner Res.* 4:137–141.
41. Boncimino, K., McMahon, D.J., Addesso, V., Bilezikian, J.P., Shane, E. (1999). Magnesium deficiency and bone loss after cardiac transplantation. *J Bone Miner Res.* 14:295–303.
42. Krieg, M.A., Seydoux, C., Sandini, L., et al. (2001). Intravenous pamidronate as treatment for osteoporosis after heart transplantation: a prospective study. *Osteoporos Int.* 12:112–116.
43. Van Cleemput, J., Daenen, W., Geusens, P., Dequeker, P., Van De Werf, F., VanHaecke, J. (1996). Prevention of bone loss in cardiac transplant recipients. A comparison of biphosphonates and vitamin D. *Transplantation.* 61:1495–1499.
44. Stempfle, H.U., Werner, C., Siebert, U., et al. (2002). The role of tacrolimus (FK506)-based immunosuppression on bone mineral density and bone turnover after cardiac transplantation: a prospective, longitudinal, randomized, double-blind trial with calcitriol. *Transplantation.* 73:547–552.
45. Henderson, K., Eisman, J., Keogh, A., et al. (2001). Protective effect of short-tem calcitriol or cyclical etidronate on bone loss after cardiac or lung transplantation. *J Bone Miner Res.* 16:565–571.
46. Sambrook, P., Henderson, N.K., Keogh, A., et al. (2000). Effect of calcitriol on bone loss after cardiac or lung transplantation. *J Bone Miner Res.* 15:1818–1824.
47. Shane, E., Rodino, M.A., McMahon, D.J., et al. (1998). Prevention of bone loss after heart transplantation with antiresorptive therapy: a pilot study. *J Heart Lung Transplant.* 17:1089–1096.
48. Addesso, V., Cohen, A., McMahon, D.J., et al. (2003). Bone density is stable after discontinuing antiresorptive therapy during the second year after cardiac transplantation. *J Bone Miner Res.* 18:S174.
49. Ippoliti, G., Pellegrini, C., Campana, C., et al. (2003). Clodronate treatment of established bone loss in cardiac recipients: a randomized study. *Transplantation.* 75:330–334.

50. Dodidou, P., Bruckner, T., Hosch, S., et al. (2003). Better late than never? Experience with intravenous pamidronate treatment in patients with low bone mass or fractures following cardiac or liver transplantation. *Osteoporos Int.* 14:82–89.
51. Braith, R.W., Magyari, P.M., Fulton, M.N., Aranda, J., Walker, T., Hill, J.A. (2003). Resistance exercise training and alendronate reverse glucocorticoid-induced osteoporosis in heart transplant recipients. *J Heart Lung Transplant.* 22:1082–1090.
52. Fahrleitner, A., Prenner, G., Tscheliessnigg, K.H., et al. (2002). Testosterone supplementation has additional benefits on bone metabolism in cardiac transplant recipients receiving intravenous bisphosphonate treatment: a prospective study. *J Bone Miner Metab.* 17:S388.
53. Rossouw, J.E., Anderson, G.L., Prentice, R.L., et al. (2002). Risks and benefits of estrogen plus progestin in healthy postmenopausal women: principal results from the Women's Health Initiative randomized controlled trial. *Jama.* 288:321–333.
54. Valimaki, M.J., Kinnunen, K., Tahtela, R., et al. (1999). A prospective study of bone loss and turnover after cardiac transplantation: effect of calcium supplementation with or without calcitonin. *Osteoporos Int.* 10:128–136.
55. Cremer, J., Struber, M., Wagenbreth, I., et al. (1999). Progression of steroid-associated osteoporosis after heart transplantation. *Ann Thorac Surg.* 67:130–133.

CHAPTER 17

Bone Loss in Patients before and after Lung Transplantation

Emily Stein, MD
Elizabeth Shane, MD
Department of Medicine, Columbia University
College of Physicians and Surgeons, New York, NY

I. INTRODUCTION

Most lung transplant recipients were exposed to high doses of glucocorticoids as therapy for their primary lung disease before transplantation. In addition, lung transplant recipients are more prone to rejection than other types of organ transplant recipients, and high doses of prednisone and other immunosuppressants must therefore be used after transplantation. At least in part for these reasons, osteoporosis and fractures are particularly common in candidates for and recipients of lung transplantation. This chapter reviews the prevalence and etiology of low bone mineral density (BMD) in patients awaiting lung transplantation, the changes in bone density and fracture incidence that develop after transplantation, and the efficacy of various treatment regimens in preventing and treating bone loss in these patients, both before and after lung transplantation. Cystic fibrosis is covered in Chapter 18, so in this chapter we focus on transplantation for other forms of pulmonary disease.

II. BONE DISEASE IN PATIENTS WITH END-STAGE PULMONARY DISEASE

Patients with end-stage lung disease are probably at higher risk for osteoporosis and fracture than patients with other types of organ failure [1]. The majority of patients with end-stage pulmonary disease who are being considered for transplantation have one or more well-known risk factors for osteoporosis, including older age, low body weight, Caucasian race, postmenopausal status, immobility, and chronic tobacco use (see Table 1). Chronic glucocorticoid therapy, used in the management of patients with end-stage chronic obstructive pulmonary disease (COPD), sarcoidosis, interstitial lung disease (ILD), and some patients with cystic fibrosis (CF), is a major pretransplantation risk factor for osteoporosis in candidates for lung transplantation. In addition, several factors specific to patients with end-stage lung disease and to the lung diseases from which they suffer may contribute to the bone loss. In patients with COPD, for example, an association has been demonstrated between hypercapnia, chronic respiratory acidosis, and biochemical evidence of increased bone resorption with resultant bone loss [2]. It has been postulated that in patients with sarcoidosis, several factors related solely to the disease process are responsible for causing bone loss, and there is evidence that even glucocorticoid-naïve subjects with sarcoidosis have lower BMD than the general public [2, 3]. Extrarenal and unregulated synthesis of $1,25(OH)_2D_3$ by alveolar macrophages and tissue macrophages at other sites results in hypercalciuria in 40–62% of patients and clinically significant hypercalcemia in approximately 5% [4]. Low BMD may also be related to high levels of $1,25(OH)_2D_3$, which may cause accelerated bone resorption. In addition, diffuse skeletal involvement with noncaseating granulomata may cause osteopenia, as may osteoclast activating factors produced by activated lymphocytes [5–8].

Several studies have found low bone mineral density and elevated fracture rates among candidates for lung transplantation [9–12]. Aris et al. performed a cross-sectional study of 100 patients before and after lung transplantation [11]. The pretransplant population consisted of 55 patients with end-stage COPD, CF, and other pulmonary diseases. BMD was measured by dual energy x-ray absorptiometry (DXA). In this group, 45% of patients had osteoporosis, as defined by a BMD greater than 2 standard deviations below the age-matched mean (Z score). The mean Z score was −1.32 at the lumbar spine and −1.55 at the femoral neck. Patients with CF and COPD had lower BMD than those with other pulmonary diseases. BMD correlated directly with body mass index (BMI) and inversely with cumulative dose of prednisone.

Shane et al. measured BMD by DXA in 70 predominantly Caucasian patients with end-stage lung disease awaiting lung transplantation [9]. The

TABLE 1 Major risk factors for osteoporosis in patients with end-stage pulmonary disease

Chronic glucocorticoid use
Low body mass index
Vitamin D deficiency
Hypogonadism
Hyperparathyroidism
Hypercapnia
Immobility
Tobacco

majority had COPD, CF, or idiopathic pulmonary fibrosis (IPF). Low bone mass was common. Osteopenia (T score between −1.0 and −2.49) was found in 35% of patients at the lumbar spine and 31% at the femoral neck. Osteoporosis (T score ≤ −2.5) was found in 30% at the lumbar spine and in 49% at the femoral neck. Vitamin D deficiency (defined as a serum 25-hydroxyvitamin D (25OHD) level ≤ 10 ng/ml) was more common in patients with CF and COPD: 36% and 20% respectively. Six of the 15 men studied had subnormal testosterone levels. No significant correlation was seen between these parameters and BMD. Although the majority of patients (66%) had significant glucocorticoid exposure, few were on any type of bone protective regimen. A significant inverse correlation was found between duration of glucocorticoid use and BMD at the lumbar spine. Patients with histories of chronic glucocorticoid use had lower BMD at both sites than their counterparts. Spinal fractures were found in 29% of patients with COPD and in 25% with CF. BMD and T scores tended to be lower in COPD patients with fractures, but this trend was not statistically significant, likely because of the small number of patients in this group.

Cahill et al. performed an osteoporosis evaluation that included BMD by DXA, spine radiographs, and biochemical indices relevant to bone health in 45 of 50 patients referred for lung transplantation between 1996 and 1999 [13]. Osteopenia was present in 49% at the lumbar spine and 62% at the total hip. Osteoporosis was present in 27% at the lumbar spine and 20% at the total hip. Only 15% of patients had normal BMD at both spine and hip. Prevalent vertebral compression deformities or hip fractures affected 29%. Fifty percent of the men and 20% of the women had untreated hypogonadism, and 15% of those in whom serum 25OHD was measured had levels below 15 ng/ml. Information on glucocorticoid use was not provided.

In a more recent study of 74 patients awaiting lung transplantation, Tschopp et al. found a similar prevalence of osteoporosis and osteopenia, as defined by World Health Organization (WHO) criteria [14]. The majority of patients studied had COPD, CF, IPF, or pulmonary hypertension. Osteopenia was found in 33% at the lumbar spine and 31% at the femoral neck. Osteoporosis was found in 50% at the lumbar spine and 61% at the femoral neck. Only 5% of the subjects had normal BMD. Osteoporosis was most common in those with COPD and CF (69% and 67%, respectively). BMI correlated directly with T score at all sites (see Figure 1). Chronic glucocorticoid use, for greater than 6 months, correlated inversely with lumbar spine T score and trended toward significance at the femoral neck. Vitamin D deficiency was observed in 25% and reduced serum osteocalcin in 28% of patients. No significant association between biochemical markers of bone turnover, serum 25-OHD, or parathyroid hormone (PTH) and BMD was found. There was a significant direct correlation between loss of lung function, as measured by forced expiratory volume over one minute (FEV-1), and BMD at all sites. The effect was most pronounced at the lumbar spine. A multivariate analysis that included age, gender, pulmonary diagnosis, BMI, glucocorticoid use, and FEV1% of predicted found that

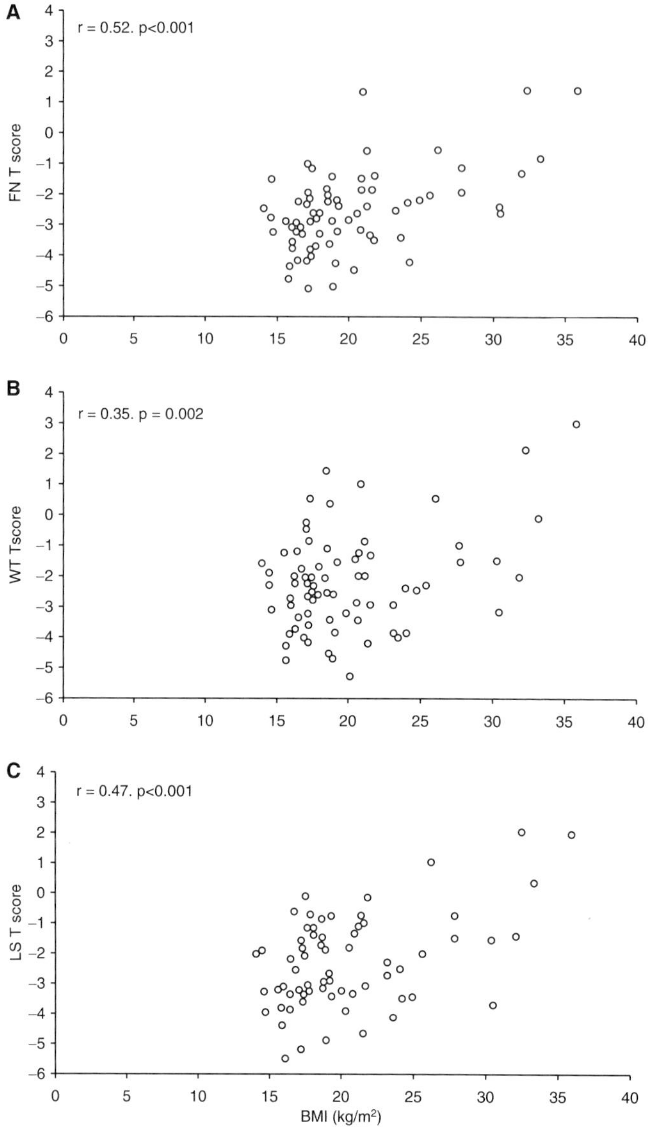

FIGURE 1 Direct relationship between body mass index and bone mineral density T score at the femoral neck (Panel A), Wards triangle (Panel B), and lumbar spine (Panel C). Reproduced from Tschopp et al. (2002). Osteoporosis before lung trasnplantation: association with low body mass index, but not with underlying disease. *American Journal of Transplantation*. 2:167-172. Reprinted with permission of Blackwell Publishing Ltd.

only BMI and FEV1% of predicted were independent risk factors for osteoporosis. This finding may have been confounded by the influence of muscle mass, and subsequently BMI, on FEV-1.

All of these studies clearly demonstrate the very high prevalence of osteoporosis in candidates for lung transplantation. Most studies clearly define the contribution of glucocorticoids to bone loss in patients with all types of severe pulmonary disease. In addition, low BMI is consistently related to BMD in the majority of these studies.

III. OSTEOPOROSIS IN PATIENTS AFTER LUNG TRANSPLANTATION

Several cross-sectional studies have evaluated lung transplant recipients at various times after grafting. In general, the prevalence of osteoporosis is even higher in lung transplant recipients than it is in lung transplant candidates. In the earliest study, Aris et al. [11] compared 55 patients with end-stage pulmonary disease before transplantation and 45 patients who had undergone transplantation in the previous 3 years. The prevalence of osteoporosis was 45% in the pretransplant group and 73% in the post-transplant group. The mean lumbar spine Z scores were −1.32 in the pretransplant group and −2.31 in the post-transplant group. The mean femoral neck Z scores were −1.55 in the pretransplant group and −2.30 in the post-transplant group. Post-transplantation Z scores were significantly lower, and the occurrence of 6 fractures before and 12 after lung transplantation suggested that transplantation was associated with considerable deterioration.

In a retrospective study of 33 patients who survived at least 1 year after lung transplantation, Aringer et al. evaluated BMD, serum 25OHD, serum PTH, serum testosterone, and markers of bone turnover [15]. The evaluation took place a mean of 23 months after transplantation (range 1–54 months). Osteoporosis (defined as a Z score below −2.0) was present in 67% at the spine and 48% at the femoral neck. There was a high prevalence of radiographic vertebral fractures (14 patients, 42%), the majority of which occurred during the first 2 years after transplantation. Only 9% of patients complained of vertebral pain prior to evaluation, indicating that the majority of fractures were asymptomatic. Patients with fractures had significantly lower BMD at all sites than those who did not have fractures, and virtually all those with fractures had T scores below −2.0 and Z scores below −1.5 (see Figure 2). Low serum levels of 25OHD (< 30 nmol/L) were found in 13 patients (39%), and elevated serum PTH levels (> 60 pg/mL) were found in 7 patients (21%). Elevated osteocalcin levels found in 12 patients (36%), despite glucocorticoid therapy, led the authors to conclude that the bone disease following transplantation is characterized by a state of high turnover. No specific risk factor was found to correlate with fracture or low BMD. Given the cross-sectional design of this study and variability in the time of the evaluation with respect to transplantation, it is unclear to what extent the low BMD and high fracture rates were influenced by conditions that existed before transplantation.

Only two small prospective studies have evaluated the natural history and pathogenesis of bone loss after lung transplantation. Ferrari et al. measured BMD in lung transplant recipients before (n = 21) and at 6 (n = 12) and 12 (n = 9) months after transplantation [12]. Initially, 60% of patients had T scores more than 2 standard deviations below the mean, and 35% of patients met WHO criteria for osteoporosis in at least 1 site. Three had already suffered osteoporotic fractures of the lumbar spine or femoral neck. By 6 months after surgery, BMD decreased by 4% at the lumbar

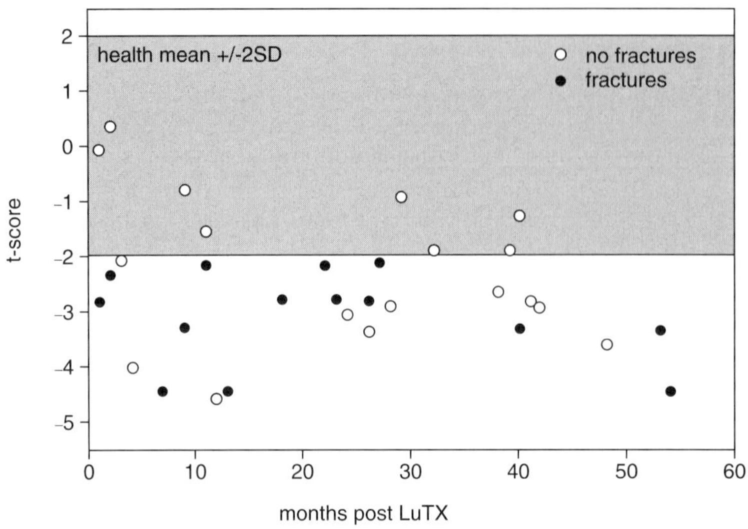

FIGURE 2 Relationship between vertebral fracture prevalence and lumbar spine T score in lung transplant recipients. Reprinted with permission from Aringer et al. (1998). High turnover bone disease following lung transplantation. *Bone*. 23(5):485–488.

spine. There were relatively minor and statistically insignificant declines at other sites, and there were no further decreases at any site in the nine patients re-evaluated at 12 months. Two patients had multiple osteoporotic vertebral fractures. All patients were taking calcium and vitamin D; 3 of the women were taking estrogen and 2 of the men were taking monofluorophosphate. After controlling for hormone replacement therapy, there was a significant positive correlation between cumulative glucocorticoid dose after transplantation and the amount of bone loss sustained.

Spira et al. conducted a prospective study of 28 patients (mean age 53.5) undergoing lung transplantation [16]. BMD was measured an average of 5 months before transplantation and again between 6 and 12 months after transplantation (22 at 6 months, 2 at 9 months and 4 at 12 months). The immunosuppressive regimen consisted of cyclosporine A, azathioprine, and prednisone. All received daily calcium (1000 mg) and vitamin D (400 IU). As observed by other investigators, the majority of patients had low BMD prior to transplantation. The prevalence of osteoporosis ($T \leq -2.5$) was 32% at the lumbar spine and 54% at the femoral neck. Furthermore, 32% had osteopenia at the spine and the femoral neck. Also consistent with previous studies, cumulative glucocorticoid dose was inversely associated and BMI directly associated with T scores at the spine and hip. Between 6 and 12 months after transplantation, mean BMD decreased by 4.8% at the lumbar spine and by 5.3% at the femoral neck. The prevalence of densitometric osteoporosis increased from 32% to 50% at the spine and from 54% to 78% at the femoral neck. Pathologic fractures occurred in 5 of the 28 patients after transplantation (18%) compared with none reported in the period prior to transplant. Cumulative prednisone dose was directly associated with the amount of bone loss at the spine and femoral neck. The main limitation of this study is that BMD was measured at different time points over the first year, making it difficult to define the evolution of bone loss. However, it remains the strongest observational study yet published.

Unusual fractures also occur after lung transplantation [17]. Sacral insufficiency fractures were identified in 4 of 71 (5.6%) patients in the first year after heart or lung transplantation. T scores, measured in 3 of the 4 patients prior to transplant, were below −4.0 at the lumbar spine, and below −2.5 at the femoral neck. All were placed on antiresorptive treatment before transplantation. The fourth patient had T scores of −1.36 at the lumbar spine and −3.38 at the femoral neck. All presented with severe back pain without a history of severe trauma, and all had tenderness to palpation over the sacroiliac joints. Plain radiographs were normal, and the diagnosis was made by a characteristic appearance on bone scan. Sacral insufficiency fractures may be a significant and underdiagnosed cause of low back pain in patients after transplantation.

IV. PREVENTION AND TREATMENT OF OSTEOPOROSIS IN PATIENTS WITH CHRONIC LUNG DISEASE

Several studies have investigated the efficacy of various treatment regimens in preventing bone loss in patients with end-stage pulmonary disease. Treatments studied include calcitriol, calcitonin, and bisphosphonates. In general, lack of randomization, small numbers of subjects, and short duration of follow-up limit these studies and make it difficult to evaluate any positive impact on the incidence of new fractures.

Sambrook et al. [18] randomized 103 patients starting glucocorticoid therapy for a variety of diseases, including sarcoidosis and ILD, to calcium alone, 1000 mg/day; calcium and calcitriol, 0.5 to 1.0 μg/day; or calcium, calcitriol, and calcitonin, 400 IU/day. The interventions were continued for 1 year, after which the subjects were followed for an additional year without any treatment. Subjects receiving calcium alone had significantly more lumbar spine bone loss (−4.3%) than those in the calcitriol and calcitonin group (−0.2%) and those in the calcitriol group (−1.3%). The amount of bone loss at the femoral neck or distal radius did not differ between groups. In the second year of the study, lumbar spine BMD increased by 0.7% in the calcitonin and calcitriol group, compared to a 2.3% decrease in the calcium group and a 3.6% decrease in the calcitriol group. The calcitriol group received significantly higher doses of prednisone than the others, however, which may have caused the higher rate of bone loss. The fracture rate did not differ significantly, likely because of the small sample size and relatively short follow-up period.

In a recent study of patients with COPD and asthma [19], 30 subjects on glucocorticoids for at least 2 years and with T scores <-1.0 by DXA received 0.25 μg daily of calcitriol, and 7 subjects with contraindications to calcitriol served as controls. After 1 year, BMD increased significantly by 0.8% at the femoral neck and 1.0% at the lumbar spine in the calcitriol group. In the control group, BMD decreased by 1.9% at the femoral neck and 0.3% at the lumbar spine. This study was not randomized, and there were significant differences between groups in baseline BMD.

Intranasal calcitonin also increases BMD in patients taking glucocorticoids [20]. Forty-four glucocorticoid-dependent asthmatics were randomized to 200 IU of intranasal calcitonin or placebo for 2 years. The average dose of prednisone (approximately 10 mg/day) was similar between the two groups. Lumbar spine BMD increased by 2.7% in the group receiving calcitonin during the first year and remained stable the second year. In contrast, the group receiving calcium alone experienced bone loss of 2.8% in the first year and an additional 5.0% the second year. There was no significant difference in fracture rate between the two groups. Unfortunately, there was a rather high attrition rate during the second year of the study (50% of each group).

Several bisphosphonates have been shown to be effective in reducing bone loss in patients with chronic lung disease who are receiving glucocorticoids [21–23]. In an open pilot study, Gallacher et al. administered intravenous pamidronate (30 mg every 3 months for 1 year) to 17 patients taking chronic oral prednisolone for treatment of sarcoidosis or asthma [21]. The subjects were taking an average of 14 mg of prednisolone daily and had been on glucocorticoids for an average of 14 years. After 1 year, lumbar spine BMD increased by 3.4%, while no change was observed at the femoral neck. Biochemical markers of bone turnover (alkaline phosphatase and hydroxyproline) decreased. This study is clearly limited by its open design and small sample size.

Alendronate has been studied in subjects taking both oral and inhaled glucocorticoids. In one study, 30 patients with sarcoidosis receiving prednisone were randomized to receive alendronate 5 mg or placebo for 12 months [22]. BMD, measured at the ultradistal radius by dual photon absorptiometry, increased by 0.8% in the alendronate group and decreased by 4.5% in the placebo group. All patients taking prednisone exhibited a decrease in markers of bone formation. Markers of bone resorption (urinary hydroxyproline and N-telopeptide) declined significantly in the alendronate group.

Lau et al. randomized 100 premenopausal and postmenopausal women taking inhaled steroids for asthma or COPD to alendronate 10 mg/day or placebo for one year [23]. Lumbar spine BMD increased by 2.99% in subjects on alendronate while control subjects lost 0.8%. At the femoral neck, the differences were smaller in magnitude but also significant; an increase of 0.97% was observed in the alendronate group and a decrease of 0.51% was observed in the controls. This study supports previous work demonstrating that significant bone loss occurs in patients treated with inhaled steroids and suggests that this loss may be prevented by bisphosphonates.

V. PREVENTION AND TREATMENT OF OSTEOPOROSIS IN PATIENTS AFTER LUNG TRANSPLANTATION

Several studies have evaluated the efficacy of different treatments in preventing bone loss in patients undergoing lung transplantation [10, 16, 24–27]. In a nonrandomized study, Shane et al. measured changes in BMD, fracture incidence, and markers of bone turnover in 30 patients during the first year after lung transplantation [24]. The immunosuppressive regimen consisted of cyclosporine or tacrolimus, azathioprine, and prednisone. All patients received calcium, vitamin D, and at least one antiresorptive drug (estrogen, calcitonin, pamidronate, cyclic etidronate, or alendronate), initiated before or shortly after transplantation. The majority of patients had very low BMD before transplantation. The average T scores at the lumbar spine and femoral neck were −2.94 and −1.96, respectively. Osteoporosis was present in 30% of patients at the lumbar spine and 40% at the femoral neck, and only 20% of patients had normal BMD at both sites (see Figure 3). Despite antiresorptive therapy, 50% of the patients sustained significant bone loss (8.6% at the spine and 11.3% at the femoral neck), and 11 patients (37%) sustained a total of 54 atraumatic fractures. The amount of bone loss observed in this study was lower than in several previous studies of other types of organ transplantation, likely because all patients received antiresorptive therapy after transplantation. The fracture rate was very high, however. Pretransplant BMD was significantly lower in patients who developed fractures (see Figure 4), and there was a trend toward an increased fracture rate in women. Patients with bone loss or fractures had greater increases in biochemical markers of bone resorption. Measurements of serum calcium, PTH, and urinary deoxypyridinoline excretion in the patients with significant reductions in BMD were consistent with secondary hyperparathyroidism, which may have contributed to increased bone loss. A significant association was found between fracture incidence and

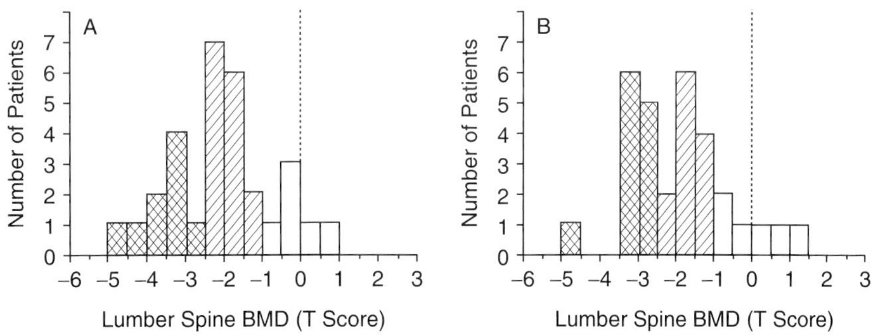

FIGURE 3 Prevalence of abnormal bone density T scores in candidates for lung transplantation. Reprinted with permission from Shane et al. (1999). *Transplantation*. 68(2):220–227.

both pretransplant glucocorticoid therapy and duration of glucocorticoid therapy. Fracture incidence tended to be lower in patients who received bisphosphonates compared to those who received other antiresorptive therapies. Since the number of patients who received each treatment was so small, however, and because several patients were exposed to a combination of therapies, no conclusions regarding efficacy of various treatments can be deduced from this trial.

The effect of calcitriol on bone loss after transplantation was evaluated by Sambrook et al. [25], who conducted a randomized, double-blind study of patients undergoing cardiac transplantation (44 patients) or lung transplantation (18 patients). Patients were stratified according to age, sex, and type of transplantation, and were managed with cyclosporine, prednisone, and either azathioprine or mycophenolate mofetil. Lung

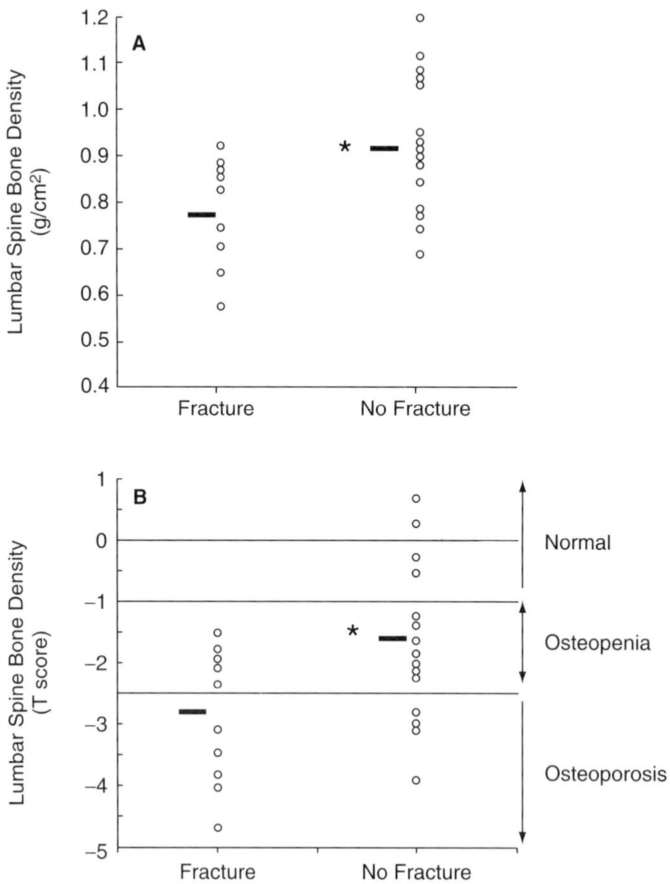

FIGURE 4 Relationship between incidence of fractures after lung transplantation and absolute bone mineral density (Panel A) and T score before transplantation. Reprinted with permission from Shane et al. (1999). *Transplantation*. 68(2):220–227.

transplantation patients with a prior history of glucocorticoid use were excluded, which may have accounted for the higher initial BMD seen in these subjects compared to most others in the literature. Treatment was initiated within 4 weeks after transplantation, and consisted of either calcitriol (0.5–0.75 μg/day; dose limited by hypercalcemia) or placebo, accompanied by calcium. After the first year, half the subjects receiving calcitriol were switched to placebo for a second year of observation. There was no significant difference between groups in femoral neck BMD at the start of the trial, although BMD at the lumbar spine was significantly lower in the placebo group. All groups received similar cumulative doses of cyclosporine and prednisone. Bone loss at the lumbar spine was not significantly different between the treatment groups after 1 or 2 years. In contrast, bone loss at the proximal femur was significantly lower in the group taking calcitriol for 2 years compared to placebo, 5.0% and 8.2% respectively. The group treated with calcitriol for 1 year and then calcium alone for 1 year exhibited similar proximal femoral bone loss to the placebo group at the end of the 2-year period, with an overall decline of 7.4%, suggesting that the protective effects of calcitriol do not persist after treatment is suspended. In the placebo group, 4 patients sustained 22 new vertebral fractures, while in the calcitriol group, 1 patient incurred 1 fracture.

In another study of patients after cardiac or lung transplantation, calcitriol was compared to cyclical etidronate [27]. Forty-one patients were treated for the first 6 months after transplantation with either calcitriol, 0.5 μg/day or 2 cycles of etidronate, 400 mg/day for 14 days followed by 76 days of calcium carbonate. Subjects were followed for 18 months after cessation of treatment. Lung transplant recipients comprised 4 of 20 in the calcitriol group and 6 of 15 in the etidronate group. The immunosuppressive regimen consisted of cyclosporine, azathioprine, and prednisone; both treatment groups received equivalent cumulative doses of cyclosporine and prednisone. Mean T scores for all groups combined were −0.82 at the lumbar spine, −0.53 for total body, and −1.64 for the femoral neck; mean T scores did not differ between groups. As there was no untreated control group, subjects were compared to a historical reference group of untreated patients who had received significantly higher doses of glucocorticoids, did not include any lung transplant recipients, and had fewer women. There was no difference in fracture rate between groups over the 2-year period. Significant decreases in BMD that did not differ between the randomized groups were observed at the lumbar spine, femoral neck, and total body over the first 12 months of the study. Although there was less bone loss in the treated groups than in the historical controls, the difference is difficult to interpret because of the known differences between the reference group and the experimental groups, as well as possible unidentified confounding differences.

Trombetti et al. also studied the effects of antiresorptive treatment on BMD in lung transplant recipients [10]. At baseline, a significant number of patients had low BMD; 55% had osteopenia and 29% had osteoporosis, as defined by WHO criteria. Prior to transplantation, several patients were taking calcium and vitamin D, and 8 were taking hormone replacement therapy (HRT). After transplantation, all subjects received calcium (1000 mg/day), and vitamin D (800–1000 IU/day). In addition, 14 subjects received pamidronate 30 mg intravenously every 3 months, and 5 received HRT. Over the 12-month study period, there was significantly less bone loss in the pamidronate and HRT groups than in the group that received only calcium and vitamin D. BMD decreased by 5.2% at the lumbar spine and 1.7% at the femoral neck in the calcium and vitamin D group. In contrast, BMD increased by 4.0% in the lumbar spine and 6.4% in the femoral neck in the HRT group. In the pamidronate group, lumbar spine BMD increased by 2.2%, while femoral neck BMD decreased by 1.0%. An 18-year-old patient probably contributed to the large differences that were observed in the HRT group. In patients receiving HRT or pamidronate, 1 vertebral fracture occurred. In the calcium and vitamin D group, 2 vertebral and 1 pelvic fracture were seen. The limitations of this study are the lack of randomization and of standardization of pretransplantation bone protective regimen (several patients were on HRT or fluoride before transplantation), and differing immunosuppressive regimens after transplantation (higher cumulative doses of prednisone during the first 6 months in the control group).

Whether initiating bisphosphonate treatment prior to transplantation is of benefit was investigated by Cahill et al. [13]. In a prospective study, candidates for lung transplantation were placed on calcium, vitamin D (400 IU/day), and HRT (if hypogonadal). After July, 1998, 13 transplant candidates with osteoporosis or osteopenia were treated with bisphosphonates, either a single 90 mg dose of intravenous pamidronate at time of listing (n = 9) or oral alendronate 10 mg daily (n = 4). After transplantation, 21 patients were treated with calcium 1500 mg/day, vitamin D 400 IU/day, and pamidronate 90 mg intravenously every 12 weeks, and followed for 1 year. Eight of 9 pamidronate-treated patients were transplanted within 6 weeks of the infusion; 1 patient, transplanted 36 weeks after the pamidronate infusion, was analyzed as though he had received only post-transplant pamidronate. Two alendronate-treated patients received the drug for 27 or 53 weeks, and 2 were treated for 3 or 10 weeks; the latter 2 subjects were also analyzed as though they had received only post-transplant pamidronate. Most of those who sustained significant bone loss had received only post-transplant bisphosphonate therapy. Those women who received bisphosphonate therapy before transplantation had greater increases in BMD than those who received only post-transplant pamidronate. In men, change in BMD was similar regardless of whether they had received pretransplant bisphosphonates. There was very little bone loss in either bisphosphonate-treated group. While this study is limited by lack of randomization, small numbers, and disparities between the groups, it does suggest benefit from pretransplant bisphosphonate therapy. Given the severity of pretransplant bone loss in lung transplant candidates and the high fracture rates observed by Shane et al., despite initiating various types of antiresorptive therapy after lung transplantation [24], it is probably reasonable to intervene while patients are on the waiting list rather than waiting until after transplantation.

Mitchell et al. investigated resistance training as a means of preventing osteoporosis in 16 lung transplant recipients [26]. Patients were randomly assigned either to receive 6 months of resistance exercise training using machines that isolated the lumbar extensor muscles or to serve as controls. Resistance training commenced 2 months after transplantation. Initially the two groups had similar BMD at the lumbar spine, and subjects met criteria for osteoporosis based upon a T score of less than 2.5. Patients in both groups lost a comparable and significant amount of bone mass, 14.5% in the first 2 months after transplantation. The control group lost an additional 5.6% over the following 6 months, resulting in a cumulative decline of 19.5%, while an increase in lumbar spine BMD of 9.2% was observed in the exercise group. Although the results of this study are quite positive, they are limited by the small population size. In addition, no assessment of the effects of mechanical loading on the reduction in fracture risk was possible, given the small size of the study and short follow-up period.

VI. CONCLUSIONS

Osteoporosis and fractures are very common in patients awaiting lung transplantation, as is hypogonadism, vitamin D deficiency, and secondary hyperparathyroidism. The most consistent risk factors for pretransplantation osteoporosis include glucocorticoid therapy, low BMI, and more severe pulmonary disease. The first year or two after lung transplantation is characterized by significant bone loss ranging between 5 and 10% and a high risk of fracture. Antiresorptive therapy is at least partially effective in reducing the bone loss that occurs in the period following transplantation, although fracture rates may be high despite such therapy. There is weak evidence of benefit in initiating antiresorptive therapy before transplantation.

There are relatively few observational and interventional studies of osteoporosis after lung transplantation, and the quality of those that do exist is often poor. In our view, placebo-controlled trials are unethical, given the severity of skeletal compromise in these patients before transplantation and the demonstrated efficacy of bisphosphonates in other forms of glucocorticoid-induced osteoporosis. The quality of the evidence could be improved by designing multicenter trials that would make larger numbers of subjects available for study, increase power to assess effects on fracture incidence, and improve generalizability of the results. Well-designed studies that address the benefit of initiating treatment before transplantation are warranted. The role for anabolic agents, particularly parathyroid hormone, to stimulate bone formation in lung transplant patients has not yet been studied. In addition, longer studies are required to determine whether and when bone loss stabilizes and the optimal duration of treatment after transplantation.

Although osteoporosis and fracture are extremely common in patients undergoing lung transplantation, they are often unrecognized. Greater vigilance and an aggressive approach to treatment are necessary to reduce morbidity and mortality related to fracture and to improve quality of life in this population.

REFERENCES

1. Cohen, A., Shane, E. (2003). Bone disease after solid organ and bone marrow transplantation. *Osteoporosis Int.* 14:617–630.
2. Dimai, H.P., Domej, W., Leb, G., Lau, K.H.W. (2001). Bone loss in patients with untreated chronic obstructive pulmonary disease is mediated by an increase in bone resorption associated with hypercapnia. *J Bone Miner Res.* 16:2132–2141.
3. Rizzato, G., Montemurro, L., Fraioli, P. (1992). Bone mineral content in sarcoidosis. *Semin Resp Med.* 13:411–423.
4. Conron, M., Young, C., Beynon, H.L. (2000). Calcium metabolism in sarcoidosis and its clinical implications. *Rheumatol (Oxford).* 39:707–713.
5. Fallon, M.D., Perry, H.M., 3rd, Teitelbaum, S.L. (1981). Skeletal sarcoidosis with osteopenia. *Metabolic Bone Disease & Related Research.* 3:171–174.
6. Rizzato, G., Fraioli, P. (1990). Natural and corticosteroid-induced osteoporosis in sarcoidosis: prevention, treatment, follow up and reversibility. *Sarcoidosis.* 7:89–92.
7. Adinoff, A.D., Hollister, J.R. (1983). Steroid-induced fractures and bone loss in patients with asthma. *New England Journal of Medicine.* 309:265–268.
8. Meyrier, A., Valeyre, D., Bouillon, R., Paillard, F., Battesti, J.P., Georges, R. (1986). Different mechanisms of hypercalciuria in sarcoidosis. Correlations with disease extension and activity. *Annals of the New York Academy of Sciences.* 465:575–586.
9. Shane, E., Silverberg, S.J., Donovan, D., Papadopoulos, A., Staron, R.B., Adesso, V., Jorgensen, B., McGregor, C., Schulman, L. (1996). Osteoporosis in lung transplantation candidates with end-stage pulmonary disease. *Am J Med.* 101:262–269.
10. Trombetti, A., Gerbase, M., Spiliopoulos, A., Slosman, D., Nicod, L., Rizzoli, R. (2000). Bone mineral density in lung-transplant recipients before and after graft: prevention of lumbra spine post-transplantation-accelerated bone loss by pamidronate. *J Heart Lung Transplant.* (19):736–743.
11. Aris, R.M., Neuringer, I.P., Weiner, M.A., Egan, T.M., Ontjes, D. (1996). Severe osteoporosis before and after lung transplantation. *Chest.* 109:1176–1183.
12. Ferrari, S.L., Nicod, L.P., Hamacher, J., Spiliopoulos, A., Slosman, D.O., Rochat, T., Bonjour, J.-P, Rizzoli, R. (1996). Osteoporosis in patients undergoing lung transplantation. *Eur Respir J.* 9:2378–2382.
13. Cahill, B.C., O'Rourke, M., Parker, S., Stringham, J.C., Karwande, S.V., Knecht, T.P. (2001). Prevention of bone loss and fracture after lung transplantation. *Transplantation.* 72:1251–1255.
14. Tschopp, O., Boehler, A., Speich, R., Weder, W., Seifert, B., Russi, E.W., Schmid, C. (2002). Osteoporosis before lung transplantation: association with low body mass index, but not with underlying disease. *American Journal of Transplantation.* 2(2):167–172.
15. Aringer, M., Kiener, H.P., Koeller, M.D., Artemiou, O., Zuckerman, A., Wieselthaler, G., Klepetko, W., Seidl, G., Kainberger, F., Bernecker, P., Smolen, J.S., Pietschmann, P. (1998). High turnover bone disease following lung transplantation. *Bone.* 23:485–488.
16. Spira, A., Gutierrez, C., Chaparro, C., Hutcheon, M.A., Chan, C.K.N. (2000). Osteoporosis and lung transplantation. *Chest.* 117:476–481.
17. Schulman, L., Adesso, V., Staron, R.B., McGregor, C., Shane, E. (1997). Insufficiency fractures of the sacrum: a cause of low back pain after lung transplantation. *J Heart Lung Transplant.* 16:1081–1085.

18. Sambrook, P., Birmingham, J., Kelly, P., Kempler, S., Nguyen, T., Pocock, N., Eisman, J. (1993). Prevention of corticosteroid osteoporosis—A comparison of calcium, calcitriol, and calcitonin. *N Eng J Med*. 328:1747–1752.
19. Mizraei, S., Zajicek, H., Knoll, P., Hahn, M., Levi, M., Kohn, H., Pohl, W. (2003). Effect of rocaltrol on bone mass in patients with pulmonary disease treated with corticosteroids. *Journal of Asthma*. 40:251–255.
20. Luengo, M., Pins, F., Martinez de Osaba, M., Picado, C. (1994). Prevention of further bone mass loss by nasal calcitonin in patients on long term glucocorticoid therapy for asthma: a two year follow-up study. *Thorax*. 49:1099–1102.
21. Gallacher, S.J., Fenner, J.A.K, Anderson, K., Bryden, F.M., Banham, S., Logue, F.C., Cowan, R.A., Boyle, I.T. (1992). Intravenous pamidronate in the treatment of osteoporosis associated with corticosteroid dependent lung disease: an open pilot study. *Thorax*. 47:932–936.
22. Gonnelli, S., Rottoli, P., Cepollaro, C., Pondrelli, C., Cappielo, V., Vagliasindi, M., Gennari, C. (1997). Prevention of corticosteroid-induced osteoporosis with alendronate in sarcoid patients. *Calcif Tissue Int*. 61:382–385.
23. Lau, E.M.C, Woo, J., Chan, Y.H., Li, M. (2001). Alendronate for the prevention of bone loss in patients on inhaled steroid therapy. *Bone*. 29:506–510.
24. Shane, E., Papadopoulos, A., Staron, R.B., Adesso, V., Donovan, D., McGregor, C., Schulman, L. (1999). Bone loss and fracture after lung transplantation. *Transplantation*. 68:220–227.
25. Sambrook, P., Henderson, K., Keogh, A., Macdonald, P., Glanville, A., Spratt, P., Bergin, P., Ebeling, P., Eisman, J. (2000). Effect of calcitriol on bone loss after cardiac or lung transplantation. *J Bone Miner Res*. 15:1818–1824.
26. Mitchell, M., Baz, M.A., Fulton, M.N., Lisor, C.F., Braith, R.W. (2003). Resistance training prevents vertebral osteoporosis in lung transplant recipients. *Transplantation*. 76:557–562.
27. Henderson, K., Eisman, J., Keogh, A., Macdonald, P., Glanville, A., Spratt, P., Sambrook, P. (2001). Protective effect of short-term calcitriol or cyclical etidronate on bone loss after cardiac or lung transplantation. *J Bone Miner Res*. 16:565–571.

CHAPTER 18

Transplantation for Cystic Fibrosis: Effect on the Skeleton

Robert M. Aris, MD
Division of Pulmonary and Critical Care Medicine,
University of North Carolina,
Chapel Hill, NC

David A. Ontjes, MD
Division of Endocrinology, University of North Carolina,
Chapel Hill, NC

I. INTRODUCTION

Cystic fibrosis (CF) is the most common recessive genetic mutation in the Caucasian population that leads to respiratory failure early in life. The prevalence of CF in the world is approximately 60,000 individuals. Advances in treating CF patients have increased the median life expectancy from approximately 2 years to over 30 in the last 3 decades [1]. Approximately 1 in 2500 children in the Caucasian population are born with CF each year in the United States and about one third of all CF individuals are currently adults. The fundamental gene defect in this disease is a mutation in the CF transmembrane conductance regulator (CFTR) protein, which is a chloride channel found in epithelial tissues in the lungs, pancreas, gastrointestinal tract, and skin. CFTR modulates the transport of salt and water across these epithelia. Mutations in CFTR lead to changes in the viscosity and hydration of epithelial tissue lining fluid, leading to alterations in host defense in the respiratory tract and ultimately chronic, progressive infection with *Pseudomonas aeruginosa, Staphaloccus aureus,* and/or other pathogens. CFTR mutations frequently lead to pancreatic duct obstruction and pancreatic insufficiency (prevalence > 80%; exocrine >> endocrine), biliary obstruction and cirrhosis (prevalence ~5%), and distal intestinal obstruction syndrome (prevalence ~5%).

Bone disease in CF patients was first described in 1979 [2, 3], years before the first successful lung transplantation was performed. Low bone density and increased fracture rates are now recognized complications of CF, especially in adults. The origin of the bone disease in CF is poorly understood and probably multifactorial (see Figure 1). Important contributing factors include delayed pubertal maturation, malabsorption of

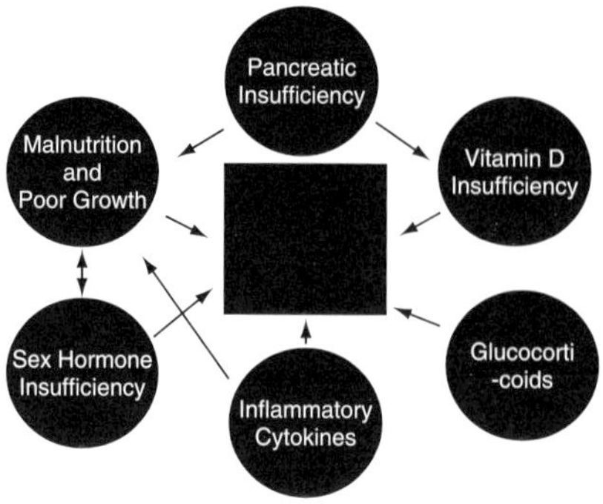

FIGURE 1 Pathogenesis of bone disease in cystic fibrosis. Factors known or thought to be involved in causing low bone density in individuals with CF.

vitamin D, poor nutritional status, physical inactivity, glucocorticoid therapy, and hypogonadism. Additionally, chronic pulmonary inflammation increases serum cytokine levels, which probably augment bone resorption and suppress bone formation. Decreased bone mineral density (BMD) resulting from these factors can lead to pathologic fractures and kyphosis decades earlier than seen in the general population. Severe bone disease can lead to exclusion from lung transplantation, often a life-saving operation for individuals with CF. Prevention, early recognition, and treatment are the most effective strategies for sustaining bone health to help maintain the quality of life of many CF patients.

II. DESCRIPTION AND PATHOPHYSIOLOGY OF BONE DISEASE IN CYSTIC FIBROSIS

A. Incidence of Bone Disease and Correlation with Lung Function and Body Mass Index

More than 50 reports from many countries have documented osteopenia, osteoporosis, and fractures in CF patients of all ages, although adults tend to be more affected. Large cross-sectional surveys of adults attending specialized CF clinics have reported the prevalence of Z-scores < -2 in 20–34% and T-scores < -2.5 in 10% [4–19]. The combined prevalence of osteopenia and osteoporosis, using the WHO criteria, has been reported to be as high as 85% in one adult CF study [5]. Younger and healthier patients tend to have higher bone density, but rarely do CF cohorts have normal BMD. Although adult CF patients suffer from small stature, corrections for bone density using bone mineral apparent density (BMAD) have confirmed that bone disease is not caused simply by small bones [18, 19]. Nonetheless, young children and adolescents may have appropriate BMD when the data are controlled for body size [20–24], suggesting that the bone disease may not be intrinsically related to the CFTR mutation but occurs as patients get older because of the contributing factors mentioned previously.

The prevalence of bone disease appears to increase with severity of lung disease and malnutrition [4–7]. Similarly, patients that are referred for lung transplantation often have severe bone disease with a high rate of kyphosis, as well as fractures of long bones, vertebrae, and ribs [4, 5]. When patients are referred for lung transplantation (FEV1 < 30%), mean Z- and T-scores at the spine and femur approximate −2, and more than 90% of the patients have osteopenia or osteoporosis by the WHO criteria [5, 9, 10]. In addition to chronic pain and debilitation, bone disease may result in rib and vertebral fractures, which cause chest wall deformities that reduce lung function, inhibit effective coughing, hinder airway clearance, and ultimately accelerate the course of CF.

B. Bone Histomorphometry in Cystic Fibrosis

One bone histomorphometric study of clinically stable adults with low BMD demonstrated significantly lower cancellous bone volume and a trend towards a decrease in cancellous bone connectivity compared to healthy controls [25]. Bone formation rates at tissue level were significantly lower as well. Wall width was significantly decreased by 50%, and the mineralizing perimeter and mineral apposition rate were significantly lower. Resorption cavities had smaller reconstructed surface lengths and were shallower, whereas eroded surface area was higher. A separate study of autopsy bone samples from a mixture of transplanted and nontransplanted CF patients demonstrated severe osteopenia in both trabecular and cortical bone [26]. At the cellular level, there was decreased osteoblastic and increased osteoclastic activity. The reduction in osteoblastic activity was a result of a decrease in both osteoblast number and the biosynthetic potential of osteoblasts. The osteoclastic changes were a result of an increase in the number of osteoclasts. The increase in osteoclasts and the uncoupling of osteoblastic and osteoclastic activity resulted in an increase in resorptive surfaces. Both cortical and trabecular bone mass tended to be lower after transplantation. The majority of these patients, however, had received high doses of glucocorticoids secondary to lung transplantation. Although there was evidence of a mineralization deficit in these studies, somewhat surprisingly only one biopsy revealed osteomalacia by strict histomorphometric criteria. Because the exact nature of low BMD in CF individuals is not clear based on the available histomorphometry, bone marker data, and natural course of illness, a consensus panel of experts chose to refer to this problem as CF bone disease rather than osteoporosis.

C. Bone Accrual and Loss in Cystic Fibrosis

Optimal bone accrual in CF patients, as in other individuals, requires adequate nutrition, body mass, physical activity, and hormone production [27, 28]. This issue is particularly germane to individuals with CF, who often suffer from delayed puberty and lower pubertal growth velocity due to chronic illness. One longitudinal study of pubertal CF children has reported that inadequate bone mineral accrual results in a lower than expected BMAD [18]. However, another small study reported normal Z-scores in prepubertal CF children with normal lung function and BMI, suggesting that a good health status during childhood and puberty may allow normal bone accrual. While growth velocity is impaired in CF adolescents, no comprehensive survey on bone accrual has been performed on a large group of children or adolescents. The small number of reports on BMD in CF children and adolescents is probably due to a relative lack of availability of BMD scanners in children's hospitals.

The majority of studies reporting abnormal BMD pertain to CF adults. Of the more than 25 published BMD surveys to date in CF adults, all have found a high prevalence of osteopenia and osteoporosis. Results from the adult studies in combination with the small database in CF children and adolescents indicate that a major problem in CF is inadequate bone acquisition during puberty. Compounding inadequate bone accrual during childhood, several longitudinal studies in young adults have unequivocally demonstrated accelerated bone loss. In fact, Haworth et al. reported mean annualized losses in BMD of 0.5%, 2.1%, and 1.8% at the lumbar spine, femoral neck, and total hip, respectively, in a cohort of 114 patients ages 15–49 (mean = 25) [29]. Aris et al. have found a similar result (annualized mean loss of 1.8% at the spine and 0.7% at the hip) in a slightly older cohort (mean age 28) treated with calcium and cholecalciferol supplements [30].

D. Bone Turnover in Cystic Fibrosis

In general, studies using bone turnover markers in clinically stable CF adults indicate a hyper-resorptive state and inadequate compensation in bone formation [7, 13, 31–33]. Baroncelli et al. found higher bone turnover, as evidenced by increased urinary carboxy-terminal propeptide of type I procollagen (two-fold higher) and N-telopeptide (NTx) in CF children and young adults [32]. Bone formation markers were significantly lower in both pubertal children and young adults. Haworth et al. found mean deoxypyridinoline (Dpd) levels of 7.4 nM/mM (normal range: 2.3–7.4nM/ mM), osteocalcin levels of 10.4 ng/ml (normal range: 3.4–10.0ng/ml), and bone-specific alkaline phosphatase (BAP) levels 20.9 U/L (normal range: 10–23 U/L) in 139 stable CF adults [7]. Aris et al. found that urinary Dpd and NTx were significantly higher (each by ~40%) in stable CF adults compared to age-matched controls [33]. Osteocalcin levels, however, were similar in CF and controls. BAP levels were also elevated. However, total alkaline phosphatase levels may also be elevated in CF due to biliary obstruction. Given the potential for cross-reactivity between BAP and liver alkaline phosphatase, BAP levels should be interpreted with caution. Taken together, the bone marker studies in CF indicate that both accelerated bone breakdown and inadequate bone formation are important in the pathogenesis of CF bone disease.

E. Pathogenesis of Bone Disease in Cystic Fibrosis

1. Pancreatic Exocrine Insufficiency and Malabsorption of Nutrients Including Vitamins D and K

Malnutrition is common in CF because of pancreatic insufficiency causing nutrient malabsorption (even with pancreatic enzyme supplementation) and increased catabolism as a result of chronic lung infection. In CF patients, a low body mass index (BMI) is a well-described risk factor for increased disease severity and adverse events. Many authors have correlated poor nutrition or reduced BMI with low BMD in CF [2, 4, 7, 11]. Nonetheless, low BMD also occurs in CF patients with pancreatic sufficiency, indicating that chronic infection may be playing an important role. Data concerning the effect of CF on the absorption and excretion of key nutrients, including calcium, phosphorus, magnesium, zinc, and copper, and vitamins D and K are conflicting [34], but a growing consensus suggests that the absorption of vitamins D and K and calcium are inadequate.

There is unequivocal evidence from more than 20 reports that vitamin D insufficiency (low or low-normal 25-hydroxy-vitamin D [25OHD] levels) is common among CF patients irrespective of latitude [35]. While frankly low 25OHD levels, seen in 5–10% of patients, are not common, the majority of adults with CF have levels in the lower part of the normal range with a mean near 20 ng/ml. Studies in non-CF populations have shown that calcium absorption efficiency declines and serum parathyroid hormone (PTH) concentrations rise progressively as serum 25OHD levels fall below 30 ng/ml (75 nmol/L) [36]. In adults with end-stage lung disease, frank vitamin D deficiency is more common and may occur in 25–33% of patients [5, 9]. Vitamin D insufficiency may result in significantly higher PTH levels in comparison to age-matched controls, but rarely do PTH levels exceed the normal range [33].

The causes of vitamin D insufficiency have just recently attracted attention. Lark et al. reported that CF adults absorbed approximately half the amount of oral vitamin D_2 (100,000 IU) given as a test dose in comparison to healthy subjects ($P < 0.001$) [37]. Absorption varied greatly, with 20% of the CF individuals having virtually undetectable vitamin D_2 levels (by HPLC) 0–36 hours after dosing. The 25OHD levels did not rise in response to vitamin D_2 in the CF group in comparison to a mean doubling of the 25OHD level in the control group ($P = 0.0012$). These results may help explain the etiology of vitamin D deficiency in CF patients. In the normal population, 90–95% of the vitamin D requirement comes from exposure to sunlight. However, some individuals in the CF population have decreased sunlight exposure because illness or the concern of photosensitivity from some antibiotics causes them to stay indoors. Many CF adults have low body fat, which may result in diminished vitamin D reserves. Exposure to sunlight could be more efficacious than oral supplementation in raising vitamin D levels, but vitamin D supplementation in CF patients may be needed, particularly during the winter months. Although bone disease in CF patients is a complex process and may well involve multiple mechanisms, perturbations in the absorption and conversion of vitamin D are very likely to be important.

A growing body of information outside of CF indicates that vitamin K also plays an important role in bone health. Even with routine supplementation, 40% of CF individuals remain vitamin K–deficient [38]. When extrapolated to the entire CF population, vitamin K deficiency and its effect on bone disease are magnified. Many adults with CF have reduced γ-carboxylated osteocalcin levels [39]. Vitamin K supplementation to improve BMD has not been studied but may be a compelling research area.

2. *Pancreatic Endocrine Insufficiency*

Diabetes mellitus, a recognized complication in approximately 10% of CF patients [1], has been associated with significant losses in trabecular and cortical bone mass in cohorts of patients without CF [40]. While CF-related diabetes may differ from classical type I or II diabetes, the abnormalities in glucose metabolism resulting from islet cell loss and peripheral insulin resistance may play a role in reduced BMD.

3. *Physical Inactivity*

Patients with CF may suffer from inactivity due to reduced lung function and the need for prolonged treatments. Most studies in CF have found that the level of physical activity or weight-bearing activity is significantly related to BMD [4, 7, 11, 18, 29], as it is in the general population.

4. *Delayed Puberty and Intermittent Hypogonadism*

Delayed puberty and hypogonadism likely play a role in bone disease in CF [5, 12, 17], but comprehensive studies on large data sets have not been performed, and these abnormalities probably have variable effects. Pubertal delay, recognized in CF for over 20 years, is related to disease status [41, 42] and retards both normal somatic development and the attainment of peak bone mass. Fortunately, as the health status and survival of CF patients has improved, more patients are currently experiencing normal development. Nonetheless, CF adults are currently 2–3 inches shorter, on average, than their age-matched peers and fall into the lowest deciles of body weight [1, 5]. Sex hormones are reduced in both adolescent girls and boys, although most values are normal when plotted for Tanner stage [43–46]. Normal levels of sex hormones (estradiol, testosterone, luteinizing hormone, and follicle-stimulating hormone) appear to be attained in most stable young adults, but intermittent menstrual dysfunction (28–73% prevalence) [43, 45] and low total testosterone levels (3–88% prevalence) are not uncommon [4, 5, 7, 11, 17]. Free testosterone levels have not been studied. Normal gonadotrophin levels suggest hypothalamic dysfunction from chronic illness. The close relationship among glucocorticoid use, physical inactivity, disease severity, and hypogonadism makes an analysis of the effect of sex-hormone deficiency on BMD difficult. Some studies have shown an association between both delayed puberty and hypogonadism and lower BMD [4, 5, 17, 23]. However, one study of teens and adults detected a high prevalence of low BMD despite few sex-hormone abnormalities [11].

5. *Chronic Infection*

In the serum and respiratory tract of CF individuals, many inflammatory factors have been identified that have been shown to stimulate osteoclastic bone resorption *in vitro*; these include tumor necrosis factor alpha (TNFα), interleukin (IL) -1, -6, and -11; PTH; and vascular endothelial growth factor (VEGF). While beyond the scope of this review, there is mounting evidence for the causal role of inflammatory cytokines in bone loss in a variety of diseases other than CF [47]. Increases in IL-6, TNFα, IL-1, parathyroid hormone related peptide (PTHrP), and receptor activator of NFkB (RANKL), for example, have been implicated in the bone loss associated with rheumatoid arthritis. Excess IL-6 has been shown to help activate osteoclastic bone resorption in hyperparathyroidism. Production of IL-1, IL-6, IL-11, TNFα, and PTHrP by tumor cells has also been shown to stimulate bone resorption. Furthermore, these cytokines may act synergistically. Finally, some inflammatory cytokines have been shown to inhibit osteoblast function. The inverse correlation between the number of intravenous antibiotic courses administered to CF patients and BMD provides indirect evidence of cytokine involvement [4]. Increased serum levels of IL-6, IL-1, and TNFα, along with increased NTx and Dpd levels and decreased osteocalcin levels, have been reported during exacerbations of lung infection in CF [8]. These abnormalities resolved almost completely when lung infection was treated with conventional care including antibiotics, chest physiotherapy, and nutrition supplementation. Lastly, by inference, BMD tends to remain more stable in CF adults after lung transplantation than in other patient groups and actually rises in healthy recipients, suggesting that the removal of the suppurative lungs has a salubrious effect on bone health despite the use of immunosuppressants.

6. *Anti-Inflammatory Therapy*

Exogenous glucocorticoids are intermittently prescribed in 20–50% of CF patients before transplantation to improve pulmonary function [5, 48]. Long-term inhaled glucocorticoid use is more common than oral use.

A myriad of adverse effects of glucocorticoids on bone metabolism and BMD has been observed and is discussed elsewhere in this book. Several studies in patients with CF have found glucocorticoid therapy to be a risk factor for low bone mass [4, 11, 29, 35], but this association has not been invariable because sicker patients tend to be prescribed glucocorticoids more frequently. The adverse effects of glucocorticoids on pediatric patients with growing bones may be even more profound than in adults. This reduced bone reservoir increases the risk for low BMD and ultimately fractures.

7. *Pathogenesis: Summary*

In conclusion, the causes of low bone mass in CF are many and include: 1) nutritional deficiencies, especially calcium and vitamin D and possibly vitamin K; 2) reduced muscle mass and physical activity; 3) delayed puberty and intermittent hypogonadism; and 4) defects in bone remodeling secondary to chronic inflammation and glucocorticoid use. Histomorphometric analysis of bone, studies of bone metabolism, and longitudinal analysis of BMD support the conclusion that bone resorption is increased and bone formation is decreased in many adult CF patients.

III. CLINICAL MANIFESTATIONS OF LOW BONE MINERAL DENSITY IN CYSTIC FIBROSIS PATIENTS

Several cross-sectional studies have indicated that CF patients (adults and children) are at higher risk for fracture compared to age-matched healthy cohorts [4, 5, 12, 49]. In 1994, Henderson and Specter first reported that female CF patients 6 to 16 years of age had a higher than normal fracture rate and a higher rate than their male counterparts in a survey of 143 patients (ages 4.7 to 21.9 years) [49]. Bachrach et al. found 12 fractures, including 1 of the femur, in 9 patients from a combined cohort of 71 children and adults [12]. In 1998, Aris et al. reported on interviews derived from a cross-sectional study of adult CF patients and found 54 fractures in 70 patients with over 1410 patient-years on analysis. Fracture rates were approximately twice as high in women with CF, ages 16–34 years ($p = 0.015$) and men with CF, ages 25–45 years ($p = 0.04$), compared to the general population [5]. Chest X-ray review demonstrated evidence of 14 additional rib fractures and 62 additional vertebral compression fractures, indicating that vertebral compression and rib fracture rates were 100 and 10 times more common than expected, respectively ($p < 0.0001$). Donovan et al. [30] studied white adults (16 women) with CF, age 30 $\pm$ 2 years (mean $\pm$ SEM) and found that vertebral fractures were present in 19% and that 41% had a confirmed history of previous fracture [19]. These results were corroborated by Elkin et al., who studied 107 adult CF patients (58 men) aged 18–60 years and found that 17% had evidence of vertebral deformity on radiography, mostly in the thoracic spine, and that 35% reported a history of fractures, of which 9% were rib fractures [4]. Numerous case reports also document fractures, sometimes severe, as, for example, bilateral femoral neck fractures associated with the trauma of grand mal seizures in a CF patient.

Erkkila et al. [50] first reported an increased prevalence of kyphosis in cystic fibrosis patients in 1978. This report was followed by others [49, 51, 52]. Early reports surveying mainly children and adolescents with CF demonstrated an unexpectedly high prevalence (9–40%) of abnormal (defined as either > 35° or > 40°) kyphosis angles, worsening kyphosis with age, and more severe kyphosis in females compared to males. In the study by Henderson and Specter, kyphosis exceeding 40°, the upper limit of normal, was found in 77% of female CF patients and 36% of male CF patients ≥ 15 years old [49]. In a cohort of 70 adults with advanced-stage CF, Aris et al. found that the mean kyphosis angle was markedly abnormal (44 ± 14° by the Cobb method; 62% were ≥ 40°) and probably contributed to a diminished stature (mean height loss in men with CF = 5.8 cm and women with CF = 5.9 cm) [5]. These data demonstrate a prevalence of kyphosis that is two times higher than the rates seen in younger CF patients and an order of magnitude higher (60% versus approximately 6%) than expected for age- and sex-matched controls.

IV. THERAPY FOR LOW BONE MINERAL DENSITY IN CYSTIC FIBROSIS PATIENTS BEFORE LUNG TRANSPLANTATION

A. Vitamin D Supplementation

Since bone disease in CF has only recently received attention, most therapeutic trials are either ongoing or have been published as preliminary observations. Several studies have assessed the efficacy of using vitamin D analogs to improve 25OHD levels or BMD. Hanley et al. demonstrated the low efficacy of 800 IU/d of vitamin D, the recommended adult supplement in the CF Clinical Practice Guidelines [53]. In a prospective trial, less than half of the vitamin D–deficient patients achieved normal serum 25OHD levels after 4–10 weeks of therapy, and only 30% had normal 25OHD levels after 1 year of therapy. In a preliminary report, Kelly et al. reported that 1800 IU of ergocalciferol daily was needed to achieve a 25OHD level above 25 ng/ml in 95% of the treated cohort (mean dose for the cohort was 843 IU) [54]. In another preliminary report, Boyle et al. were rarely successful in achieving the targeted 25OHD level of 30 ng/ml in 58 adult CF patients treated with ergocalciferol (50,000 IU weekly or twice weekly for up to 4 months) [55]. A poor response to intramuscular ergocalciferol in one trial should not preclude other studies in this area, however, especially if oral supplementation remains problematic [56]. Since some of these reports have been published in preliminary form, seasonal effects, product reliability, and measurement methods may have resulted in some of the variability reported.

In preliminary results from another case-control trial with 73 CF patients, calcifediol and calcium supplementation was beneficial in improving BMD. Children or adults with CF with Z-scores < -1.5 or < -2.0, respectively, were treated with calcifediol (0.7 mg/kg/d) and 1 g of calcium or with calcium alone [57]. Confounding factors such as vitamin D levels, calcium intake, FEV_1, weight/height index, and glucocorticoid usage were included in the analysis. Based on annual DXA results, 69% of calcifediol-treated patients experienced an increase in BMD, whereas only 32% of the control patients experienced increases (mean BMD increase: calcifediol 9.3% versus control 3.6%, $p = 0.004$). In a short-term study, Brown et al. reported that calcitriol (0.5 mcg po once daily for 2 weeks) significantly increased the fractional gastrointestinal absorption of ^{45}Ca ($p = 0.015$), reduced the serum PTH concentration ($p = 0.03$), decreased urinary NTx levels ($p = 0.01$), and trended toward increasing urinary calcium excretion ($p = 0.10$) in 10 adults with CF [58]. Serum calcium levels did not change. Thus, oral calcitriol improved measures of calcium balance in adults with CF and provides another treatment option for vitamin D supplementation.

While vitamin D supplementation is probably important in the management of CF bone disease, further research is needed to determine the optimal vitamin D analog and dose. Current recommendations from a consensus panel are shown in Figure 2 and target 25OHD levels of 30–60 ng/ml (70–150 nmol/L). It is likely that each of the available analogs (ergocalciferol, cholecalciferol, calcifediol [25-hydroxyvitamin D], or calcitriol [$1,25OH_2D$]), when dosed appropriately, can improve serum vitamin D levels and measures of calcium homeostasis and ultimately help improve BMD in CF patients. Drug cost and safety favor the least polar analog, ergocalciferol or cholecalciferol, but commercially available capsule doses (400 IU or 50,000 IU) may be inadequate for CF patients. The type and dose that will be suitable for chronic therapy by maintaining or improving BMD require further research.

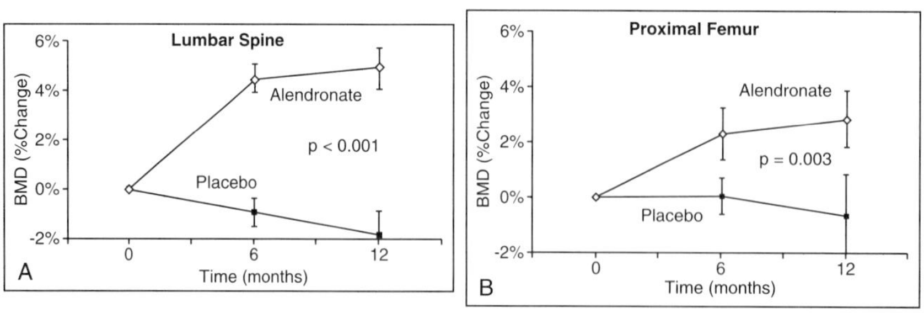

FIGURE 2 Effect of alendronate on bone mineral density in patients with cystic fibrosis. Mean ± SE change in (A) lumbar spine and (B) proximal femur BMD over time in subjects on alendronate plus calcium and vitamin D (open diamonds) compared to placebo and calcium and vitamin D (solid squares), demonstrating significantly greater improvements at the lumbar spine and proximal femur with alendronate.

B. Calcium and Vitamin K Supplementation

To date, no studies have been performed in CF. Calcium and vitamin K supplementation should follow the Dietary Reference Intakes.

C. Hormone Replacement Therapy (HRT)

The efficacy of short-term androgen therapy in promoting growth and pubertal development has been assessed in 54 adolescent and young adult men between the ages of 14 and 18 with CF [42]. In this cohort, 39% were below the fifth percentile in height and 8/28 (28%) of the cohort had delays in pubertal development. Five male adolescents aged 13–18 years were treated with testosterone supplementation (200 mg testosterone enanthate intramuscularly every 3 weeks) in a year-long intervention. Growth rates increased from an entry mean of 2.2 cm/yr (range 0 to 4 cm/yr) to 7.2 cm/yr (range 3 to 10 cm/yr). All participants, while achieving advancement in sexual maturation, only trended towards obtaining normal serum testosterone concentrations. Estrogen replacement therapy trials in female CF patients with delayed puberty or following menopause have not been conducted. Ultimately, HRT may be of benefit in CF patients because chronic illness and the associated glucocorticoid therapy often lead to hypogonadism, resulting in reduced sex-hormone production, oligomenorrhea, and premature menopause. Nonetheless, the complicated nature of CF bone disease and the risk/benefit ratio for HRT in any given patient makes individualization of therapy very important. The early identification of pubertal delays in children or hypogonadism in adults may be best treated with specialist referral.

D. Antiresorptive Agents

Bisphosphonates reduce bone resorption by inhibiting the recruitment and function of osteoclasts, shortening osteoclast lifespan, and slowing osteoblast apoptosis. Intravenous pamidronate (30 mg IV every 3 months) was the first bisphosphonate used in CF patients because it circumvented the potential problems related to malabsorption of an oral bisphosphonate [59]. It has been shown to be effective in adults with CF, resulting in significant gains in lumbar spine BMD (mean difference between arms of 5.8% [$p < 0.001$] and total hip [mean difference 5.0%, $p < 0.05$]) after 6 months. Unfortunately, significant adverse events have occurred with pamidronate use despite adequate 25OHD levels. These included moderate to severe bone pain, in fever, and phlebitis 73% of the patients, that required hospitalization in some [60]. None of the patients taking oral glucocorticoid therapy at the time of pamidronate infusion developed bone pain, suggesting that prednisone therapy had a protective effect. Thus a 3- to 5-day course of prednisone may be useful before the pamidronate infusion.

Alendronate has also shown promise for treating bone disease in CF patients despite early concerns that pancreatic insufficiency would limit absorption [30]. A placebo-controlled, randomized, double-blinded trial of alendronate (10 mg/day orally) ($n = 24$, the treatment group) compared to placebo ($n = 24$, the controls) was conducted for 1 year in 48 patients to improve BMD using spine BMD as the primary endpoint. The alendronate-treated patients gained (mean ± SD) 4.9 ± 3.0% and 2.8 ± 3.2% BMD ($p<0.003$) after 1 year, versus controls, who lost (mean ± SD) 1.8 ± 4.0% and 0.7 ± 4.7%, in spine and femur BMD respectively (see Figure 2). Urine N-telopeptide levels, a bone resorption marker, declined from baseline to the 45- and 90-day time points in the treatment group more than in the controls (−36 ± 23% and −28 ± 13% versus −12 ± 20% and 6 ± 17%, $p = 0.002$), consistent with the known antiresorptive effects of bisphosphonates.

Several potential safety issues with oral bisphosphonates may occur in CF patients if this therapy is used more widely. The incidence of erosive "pill" esophagitis may be higher since patients with CF have a high incidence of gastroesophageal reflux. Furthermore, a minority of CF patients will develop cirrhosis with esophageal varices, which form a contraindication to oral bisphosphonate therapy. Last, adherence to oral bisphosphonate may be suboptimal in CF patients because of their already demanding medical regimens. Once-weekly oral bisphosphonate dosing may improve compliance, however. The efficacy of oral bisphosphonates in CF patients is being investigated in several large multicenter trials. Data from these trials will be available in several years.

E. Anabolic Agents

Anabolic agents such as PTH and statins generally have favorable effects on bone formation and improve bone density, but these medications have not been studied in CF. A study with recombinant human PTH (1-34) (teriparatide) has just been started and may prove valuable since individuals with CF have depressed bone formation.

Human recombinant growth hormone (GH) is another anabolic agent currently demonstrating promise for use in CF. Several studies [61, 62] have demonstrated improvements in linear growth, weight, and lean tissue mass in prepubertal CF children and adolescents treated with GH. New data from a study of children and teens with CF demonstrated that the GH-treated group had statistically greater accretion of bone mineral content than the untreated, age-matched controls.

V. LUNG TRANSPLANTATION FOR CYSTIC FIBROSIS PATIENTS

Approximately one-third of patients with CF in the United States undergo lung transplantation to prolong and improve the quality of their lives [1].

When CF patients were referred to lung transplantation centers, the vast majority had advanced bone disease with mean T (or Z) scores at or below the fracture threshold defined by the WHO diagnostic category for osteoporosis (T score < −2.5) at one or more sites [63–65]. Spine and proximal femur sites were equally affected. BMD was lowest in patients with a low BMI or vitamin D level or a high cumulative exposure to glucocoritcoids. Immunosuppression is mandatory after lung transplantation and may exacerbate the low BMD that exists because of CF itself. For this reason, CF patients with very low BMD and a history of prior fractures may be considered at high risk of developing further fractures and may be turned down for this vital operation. Similar to data after kidney, heart, and liver transplantation, longitudinal studies of lung transplant recipients with various diagnoses (approximately 20% had CF) have shown that spine and femur BMD decreases 2–5% in the first 6–12 months after transplant due to immunosuppressant therapy and decreased physical activity [66, 67]. The BMD losses that occur after the first post-transplant year are variable. More important, patients (including CF and non-CF) who have received lung transplants have alarmingly high rates of pathologic fractures, ranging from 27 to 42% of studied cohorts, with some patients having multiple fractures [63, 64]. CF patients also seem to suffer from post-transplant osteonecrosis, a disorder that affects bone and quality of life, but one with a different pathogenesis [65].

A. Biological Effects of Transplant: Change in BMI and Activity Level

The biological effects of lung transplantation are discussed in Chapter 17, and the effects of immunosuppressants are discussed in Chapters 3, 4, and 5. Patients with CF may differ from other patients after transplantation in that they gain significant weight as a result of the removal of chronically infected lungs, which had a deleterious effect on their lean and total body weight [69]. While clinical experience at many centers indicates that the majority of CF patients will gain weight after lung transplantation, the only published study has reported average BMI gains of 1.5 kg/m^2 over a 2-year period. This weight gain and the increased activity after transplant may mitigate the deleterious effects of immunosuppressants on bone health.

B. Changes in Vitamin D, PTH, and Bone Biomarkers after Lung Transplantation

Serum 25OHD, 1,25(OH$_2$)D, and PTH levels have been measured in the context of a clinical trial using pamidronate to improve BMD in CF patients after lung transplantation. Both vitamin D metabolites and serum PTH rose significantly, while serum calcium levels remained stable, over the first two post-transplant years, and none of the levels were affected by treatment with pamidronate [69]. Mean (± SD) serum 25OHD levels rose significantly from 26 ± 8 to 40 ± 9 ng/ml by the end of 2 years, suggesting that the healthier lung transplant recipients were synthesizing more vitamin D cutaneously from sunlight exposure related to outdoor activities, or that the biotransformation of vitamin D improved after transplant. The $1,25(OH)_2D$ levels rose significantly from 20 ± 3 to 31 ± 4 pg/ml. The rise in PTH from 40 ± 20 to 74 ± 28 U/l was probably due to worsening kidney function from calcineurin inhibitor–based immunosuppression. For the group as a whole, mean (± SD) serum creatinine levels, as a result of cyclosporin treatment, increased over the study (0.9 ± 0.3 to 1.8 ± 0.4 mg/dl, $p < 0.001$).

Bone biomarkers have been studied in the context of the aforementioned trial. As expected, markers of bone resorption were very high in CF patients immediately after lung transplantation (mean urine NTx > 100 nmol/mmol creatinine and mean urine Dpd > 10 nmol/mmole creatinine) and remained unchanged over the first post-transplant year in patients receiving calcium and vitamin D supplements alone [69]. Osteocalcin levels were very low (mean level < 10 ng/ml) immediately after transplantation and rose dramatically after 1 year to mean levels > 50 ng/ml ($p < 0.001$ for effect of time; $p > 0.1$ for effect of treatment). Mean serum bone-specific alkaline phosphatase levels were in the normal range and did not change significantly based on treatment or time. Transplant patients in general, and those patients with CF in particular, appear to develop high-turnover osteoporosis and the associated sequelae in the early post-transplant period [70].

C. Post-Transplant Therapy

Aris et al. conducted the only published controlled, randomized, nonblinded trial of a bisphosphonate (pamidronate: 30 mg IV every 3 months) with vitamin D (800 IU/day) and calcium (1 g/day) (n = 16) compared to vitamin D and calcium alone in CF patients [70]. Pamidronate was used to ensure drug bioavailability and because newer oral and intravenous bisphosphonates were not yet on the U.S. market. Thirty-four CF patients were treated for 2 years after lung transplantation in an effort to improve bone mineral density (BMD). The treatment groups were similar in age, gender, renal function, hospitalization rates, immunosuppressant levels, and change in lung function and BMI over the study period. Baseline T scores for the pamidronate group (spine −3.00 ± 1.00; femur −2.61 ± 0.95) and control group (spine −2.78 ± 1.05; femur −2.36 ± 1.05) were similar, with all patients osteopenic or osteoporotic at one or more sites by the WHO criteria. The patients treated with pamidronate gained 8.8 ± 2.5% and 8.2 ± 3.8% in spine and femur BMD after 2 years in comparison to controls, who gained on average (± SD) 2.6 ± 3.2% and 0.3 ± 2.2%, respectively ($p < 0.015$ for both) (see Figure 3). Seven and six fractures occurred in the control and pamidronate groups, respectively ($p > 0.2$). Thus, pamidronate was

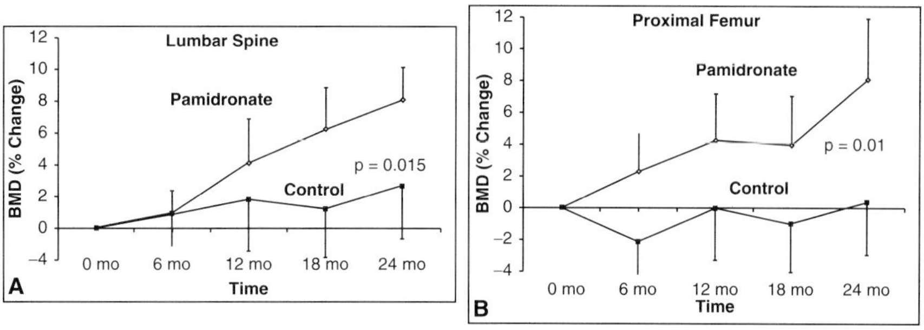

FIGURE 3 Effect of pamidronate on bone mineral density incystic fibrosis patients following lung transplantation. Mean ± SE change in BMD over time in subjects on pamidronate plus calcium and vitamin D (open diamonds) compared to calcium and vitamin D alone (solid squares) for **(A)** spine and **(B)** proximal femur, demonstrating significantly greater improvements with pamidronate.

more effective than control in improving BMD after lung transplantation in CF patients. None of the post-transplant patients treated with pamidronate developed bone pain, in contrast to the experience of Haworth et al. [60]; the use of prednisone and other immunosuppressants in the post-transplant patients may have prevented infusion-related bone pain.

VI. CONCLUSIONS

Low bone density, fractures, and kyphosis have become common in adult CF patients. The multifaceted nature of bone disease in CF makes it a particularly difficult problem to manage. Aggressive fat-soluble vitamin, calcium, and nutritional supplementation during childhood may allow the greatest accrual of bone mass and provide some protection from fractures as post-pubertal bone losses from chronic infection, intermittent immobility, and treatments take their toll. Maintenance of body weight and regular weight-bearing exercise are likely to improve bone health. Bisphosphonates, such as alendronate and pamidronate, are useful to improve BMD. Hormone replacement therapy and teriaparatide offer potential, but unproven, treatment options. In a relatively short time, the management and treatment of bone disease in CF patients have significantly improved the quality of life for these patients.

Acknowledgments

This work was supported in part by the U.S. Food and Drug Administration (FD-R-001518-01), Merck and Co, Inc. (Medical School Grants Program), the Clinical Nutrition Research Unit (NIDDK 56350), the Verne Caviness General Center for Clinical Research (NIH RR00046), the Cystic Fibrosis Foundation (A936), and a Medical Student Training Grant (5 T35 DK07386).

REFERENCES

1. Cystic Fibrosis Foundation, Patient Registry 2002 Annual Report. Bethesda, MD: Cystic Fibrosis Foundation, 2003.
2. Mischler, E.H., Chesney P.J., Chesney R.W., Mazess, R.B. (1979). Demineralization in cystic fibrosis detected by direct photon absorptiometry. *Am J Dis Child.* 133:632–635.
3. Hahn, T.J., et al. (1979). Reduced serum 25-hydroxyvitamin D concentration and disordered mineral metabolism in patients with cystic fibrosis. *J Pediatr.* 94(1):38–42.
4. Elkin, S.L., Fairney A., Burnett S., Kemp M., Kyd P., Burgess J., Compston J.E., Hodson M.E. (2001). Vertebral deformities and low bone mineral density in adults with cystic fibrosis: a cross-sectional study. *Osteoporos Int.* 12:366–372.
5. Aris, R.M., Renner, J.B., Winders, A.D., Buell, H.E., Riggs, D.B., Lester, G.E., Ontjes, D.A. (1998). Increased rate of fractures and severe kyphosis: sequelae of living to adulthood with cystic fibrosis. *Ann Intern Med.* 128:186–193.
6. Henderson, R.C., Madsen C.D. (1999). Bone mineral content and body composition in children and young adults with cystic fibrosis. *Pediatr Pulmonol.* 27:80–84.
7. Haworth, C.S., Selby, P.L., Webb, A.K., Dodd, M.E., Musson, H., McL Niven, R., Economou, G., Horrocks, A.W., Freemont, A.J., Mawer, E.B., Adams, J.E. (1999). Low bone mineral density in adults with cystic fibrosis. *Thorax.* 54:961–967.
8. Moran, C.E., Sosa, E.G., Martinez, S.M., Geldern, P., Messina, D., Russo, A., Boerr, L., Bai, J.C. (1997). Bone mineral density in patients with pancreatic insufficiency and steatorrhea. *Am J Gastroenterol.* 92:867–871.
9. Shane, E., Silverberg, S.J., Donovan, D., Papadopoulos, A., Staron, R.B., Addesso, V., Jorgesen, B., McGregor, C., Schulman, L. (1996). Osteoporosis in lung transplantation candidates with end-stage pulmonary disease. *Am J Med.* 101:262–269.
10. Tschopp, O., Boehler, A., Speich, R., Weder, W., Seifert, B., Russi, E.W., Schmid, C. (2002). Osteoporosis before lung transplantation: association with low body mass index, but not with underlying disease. *Am J Transplant.* 2(2):167–172.

10a. Gibbens, D.T., et al. (1988). Osteoporosis in cystic fibrosis. *J Pediatr.* 113:295–300.

11. Conway, S.P., Morton, A.M., Oldroyd, B., Truscott, J.G., White, H., Smith, A.H., Haigh, I. (2000). Osteoporosis and osteopenia in adults and adolescents with cystic fibrosis: prevalence and associated factors. *Thorax.* 55:798–804.
12. Bachrach, L.K., Loutit, C.W., Moss, R.B. (1994). Osteopenia in adults with cystic fibrosis. *Am J Med.* 96:27–34.
13. Grey, A.B., Ames, R.W., Matthews, R.D., Reid, I.R. (1993). Bone mineral density and body composition in adult patients with cystic fibrosis. *Thorax.* 48:589–593.
14. Shaw, N., Bedford, C., Heaf, D., Carty, H., Dutton, J. (1995). Osteopenia in adults with cystic fibrosis. *Am J Med.* 99:690–692.
15. Rochat, T., Slosman, D.O., Pichard, C., Belli, D.C. (1994). Body composition analysis by dual-energy x-ray absorptiometry in adults with cystic fibrosis. *Chest.* 106:800–805.
16. Henderson, R.C., Madsen, C.D. (1996). Bone density in children and adolescents with cystic fibrosis. *J Pediatr.* 128:28–34.
17. Bhudhikanok, G.S., Lim, J., Marcus, R., Harkins, A., Moss, R.B., Bachrach, L.K. (1996). Correlates of osteopenia in patients with cystic fibrosis. *Pediatrics.* 97:103–111.
18. Bhudhikanok, G.S., Wang, M.C., Marcus, R., Harkins, A., Moss, R.B., Bachrach, L.K. (1998). Bone acquisition and loss in children and adults with cystic fibrosis: a longitudinal study. *J Pediatr.* 133:18–27.
19. Donovan, D.S. Jr, Papadopoulos, A., Staron, R.B., Addesso, V., Schulman, L., McGregor, C., Cosman, F., Lindsay, R.L., Shane, E. (1998). Bone mass and vitamin D deficiency in adults with advanced cystic fibrosis lung disease. *Am J Respir Crit Care Med.* 157 (6 Pt 1):1892–1899.
20. Salamoni, F., Roulet, M., Gudinchet, F., Pilet, M., Thiebaud, D., Burckhardt, P. (1996). Bone mineral content in cystic fibrosis patients: correlation with fat-free mass. *Arch Dis Child.* 74:314–318.

21. Hardin, D.S., Arumugam, R., Seilheimer, D.K., LeBlanc, A., Ellis, K.J. (2001). Normal bone mineral density in cystic fibrosis. *Arch Dis Child.* 84:363–368.
22. Humphries, I.R., Allen, J.R., Waters, D.L., Howman-Giles, R., Gaskin, K.J. (1998). Volumetric bone mineral density in children with cystic fibrosis. *Appl Radiat Isot.* 49:593–595.
23. Laursen, E.M., Molgaard, C., Michaelsen, K.F., Koch, C., Muller, J. (1999). Bone mineral status in 134 patients with cystic fibrosis. *Arch Dis Child.* 81(3):235–240.
24. Sood, M., Hambleton, G., Super, M., Fraser, W.D., Adams, J.E., Mughal, M.Z. (2001). Bone status in cystic fibrosis. *Arch Dis Child.* 84:516–520.
25. Elkin, S.L., Vedi, S., Bord, S., Garrahan, N.J., Hodson, M.E., Compston, J.E. (2002). Histomorphometric analysis of bone biopsies from the iliac crest of adults with cystic fibrosis. *Am J Resp Crit Care Med.* 166:1470–1474.
26. Haworth, C.S., Webb, A.K., Egan, J.J., Selby, P.L., Hasleton, P.S., Bishop, P.W., Freemont, T.J. (2000). Bone histomorphometry in adult patients with cystic fibrosis. *Chest.* 118:434–439.
27. Bachrach, L.K. (2001). Acquisition of optimal bone mass in childhood and adolescence. *Trends in Endocrinol Metab.* 12:22–27.
28. Bailey, D.A., McKay, H.A., Mirwald, R.L., Crocker, P.R., Faulkner, R.A. (1999). A six-year longitudinal study of the relationship of physical activity to bone mineral accrual in growing children; The University of Saskatchewan Bone Mineral Accrual Study. *J Bone Miner Res.* 14:1672–1679.
29. Haworth, C.S., Selby, P.L., Horrocks, A.W., Mawer, E.B., Adams, J.E., Webb, A.K. (2002). A prospective study of change in bone mineral density over one year in adults with cystic fibrosis. *Thorax.* 57(8):719–723.
30. Aris, R.M., Lester, G.E., Caminiti, M., Blackwood, A.D., Hensler, M., Lark, R.K., Hecker, T.M., Renner, J.B., Guillen, U., Brown, S.A., Neuringer, I.P., Chalermskulrat, W., Ontjes, D.A. (2004). Efficacy of alendronate in adults with cystic fibrosis with low bone density. *Am J Respir Crit Care Med.* 169(1):77–82.
31. De Schepper, J., Smitz, J., Dab, I., Piepsz, A., Jonckheer, M., Bergmann, P. (1993). Low serum bone gamma-carboxyglutamic acid protein concentrations in patients with cystic fibrosis: correlation with hormonal parameters and bone mineral density. *Horm Res.* 39:197–201.
32. Baroncelli, G.I., De Luca, F., Magazzu, G., Arrigo, T., Sferlazzas, C., Catena, C., Bertelloni, S., Saggese, G. (1997). Bone demineralization in cystic fibrosis: evidence of imbalance between bone formation and degradation. *Pediatr Res.* 41:397–403.
33. Aris, R.M., Ontjes, D.A., Buell, H.E., Blackwood, A.D., Lark, R.K., Brown, S.A., Caminiti, M., Chalermskulrat, W., Renner, J.B., Lester, G.E. (2002). Abnormal bone turnover in cystic fibrosis adults. *Osteoporosis Int.* 13(2):151–157.
34. Borowitz, D., Baker, R.D., Stallings, V. (2002). Consensus Report on Nutrition for Pediatric patients with Cystic Fibrosis. *J Pediatr Gastroenterol Nutr.* 35:246–259.
35. Ott, S.M., Aitken, M.L. (1998). Osteoporosis in patients with cystic fibrosis. *Clin Chest Med.* 19(3):555–567.
36. Heaney, R.P., Dowell, M.S., Hale, C.A. Bendich, A. (2003). Calcium absorption varies within the reference range for serum 25-hydroxyvitamin D. *J Am Coll Nutr.* 22(2):142–146.
37. Lark, R.K., Lester, G.E., Ontjes, D.A., Blackwood, A.D., Hollis, B.W., Hensler, M.M., Aris, R.M. (2001). Diminished and erratic absorption of ergocalciferol in adult cystic fibrosis patients. *Am J Clin Nutr.* 73(3):602–606.
38. Wilson, D.C., Rashid, M., Durie, P.R., Tsang, A., Kalnins, D., Andrew, M., Corey, M., Shin, J., Tullis, E., Pencharz, P.B. (2001). Treatment of vitamin K deficiency in cystic fibrosis: effectiveness of a daily fat-soluble vitamin combination. *J Pediatr.* 138(6):851–855.
39. Aris, R.M., Brown, S.A., Ontjes, D.A., Chalermskulrat, W., Neuringer, I.P., Lester, G.E. (2003). Reduced carboxylated osteocalcin levels in cystic fibrosis. *Am J Respir Crit Care Med.* 168(9):1129.

40. Levin, M.E., V.C. Boisseau, and, L.V. Avioli. (1976). Effects of diabetes mellitus on bone mass in juvenile and adult-onset diabetes. *N Engl J Med.* 294(5):241–245.
41. Stead, R.J., Hodson, M.E., Batten, J.C., Adams, J., Jacobs, H.S. (1987). Amenorrhoea in cystic fibrosis. *Clin Endocrinol (Oxf).* 26(2):187–195.
42. Landon, C., Rosenfeld, R.G. (1984). Short stature and pubertal delay in male adolescents with cystic fibrosis. Androgen treatment. *Am J Dis Child.* 138(4):388–391.
43. Moshang, T., Holsclaw, D.S. Jr. (1980). Menarchal determinants in cystic fibrosis. *Am J Dis Child.* 134(12):1139–1142.
44. Johannesson, M., Landgren, B.M., Csemiczky, G., Hjelte, L., Gottlieb, C. (1998). Female patients with cystic fibrosis suffer from reproductive endocrinological disorders despite good clinical status. *Hum Reprod.* 13(8):2092–2097.
45. Weltman, E.A., Stern, R.C., Doershuk, C.F., Moir, R.N., Palmer, K., Jaffe, A.C. (1990). Weight and menstrual function in patients with eating disorders and cystic fibrosis. *Pediatrics.* 85(3):282–287.
46. Boas, S.R., Cleary, D.A., Lee, P.A., Orenstein, D.M. (1996). Salivary testosterone levels in male adolescents with cystic fibrosis. *Pediatrics.* 97(3):361–363.
47. Manolagas, S.C., Jilka, R.L. (1995). Bone marrow, cytokines, and bone remodeling. Emerging insights into the pathophysiology of osteoporosis. *N Engl J Med.* 332(5):305–311.
48. Aris, R.M., Stevens, A., Ontjes, D.A., Blackwood, A.D., Lark, R.K., Hensler, M., Neuringer, I.P., Lester, G.E. (2000). Adverse alterations in bone metabolism are associated with lung infection in adults with cystic fibrosis. *Am J Respir Crit Care Med.* 162(5):1674–1678.
49. Henderson, R.C., Specter, B.B. (1994). Kyphosis and fractures in children and young adults with cystic fibrosis. *J Pediatr.* 125(2):208–212.
50. Erkkila, J., Warwick, W., Bradford, D. (1978). Spine deformities and cystic fibrosis. *Clin Orthop.* 131:146–149.
51. Denton, J.R., Tietjen, R., Gaerlan, P.F. (1979). Thoracic kyphosis in cystic fibrosis. *Clin Orthop.* 155:71–74.
52. Logvinoff, M., Fon, G., Taussig, L.M., Pitt, M.J. (1984). Kyphosis and pulmonary function cystic fibrosis. *Clin Pediatr.* 23:389–392.
53. Hanly, J.G., McKenna, M.J., Quigley, C., Freaney, R., Muldowney, F.P., FitzGerald, M.X. (1985). Hypovitaminosis D and response to supplementation in older patients with cystic fibrosis. *Q J Med.* 56(219):377–385.
54. Kelly, E., Marsh, R., Pencharz, P., Tullis, E. (2002). Effect of vitamin D supplementation on low serum 25-hydroxyvitamin D in adults with cystic fibrosis. *Pediatr Pulmonol.* Suppl 24:344 (abstr).
55. Boyle, M.P., Noschese, M.L., Watts, S.L., Davis, M.E., Lechtzin, N. (2003). Prevalence of 25-hydroxyvitamin D defeciency in adults with CF and effect of high dose ergocalciferol supplementation. *Ped Pulmonol.* Suppl 25:350 (abstract).
56. Ontjes, D.A., Lark, R.K., Lester, G.E., Aris, R.M. Vitamin D depletion and replacement in patients with cystic fibrosis, in vitamin D endocrine system: structural, biological, genetic and clinical aspects, A.W. Norman, R. Bouillon, and M. Thomasset, eds. (2000), pp. 893–896, University of California, Riverside Press.
57. Enfissi L., Bianchi M.L., Galbiati E., et al. (2001). Osteoporosis in CF: calcifediol therapy increases bone mineral density (BMD). *Pediatric Pulm.* Supp 22 A475:334.
58. Brown, S.A., Ontjes, D.A., Lark, R.K., Blackwood, A.D., Hensler, M., Caminiti, M., Aris, R.M. (2003). Short-term calcitriol administration improves calcium homeostasis in adults with CF. *Osteoporosis Int.* 14(5):442–449.
59. Haworth, C.S., Selby, P.L., Adams, J.E., Mawer, E.B., Horrocks, A.W., Webb, A.K. (2001). Effect of intravenous pamidronate on bone mineral density in adults with cystic fibrosis. *Thorax.* 56(4):314–316.
60. Haworth, C.S., Selby, P.L., Webb, A.K., Mawer, E.B., Adams, J.E., Freemont, T.J. (1998). Severe bone pain after intravenous pamidronate in adult patients with cystic fibrosis. *Lancet.* 352(9142):1753–1754.

61. Hardin, D.S., Ellis, K.J., Dyson, M., Rice, J., McConnell, R., Seilheimer, D.K. (2001). Growth hormone decreases protein catabolism in children with cystic fibrosis. *J Clin Endocrinol Metab.* 86(9):4424–4428.
62. Hardin, D.S., Ellis, K.J., Dyson, M., Rice, J., McConnell, R., Seilheimer, D.K. (2001). Growth hormone improves clinical status in prepubertal children with cystic fibrosis: results of a randomized controlled trial. *J Pediatr.* 139(5):636–642.
63. Aris, R.M., Neuringer, I.P., Egan, T.M., Weiner, M., Ontjes, D. (1996). Severe osteoporosis before and after lung transplantation. *Chest.* 109:1176–1183.
64. Shane, E., Papadopoulos, A., Staron, R.B., Addesso, V., Donovan, D.S., McGregor, C., Schulman, L.L. (1999). Bone loss and fracture after lung transplantation. *Transplantation.* 68(2):220–227.
65. Tschopp, O., Boehler, A., Speich, R., Weder, W., Seifert, B., Russi, E.W., Schmid, C. (2002). Osteoporosis before lung transplantation: association with low body mass index, but not with underlying disease. *Am J Transplant.* 2(2):167–172.
66. Ferrari, S.L., Nicod, L.P., Hamacher, J., Spiliopoulos, A., Slosman, D.O., Rochat, T., Bonjour, J.P., Rizzoli, R. (1996). Osteoporosis in patients undergoing lung transplantation. *Eur Respir J.* 9(11):2378–2382.
67. Spira, A., Gutierrez, C., Chaparro, C., Hutcheon, M.A., Chan, C.K. (2000). Osteoporosis and lung transplantation: a prospective study. *Chest.* 117(2):476–481.
68. Schoch, O.D., Speich, R., Schmid, C., Tschopp, O., Russi, E.W., Weder, W., Boehler, A. (2000). Osteonecrosis after lung transplantation: cystic fibrosis as a potential risk factor. *Transplantation.* 69(8):1629–1632.
69. Aris, R.M., Lester, G.E., Renner, J.B., Winders, A.W., Blackwood, A.D., Lark, R.K., and Ontjes, D.A. (2000). Efficacy of pamidronate for osteoporosis in patients with cystic fibrosis following lung transplantation. *Am J Respir Crit Care Med.* 162(3 Pt 1):941–946.
70. Aringer, M., Kiener, H.P., Koeller, M.D., Artemiou, O., Zuckermann, A., Wieselthaler, G., Klepetko, W., Seidl, G., Kainberger, F., Bernecker, P., Smolen, J.S., Pietschmann, P. (1998). High turnover bone disease following lung transplantation. *Bone.* 23(5):485–488.

CHAPTER 19

Bone Disease after Bone Marrow Transplantation

Peter R. Ebeling, MD, FRACP
Departments of Diabetes and Endocrinology and Medicine,
The Royal Melbourne Hospital, Victoria, Australia

I. INTRODUCTION

Bone marrow, or peripheral blood progenitor cell, transplantation (BMT) is the treatment of choice for patients with certain hematological malignancies, the majority of whom will survive many years thereafter. Bone disease is a common long-term complication [1, 2]. Osteoporosis after BMT has a complex pathogenesis, related to the effects of both immunosuppressive therapy and effects on the stromal cell compartment of the bone marrow peculiar to BMT [3]. This results in reduced bone formation in the face of increased bone resorption [4]. Rapid and early bone loss, most severe at the femoral neck, is characteristic. In addition to osteopenia and osteoporosis, osteomalacia, fragility fractures, and avascular necrosis of bone may also complicate BMT.

Bone disease after BMT therefore differs from that following solid-organ transplantation. In addition to effects on bone marrow stromal cells, differences also relate to patients being younger, a short interval between diagnosis and BMT, and effects of pre-BMT treatment on bone.

II. CANDIDATES FOR BONE MARROW TRANSPLANTATION

Bone loss in BMT recipients is related both to the underlying diseases and to the agents used to treat them. These include glucocorticoid-induced decreases in bone formation and serum 1,25-dihydroxyvitamin D_3 (1,25-$(OH)_2D_3$), hypogonadism secondary to the effects of high-dose chemotherapy, total body irradiation (TBI), and physical inactivity. Women are particularly sensitive to the adverse effects of TBI and myeloablative chemotherapy on gonadal function. Ovarian insufficiency occurs in the majority [5, 6], although young, premenarchal women may recover ovarian function. After allogeneic BMT in women, treatment for graft-versus-host disease can decrease estradiol and androgen levels further [7]. Testosterone levels decline acutely after BMT then return to normal in most men [8]. There may be long-term impairment of spermatogenesis with elevated FSH occurring in 47% of men [9, 10]. In adult patients, hypothalamic-pituitary function is normal [11]. Growth hormone deficiency has been documented in children before and after BMT [12] and may contribute to low BMD. Growth hormone secretion is decreased by TBI, resulting in low body mass index and increased serum leptin concentrations [13]. In patients studied after chemotherapy but before BMT, osteopenia was present in 24% and osteoporosis in 4% [14].

III. BONE LOSS AFTER BONE MARROW TRANSPLANT

A. Skeletal Effects of Immunosuppressive Drugs

1. Glucocorticoids

High doses of glucocorticoids (e.g., > 50 mg/day of prednisone or prednisolone) are commonly prescribed immediately after BMT, with subsequent dose reduction over several weeks and transient increases during episodes of graft-versus-host disease. Exposure also varies with the practice of transplantation programs. The introduction of cyclosporine A has reduced glucocorticoid requirements, but exposure is still sufficient, particularly during the first few months after transplantation, to cause substantial bone loss.

Glucocorticoids reduce BMD predominantly at trabecular sites, and even small doses are associated with markedly increased fracture risk. Glucocorticoids cause direct and profound reductions in bone formation by decreasing osteoblast replication, differentiation, and lifespan, and by inhibiting genes for type I collagen, osteocalcin, insulin-like growth factors, bone morphogenetic proteins and other bone matrix proteins, transforming growth factor β (TGFβ), and receptor activator for NFκ B-ligand (RANK-L). Direct effects of glucocorticoids on bone resorption are minor relative to formation. Glucocorticoids may increase bone resorption indirectly, however, by inhibiting synthesis of gonadal steroids and inducing secondary hyperparathyroidism from reduced intestinal and renal calcium absorption, although hyperparathyroidism (HPT) is thought to be of minor importance in the pathogenesis of steroid-induced bone loss [15]. Glucocorticoids also decrease serum $1,25(OH)_2D_3$ concentrations.

2. *Calcineurin Inhibitors: Cyclosporine A*

The introduction of cyclosporine (CsA) to transplantation regimens was associated with a marked reduction in rejection episodes and improved survival. CsA inhibits calcineurin, a T-cell phosphatase, and reduces T-cell function [2]. In the rat, CsA administration caused severe bone loss, particularly in trabecular bone, that was associated with marked increases in resorption and formation and with increased levels of osteocalcin and $1{,}25(OH)_2D_3$ [2, 16]. The CsA-mediated bone loss was associated with testosterone deficiency [17], independent of renal function [2], and attenuated by parathyroidectomy [18]. Antiresorptive agents such as estrogen, raloxifene, calcitonin, and alendronate prevented CsA-induced bone loss [2]. These animal studies suggest that CsA could be responsible for the high-turnover aspects of post-transplantation bone disease. The effects of CsA on the human skeleton after BMT are still unclear, however. Bone loss post-BMT has been related to duration of CsA exposure [19, 20], and hypomagnesemia is potentiated by cyclosporin, causing hypocalcaemia.

IV. BONE MARROW TRANSPLANTATION

A. Autologous BMT

The effects of autologous stem-cell transplantation on bone and mineral metabolism are less well characterized than those of allogeneic BMT. In 68 consecutive autologous BMT survivors, evaluated a median of 4.2 years after BMT, 26 and 46% of patients had osteopenia, and 2 and 8% had osteoporosis, at the spine and femoral neck, respectively [21]. However, only mean femoral neck BMD was lower than in age- and sex-matched controls. Older age was predictive for lower BMD.

The largest prospective study of 38 autologous stem-cell transplants showed femoral neck bone loss occurred as early as 3 months post-BMT and persisted at 2 years, while, after an initial decrease at the spine, BMD had returned to baseline at 2 years [22]. The decrease in femoral neck BMD of about 4% was less than that seen after allogeneic BMT (see Figure 1). Bone specific alkaline phosphatase, a marker of bone formation, also declined 1 month after BMT. Another smaller study of 10 patients after autologous stem-cell transplant showed no change in spinal or femoral neck BMD after 30 months [19]. Differences may relate to a longer time interval between BMD scans, different preparative regimens, variable use of HRT in female autologous BMT recipients, and small study numbers in each control group. Nevertheless, it seems likely that significant bone loss from the femoral neck may occur after autologous BMT, and the implications for future fracture risk in these patients require further investigation.

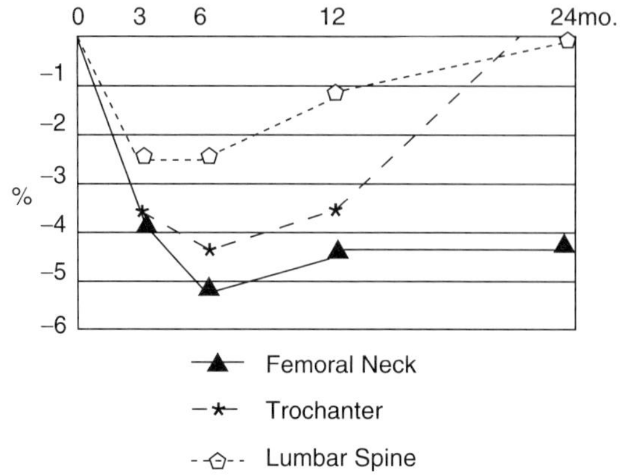

FIGURE 1 Cumulative percentage changes in spine, femoral neck, and trochanter BMD from baseline to 24 months after autologous BMT. Reproduced from Ghandi et al. (2003), Significant and persistent loss of bone mineral density in the femoral neck after haematopoetic stem cell transplantation: long-term follow-up of a prospective study. Br J. Haematol. 121(3): 462–468 with permission of Blackwell Publishing Ltd.

B. Allogeneic BMT

Small cross-sectional studies have shown decreased femoral neck and lumbar spine BMD in adults and children following allogeneic (allo) BMT [23–27]. Up to 29 and 52% of survivors have T scores < −1.0 at the lumbar spine and femoral neck, respectively, post-allo BMT [23]. Osteoporosis is more common at proximal femur sites than at the spine [24]. Patients who are younger than 18 at the time of BMT may fail to achieve peak bone mass, and low BMD in this population may also be related to smaller bone size secondary to reduced height for age [25]. Longitudinal studies [8, 19, 28–33] have shown rapid bone loss in the first 6–12 months after BMT that is greater at the proximal femur than the spine and total body (see Table 1) and is highly variable (see Figure 2). Rates of bone loss in the first year post-BMT from the proximal femur were consistently 8.5-12%, compared with 3-5.9% at the spine and 3.1-3.8% at the total body. In general, most of the bone loss occurs in the first six months with little additional bone loss after this time. Studies of long-term survivors of BMT have shown that losses from the proximal femur are not regained 3 to 10 years later [23, 34, 35].

The pathogenesis of BMT-related bone loss is quite complex (see Table 2). A reduction in bone formation in the face of ongoing or increased bone resorption is a hallmark of this condition. Contributing factors include cumulative glucocorticoid exposure, whether given before BMT or for treatment of graft-versus-host disease (GVHD). Bone loss has also been related to duration of CsA exposure [19, 20] and tacrolimus therapy [20], and it may also be a direct effect of GVHD itself on bone cells [36].

TABLE 1 Changes in LS and FN BMD and total body bone mineral content (TBBMC) 12 months after BMT

Study	n	LS-BMD	FN-BMD	TBBMC
Stern, J. M., et al., 1996	9	−9.5%	–	–
Ebeling, P. R., et al., 1999	39	−3.9%	−11.7%	−3.5%
Valimaki, M.J. et al., 1999	22	−5.7%	−8.0	–
Kashyap, A. et al., 2000	21	−3.0%	−11.6%	–
Schulte, C. et al., 2000	81	−7.2%	−11.9%	−3.8%
Kang, M.I. et al., 2000	31	−2.2%*	−6.2%	–
Buchs, N. et al., 2001**	23	0	−5.6%	−3.1%
Lee, W. L. et al., 2002	67	−3.3%	−8.9% (total hip)	–

*Not significant

**75% treated with intravenous pamidronate

Reproduced from Cohen, A., Ebeling, P., Sprague, S., Shane, E. 2003 Transplantation Osteoporosis. In: Favus, M. (ed.) The Primer on the Metabolic Bone Diseases and Disorders of Mineral Metabolism, 5th ed. American Society for Bone and Mineral Research, Washington, DC, USA, pp. 370–379, table 2.

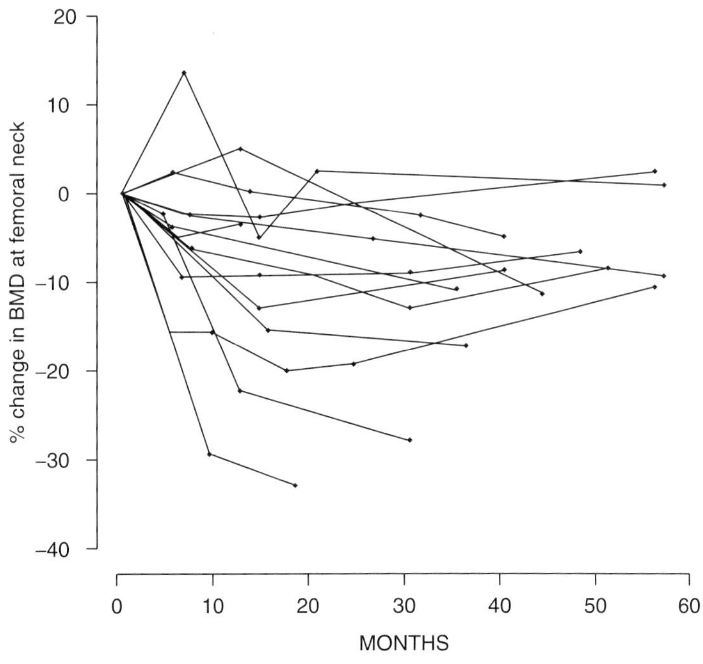

FIGURE 2 Cumulative percentage changes in femoral neck BMD in patients with three or more BMD measurements following allogeneic BMT. Reproduced from *J Bone Miner Res* 1999:14:342–350 with permission of the American Society for Bone and Mineral Research.

TABLE 2 Causes of decreased bone formation following bone marrow transplantation

Causes of decreased bone formation post-BMT
Glucocorticoids
Effects of cytokines
Effect of chemotherapy on bone marrow stromal cells to reduce osteoprogenitor cells

C. Effects of BMT on Cytokines and Bone Marrow Stromal Cells

Abnormal cellular or cytokine-mediated bone marrow function may affect bone turnover and BMD after BMT [37, 38, 39]. Both myeloablative treatment and BMT stimulate the early release of cytokines, including interleukin-6 (IL-6), tumor necrosis factor α (TNFα), and granulocyte-macrophage colony stimulating factor (GM-CSF) [37]. Serum levels of both IL-6 and TNFα peak at about the time of maximal bone resorption, but only bone marrow IL-6 concentrations are positively related to bone resorption markers. Serum growth factors levels also decline early after BMT [34]. Serum insulin-like growth factor-I (IGF-I) and fibroblast growth factor-2 (FGF-2) decrease at 1–3 weeks and return to baseline levels at 3 months. At the same time, serum levels of osteoprotegerin (OPG), a decoy receptor for RANK ligand and a potent inhibitor of osteoclast function and differentiation, increase. Serum IGF-I levels within 3 months of BMT are related to post-BMT changes in femoral neck BMD [38]. After 3 months post-BMT, glucocorticoid effects on bone formation markers predominate.

BMT also has adverse effects on bone marrow osteoprogenitors, reducing their numbers and function. Osteocyte viability is decreased after BMT [40], and osteocytes are replaced by differentiation of host stromal cells comprising precursor cells for adipocytes, fibroblasts, endothelial cells, osteoblasts, and osteocytes [41]. Bone marrow stromal cells are damaged by high-dose chemotherapy, TBI, glucocorticoids, and CsA, reducing osteoblastic differentiation from osteoprogenitor cells. Colony forming units-fibroblasts (CFU-F) are reduced for up to 12 years after allo-BMT [3, 23, 42]. In this regard, high-dose chemotherapy is an important factor, irrespective of gonadal status [3]. The relative importance of this mechanism is highlighted by the decrease in femoral neck BMD following auto BMT [22]. More recently, a study has shown reduced differentiation of bone marrow stromal cells into osteoblasts from BMT recipients compared with those from BMT donors [33]. Mineralization was also delayed in recipient cells compared with donor cells.

D. Other Considerations

Mild, moderate, or severe vitamin D deficiency is common after BMT, particularly in some northern European studies where it was universal and prolonged, lasting more than 6 months [43]. Treatment with vitamin D improves BMD in patients with vitamin D deficiency and intestinal GVHD [44, 45]. Serum vitamin D concentrations should be assessed before and after BMT, and deficits require replacement.

The incidence of fragility fractures has not been well studied after BMT. One study reported an incidence of 10.6% within 3 years of BMT [20]. Significant height loss also occurs in the first 12 months after BMT. Avascular necrosis is the most serious complication and develops in 10 to 20% of allo-BMT survivors, a median of 12 months after BMT [19, 20, 23, 46, 47]. The femoral head is most often affected and frequently more than one site per patient may be affected. It is less common after autologous BMT, occurring in 1.9% of patients. The cumulative dose of glucocorticoids used in treatment of chronic GVHD is the most important risk factor. Age, but not sex, was also important. Femoral neck bone loss was also greater in men with avascular necrosis of the femoral head in one study [19]. Another study showed avascular necrosis was related to the decreased number of bone marrow colony forming units-fibroblasts (CFU-F) colonies in vitro, but not to BMD values [47]. Avascular necrosis may be facilitated by a deficit in regeneration of bone marrow stromal stem cells after BMT.

V. PREVENTION AND MANAGEMENT OF OSTEOPOROSIS AFTER BONE MARROW TRANSPLANT

A. Before BMT

Because of the high prevalence of osteoporosis, osteopenia, and abnormal bone and mineral metabolism in patients awaiting BMT and the morbidity caused by osteoporosis after transplantation, all candidates for BMT would benefit from an evaluation of bone health. BMD of the hip and spine should be measured before transplantation, preferably at the time of acceptance to the waiting list. Spine radiographs should be performed to detect prevalent fractures. If BMD is low, an evaluation for secondary causes of osteoporosis should be undertaken, and if osteoporosis is detected, it should be treated specifically. Most cases will be related to myeloablative chemotherapy and glucocorticoids, however. All patients should receive the recommended daily allowance for calcium and vitamin D (1000–1500 mg of calcium and 400–800 IU of vitamin D).

Whether therapy for osteoporosis before transplantation reduces fracture risk after transplantation is presently unclear. Bisphosphonates, in particular, suppress bone resorption for up to 12 months after discontinuation of therapy.

Transplantation with bisphosphonates already "on board" may prevent the increase in resorption that develops immediately after grafting and could theoretically mitigate post-transplant bone loss. Moreover, antiresorptive therapy clearly increases BMD and reduces fractures in other populations.

B. After BMT

Bone loss is most rapid immediately after BMT. Patients with both low and normal pretransplant BMD may be affected by skeletal complications. Most patients (even those with normal BMD) will therefore require preventive therapy instituted at the time of BMT. In addition, there are many patients who received BMT months or years before, yet were never evaluated or treated for osteoporosis.

1. Vitamin D and Analogues

Vitamin D metabolites may reduce post-transplantation bone loss by reversing glucocorticoid-induced decreases in intestinal calcium absorption and by mitigating secondary hyperparathyroidism [48]. Theoretically, they could also reduce glucocorticoid exposure by virtue of their immunomodulatory effects [48].

Parent vitamin D, in doses of 400–1000 IU, does not prevent significant post-transplantation bone loss. However, 25-OHD (calcidiol) treatment has been associated with significant increases in lumbar spine BMD after cardiac transplantation and prevents bone loss in long-term cardiac transplant recipients [49]. 1,25-$(OH)_2D_3$ (calcitriol) has been studied in heart, lung, liver, and kidney transplant recipients. The results of these trials have been contradictory. There are no studies of vitamin D treatment following BMT.

Hypercalcemia and hypercalciuria, common side effects of vitamin D metabolites, may develop at any point during treatment. Frequent monitoring of urine and serum is required. Thus, active vitamin D metabolites should not be selected as first-line treatment because of their limited effectiveness and narrow therapeutic window.

2. Bisphosphonates

Several studies suggest that oral or intravenous bisphosphonates prevent bone loss and fractures after transplantation. The experience with bisphosphonates after BMT has been more limited. Intravenous bisphosphonates would be advantageous given the high prevalence of gastrointestinal graft-versus-host disease post allo-BMT and likely decreased oral bioavailability of oral bisphosphonates.

In a prospective randomized 12-month study of risedronate on bone mass and turnover in patients who had undergone allogeneic BMT at least 6 months before, spine BMD increased in patients on risedronate and decreased in those taking placebo [50]. All patients received calcium and vitamin D. At the femoral neck, BMD did not change significantly in patients on risedronate, but decreased in those on placebo. However, it is not clear from this study whether risedronate prevents the rapid early bone loss from the femoral neck occurring after BMT. In an uncontrolled observational study, three monthly intravenous pamidronate infusions attenuated femoral neck bone loss in the first six months after allo BMT [32]. Bisphosphonates predominantly act to inhibit the action of osteoclasts and induce their apoptosis. However, they may also reduce osteoblast apoptosis [51]. It is not currently known whether bisphosphonates may also promote differentiation of bone marrow stromal cells into osteoblasts.

Bisphosphonates are the most promising approach for the management of osteoporosis after BMT. However, controversies remain regarding optimal administration of bisphosphonates. These include whether continuous or intermittent therapy should be used, the route of administration and duration of therapy, and the level of renal impairment at which bisphosphonates should be avoided.

3. *Calcium and Calcitonin*

Calcium supplementation given with or without calcitonin is ineffective in preventing bone loss after BMT [8].

4. *Hormone Replacement Therapy (HRT)*

HRT protects the skeleton in women treated with glucocorticoids, as well as in women undergoing liver, lung, and bone marrow transplantation. Because amenorrhea is a common sequel of BMT in young women, they should receive HRT whenever possible. In one study of HRT with a progestagen initially then combined estrogen and progestagen, bone loss was not prevented [19]. This may be related to the failure of progestagen to prevent bone loss initially or because estrogen was also unable to prevent rapid bone loss at the femoral neck after BMT. The latter is likely given that bone loss continued for 3 months after BMT. A small study of cyclical combined HRT commencing 13 months after BMT showed that spinal BMD increased, but the proximal femur was not studied [52]. It is not known whether treatment with testosterone in men prevents bone loss after BMT. In general, testosterone replacement should be reserved for men with true hypogonadism. Potential risks of testosterone therapy, such as prostatic hypertrophy, hyperlipidemia, and abnormal liver enzymes, may have particular relevance for this population.

5. *Parathyroid Hormone*

Teriparatide or hPTH(1-34) administration increases BMD and prevents fractures in postmenopusal women with osteoporosis [53] by increasing new bone formation. A key contributor to post-BMT bone loss is a reduction in bone formation and bone marrow osteoprogenitor cells. Because teriparatide stimulates the maturation of osteoblasts from progenitors, it would seem to be a potential candidate to increase bone formation in patients post-BMT. However, no studies have yet been performed of the safety and efficacy of PTH treatment following BMT.

VI. SUMMARY

Bone marrow transplantation is used with increasing frequency and now outnumbers other forms of transplants. Osteoporosis is more common after allo-BMT than auto-BMT and has a complex pathogenesis, related both to immunosuppressive therapy and effects on the stromal cell compartment of the bone marrow peculiar to BMT. This results in reduced bone formation in the face of increased bone resorption. Rapid and early bone loss, most severe at the femoral neck, is characteristic. The risk of osteoporosis, osteomalacia, fragility fractures, and avascular necrosis is increased. Further studies are required to determine whether bone loss and the skeletal complications of BMT can be prevented.

Acknowledgments

I gratefully acknowledge Drs. Elizabeth Shane, Sol Epstein, Jeffrey Szer, and Andrew Grigg for their expertise and enthusiastic encouragement.

REFERENCES

1. Shane, E. Transplantation osteoporosis, in Osteoporosis: Pathophysiology and Clinical Management, Orwoll, E., Bliziotes, M., eds. 2003, pp. 537–567. Totowa, NJ: Humana Press.
2. Epstein S. (1996). Post-transplantation bone disease: the role of immunosuppressive agents on the skeleton. *J Bone Miner Res.* 11:1–7.
3. Banfi, A., Podesta, M., Fazzuoli, L., Sertoli, M.R., Venturini, M., Santini, G., Cancedda, R., Quarto, R. (2001). High-dose chemotherapy shows a dose-dependent toxicity to bone marrow osteoprogenitors: a mechanism for post-bone marrow transplantation osteopenia. *Cancer.* 92(9):2419–2428.
4. Carlson, K., Simonsson, B., Ljunghall, S. (1994). Acute effects of high-dose chemotherapy followed by bone marrow transplantation on serum markers of bone metabolism. *Calcif Tissue Int.* 55:408–411.
5. Chaterjee, R., Goldstone, A.H. (1996). Gonadal damage and effects on fertility in adult patients with haematological malignancy undergoing stem cell transplantation. *Bone Marrow Transplant.* 17:5–11.
6. Spinelli, S., Chiodi, S., Bacigalupo, A., Brasca, A., Menada, M.V., Petti, A.R., Ravera, G., Gualandi, F., VanLint, M.T., Sessarego, M., Frassoni, F., Occini, D., Lamparelli, T., Valeriani, A., Oneto, R., Vitale, V., Corvo, R., Marmount, A.M. (1994). Ovarian recovery after total body irradiation and allogeneic bone marrow transplantation: long-term follow up of 79 females. *Bone Marrow Transplant.* 14(3):373–380.

7. Tauchmanova, L., Selleri, C., De Rosa, G., Esposito, M., Orio, F. Jr, Palomba, S., Bifulco, G., Nappi, C., Lombardi, G., Rotoli, B., Colao, A. (2003). Gonadal status in reproductive age women after haematopoietic stem cell transplantation for haematological malignancies. *Hum Reprod.* 18(7):1410–1416.
8. Valimaki, M., Kinnunen, K., Volin, L., Tahtela, R., Loyttniemi, E., Laitinen, K., Makela, P., Keto, P., Ruutu, T. (1999). A prospective study of bone loss and turnover after allogeneic bone marrow transplantation: effect of calcium supplementation with or without calcitonin. *Bone Marrow Transplantation.* 23:355–361.
9. Keilholz, U., Max, R., Scheibenbogen, C., Wuster, C., Korbling, M., Haas, R. (1997). Endocrine function and bone metabolism 5 years after autologous bone marrow/blood-derived progenitor cell transplantation. *Cancer.* 79:1617–1622.
10. Tauchmanova, L., Selleri, C., Rosa, G.D., Pagano, L., Orio, F., Lombardi, G., Rotoli, B., Colao, A. (2002). High prevalence of endocrine dysfunction in long-term survivors after allogeneic bone marrow transplantation for hematologic diseases. *Cancer.* 95(5):1076–1084.
11. Chatterjee, R., Mills, W., Katz, M., McGarrigle, H.H., Goldstone, A.H. (1994). Prospective study of pituitary-gonadal function to evaluate short-term effects of ablative chemotherapy or total body irradiation with autologous or allogenic marrow transplantation in post-menarcheal female patients. *Bone Marrow Transplant.* 13(5):511–517.
12. Shalet, S.M., Didi, M., Ogilvy-Stuart, A.L., Schulga, J., Donaldson, M.D. (1995). Growth and endocrine function after bone marrow transplantation. *Clin Endocrinol (Oxf).* 42(4):333–339.
13. Couto-Silva, A.C., Trivin, C., Esperou, H., Michon, J., Fischer, A., Brauner, R. (2000). Changes in height, weight and plasma leptin after bone marrow transplantation. *Bone Marrow Transplant.* 26(11):1205–1210.
14. Schulte, C., Beelen, D., Schaefer, U., Mann, K. (2000). Bone loss in long-term survivors after transplantation of hematopoietic stem cells: a prospective study. *Osteoporos Int.* 11:344–353.
15. Rubin, M.R., Bilezikian, J.P. (2002). Clinical review 151: The role of parathyroid hormone in the pathogenesis of glucocorticoid-induced osteoporosis: a re-examination of the evidence. *J Clin Endocrinol Metab.* 87(9):4033–4115
16. Movsowitz, C., Epstein, S., Fallon, M., Ismail, F., Thomas, S. (1988). Cyclosporin-A in vivo produces severe osteopaenia in the rat: effect of dose and duration of administration. *Endocrinology.* 123:2571–2577.
17. Bowman, A.R., Sass, D.A., Dissanayake, I.R., Ma, Y.F., Liang, H., Yuan, Z., Jee, W.S., Epstein, S. (1997). The role of testosterone in cyclosporine-induced osteopenia. *J Bone Miner Res.* 12(4):607–615.
18. Epstein, S., Dissanayake, A., Goodman, G.R., Bowman, A., Zhou, H., Ma, Y., Jee, W.S. (2001). Effect of the interaction of parathyroid hormone and cyclosporine A on bone mineral metabolism in the rat. *Calcif Tissue Int.* 68:240–247.
19. Ebeling, P., Thomas, D., Erbas, B., Hopper, L., Szer, J., Grigg, A. (1999). Mechanism of bone loss following allogeneic and autologous hematopoeitic stem cell transplantation. *J Bone Miner Res.* 14:342–350.
20. Stern, J.M., Sullivan, K.M., Ott, S.M., Seidel, K., Fink, J.C., Longton, G., Sherrard, D.J. (2001). Bone density loss after allogeneic hematopoietic stem cell transplantation: a prospective study. *Biol Blood Marrow Transplant.* 7(5):257–264.
21. Schimmer, A.D., Mah, K., Bordeleau, L., Cheung, A., Ali, V., Falconer, M., Trus, M., Keating, A. (2001). Decreased bone mineral density is common after autologous blood or marrow transplantation. *Bone Marrow Transplant.* 28(4):387–391.
22. Gandhi, M.K., Lekamwasam, S., Inman, I., Kaptoge, S., Sizer, L., Love, S., Bearcroft, P.W., Milligan, T.P., Price, C.P., Marcus, R.E., Compston, J.E. (2003). Significant and persistent loss of bone mineral density in the femoral neck after haematopoietic stem cell transplantation: long-term follow-up of a prospective study. *Br J Haematol.* 121(3):462–468.
23. Tauchmanova, L., Serio, B., Del Puente, A., Risitano, A.M., Esposito, A., De Rosa, G., Lombardi, G., Colao, A., Rotoli, B., Selleri, C. (2002). Long-lasting bone damage

detected by dual-energy x-ray absorptiometry, phalangeal osteosonogrammetry, and in vitro growth of marrow stromal cells after allogeneic stem cell transplantation. *J Clin Endocrinol Metab.* 87(11):5058–5065.

24. Kelly, P.J., Atkinson, K., Ward, R.L., Sambrook, P.N., Biggs, J.C., Eisman, J.A. (1990). Reduced bone mineral density in men and women with allogeneic bone marrow transplantation. *Transplantation.* 50(5):881–883.
25. Nysom, K., Holm, K., Michaelsen, K.F., Hertz, H., Jacobsen, N., Muller, J., Molgaard, C. (2000). Bone mass after allogeneic BMT for childhood leukaemia or lymphoma. *Bone Marrow Transplant.* 25(2):191–196.
26. Bhatia, S., Ramsay, N.K., Weisdorf, D., Griffiths, H., Robison, L.L. (1998). Bone mineral density in patients undergoing bone marrow transplantation for myeloid malignancies. *Bone Marrow Transplant.* 22(1):87–90.
27. Kauppila, M., Irjala, K., Koskinen, P., Pulkki, K., Sonninen, P., Viikari, J., Remes, K. (1999). Bone mineral density after allogeneic bone marrow transplantation. *Bone Marrow Transplant.* 24(8):885–889.
28. Stern, J.M., Chesnut, C.H. 3rd, Bruemmer, B., Sullivan, K.M., Lenssen, P.S., Aker, S.N., Sanders, J. (1996). Bone density loss during treatment of chronic GVHD. *Bone Marrow Transplant.* 17(3):395–400.
29. Kashyap, A., Kandeel, F., Yamauchi, D., Palmer, J.M., Niland, J.C., Molina, A., Fung, H., Bhatia, R., Krishnan, A., Nademanee, A.,, O.'Donnell, M.R., Parker, P., Rodriguez, R., Snyder, D., Spielberger, R., Stein, A., Nadler, J., Forman, S.J. (2000). Effects of allogeneic bone marrow transplantation on recipient bone mineral density: A prospective study. *Biol Blood Marrow Transplant.* 6(3A):344–351.
30. Schulte, C., Beelen, D., Schaefer, U., Mann, K. (2000). Bone loss in long-term survivors after transplantation of hematopoietic stem cells: a prospectiv estudy. *Osteoporosis International.* 11:344–353.
31. Kang, M.I., Lee, W.Y., Oh, K.W., Han, J.H., Song, K.H., Cha, B.Y., Lee, K.W., Son, H.Y., Kang, S.K., Kim, C.C. (2000). The short-term changes of bone mineral metabolism following bone marrow transplantation. *Bone.* 26(3):275–279.
32. Buchs, N., Helg, C., Collao, C., Chapuis, B., Slosman, D., Bonjour, J.P., Rizzoli, R. (2001). Allogeneic bone marrow transplantation is associated with a preferential femoral neck bone loss. *Osteoporos Int.* 12(10):880–886.
33. Lee, W.Y., Cho, S.W., Oh, E.S., Oh, K.W., Lee, J.M., Yoon, K.H., Kang, M.I., Cha, B.Y., Lee, K.W., Son, H.Y., Kang, S.K., Kim, C.C. (2002). The effect of bone marrow transplantation on the osteoblastic differentiation of human bone marrow stromal cells. *J Clin Endocrinol Metab.* 87(1):329–335.
34. Lee, W.Y., Kang, M.I., Baek, K.H., Oh, E.S., Oh, K.W., Lee, K.W., Kim, S.W., Kim, C.C. (2002). The skeletal site-differential changes in bone mineral density following bone marrow transplantation: 3-year prospective study. *J Korean Med Sci.* 17(6):749–754.
35. Kananen, K., Volin, L., Tahtela, R., Laitinen, K., Ruutu, T., Valimaki, M.J. (2002). Recovery of bone mass and normalization of bone turnover in long-term survivors of allogeneic bone marrow transplantation. *Bone Marrow Transplant.* 29(1):33–39.
36. Withold, W., Wolf, H.H., Kollbach, S., Heyll, A., Schneider, W., Reinauer, H. (1996). Relationship between bone metabolism and plasma cytokine levels in patients at risk of post-transplantation bone disease after bone marrow transplantation. *Eur J Clin Chem Clin Biochem.* 34(4):295–259.
37. Lee, W.Y., Kang, M.I., Oh, E.S., Oh, K.W., Han, J.H., Cha, B.Y., Lee, K.W., Son, H.Y., Kang, S.K., Kim, C.C. (2002). The role of cytokines in the changes in bone turnover following bone marrow transplantation. *Osteoporos Int.* 13(1):62–68.
38. Baek, K.H., Lee, W.Y., Oh, K.W., Kim, H.S., Han, J.H., Kang, M.I., Cha, B.Y., Lee, K.W., Son, H.Y., Kang, S.K., Kim, C.C. (2004). Changes in the serum growth factors and osteoprotegerin after bone marrow transplantation: impact on bone and mineral metabolism. *J Clin Endocrinol Metab.* 89(3):1246–1254.

39. Hamanishi, C., Yoshii, T., Totani, Y., Tanaka, S. (1994). Bone mineral density of lengthened rabbit tibia is enhanced by transplantation of fresh autologous bone marrow cells. An experimental study using dual X-ray absorptiometry. *Clin Orthop.* 303:250–255.
40. Michelson, J.D., Gornet, M., Codd, T., Torres, J., Lanighan, K., Jones, R. (1993). Bone morphology after bone marrow transplantation for Hodgkin's and non-Hodgkin's lymphoma. *Exp Hematol.* 21(3):475–482.
41. Athanasou, N.A., Quinn, J., Brenner, M.K., Prentice, H.G., Graham, A., Taylor, S., Flannery, D., McGee, J.O. (1990). Origin of marrow stromal cells and haemopoietic chimaerism following bone marrow transplantation determined by in situ hybridisation. *Br J Cancer.* 61(3):385–389.
42. Galotto, M., Berisso, G., Delfino, L., Podesta, M., Ottaggio, L., Dallorso, S., Dufour, C., Ferrara, G.B., Abbondandolo, A., Dini, G., Bacigalupo, A., Cancedda, R., Quarto, R. (1999). Stromal damage as consequence of high-dose chemo/radiotherapy in bone marrow transplant recipients. *Exp Hematol.* 27(9):1460–1466.
43. Massenkeil, G., Fiene, C., Rosen, O., Michael, R., Reisinger, W., Arnold, R. (2001). Loss of bone mass and vitamin D deficiency after hematopoietic stem cell transplantation: standard prophylactic measures fail to prevent osteoporosis. *Leukemia.* 15(11):1701–1705.
44. Arekat, M.R., And, G., Lemke, S., Moses, A.M. (2002). Dramatic improvement of BMD following vitamin D therapy in a bone marrow transplant recipient. *J Clin Densitom.* 5(3):267–271.
45. Hattori, M., Morita, N., Tsujino, Y., Yamamoto, M., Tanizawa, T. (2001). Vitamins D and K in the treatment of osteoporosis secondary to graft-versus-host disease following bone-marrow transplantation. *J Int Med Res.* 29(4):381–384.
46. Enright, H., Haake, R., Weisdorf, D. (1990). Avascular necrosis of bone: a common serious complication of allogeneic bone marrow transplantation. *Am J Med.* 89(6):733–738.
47. Tauchmanova, L., De Rosa, G., Serio, B., Fazioli, F., Mainolfi, C., Lombardi, G., Colao, A., Salvatore, M., Rotoli, B., Selleri, C. (2003). Avascular necrosis in long-term survivors after allogeneic or autologous stem cell transplantation: a single center experience and a review. *Cancer.* 97(10):2453–2461.
48. Sambrook P. (1999). Alfacalcidol and calcitriol in the prevention of bone loss after organ transplantation. *Calcif Tissue Int.* 65(4):341–343.
49. Meys, E., Terreaux-Duvert, F., Beaume-Six, T., Dureau, G., Meunier, P.J. (1993). Effects of calcium, calcidiol, and monofluorophosphate on lumbar bone mass and parathyroid function in patients after cardiac transplantation. *Osteoporosis Int.* 3:329–332.
50. Tauchmanova, L., Selleri, C., Esposito, M., Di Somma, C., Orio, F. Jr, Bifulco, G., Palomba, S., Lombardi, G., Rotoli, B., Colao, A. (2003). Beneficial treatment with risedronate in long-term survivors after allogeneic stem cell transplantation for hematological malignancies. *Osteoporos Int.* 14(12):1013–1019.
51. Plotkin, L.I., Weinstein, R.S., Parfitt, A.M., Roberson, P.I.C. Manolagos, S.C., Bellido, T. (1999). Prevention of osteocyte and osteoblast apoptosis by bisphosphonates and calcitonin. *J Clin Invest.* 104:1363–1374.
52. Castelo-Branco, C., Rovira, M., Pons, F., Duran, M., Sierra, J., Vives, A., Balasch, J., Fortuny, A., Vanrell, J. (1996). The effect of hormone replacement therapy on bone mass in patients with ovarian failure due to bone marrow transplantation. *Maturitas.* 23(3):307–312.
53. Ebeling, P.R., Russell R.G.G. (2003). Teriparatide (rhPTH 1-34) treatment of osteoporosis. *Inter J Clinical Pract.* 57:710–718.

CHAPTER 20

Osteonecrosis and Organ Transplantation

Neveen A.T. Hamdy, MD, MRCP
Department of Endocrinology and Metabolic Diseases,
Leiden University Medical Center, Leiden, The Netherlands

I. INTRODUCTION

Osteonecrosis is a pathological process characterized by death of the cellular constituents of bone and marrow. The process of aseptic bone necrosis was first described nearly a century ago [1, 2], and its association with glucocorticoid use has been recognized for more than 50 years. Rates are particularly high in patients with systemic lupus erythematosus [3, 4]. The incidence of osteonecrosis is increased in patients on dialysis [5–8]. It is also a well-recognized complication of kidney transplantation, with patients on long-term maintenance dialysis before transplantation more likely to develop this complication after transplantation [9]. The exact prevalence of osteonecrosis after organ transplantation is, however, difficult to assess as many cases are clinically silent.

II. CLINICAL FEATURES OF OSTEONECROSIS

The most common presenting symptom of osteonecrosis is pain, although many cases may be asymptomatic. The pain is usually deep in nature, localized to the groin with occasional radiation down the thigh to the knee. Symptoms are usually exacerbated by physical activity and weight bearing and relieved by rest. In the late stages of osteonecrosis, pain is often present at rest, and patients may develop a limp, as they are no longer able to bear weight on the affected joint. Osteonecrosis affecting the bone beneath a weight-bearing joint surface is associated with a significant risk of developing a subarticular fracture, which appears to initiate the symptoms [10].

Resulting joint incongruity and premature arthrosis lead to more chronic symptoms. In contrast, when the process affects the metaphyseal region of a bone, it is typically clinically silent and without sequelae.

On physical examination, the range of movement of the affected hip is often limited and painful (especially on flexion and internal rotation), and local tenderness is occasionally elicited. The gait pattern may be antalgic. The femoral head is the most commonly and severely affected site, followed by the head of the humerus, distal femur, and small bones of the wrist and foot. Other weight-bearing joints are frequently involved [11].

III. OSTEONECROSIS AND ORGAN TRANSPLANTATION

A. Prevalence of Osteonecrosis after Organ Transplantation

The first reports of osteonecrosis occurring after renal transplantation date from the early 1960s [12]. Since then, the reported incidence of post-transplantation osteonecrosis has varied between 3 and 50%, depending on the method used to diagnose osteonecrosis and the length of follow-up [13–21]. Osteonecrosis appears to be less common after cardiac transplantation [22, 23] or liver transplantation [24, 25].

In a large study addressing the prevalence of osteonecrosis in renal transplant recipients in whom radiological skeletal surveys were performed yearly, 115 lesions of osteonecrosis were identified in 36 patients, with 2 further patients diagnosed at autopsy, amounting to a total incidence of about 24% at a mean interval of 19 months after transplantation. Lesions were frequently multiple and bilateral, and structural failure was the most common initial abnormality. The femoral head was the most frequent site affected. Many of the lesions were symptom-free. Osteonecrosis was more frequent in women and in high-dose versus low-dose glucocorticoid users [15]. Screening MRI studies of asymptomatic renal transplant recipients receiving glucocorticoids further identified a prevalence of osteonecrosis of the hip of 6 to 14%. Only 0 to 4% of cases became symptomatic, and 30% of asymptomatic lesions tended to heal spontaneously [26]. The lesions appear most often during the first 2 years after transplantation [14, 27–30]. The time interval between organ transplantation and osteonecrosis varies widely between 5 and 75 months after transplantation [9, 15, 31–33].

B. Risk Factors for Osteonecrosis after Organ Tranplantation

1. Glucocorticoid Use and the Risk of Osteonecrosis

Osteonecrosis occurs in up to 52% of patients using glucocorticoids [34–36]. Reports on the relationship between cumulative dose of prednisone and incidence of osteonecrosis were initially conflicting, some studies demonstrating no correlation [29, 33, 37, 38], while others did [15, 27, 39–42]. The clear relationship between total dose of glucocorticoids and incidence of osteonecrosis was eventually established in a quantitative review of 22 studies [17]. Although the risk of osteonecrosis increases with both dose and duration of treatment with glucocorticoids, it is still difficult to predict which patient will develop osteonecrosis [17, 35, 36]. Osteonecrosis has been shown to develop after high-dose glucocorticoids given for a short time [34, 43–47], after moderate doses given for a long time [48], or just after intra-articular or epidural injection of glucocorticoids [49].

2. Glucocorticoid Use and the Risk of Osteonecrosis after Organ Transplantation

Until the introduction of cyclosporin in the early 1980s and its subsequent widespread use, a combination of glucocorticoids and azathioprine represented the cornerstone of immunosuppressive therapy in human organ transplantation [50]. Initial doses of glucocorticoids were selected empirically, with original predilection for high doses on the basis of "more is better" to minimize potential graft rejection. The controversy over high-dose versus low-dose glucocorticoids, particularly as administered in the early post-transplant period, raged for years before the issue was definitively resolved by prospective studies comparing both regimens [51–53]. By the mid-1980s, a number of studies had further established that similar patient and graft survival could be achieved by high- or low-dose methylprednisolone after transplantation [51–57]. This further consolidated the practice of using lower doses of glucocorticoids, which are sufficient to prevent graft rejection while carrying less risk for systemic side effects.

There is no identifiable "threshold" cumulative dose associated with osteonecrosis. In a retrospective study of 750 transplant recipients over a period of 27 years, a significantly higher incidence of osteonecrosis was documented in patients receiving a high (12.5 g) versus a low (6.5 g) cumulative dose of glucocorticoids during the first month and year post-transplantation: 11.2% versus 5.1%, $p<0.005$. The low-dose group had received cyclosporin A in addition to glucocorticoids [58]. The interval between start of glucocorticoids and osteonecrosis is variable, rarely being less than 6 months, occasionally being as long as 3 years after transplantation [15, 48]. Not all patients treated with glucocorticoids after transplantation develop osteonecrosis, however, suggesting individual differences in susceptibility to these agents [59].

The role of glucocorticoids in the pathogenesis of osteonecrosis after renal transplantation has been addressed to date in seven studies including a total of 1471 patients [15, 52, 53, 57, 58, 60, 61]. A meta-analysis of 5 of these studies, which were controlled and compared high-dose versus low-dose glucocorticoids in conjunction with azathioprine, was recently undertaken [62]. Patients using the high-dose glucocorticoid regimen had a significant 1.5-fold greater risk of developing osteonecrosis than patients treated with the low-dose combination ($p < 0.001$). Calcineurin inhibitors were used in only 2 of the 5 studies [60, 61], however, so results cannot be extrapolated to currently used immunosuppressive regimens. In organ transplantation, the optimization of the dose of glucocorticoids had clear implications on early and late high-dose glucocorticoid-related effects, including the incidence of osteonecrosis.

3. Calcineurin Inhibitors and the Risk of Osteonecrosis after Organ Transplantation

Originally thought to potentially protect bone against glucocorticoid effects, the use of cyclosporin is more likely to be associated with a low incidence of osteonecrosis by allowing lower doses of glucocorticoids to be used [65]. With the more widespread use of cyclosporin, the incidence of osteonecrosis was indeed observed to further decrease in renal transplant recipients in whom prednisone had been partially substituted by the new immunosuppressive agent [60]. More recent data suggest an even lower incidence of osteonecrosis with the use of tacrolimus as compared to cyclosporin because of the lower doses of glucocorticoids used with the former [66]. On the other hand, the incidence of osteonecrosis appears to be increased with the use of sirolimus, possibly attributable to the adverse lipid profile of sirolimus, its potent bone marrow suppressive effect, or an idiosyncratic effect [67].

4. Other Risk Factors for Osteonecrosis after Organ Transplantation

Risk factors for osteonecrosis were examined in a large historical cohort study of 42,096 renal transplant recipients conducted in the United States. The incidence of osteonecrosis requiring hospitalization was 7.1 episodes/1000 person-years, and femoral head pathology was responsible for 89% of admissions [68]. Patients with allograft rejection, African-American race, peritoneal dialysis, and earlier date of transplant were at higher risk of osteonecrosis. A lower risk was found in patients with diabetes mellitus. One of the study's main limitations, however, is that the cases studied were restricted to those hospitalized, and thus to the more severe and disabling cases of osteonecrosis.

Of the risks cited, allograft rejection is likely to be related to transplant recipients receiving substantially higher cumulative doses of glucocorticoids [69–71]. The increased risk observed in African-Americans [68–70] may be due to the generally higher cumulative doses of immunosuppression required due to poorer HLA matching and sensitization leading to higher risk of graft loss [70]. The more rapid tapering of glucocorticoids and thus lower cumulative exposure after transplantation may explain the decreased risk for osteonecrosis associated with diabetes mellitus [20, 68].

In a large ethnic Chinese population of transplant recipients ($n = 397$) studied over a period of 25 years, post-transplant body weight gain was an independent risk factor for osteonecrosis, although weight gain may again be related to glucocorticoid use [63].

Both hyperparathyroidism, which is associated with high bone turnover [39, 71, 72], and low turnover states [9] have been cited as risk factors for osteonecrosis after transplantation.

Finally, an association has recently been found between plasminogen activator inhibitor-1 genotype and avascular osteonecrosis in glucocorticoid-treated renal allograft recipients. It has been postulated that hypofibrinolysis, conferred by this genotype, may represent a predisposing factor for osteonecrosis, particularly in obese patients or patients with persistent hyperparathyroidism [73].

IV. PATHOPHYSIOLOGY OF OSTEONECROSIS

A. General Considerations

The pathologic picture and clinical course of osteonecrosis is characteristic despite its variable etiology. In femoral head osteonecrosis, the process usually begins at the weight-bearing surface, leading to gradual collapse of surface bone and cartilage. In time, the area of collapse spreads to involve a large proportion of the femoral head. Other weight-bearing joints are frequently involved [11]. Under certain pathologic conditions, intra-osseous bone marrow pressure rises at the involved site [11, 74]. The increased pressure is transmitted to small venules and capillaries within bone, causing a decrease in blood flow and eventually resulting in irreversible circulatory disturbances and subsequent tissue damage. Tissue damage results in edema, which further increases intra-osseous bone marrow pressure in the closed compartment, perpetuating the cycle of ischemia. This forms the rationale for the management of early osteonecrosis by decompression of bone to break the cycle of ischemia and increased marrow pressure before the damage becomes irreversible (see Section 20.VII.B.1).

B. Pathogenetic Mechanisms for Osteonecrosis

A number of theories have been postulated to explain the pathogenetic events eventually leading to the death of a segment of bone.

1. *Mechanical Theory*

Ischemia and necrosis of a segment of bone may result from the interruption of a blood vessel with limited collateral circulation that feeds a portion of medullary cavity or cortex. Damage to the blood vessel may be due to fracture, dislocation, or accumulation of unhealed trabecular microcracks resulting in fatigue fractures [75–76].

2. *Vascular Theory*

The vascular theory proposes that ischemia may be caused by microscopic fat emboli. However, recent studies suggest no contribution of vascular changes, thrombi, or necrosis of marrow cells to the pathophysiology of osteonecrosis [77].

3. *Fat Accumulation Theory*

This theory is based on the finding of deformed fat globules, which appear to be intravascular, in the subchondral bone of necrotic femoral heads in patients on high-dose glucocorticoids [34, 78]. Proliferation of fat cells may be the cause of the high intra-osseous pressure, which subsequently interferes with perfusion of the affected bone segment by mechanical impingement on the sinusoidal vascular bed [11]. This is the mechanism put forward for the high incidence of osteonecrosis in patients with Cushing's disease [36].

4. *Osteocyte Apopotosis*

After completion of its active life span, an osteoblast becomes either a bone-lining cell or an osteocyte when it becomes embedded in the bone matrix it has secreted. It may also undergo apoptosis. The lifespan of an osteocyte is estimated to be at least 20 years in human rib cortical bone [79]. Osteocytes also die, as evidenced by empty lacunae and hypermineralized perilacunar areas in inactive bone known as "micropetrosis" [80]. A relationship between glucocorticoid use and osteocyte apoptosis was first suggested in the late 1990s [81]. A clear increase in osteoblast and osteocyte apoptosis was observed in a murine model of glucocorticoid excess, representative of the human disease [81]. Similar apoptotic changes were also observed in bone biopsy specimens of patients with glucocorticoid-induced osteoporosis [81]. An unusual pattern of tetracycline uptake in the extracellular matrix was further described, deep in the trabeculae of femora of rabbits early after exposure to high doses of glucocorticoids. This unusual uptake was correlated with an increase in osteocyte apoptosis in subarticular trabecular bone. The timing of these changes early after exposure to glucocorticoids suggests that osteocytic matrix damage and apoptosis are early events in glucocorticoid-mediated skeletal changes [77]. The role of glucocorticoids in the pathogenesis of osteonecrosis was further confirmed by the discovery of abundant apoptotic osteocytes and bone lining cells in areas adjacent to the subchondral fracture crescent in whole femoral heads in patients who underwent prosthetic total hip replacement for glucocorticoid-induced osteonecrosis, compared to femoral heads from patients with osteonecrosis caused by other etiologies such as alcoholism, trauma, or sickle cell anaemia [82]. Contrary to the commonly held view that vascular ischemia plays the central role in the pathogenesis of osteonecrosis, regardless of its etiology, it appears that induction of early osteocyte cell death is the predominant pathophysiologic mechanism in glucocorticoid-induced osteonecrosis.

The network of osteocytes probably participates in microdamage detection and in the transmission of signals for its repair by bone remodeling [83]. Disruption of this system by osteocyte apoptosis would compromise bone integrity, resulting in microdamage accumulation and increased bone fragility [84]. "The cumulative and irreparable defect resulting from glucocorticoid-induced osteocyte apoptosis would in turn result in unique disruption of the mechano-sensory function of the osteocyte network starting the inexorable sequence of events leading to collapse of the femoral head" [82]. The exact molecular mechanism by which glucocorticoids induce osteocyte apoptosis remains to be clarified, but it has been suggested that this process may be mediated by a mechanism requiring the dimerization of the glucocorticoid receptor and direct binding to glucocorticoid response elements (GRE) [85]. It has also been suggested that the pro-apoptotic effect of glucocorticoids may be mediated through inhibition of collagenase gene transcription, which is responsible for collagenase production by osteoblasts and stromal cells, resulting in decreased cleavage of type I collagen in the extracellular matrix of bone [86].

V. DIAGNOSIS OF OSTEONECROSIS

Establishing the diagnosis of osteonecrosis early is critical for therapeutic outcome, since treatment options for advanced disease are limited and largely unsuccessful. The diagnosis relies heavily on radiological studies. Radiographs may be normal at early stages but show typical abnormalities in late stages. MRI is especially useful in early stages. Both extent and location of the necrotic area as appraised by radiographs and MRI are important in predicting the evolution toward collapse.

A. Plain Radiographs

Radiographic evidence of necrosis may not occur for 6 to 10 weeks after onset of symptoms. In osteonecrosis of the femoral head, the most common initial radiological feature is structural failure of the articular surface, appearing as a translucent subcortical band sometimes described as "radiolucent crescent sign," and loss of the head's spherical shape. In time, radiographic appearances reflect changes occurring in the mechanically weakened weight-bearing bone, which, after flattening, eventually collapses (see Figure 1). Different views of the hips must be obtained.

Depression of the articular surface is sometimes associated with sequestrated segments, which may resemble osteochondritis dissecans. Osteoarthritis occurs as a late radiological abnormality as a consequence of structural failure of the joint surfaces (see Figures 1 and 2). Lesions may occur away from joint surfaces and appear as sequestrated dense segments. These lesions are found incidentally as they are usually asymptomatic. Symptomatic fractures may occur at the site of a lesion.

B. Technetium-99m Bone Scintigraphy

Very early in the course of osteonecrosis, a dead central area surrounded by a region of increased activity (the "doughnut sign") can be seen on technetium-99m bone scintigraphy [87]. Within weeks, there is a uniform increase in radioactive isotope uptake, which remains increased throughout the course of the disease [88].

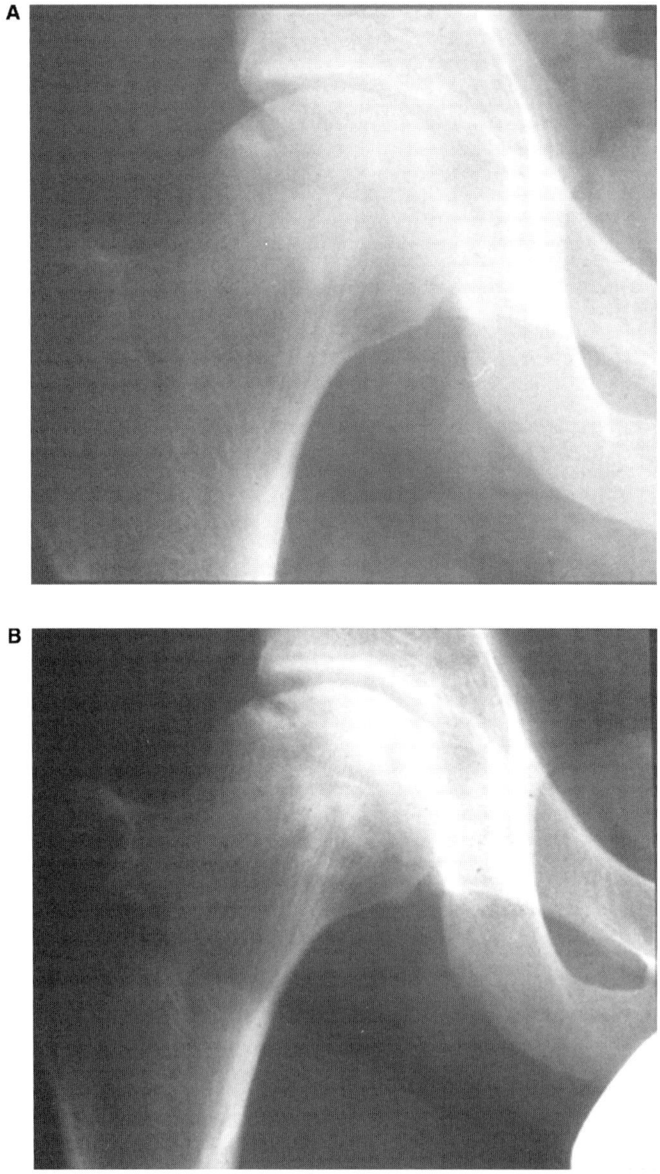

FIGURE 1 Follow-Up AP Radiographs of the Right Femoral Head showing Osteonecrosis Developing in a 66-year-old man 6 Months **(A)**, 13 Months **(B)**, and 20 Months **(C)** after Renal Transplantation. The last radiograph shows structural failure and markedly increased density and deformity of the femoral head.

c

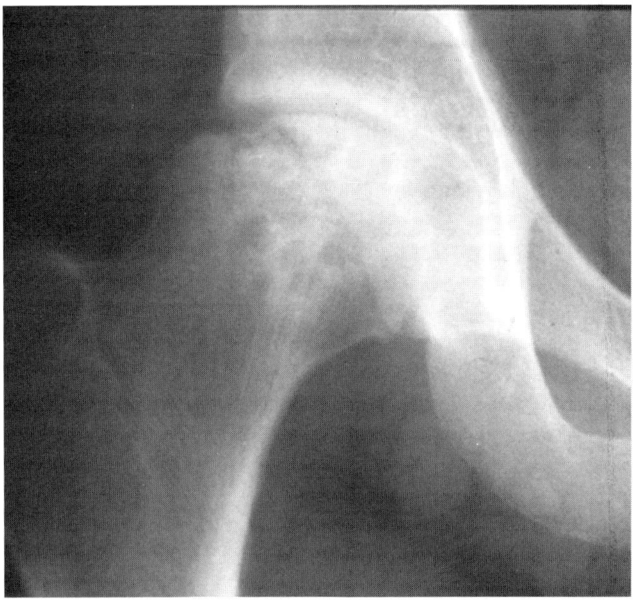

FIGURE 1 *(Continued)*

C. Magnetic Resonance Imaging (MRI)

Magnetic resonance imaging (MRI) is the most sensitive method and the current widely accepted standard for the noninvasive diagnosis of osteonecrosis. This imaging technique has a sensitivity of 97% for differentiating osteonecrosis from a normal hip and 85% sensitivity for differentiating osteonecrosis from other hip disorders, with an overall sensitivity of 91% for diagnosing the pathologic process [89]. T1- and T2-weighted acquisition images in both coronal and sagittal planes should be included as these provide different and complementary data (see Figure 3).

Diagnostic MRI features of osteonecrosis are the presence of foci of low signal intensity in the bone marrow (focal bone marrow edema) on T1-weighted images, typically in the superior portion of the femoral head (diagnostic in 95% of cases), and the pathognomonic "double-line" sign on fat-suppressed T2-weighted images [90]. T2-weighted images are also necessary to exclude other potential diagnoses such as septic arthritis and insufficiency or stress fractures, relatively common in patients using glucocorticoids.

VI. NATURAL HISTORY OF OSTEONECROSIS

The prognosis of osteonecrosis depends on the size of the lesion, its localization, and the degree of collapse at the time of diagnosis [91, 92]. In femoral head osteonecrosis, large lesions (> 40% involvement of the femoral head) and lesions located under the lateral and central weight-bearing

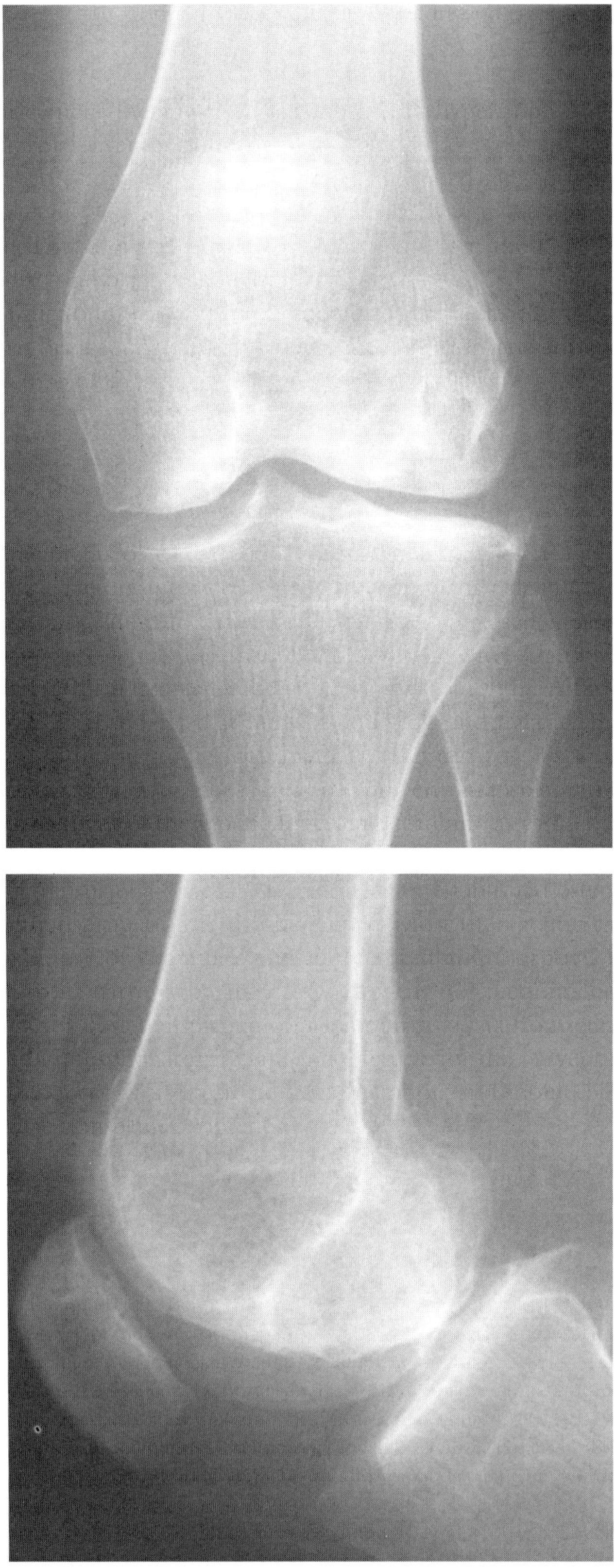

FIGURE 2 Plain radiographs of the left knee demonstrating osteonecrosis of the distal end of the femur in a 55-year-old transplant recipient 10 years after kidney transplantation. She had already had bilateral hip arthroplasty for extensive necrosis of the femoral heads. She has since had bilateral knee arthroplasty.

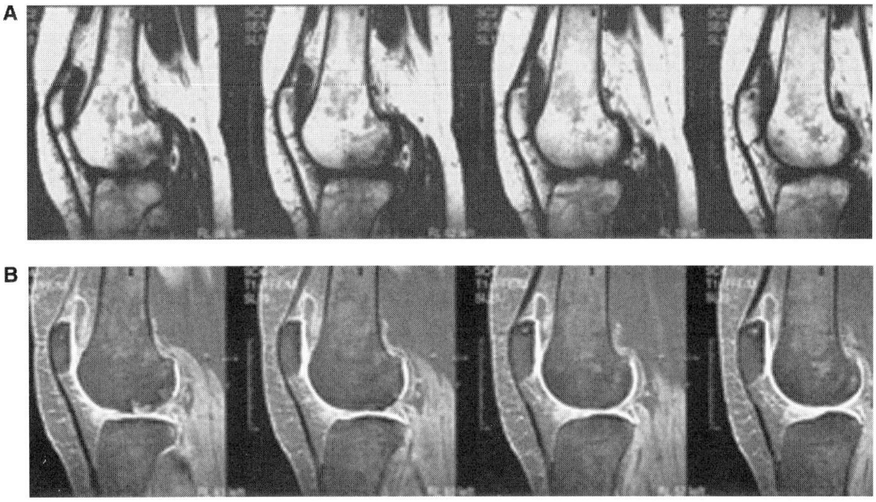

FIGURE 3 T1-weighted (a) and T2-weighted (b) images of the left knee corresponding to the plain radiographs shown in Figure 2.

portion of the acetabulum have a greater tendency to progress to collapse than smaller lesions and those located under the medial non-weight-bearing portion of the acetabulum. In the absence of surgical intervention, 80% of patients who present with symptomatic osteonecrosis of the hip progress to end-stage osteonecrosis over the following 3 to 5 years [93, 94]. MRI findings are predictive of prognosis [95].

VII. MANAGEMENT OF OSTEONECROSIS

The foremost aim of any successful management of osteonecrosis is early diagnosis by maintaining a high level of suspicion in patients at risk. Once the diagnosis is made, treatment should be initiated without delay to prevent disease progression and, if possible, reverse the disease process. For patients with asymptomatic disease, close follow-up is recommended, with plain radiographs and/or MRI scans every 6 to 12 months to monitor disease progression. Surgical treatment in the form of core decompression, bone grafting, or vascularized fibular grafts may be considered (see Section 20.VII.B). In symptomatic patients, the ideal treatment would provide complete relief of pain and preservation of a stable joint for the duration of the patient's lifespan. In general, conservative treatment of osteonecrosis does not alter the natural history of progressive collapse and arthrosis.

A. Nonsurgical Management of Osteonecrosis

1. Limitation of Weight Bearing

Limitation of weight bearing may be complete or partial, using crutches, or weight bearing may be limited to what is tolerated. Conservative management consisting of limitation of weight bearing and nonsteroidal anti-inflammatory drugs may be effective in early and localized disease of the distal end of tibia or femur [96], but outcome is generally unsatisfactory. A meta-analysis of 21 studies from 1960 to 1993 reports a successful clinical result in only 22.7% of hips with osteonecrosis after an average follow-up of 34 months, with no difference in outcome between different degrees of weight bearing [93].

2. *Electrical Stimulation*

Electrical stimulation can be applied in the form of direct current, pulse electromagnetic field (PEMF), or capacitance coupled current. Electrical stimulation is used as a primary treatment modality or as adjunctive therapy in combination with core decompression and bone grafting. Electrical current stimulation may enhance osteogenesis and neovascularisation of the affected area [97, 98].

3. *Pharmacological Agents*

The use of pharmacological agents such as vasodilators or anticoagulants has met with very limited or no success. It has been suggested that the use of statins may reduce the risk of osteonecrosis in patients receiving glucocorticoid therapy [99]. The potential beneficial effect of these agents has not been examined in organ transplant recipients.

B. Surgical Management of Osteonecrosis

1. *Core Decompression*

This procedure, in which a core of bone is removed from the femoral neck and head, provides pain relief by decreasing intra-osseous pressure in the femoral head. A further aim of the procedure is to stimulate angiogenesis by providing a channel for vascular ingrowth, thereby improving revascularisation of the necrotic lesion [100–102]. Core decompression almost uniformly provides pain relief, but its clinical efficacy in preventing disease progression remains questionable. The rate of clinical success varies widely from 33 to 95% [36, 100, 102–106]. A meta-analysis of studies published between 1960 and 1995 indicates a successful result in 63.5% of hips after an average follow-up of 30 months. Success was directly related to stage of disease, with an average hip survival of 84% in patients with stage I disease compared to 47% for the more advanced stages [101].

2. *Bone Grafting Procedures*

Bone grafting is a surgical technique in which a bone graft is inserted into the necrotic lesion of the femoral head through a core decompression tract. An allograft, cancellous autograft, or cortical autograft can be used to replace the removed necrotic segment. The bone graft provides structural support to the overlying subchondral bone, thereby preventing its collapse. The technique can also be performed through windows made in the femoral neck or femoral head (trapdoor procedure) [107–108]. Variable success has been reported depending on disease stage at the time of the procedure [109–110]. A major drawback of bone grafting is that it requires extended periods of restricted weight bearing. Vascularised structural fibular bone grafts have an additional vascular pedicle, which is anastomosed to a nearby vessel after inserting the graft into the core decompression tract. These bone grafts are preferred by several groups because revascularization and union are more likely to be enhanced by the addition of blood supply to the structural graft than would be the case with nonvascularized grafts [111–113]. Drawbacks to this procedure exist, however: The procedure requires microvascular surgical skills, donor-site morbidity is relatively high after harvesting of the graft, and there is a significant rate of conversion to total hip arthroplasty [108–114]. Combining bone grafting with electrical stimulation may improve outcome.

3. Femoral Osteotomy

Femoral osteotomy is a surgical procedure in which a cut is made in the proximal femur, allowing the necrotic segment of bone to be rotated away from the weight-bearing area of the acetabulum. This procedure facilitates healing of osteonecrosis by eliminating direct shear forces on the necrotic lesion [115–117]. An extended period of restrictions on weight bearing is also required postoperatively. The outcome is variable, depending on stage of disease and current use of glucocorticoids. Subsequent total hip arthroplasty may be technically more difficult.

4. Hemisurfacing Procedures and Hemiarthroplasty

Resurfacing arthroplasty is a procedure in which a metal or ceramic shell is cemented over the surface of a femoral head after debridement of the necrotic material. The procedure is used to treat the advanced stages of osteonecrosis in which the acetabulum is not affected. Hemiarthroplasty is a procedure in which the femoral head is replaced by a prosthetic head. In most cases, both procedures represent temporary measures until total hip arthroplasty is required [118–119].

5. Total Hip Arthroplasty

In total hip arthroplasty, both the femoral head and acetabular surface are replaced by prosthetic components. It is the most frequent procedure performed in advanced osteonecrosis of the hip or knee, providing predictable pain relief and good joint function [65, 120–122]. In older patients, long-term results are excellent, but results are more disappointing in younger patients, in whom frequent revision surgery is required. In these younger patients, various treatment approaches are preferred to maintain the native hip for as long as possible. With the use of modern cementing techniques, newer prosthetic designs, and alternative bearing surfaces, success rate is projected to improve significantly.

VIII. CONCLUSION

Osteonecrosis is a well-recognized complication of organ transplantation and one that is associated with a significant degree of morbidity. Glucocorticoid excess has been identified as its main risk factor, and the mechanism by which glucocorticoids initiate the pathologic process has recently been elucidated. Optimizing the dose of glucocorticoids has already led to a significant reduction in the incidence of osteonecrosis post-transplantation. Substituting these agents entirely with calcineurin inhibitors may decrease this complication of the transplantation process even further. Early diagnosis using magnetic resonance imaging is essential for the success of available surgical interventions.

REFERENCES

1. Schmorl, G. (1920). Anaemische nekrose in schenkelkopf. *Zentralbl Allg Pathol.* 35:261–264.
2. Freund, E. (1926). Frage der asptischen knochennekrose. *Virchows Arch [Pathol Anat].* 261:287–291.
3. Weiner, E.S., Abeles, M. (1989). Aseptic necrosis and glucoglucocorticoids in systemic lupus erythematosus: a reevaluation. *J Rheumatol.* 16:604–608.
4. Fishel, B., Caspi, D., Eventov, I., Avrahami, E., Yaron, M. (1987). Multiple osteonecrotic lesions in systemic lupus erythematosus. *J Rheumatol.* 14:601–604.
5. Mehls, O., Ritz, E., Opperman, H.C., et al. (1981). Femoral head necrosis in uremic children without steroid treatment or transplantation. *J Pediatr.* 99:926–929.
6. Brown, E.A., Vower, P.E. (1982). Joint problems in patients on maintenance hemodialysis. *Clin Nephrol.* 18:247–250.
7. Menerey, K., Braunstein, E., Brown, M., et al. (1988). Musculoskeletal symptoms related to arthropathy in patients receiving dialysis. *J Rheumatol.* 15:1848–1854.
8. Langevitz, P., Buskila, D., Stewart, J., Sherrard, D.J., Hercz, G. (1990). Osteonecrosis in patients receiving dialysis: report of two cases and review of the literature. *J Rheumatol.* 17:402–406.
9. Nielsen, H.E., Melsen, F., Christensen, M.S. (1977). Aseptic necrosis of bone following kidney transplantation. Clinical and biochemical aspects and bone morphometry. *Acta Med Scand.* 202:27–32.
10. Maldague, B., Malghem, J., de Deuxchaines, C. (1984). Radiologic aspects of glucocorticoid-induced bone disease. *Adv Exp Med Biol.* 171:155–190.
11. Ficat, R.P. (1985). Idiopathic bone necrosis of the femoral head. Early diagnosis and treatment. *J Bone Joint Surg Br.* 67:3-9.

12. Startzl, T.E., Marchioso, T.L., Porter, K.A., et al. (1964). Renal homotransplantations. Late function and complications. *Ann Intern Med.* 61:470–497.
13. Griffiths, H.J., Ennis, J.T., Bailey, G. (1974). Skeletal changes following renal transplantation. *Radiology.* 113:621-626.
14. Hawking, K.M.,van den Bosch, B.F., Wilmink, J.M. (1976). Avascular necrosis of bone after renal transplantation [Letter]. *N Engl J Med.* 294:397.
15. Davidson, J.K., Tsakiris, D., Briggs, J.D., Junor, B.J. (1985). Osteonecrosis and fractures following renal transplantation. *Clin Radiol.* 36:27–35.
16. Brazil, M., Linderer, R.J., Dickhans, M.J., Garvin, P.J. (1986). Aseptic hip necrosis after renal transplantation. *Arch Surg.* 121:803–805.
17. Felson, D.T., Anderson, J.J. (1987). A cross-study evaluation of association between steroid dose and bolus steroids and avascular necrosis of bone. *Lancet.* 1:902–906.
18. Fryer, J.P., Granger, D.K., Leventhal, J.R., et al. (1994). Steroid-related complications in the cyclosporin era. *Clin Transplant.* 8:224–229.
19. Tuncay, I.C., Demirors, H., Tandogan, R., Isiklar, U., Bilgin, N. (1998). Femoral head necrosis after kidney transplantation. *Transplant Proc.* 30:800–801.
20. Veenstra, D.L., Best, J.H., Hornberger, J., et al. (1999). Incidence and long-term cost of steroid-related side-effects after renal transplantation. *Am J Kidney Dis.* 33:829–839.
21. Tang, S., Lui, S.L., Li, F.K., et al. (1999). Long-term renal allograft recipients from South-East Asia in the pre-cyclosporin era. *Int J Artif Org.* 22:131–137.
22. Bradbury, G., Benjamin, J., Thompson, J., Klees, E., Copeland, J. (1994). Avascular necrosis of bone after cardiac transplantation. *J Bone Joint Surg Am.* 76:1385–1388.
23. Pavie, A., Dorent, R., Reagan, M., et al. (1998). La Pitié heart transplantation: 30-year single center clinical experience. *Clin Transpl.* 12:311-314.
24. Lieberman, J.R., Scaduto, A.A., Wellmeyer, E. (2000). Symptomatic osteonecrosis of the hip after orthotopic liver transplantation. *J Arthroplasty.* 15:767–771.
25. Horuchi, H., Hashikura, Y., Hisa, K., et al. (2004). Osteonecrosis of the femoral heads in Japanese adults after liver transplantation: a preliminary report. *J Orthop Sci.* 9:119–121.
26. Kopecky, K.K., Braunstein, E.M., Brandt, K.D., et al. (1991). Apparent avascular necrosis of the hip: Appearance and spontaneous resolution of MR findings in renal allograft recipients. *Radiology.* 179:523–527.
27. Harrington, K.D., Murray, W.R., Kountz, S.L., Belzer, F.O. (1971). Avascular necrosis of bone after renal transplantation. *J Bone Joint Surg Am.* 53:203–215.
28. Bewick, M., Stewart, P.H., Rudge, C., Farrand, C., McColl, I. (1976). Avascular necrosis of bone in patients undergoing renal allo-transplantation. *Clin Nephrol.* 5:66–72.
29. Ibels, L.S., Alfrey, A., Huffer, W.E., Weil, R. III. (1978). Aseptic necrosis of bone following renal transplantation: Experience in 194 transplant recipients and review of the literature. *Medicine.* 57:25–45.
30. Siddiqui, A.R., Kopecky, K.K., Weeman, H.N., et al. (1993). Prospective study of magnetic resonance imaging and SPECT bone scans in renal allograft recipients: Evidence for a self-limited subclinical abnormality of the hip. *J Nucl Med.* 34:381–386.
31. Levine, F., Erken, E.H., Price, H.I., Meyers, A.M., Solomon, L. (1977). Osteonecrosis following renal transplantation. *Am J Roentgen.* 128:985–991.
32. Stern, P.J., Watts, H.G. (1979). Osteonecrosis after renal transplantation in children. *J Bone Joint Surg Am.* 61:851–856.
33. Elmstedt, E. (1981). Avascular bone necrosis in the renal transplant patients: a discriminant analysis of 144 cases. *Clin Orthop Rel Res.* 158:149–157.
34. Fisher, D.E., Bickel, W.H. (1971). Glucocorticoid-induced avascular necrosis: a clinical study of seventy-seven patients. *J Bone Joint Surg Am.* 53:859–873.
35. Zizic, T.M., Marcoux, C., Hungerford, D.S., Dansereau, J.V., Stevens, M.B. (1985). Glucocorticoid therapy associated with ischemic necrosis of bone in systemic lupus erythematosus. *Am J Med.* 79:596–604.

36. Mankin, H.J. (1992). Non-traumatic necrosis of bone (Osteonecrosis). *N Engl J Med.* 326:1473–1479.
37. Arfi, S., Moreau, F., Heuclin, C., et al. (1975). L'osteonecrose aseptique de la transplantation renale. A propos de 29 cas. *Rev Rheum.* 42:167–176.
38. Susan, L.P., Braun, W.E., Banowsky, L.H., Straffon, R.A., Bergfeld, J.A. (1978). Avascular necrosis following renal transplantation. Experience with 449 allografts with and without high-dose steroid therapy. *Urology.* 11:225–229.
39. Briggs, W.A., Hampers, C.L., Merrill, et al. (1972). Aseptic necrosis in the femur after renal transplantation. *Ann Surg.* 175:282–289.
40. Murray, W.R. (1973). Hip problems associated with renal transplantation. *Clin Orthop Rel Res.* 90:57–69.
41. Pierides, A.M., Simpson, W., Stainsby, D., Alvarez-Ude, F., Uldall, P.R. (1975). Avascular necrosis of bone following renal transplantation. *Quart J Med.* 44:459–480.
42. de Graaf, P., van Hooff, J.P., Boekhout, M., et al. (1982). Hyperparathyroidism and avascular necrosis of bone after kidney transplantation. *Neth J Med.* 25:230–236.
43. Good, A.E. (1974). Bilateral aseptic necrosis of the femur following a 16-day course of corticotropin. *JAMA.* 228:497.
44. Anderton, J.M., Helm, R. Multiple joint osteonecrosis following short-term steroid therapy: case report. *J Bone Joint Surg Am.* 228:497.
45. McCluskey, J., Gutteridge, D.H. (1982). Avascular necrosis of bone after high doses of dexamethasone during neurosurgery. *Br Med J.* 284:333–334.
46. Taylor, L.J. (1984). Multifocal avascular necrosis after short-term high-dose steroid therapy: a report of three cases. *J Bone Joint Surg Br.* 66:431–433.
47. Haajanen, J., Saarinen, O., Laasonen, L., et al. (1984). Steroid treatment and aseptic necrosis of the femoral head in renal transplant recipients. *Transplant Proc.* 16:1316–1319.
48. Metselaar, H.J., van Steenberge, E.J.P., Bijnen, A.B., Jeekel, J.J., van Lingen, B., Weimar, W. (1985). Incidence of osteonecrosis after renal transplantation. *Acta Orthop Scand.* 56:413–415.
49. Laroche, H., Arlet, J., Mazieres, B. (1990). Osteonecrosis of the femoral and humeral heads after intraarticular glucocorticoid injections. *J Rheumatol.* 17:549–551.
50. Goodwin, W.E., Kaufman, J.J., Mims, M.M., et al. (1963). Human renal transplantation. I. Clinical experience with six cases of renal homotransplantation. *J Urol.* 89:13–24.
51. Buckels, J.A.C., Mackintosh, P., Barnes, A.D. (1981). Controlled trial of low versus high dose oral steroid therapy in 100 cadaveric renal transplants. *Proc Eur Dial Transplant Assoc.* 18:394-398.
52. Morris, P.J., Chan, L., French, M.E., Ting, A. (1982). Low dose oral prednisolone in renal transplantation. *Lancet.* 1:525–527.
53. Papadakis, J., Brown, C.B., Cameron, J.S., et al. (1983). High versus "low" dose glucocorticoids in recipients of cadaveric kidneys: Prospective controlled trial. *Br Med J.* 286:1097–1100.
54. McGeown, M.G. (1973). Immunosuppression for kidney transplantation. *Lancet.* 2:310-312.
55. McGeown, M.G., Douglas, J.F., Brown, W.A., et al. (1980). Advantages of low dose steroid from the day after renal transplantation. *Transplantation.* B29:287–289.
56. Salaman, J.R., Griffin, P.J.A., Price, K. (1983). High or low dose steroids for immunosuppression. *Transplant Proc.* 15:1086–1088.
57. de Vecchi, A., Rivolta, E., Tarantino, A., et al. (1985). Controlled trial of two different methylprednisolone doses in cadaveric renal transplantation. *Nephron.* 41:262–266.
58. Lausten, G.S., Lemser, T., Jensen, P.K., Egfjord, M. (1998). Necrosis of the femoral head after kidney transplantation. *Clin Transplant.* 12:572–574.
59. Lausten, G.S., Egfjord, M., Olgaard, K. (1993). Metabolism of prednisone in kidney transplanted patients with necrosis of the femoral head. *Pharmacol Toxicol.* 72:78–83.
60. Landmann, J., Renner, N., Gatcher, A., Thiel, G., Harder, F. (1987). Cyclosporin A and osteonecrosis of the femoral head. *J Bone Joint Surg Am.* 69:1226–1228.

61. Ponticelli, C., Civati, G., Tarantino, A., et al. (1996). Randomized study with cyclosporin in kidney transplantation: 10-year follow-up. *J Am Soc Nephrol*. 7:792–797.
62. Clinical Practice Guidelines for Bone Metabolism and Disease in Chronic Kidney Disease. (2003). *Am J Kid Dis*. 42:S138-140.
63. Tang, S., Chan, T.M., Lui, S.L., et al. (2000). Risk factors for avascular bone necrosis after renal transplantation. *Transpl Proc*. 32:1873–1875.
64. Han, D., Kim, S., Chang, J., Kim, S. (1998). Avascular necrosis following renal transplantation. *Transplant Proc*. 30:3034–3035.
65. Kelly, P.J., Sambrook, P.N., Eisman, J.A. (1989). Potential protection by cyclosporin against glucocorticoid effects on bone. *Lancet*. 2:1388
66. Sakai, T., Sugano, N., Kokado, Y., et al. (2003). Tacrolimus may be associated with lower osteonecrosis rates in renal transplantation. *Clin Orthop*. 415:163–170.
67. Bhandari, S., Eris, J. (2001). Drug points: Premature osteonecrosis and sirolimus treatment in renal transplantation. *BMJ*. 323:665.
68. Abbott, K.C., Oglesby, R.J., Ogodoa, L.Y. (2002). Hospitalized avascular necrosis after renal transplantation in the United States. *Kidney Int*. 62:2250–2256.
69. Patton, P.R., Peaff, W.W. (1988). Aseptic bone necrosis after renal transplantation. *Surgery*. 103:63–68.
70. Koyama, H., Cecka, J.M., Terasaki, P.I. (1994). Kidney transplants in black recipients. HLA-matching and other factors affecting long-term graft survival. *Transplantation*. 57:1064–1068.
71. Chatterjee, S.N., Friedler, R.M., Berne, T.V., et al. (1976). Persistent hypercalcemia after successful renal transplanatation. *Nephron*. 17:1-7.
72. Nehme, D., Rondeau, E., Paillard F., et al. (1989). Aseptic necrosis of bone following renal transplantation: Relationship with hyperparathyroidism. *Nephrol Dial Transplant*. 4:123–128.
73. Ferrari, P., Schroeder, V., Anderson, S., et al. (2002). Association of plasminogen activator inhibitor-1 genotype with avascular necrosis in steroid-treated renal allograft recipients. *Transplantation*. 74:1147-1152.
74. Hungerford, D.S., Zizic, T.M. (1983). Pathogenesis of ischemic necrosis of the femoral head, in *The Hip*. Proceedings of the open scientific meeting of the Hip Society, Hunger Ford, D.S., ed. 1983, pp. 249–262, The C.V. Mosby Co.
75. Glimcher, M.J., Kenzora, J.E. (1979). The biology of osteonecrosis of the human femoral head and its clinical implications. I. Tissue biology. *Clin Orthop*. 138:284–309.
76. Cruess RL. (1986). Osteonecrosis of bone: current concepts as to etiology and pathogenesis. *Clin Orthop*. 208:30–39.
77. Eberhardt, A.W., Yeager-Jones, A., Blair, H.C. (2001). Regional trabecular bone matrix degeneration and osteocyte death in femora of glucocorticoid-treated rabbits. *Endocrinology*. 142:1333–1340.
78. Jones, J.P. Alcoholism, hypercortisonism, fat embolism and osseous avascular necrosis, in Idiopathic ischemic necrosis of the femoral head in adults, Zinn, W.M., ed. 1971, pp.112–132, Stuttgart: Georg Thieme.
79. Frost, H.M. (1960). In vivo osteocyte cell death. *J Bone Joint Surg Am*. 42:138–143.
80. Frost, H.M. (1960). Micropetrosis. *J Bone Joint Surg Am*. 42:144–150.
81. Weinstein, R.S., Jilka, R.L., Parfitt, A.M., Manolagas, S.C. (1998). Inhibition of osteoblastogenesis and promotion of apoptosis of osteoblasts and osteocytes by glucocorticoids. Potential mechanisms of their deleterious effects on bone. *J Clin Invest*. 102:274–282.
82. Weinstein, R.S., Nicholas, R.W., Manolagas, S.C. (2000). Apoptosis of osteocytes in glucocorticoid-induced osteonecrosis of the hip. *J Clin Endocrinol Metab*. 85:2907-2912.
83. Aarden, E.M., Burger, E.H., Nijweide, P.J. (1994). Function of osteocytes in bone. *J Cell Biochem*. 55:287–299.
84. Noble, B.S., Stevens, H., Loveridge, N. Reeve, J. (1997). Identification of apoptotic osteocytes in normal and pathological human bone. *Bone*. 20:273–282.

85. Reichardt, H.M., Schutz, G. (1998). Glucocorticoid signalling – multiple variations of a common theme. *Mol Cell Endocrinol.* 146:1–6.
86. Zhao, W., Byrne, M.H., Wang, Y., Krane, S.M. (2000). Osteocyte and osteoblast apoptosis and excessive bone deposition accompany failure of collagenase cleavage of collagen. *J Clin Invest.* 106:941-949.
87. Dumont, M., Danais, S., Taillefer, R. (1983). "Doughnut" sign in avascular necrosis of the bone. *Clin Nucl Med.* 9:44.
88. Tawn, D.J., Watt, I. (1989). Bone marrow scintigraphy in the diagnosis of post-traumatic avascular necrosis of bone. *Br J Radiol.* 62:790–795.
89. Glickstein, M.F., Benk, D.L., Schreibber, M.L., et al. (1988). Avascular necrosis versus other diseases of the hip: sensitivity of MR imaging. *Radiology.* 166:215–220.
90. Mitchell, D.G., Rao, V.M., Dalinka, M.K., et al. (1987). Femoral head avascular necrosis: correlation of MR imaging, radiographic staging, radionuclide imaging and clinical findings. *Radiology.* 162:709–715.
91. Steinberg, M.E., Hayken, G.D., Steinberg, D.R. (1995). A quantitative system for staging avascular necrosis. *J Bone Joint Surg Br.* 77:34–38
92. Sugano, N., Takaoka, K., Ohaono, K., et al. (1994). Prognostication of non-traumatic avascular necrosis of the femoral head. *Clin Orthop Rel Res.* 303:155–162.
93. Mont, M.A., Carbone, J.J., Fairbank, A.C. (1996). Core decompression versus nonoperative management for osteonecrosis of the hip. *Clin Orthop Rel Res.* 324:169–178.
94. Churchill, M.A., Spencer, J.D. (1991). End-stage AVN in renal transplant patients. The natural history. *J. Bone Joint Surg Br.* 73:618–620.
95. Lafforgue, P., Dahan, E.,Chagnaud, C., Schiano, A., Kasbarian, M., Acquaviva, P.C. (1993). Early stage avascular necrosis of the femoral head: MR imaging for prognosis in 31 cases with at least 2 years of follow-up. *Radiology.* 187:199–204.
96. Motohashi, M., Morii, T., Koshino, T. (1991). Clinical course of roentgenographic changes of osteonecrosis of the femoral condyle under conservative treatment. *Clin Orthop.* 266:156–161.
97. Steinberg, M.E., Brighton, C.T., Bands, R.E., et al. (1990). Capacitive coupling as an adjunctive treatment for avascular necrosis. *Clin Orthop.* 261:11.
98. Aaron, R.K, Cimobor, D.M. Electrical stimulation of bone induction and grafting, in Bone grafts and bone substitutes, Habal, M.B., Reddi, A.H., eds. 1992, pp. 192–205, Philadelphia: W.B. Saunders.
99. Pritchett, J.W. (2001). Statin therapy decreases the risk of osteonecrosis in patients receiving steroids. *Clin Orthop.* 386:173–178.
100. Koo, K.H., Kim, R., Ko, G.H., et al.(1995). Preventing collapse in early osteonecrosis of the femoral head: A randomized clinical trial of core decompression. *J Bone Joint Surg Br.* 77:870–874.
101. Mont, M.A., Hungerford, D.S. (1995). Non-traumatic avascular necrosis of the femoral head. *J Bone Joint Surg Am.* 77:459–474.
102. Hungerford, D.S. (1989). The role of core decompression in the treatment of ischemic necrosis of the femoral head. *Arthritis Rheum.* 32:801–806.
103. Learmonth, I.D., Maloon, S., Dall, G. (1990). Core decompression for early atraumatic osteonecrosis of the femoral head. *J Bone Joint Surg Br.* 72:387–390.
104. Hopson, C.N., Siverhus, S.W. (1988). Ischemic necrosis of the femoral head: treatment by core decompression. *J Bone Joint Surg Am.* 70:1048–1051.
105. Mont, M.A., Tomek, I.M., Hungerford, D.S. (1997). Core decompression for avascular necrosis of the distal femur: long-term follow-up. *Clin Orthop.* 334:124–130.
106. Stulberg, B.N., Dais, A.W., Bauer, T.W., Levine, M., Easley, K. (1991). Osteonecrosis of the femoral head: A prospective randomised treatment protocol. *Clin Orthop.* 268:140–151.
107. Rosenwasser, M.P., Garino, J.P., Kierman, H.A., Michelsen, C.B. (1994). Long-term follow-up of thorough debridement and cancellous bone grafting of the femoral head for avascular necrosis. *Clin Orthop.* 306:17–27.

108. Urbaniak, J.R., Coogan, P.G., Gunneson, E.B., et al. (1995). Treatment of osteonecrosis of the femoral head with free vascularized fibular grafting: A long-term follow-up study of one hundred and three hips. *J Bone Joint Surg Am.* 77:681–694.
109. Marcus, N.D., Enneking, W.F., Massam, R.A. (1973). The silent hip in idiopathic aseptic necrosis: Treatment by bone grafting. *J Bone Joint Surg Am.* 55:1351–1366.
110. Buckley, P.D., Gearin, P.F., Petty, R.W. (1991). Structural bone grafting for early atraumatic avascular necrosis of the femoral head. *J Bone Joint Surg Am.* 73:1357–1364.
111. Sotereanos, D.G., Plaksychuck, A.Y., Rubash, H.E. (1997). Free vascularized fibula grafting for the treatment of osteonecrosis of the femoral head. *Clin Orthop.* 344:243–256.
112. Scully, S.P., Aaron, R.K., Urbaniak, J.R. (1998). Survival analysis of hips treated with core decompression or vascularized fibular grafting because of avascular necrosis. *J Bone Joint Surg Am.* 80:1270– 1275.
113. Urbaniak, J.R., Harvey, E.J. (1998). Revascularisation of the femoral head in osteonecrosis. *J Am Acad Orthop Surg.* 6:44–54.
114. Vail, T.P., Urbaniak, J.R. (1996). Donor-site morbidity with use of vascularized autogenous fibular grafts. *J Bone Joint Surg Am.* 78:204–211.
115. Mont, M.A., Fairbank, A.C., Drackow, D.A., et al. (1996). Corrective osteotomy for osteonecrosis of the femoral head. *J Bone Joint Surg Am.* 78:1032–1041.
116. Scher, M.A., Jakim, I. (1993). Intertrochanteric osteotomy and the autogenous bone-grafting for avascular necrosis of the femoral head. *J Bone Joint Surg Am.* 75:1119–1133.
117. Hosokawa, A., Mohtai, M., Hotokebuchi, T., et al. Transtrochanteric rotational osteotomy for idiopathic and steroid-induced osteonecrosis of the femoral head, in Osteonecrosis: etiology, diagnosis and treatment, Urbaniak, J.R., Jones, J.P. Jr., eds. 1997, pp. 309–314. Rosemont IL, American Academy of Orthopaedic Surgeons.
118. Amstutz, H.C., Noordin, S., Campbell, P.A., et al. Precision fit surface hemiarthroplasty for femoral head osteonecrosis, in Osteonecrosis: etiology, diagnosis and treatment, Urbaniak, J.R., Jones, J.P. Jr., eds. 1997, pp. 373–383. Rosemont IL, American Academy of Orthopaedic Surgeons.
119. Hungerford, M.W., Mont, M.A., Scott, R., et al. (1998). Surface replacement hemiarthroplasty for the treatment of osteonecrosis of the femoral head. *J Bone Joint Surg Am.* 80:1656–1664.
120. Cornell, C.N., Salvati, E.A., Pellicci, P.M. (1986). Long-term follow-up of total hip replacement in patients with osteonecrosis. *Orthop Clin North Am.* 16:757–769.
121. Radford, P.J., Doran, A., Greatorex, R.A., Rushton, N. (1989). Total hip replacement in the renal transplant recipient. *J Bone Joint Surg Br.* 71:456–459.
122. Orwin, J.F., Fisher, R.C., Wiedel, J.D. (1991). Use of the cemented bipolar endoprosthesis for the treatment of steroid-induced osteonecrosis of the hip in renal transplant patients. *J Arthroplasty.* 6:1–9.

CHAPTER 21

Pediatric Transplant Bone Disease

Mary B. Leonard, MD, MSCE
Division of Pediatrics and Epidemiology, The Children's Hospital of Philadelphia,
Department of Biostatistics and Epidemiology, University of Pennsylvania School of Medicine,
Philadelphia, PA

Craig B. Langman, MD
Feinberg School of Medicine, Northwestern University,
Division of Kidney Diseases, Children's Memorial Medical Center, Chicago, IL

I. INTRODUCTION

Throughout childhood and adolescence, bone mineral accrual results in ethnic-, gender-, maturation-, and site-specific increases in bone dimensions and density. During the critical 2-year interval surrounding the time of peak height velocity, approximately 25% of skeletal mass is laid down, and 90% of peak bone mass is established by 18 years of age [1]. This rapid accumulation of bone mass correlates with the rate of growth and requires the coordinated actions of growth hormone, insulin-like growth factor-I (IGF-I), and sex steroids. Individuals with higher peak bone mass in early adulthood have a protective advantage against fracture when the inexorable decline in bone mass associated with older age or menopause occurs. Accordingly, the NIH Consensus Statement on Osteoporosis Prevention, Diagnosis and Therapy concluded "bone mass attained early in life is perhaps the most important determinant of life-long skeletal health" [2].

Pediatric transplant recipients have multiple risk factors for impaired bone development, including preexisting metabolic bone disease, poor growth, delayed development, malnutrition, decreased weight-bearing activity, chronic inflammation, and immunosuppressive therapies. The impact of these threats to bone health may be immediate, resulting in fragility fractures, or delayed, resulting from suboptimal peak bone mass accrual. Recent years have seen an increased interest in the effects of pediatric solid-organ transplantation on bone mineral accrual; the short- and long-term implications for fracture risk are poorly understood, however.

This review summarizes the organ-specific epidemiology of pediatric solid-organ transplantation, including the age at transplantation, allograft and patient survival rates, and indications for transplantation. The skeletal impacts of the underlying disease and subsequent transplant complications are also reviewed. The classification of bone health in children and adolescents is discussed, as are the advantages and disadvantages of available technologies for the assessment of bone in children and adolescents. The difficulties in assessing and interpreting bone measures in pediatric transplantation are underscored in a review of selected studies. Two recent studies demonstrating recovery of bone in liver transplant recipients are highlighted. Finally, potential therapies are considered.

II. EPIDEMIOLOGY OF SOLID–ORGAN TRANSPLANTATION IN CHILDREN

A. Age at Transplantation

In the year 2002, a total of 1,751 solid-organ transplants were performed in children and adolescents less than 18 years old [3]. The majority of these were kidney transplants in adolescent patients, as shown in Table 1. Transplantation rates, expressed as transplants per million population per year, were greatest in infants requiring liver transplantation [3]. Figure 1 illustrates the marked differences in transplantation rates according to age and allograft type in children, adolescents, and young adults. The timing of transplantation may have important implications for the severity of bone loss and potential for recovery throughout growth and development.

B. Patient and Allograft Survival

A comprehensive description of age-, organ-, and donor-specific patient and graft survival rates in pediatric transplantation is beyond the scope of the chapter and was recently summarized by Colambani et al. [4]. The 3-year patient and allograft survival rates reported by the Scientific Registry of Transplant Recipients in children and adolescents less than 18 years of age are summarized in Figure 2. Patient and allograft survival rates

TABLE 1 Pediatric Transplants in the U.S. in 2002 [3]

Age (yr)	Kidney	Liver	Heart	Intestine	Lung	Pancreas	Heart-lung	Kidney-pancreas
< 1	5	154	71	15	3	8	1	0
1 to 5	140	210	79	30	5	9	0	0
6 to 10	157	59	41	10	8	2	0	0
11 to 17	464	132	97	13	28	4	5	1

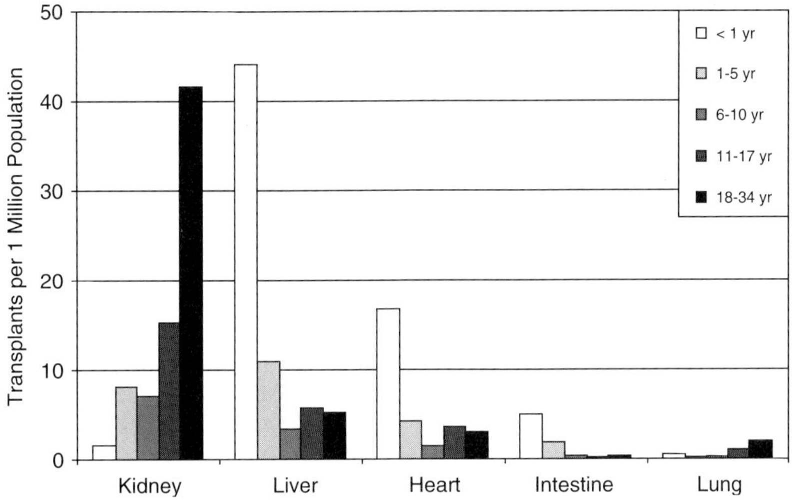

FIGURE 1 Incidence of transplantation in children and young adults in 2001, according to age and organ (from Scientific Registry of Transplant Recipients).

are highest among kidney transplant recipients, exceeding adult rates with one notable exception: Adolescent recipients of cadaveric grafts had a 3-year graft survival rate of only 75% and 5-year graft survival rate of 54%. Adolescents suffered increased late acute rejection, incomplete reversal of acute rejection, and increased allograft loss compared with younger children [5]. Adolescent liver recipients exhibited a similar trend towards worse graft survival 3 and 5 years after transplantation [4]. Noncompliance with immunosuppression regimens likely contributed to allograft loss in these

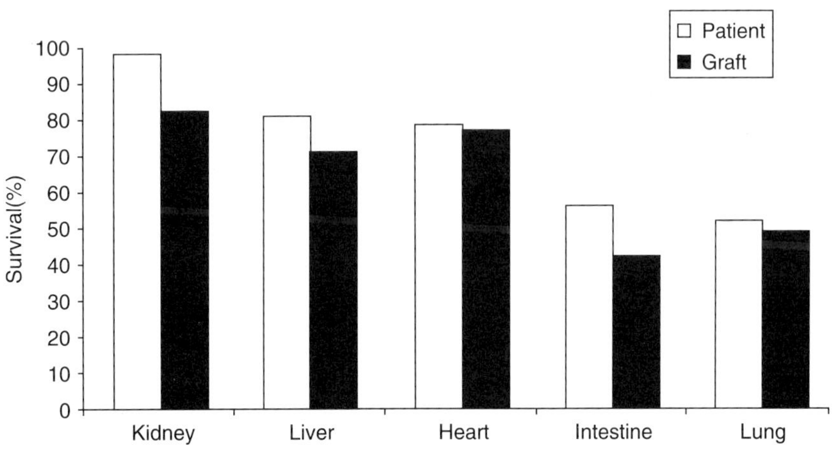

FIGURE 2 Patient and allograft survival at 3 years among patients less than 18 years of age at the time of transplant (from Scientific Registry of Transplant Recipients, for patients receiving their first transplant of this type between 01/01/1998 and 12/31/1999).

high-risk groups [6]. Because adolescence is a critical time for bone mass accrual, allograft failure and treatment of rejection with high-dose glutocorticoids may have negative effects on peak bone mass.

C. Indications for Transplantation

The indications for solid-organ transplantation differ according to the age of transplantation. For example, among lung transplant recipients less than 1 year of age, a congenital lung abnormality is the most frequent indication for transplantation [7]. However, in older children and adolescents, cystic fibrosis accounts for over 60% of lung transplants. The leading indications for each type of transplant are summarized in Table 2. While any end-organ disease may impair bone mineral accrual through decreased physical activity and poor growth, many of the underlying pulmonary, hepatic, intestinal, cardiac, and renal diseases have independent detrimental effects on bone mineral accrual in childhood.

III. IMPACT OF THE UNDERLYING PRIMARY DISEASE ON BONE

A. Kidney Disease

Renal osteodystrophy is an early and pervasive consequence of chronic kidney disease. The effects on endochondral ossification during growth result in complications in the epiphyseal region that are unique to children

TABLE 2 Leading indications for organ transplantation

	Infants and young children	Older children and adolescents
Kidney [8]	Aplasia/hypoplasia/dysplasia	Aplasia/hypoplasia/dysplasia
	Obstructive uropathy	Obstructive uropathy
		FSGS
Liver [63]	Biliary atresia	Cirrhosis
	Other cholestatic disease	Fulminant liver failure
	Fulminant liver failure	Other metabolic
	Metabolic	Biliary atresia
Heart [7]	Congenital cardiac abnormality	Cardiomyopathy
	Cardiomyopathy	Congenital cardiac abnormality
	Retransplant	Retransplant
Intestine [155]	Short gut syndrome	Short gut syndrome
Lung [7]	Congenital pulmonary abnormality	Cystic fibrosis
	Primary pulmonary hypertension	Primary pulmonary hypertension
	Retransplant	Retransplant

with chronic kidney disease. Severe growth retardation and delayed maturation complicate chronic kidney disease in children. At the time of transplantation, height is equivalent to the 3rd percentile for age [height Z-score (standard deviation score) of −1.88], on average [8]. Height deficits are greatest among children with early-onset and long-standing chronic kidney disease. Potential contributing factors include prior glucocorticoid therapy; chronic acidosis; anorexia; inadequate nutrient (vitamins, trace minerals) and caloric intakes; hyposthenuria and sodium depletion; alterations of the normal physiology of the growth hormone–IGF axis, including increased serum IGFBP-3 levels with inadequate IGF-1 availability; inadequate testosterone or estrogen production during puberty; and bone disease, including severe rachitic-like lesions. Bone disease likely contributes to growth failure; a study of 25-hydroxyvitamin D therapy in children with chronic kidney disease resulted in improved growth [9].

An underexplored aspect of chronic kidney disease in children is impaired vitamin D metabolism, including nutritional deficiency. These disorders result in skeletal deformities resembling vitamin D–deficient rickets. Histologically, disorganization occurs in the growth plate and subjacent metaphysis. The growth plate in children with chronic kidney disease is vulnerable to injury. These abnormalities, along with hyperparathyroid erosions of bone, result in increased risk for slipped epiphyses and genu valgum or varus deformities, osteonecrosis, chondrolysis, and degenerative joint disease. Adynamic bone disease occurs with increasing frequency in maintenance dialysis patients [10]. This disease contributes to linear growth failure and fractures.

B. Liver Disease

Growth retardation in end-stage liver disease is significant, but less severe than in children with end-stage renal disease. At the time of transplantation, height is equivalent to the 10th percentile for age, on average [11]. As is the case with children with chronic kidney disease, the height deficits are significantly greater in infants and young children, when compared to adolescents. Patients with cirrhosis and cholestasis manifest growth hormone insensitivity, as seen by low circulating IGF-I levels in the face of elevated serum growth hormone concentrations [12, 13].

Chronic liver disease (cirrhosis or severe cholestatic liver disease) is associated with decreased serum levels of 25-hydroxyvitamin D, and levels fall as liver disease progresses to cirrhosis [14]. Adults with chronic liver disease demonstrated an appropriate increase in serum 25-hydroxyvitamin D levels following administration of ergocalciferol, indicating preservation of sufficient hepatic enzymatic function [15]. Therefore, the vitamin D deficiency is likely related to decreased dietary vitamin D, malabsorption of fat-soluble vitamins secondary to cholestasis, and decreased sun exposure with a reduction in the cutaneous synthesis of vitamin D [14]. Vitamin K, another fat-soluble vitamin, is required for the gamma-carboxylation of the bone matrix protein osteocalcin. Vitamin K supplementation has prevented bone loss in adults with cirrhosis [16].

In children with cholestasis, osteopenia is present early and worsens rapidly [17]. Deficiencies in fat-soluble vitamins and magnesium have been documented [17, 18]. Decreased bone mineral density (BMD) has also been reported in children with biliary atresia [19–21], and was associated with jaundice and decreased 25-hydroxyvitamin D levels in one study [20]. Hepatic osteodystrophy in children with biliary atresia results in radiologic evidence of rickets, widespread skeletal demineralization, and recurrent fragility fractures before transplantation [18, 22, 23].

Children also undergo liver transplantation for inborn errors of metabolism that do not cause liver failure [24], but may affect bone. The most frequent example of this type of disorder is primary hyperoxaluria type 1 (OMIM # 259900). Primary hyperoxaluria results from a functional or real deficiency of hepatic peroxisomal alanine glyoxylate aminotransferase activity. The resultant deficiency leads to overproduction of oxalate from glyoxylate. Overproduction of oxalate results in accumulation in the kidneys, small arteries, eyes, soft tissues, and bone. Deposition of calcium oxalate crystals in the bone marrow of children results in irregular transverse sclerotic bands in the metaphyseal segments of tubular bones that can be seen radiographically. Further evidence of disordered skeletal growth includes wide areas of rarefaction at the ends of the long bones, and translucent rims around the epiphyses [25]. Additional changes secondary to renal osteodystrophy are superimposed on oxalate bone disease as oxalate accumulation results in chronic kidney disease and kidney failure. (see Table 3).

TABLE 3 Potential musculoskeletal complication of kidney and liver disease

Kidney	Severe growth failure
	Delayed skeletal maturation
	Atraumatic fractures
	Deformities: slipped epiphyses, genu valgum, varus deformity
	Vitamin D deficiency: rachitic rosary, wide metaphysis, frontal bossing, craniotabes, ulnar deviation, and pes varus
	Secondary hyperparathyroidism: osteitis fibrosa, subperisoteal resorption
	Bone pain
	Avascular necrosis
	Myopathy
Liver	Growth failure
	Delayed skeletal maturation
	Atraumatic fractures
	Vitamin D deficiency and rickets
	Vitamin K and magnesium deficiency
	Generalized skeletal demineralization
	Metabolic bone disease (e.g., oxalosis)

C. Cardiac Disease

Children with isolated congenital cardiac defects that are amenable to definitive surgical correction may not have alterations of bone accrual. A study in adolescents with a history of surgical repair of tetralogy of Fallot did not demonstrate deficits in height, weight, nutritional status, body composition, or bone mineral density (BMD) [26]. In contrast, infants and young children with single-ventricle physiology undergo repetitive palliative surgery and suffer numerous morbidities that may impact bone accrual, including diminished exercise capacity, protein-losing enteropathy, growth retardation, and the need for chronic diuretic therapy [27]. A recent review of 62 children treated with such staged surgeries reported that 43% of children weighed below the 3rd percentile for age, and the median height was at the 10th percentile for age [28]. Only 49% of children reported normal physical activity. Patients with cardiomyopathies associated with skeletal myopathies, such as Duchenne's muscular dystrophy, may have localized or systemic reductions in BMD and increased fracture rates related to decreased weight-bearing activity [29].

D. Short Gut Syndrome and TPN Dependence

Short gut syndrome requiring intestinal transplantation in children is most frequently caused by neonatally acquired or recognized disorders that include volvulus, gastroschisis, necrotizing enterocolitis, intestinal atresia, intestinal stenosis, or functional pseudo-obstruction. Such patients develop severe malabsorption of macronutrients, micronutrients, and electrolytes. Children with short gut syndrome requiring long-term total parental nutrition (TPN) exhibit poor growth and decreased circulating levels of IGF-1 and IGFBP-3 [30, 31]. Vitamin D–deficiency rickets has been described [32]. Cholestasis, a major complication of chronic TPN therapy in short bowel syndrome, accounts for the majority of morbidity and mortality in this group of patients [33]. While osteoporosis frequently complicates chronic TPN therapy in adults [34], a study in 18 children with short gut syndrome demonstrated normal whole-body bone mineral content (BMC) relative to weight and height after discontinuation of the TPN [35].

E. Pulmonary Disease

Cystic fibrosis (CF) is the most common indication for lung transplantation in children and adolescents. Concern about osteoporosis in CF became widespread when adolescent and young adult patients who were awaiting lung transplants were found to have rib and spine fractures, kyphosis, and osteoporosis [36, 37]. In a series of 70 adults with cystic fibrosis and end-stage lung disease, fracture rates were 10- and 100-fold greater than expected for rib fractures and vertebral compression, respectively [36]. Studies have demonstrated that markers of bone formation were decreased relative to resorption in children and adolescents with CF [38, 39]. Delayed puberty, malabsorption, reduced weight-bearing exercise, corticosteroid therapy, and the presence of pro-inflammatory cytokines associated with infective respiratory exacerbations may impair bone mineral accrual in children and adolescents with CF [40–43].

IV. THREATS TO BONE HEALTH FOLLOWING TRANSPLANTATION

Successful solid-organ transplantation corrects many of the underlying abnormalities contributing to bone disease in children and adolescents. Following organ transplantation, however, subsequent decreased physical activity, allograft failure, and immunosuppression regimens may impair recovery of bone disease and lead to further bone loss.

A. Growth

Fine reviewed changes in height Z-scores following solid-organ transplantation, and noted similar factors that impacted growth post-transplant in pediatric liver, kidney, or heart transplant recipients [11]. These include the findings that younger patients and those with the most severe pretransplant growth retardation had the greatest potential for catch-up growth, allograft failure was associated with faltering growth, and daily corticosteroid therapy was associated with worse growth compared to alternate-day therapy.

During the first two years following renal transplantation, infants and young children exhibited catch-up growth [11], but this population forms a small percentage of the kidney transplant population (see Table 1). In contrast, the majority of renal transplant recipients greater than six years of age failed to undergo catch-up growth, or suffered further reductions in height percentiles [11]. Among liver transplant recipients, patients with biliary atresia manifested the greatest catch-up growth following transplantation [11, 21, 44]. Data in heart transplant recipients demonstrated greatest catch-up in growth in infants that did not receive maintenance corticosteroid therapy [11, 45]. In contrast, adolescent heart transplant recipients failed to demonstrate increased linear growth post-transplant [7, 46]. Insufficient data are available at this time in the small cohorts of lung and small intestine transplant recipients to address the risk factors for poor growth [11].

Factors that delay successful linear growth in transplant recipients, such as corticosteroids, alterations in the IGF–growth hormone axis, and allograft failure, likely have parallel adverse consequences for bone mineralization. In addition, as detailed later in this chapter, short stature confounds the assessment of dual energy x-ray absorptiometry (DXA) measures in children, and requires careful consideration in the interpretation of DXA results in studies of pediatric solid-organ transplantation.

B. Allograft Failure

Allograft failure may reintroduce or exacerbate the adverse bone effects of the primary disease in transplant recipients, such as renal osteodystrophy or hepatic osteodystrophy. Furthermore, cardiac, liver, and lung transplant recipients may develop chronic kidney disease as a sequelae of nephrotoxic immunosuppressive medications [47, 48], and suffer from superimposed renal osteodystrophy.

C. Decreased Physical Activity

Weight-bearing physical activity and biomechanical loading of bone are critical determinants of bone mass in growing, normal children [49]. The influence of skeletal loading on bone accretion is illustrated in two exercise trials in healthy children. An easily implemented school-based jumping intervention augmented cortical thickness in the femoral neck of healthy children [50]. A randomized clinical trial of physical activity and calcium supplementation in prepubertal children resulted in a significant, positive interaction between calcium supplements and physical activity in both cortical thickness and cortical area [51].

Decreased exercise capacity and markedly reduced muscle strength complicate transplantation in adults, because of chronic deconditioning and a myopathy related to immunosuppressive medications [52–55]. A randomized trial of exercise training in adult renal transplant patients resulted in greater gains in exercise capacity and muscle strength, and higher self-reported physical functioning [56]. A recent small, randomized clinical trial in adult lung transplant recipients demonstrated that mechanical loading was associated with a 9.2% increase in lumbar spine BMC, compared to progressive bone loss in the controls [57]. Similarly, resistance exercise plus alendronate was more efficacious than alendronate alone in restoring BMD in adult heart transplant recipients [58].

Decreased strength and markedly decreased exercise capacity have been demonstrated in pediatric liver, heart, and lung transplant recipients [59–61]. In pediatric renal transplant recipients, an inverse relationship was found between fat body mass and physical performance [62]. Pastore et al. concluded that few transplant recipients undertake physical activity after surgery, possibly owing to "over-protective parents and teachers and to lack of suitable supervised facilities" [60]. Of note, the Registry of the

International Society for Heart and Lung Transplantation Pediatric Report stated that 94% of heart transplant recipients and 86% of lung transplant recipients reported "no activity limitation" one year after transplantation [7]. While the authors conclude that patients' function status was excellent, these data may belie suboptimal exercise capacity and strength, with implications for bone accrual.

D. Immunosuppressive Therapies

Immunosuppression use varies considerably across centers, and the patterns of therapy continue to evolve. Because of the differences in the format of annual reports and published registry data, it is difficult to compare protocols across the different solid organ types. Trends are apparent, however, in comparing three resources [7, 8, 63]. In general, more than 95% of renal, liver, heart, and lung recipients receive a calcineurin inhibitor, either cyclosporine or tacrolimus, through 3 years of follow-up. The most notable differences across organ types are observed in the patterns of corticosteroid use. Table 4 summarizes glucocorticoid use in the early years following transplantation. Of note, a substantial portion of heart and liver recipients discontinue glucocorticoid use in the first 2 to 3 years, while the majority of renal transplant recipients continue daily glucocorticoids. Recent protocols for glucocorticoid avoidance in pediatric renal transplantation have been promulgated [64].

The effects of glucocorticoids and calcineurin inhibitors on trabecular bone turnover in the *remodeling* adult skeleton are well known [65, 66]. However, the impact of corticosteroid-induced suppression of bone formation on cortical and trabecular bone dimensions and density in the

TABLE 4 Glucocorticoid use in pediatric solid-organ transplantation

Kidney [8] **1996–2003**	Used in approximately:
	> 95% at hospital discharge
	> 90% at year 1 (15% on alternate day)
	> 88% at year 2 (25% on alternate day)
	> 85% at year 3 (33% on alternate day)
Liver [63] **1995–2003**	Used in:
	96% at hospital discharge
	64% at year 1
	42% at year 2
Heart [7] **1983–1999**	Used in approximately:
	80% at hospital discharge
	70% at year 1
	50% at year 3
Lung [7] **1983–1999**	Essentially all lung transplant recipients continue prednisone throughout follow-up.

Data estimated from tables and figures in registry reports.

modeling skeleton during critical growth periods is not known. While numerous studies have documented decreased BMD by DXA in children receiving glucocorticoids for various conditions, DXA is a two-dimensional technique that fails to discriminate between differences in trabecular and cortical bone, or in differences in bone density and geometry. An animal study addressed the structural effects of glucocorticoids in young growing rats [67]. In a dose-dependent manner, glucocorticoid administration decreased the ultimate load capacity and the ultimate stiffness of the femoral diaphysis. The decrease in ultimate load was explained by a glucocorticoid-induced decrease in the cross-sectional area of the femoral diaphysis secondary to reduced bone formation rates on the periosteal surface. Glucocorticoids also decreased the trabecular bone volume and mineralizing surface. These findings raise the concern that glucocorticoids adversely impact bone dimensions in the growing skeleton.

V. ASSESSMENT OF BONE STATUS IN CHILDREN AND ADOLESCENTS

A. Classification of Bone Health

DXA is widely accepted as a quantitative measurement technique for assessing skeletal status. In elderly adults, DXA BMD is a sufficiently robust predictor of osteoporotic fractures that it can be used to define the disease. The World Health Organization criteria for the diagnosis of osteoporosis in adults is based on a T-score, the comparison of a measured BMD result with the average BMD of young adults at the time of peak bone mass [68]. A T-score ≤ -2.5 SD below the mean peak bone mass is used for the diagnosis of osteoporosis, and a T-score ≤ -2.5 SD with a history of a low-impact fracture is classified as severe osteoporosis. While the T-score is a standard component of DXA BMD results, it is clearly inappropriate to assess skeletal health in children through comparison with peak adult bone mass. Rather, children are assessed relative to age or body size, expressed as a Z-score. In adults, low-impact fractures are defined as fractures that occur after a fall from standing height or less. This definition is often difficult to apply to fractures in children that occur during play or sports activities.

Despite the growing body of published normative data utilizing DXA in children, there are no evidence-based guidelines for the definition of osteoporosis in children. Fractures occur commonly in otherwise healthy children with a peak incidence during early adolescence around the time of the pubertal growth spurt [69]. This pattern has been attributed to a transient deficit in cortical bone mass due to an increased calcium demand during maximal skeletal growth. Khosla et al. recently reported that forearm (the most common site) fracture rates have increased significantly in males and females over the last 30 years; the peak incidence and greatest increase occurred between ages 11 and 14 years in boys and 8 and 11 years in girls [69]. Possible explanations include changing patterns of physical activity or decreased bone acquisition due to poor calcium intake.

Several studies have compared the DXA BMD of normal children and adolescents with forearm fractures to that of age-matched controls without fractures. Most [70–74], but not all [75, 76], found that mean DXA BMD was significantly lower in children with forearm fractures than in controls. One study reported that 69% of fractures were due to low-energy falls at home [75]; the authors did not provide their definition of a low-energy fall, however. Studies using quantitative computed tomography or metacarpal morphometry to characterize cortical geometry showed that decreased cortical thickness was associated with significantly increased fracture risk [74, 77]. Finally, television, computer, and video viewing had a dose-dependent association with wrist and forearm fractures [78].

These data suggest that low DXA BMD can be a contributing factor for pediatric fracture in healthy children, but bone geometry and nonskeletal factors such as sports participation, body size, and sedentary activities also contribute to fracture risk. Importantly, the relationships between DXA BMD, bone geometry, and fracture risk in children with chronic illness may be different from those observed in healthy children.

Comparisons to appropriate pediatric reference data are essential to describe accurately the clinical impact of childhood disease on bone development, to monitor changes in bone mineralization, and to identify patients for treatment protocols. Multiple sources of pediatric DXA reference data are now available for the calculation of DXA Z-scores. These include varied approaches, such as gender-specific centile curves; age- and height-specific means and standard deviations; Tanner- and weight-specific percentiles; age-, sex-, weight-, and height-adjusted curves; and Z-score prediction models [42, 79–91]. Differences in reference data have a significant impact on the diagnosis of osteopenia in children with chronic disease [92]. For example, use of reference data that are not gender-specific resulted in significantly greater misclassification of males as osteopenic [92]. In addition, use of published pediatric reference ranges has been complicated by differences in scanner manufacturers and frequent changes in hardware and software technology, including fan-beam technology, low-density software analysis modes, and specialized pediatric software. These technical changes result in clinically significant alterations in DXA results [93].

Therefore, despite the widespread availability of data on normal children, the prevalences of reduced bone mass, osteopenia, or osteoporosis in many childhood diseases are not known. Further effort is needed to develop adequate reference data and validate classification schemes of bone health in children.

B. DXA

DXA is, by far, the most common method for the assessment of bone health in children. Unfortunately, a significant limitation of DXA is the reliance on measurement of areal rather than volumetric BMD. DXA provides an estimate of BMD expressed as grams per anatomical region (e.g., individual vertebrae, whole body, or hip). Dividing the BMC within the defined anatomical region (g) by the projected area of the bone (cm^2) then derives "areal-BMD" (g/cm^2). This BMD is not a measure of volumetric density (g/cm^3) because it provides no information about the depth of bone. Bones of larger width and height also tend to be thicker. Since bone thickness is not factored into DXA estimates of BMD, reliance on areal-BMD inherently underestimates the bone density of short people. Despite identical volumetric bone density, the child with smaller bones appears to have a mineralization disorder (decreased areal-BMD). This is clearly an important artifact in children with chronic diseases associated with growth delay and short stature.

The confounding effect of skeletal geometry on DXA measures is now well recognized and multiple analytic strategies have been proposed to express DXA bone mass in a form that is less sensitive to differences in skeletal size [79, 80, 94–96]. Further studies are indicated to compare the sensitivity and specificity of varied approaches in the assessment of fracture risk.

An additional shortcoming of DXA is that the integrated measure of bone mass in a given projected area does not allow distinction between cortical and trabecular bone. DXA-based measures provide no information on bone architecture, and are limited in their usefulness to differentiate the spectrum of bone accrual during growth.

1. *DXA and Renal Osteodystrophy*

DXA has been used extensively to evaluate renal osteodystrophy. Since trabecular and cortical bone behave differently in response to chronically increased circulating levels of parathyroid hormone (increases and decreases, respectively), and DXA does not allow distinction of the effects of renal osteodystrophy on the two types of bone, DXA is inherently limited in these patients. The conflicting data on DXA-derived measures of areal-BMD in adults with renal osteodystrophy are consistent with these limitations. DXA results have been quite variable, with mean areal-BMD values that are higher than, the same as, or lower than controls subjects (reviewed in [97]). Predictably, fracture risk correlates poorly with DXA measures of trabecular areal-BMD in adults with renal disease [98, 99]. The limitations of DXA are summarized in Table 5.

C. Peripheral Quantitative Computed Tomography

A three-dimensional structural analysis of trabecular architecture and cortical bone dimensions can be obtained by computed tomography (CT). This technique offers an opportunity to overcome the limitations of DXA and advance our understanding of bone mineralization in children. CT

TABLE 5 Limitations of DXA in the assessment of bone status in children with chronic disease

Scan Acquisition	Fan beam results in magnification error with apparent differences in bone area and BMC as body size varies [156]
Scan Analysis	Pediatric software (Hologic, Inc.) results in underestimation of spine BMD [93]
	Difficult to define landmarks and region of interest in the immature hip [157]
Reference Data [42, 79–91]	Limited data in infants and young children
	Analysis methods not standardized
	Variable hardware and software
	Some are not gender-specific [92]
	Some presented relative to age, others relative to height, Tanner stage, and weight
Interpretation	Underestimates volumetric density in children with short stature
	Unable to distinguish between changes in bone dimensions and density
	Unable to distinguish between cortical and trabecular bone

provides an image unobscured by overlying structures [100]. The CT attenuation of different bone tissues provides quantitative information, referred to as quantitative CT (QCT). In contrast to DXA, this technique describes authentic volumetric BMD, accurately measures bone dimensions, and distinguishes between cortical and trabecular bone. To minimize radiation exposure, special high-resolution scanners were developed for the peripheral skeleton (pQCT), specifically, the radius or tibia. The distal site is largely trabecular bone, while the midshaft is almost entirely cortical bone. The volume of each component is calculated from the scan thickness and cross-sectional area, and the density by attenuation of the x-ray beam. Bone strength can also be estimated by pQCT from the total bone area and cortical thickness and density [101]. For example, QCT studies of bone mineral accretion and bone strength demonstrated gender-, maturation-, and ethnic-specific patterns of development of bone strength during childhood and adolescence (reviewed in [102]).

VI. CLINICAL STUDIES OF BONE HEALTH IN PEDIATRIC TRANSPLANT RECIPIENTS

A. Liver Transplantation

Three early reports evaluated bone mineralization in small series (6 to 9 patients) of liver transplant recipients and documented significant increases in BMC or BMD following transplantation [103–105]. Improved BMC was associated with normalization of vitamin D levels [103].

However, these increases are likely explained, at least in part, by linear growth over the study interval. In the series by D'Antiga, height gain and whole-body areal-BMD gain were highly correlated (r = 0.93) [105]. Of note, 1 postpubertal patient with no linear growth after transplant still exhibited increased spine and whole-body areal-BMD [105].

More recently, Okajima et al. reported the results of a prospective study of lumbar spine areal-BMD in 30 children (15 male), ages 7 months to 15 years, undergoing liver transplantation for biliary atresia [21]. At 6 months post-transplant, the patients were weaned off glucocorticoids, and all had stable liver function. The lumbar spine BMD for age Z-scores were calculated using non-gender-specific French data [87]. During the 2-year interval following transplantation, height Z-scores increased from a mean of −2.0 to −0.29, while areal-BMD Z-scores increased from a mean of −3.4 to +0.16. These dramatic increases were accompanied by significant increases in serum vitamin D and IGF-I levels. Three patients suffered fractures prior to transplantation, and none post-transplantation. A particularly notable finding of this study is that there was no reduction in BMD in the early post-operative phase. Rather, BMD increased significantly in the first 3 months despite the fact that height Z-scores did not increase until 3 to 6 months after the transplant.

A subsequent study evaluated BMD in children at least 1 year after liver transplantation [106]. A total of 109 patients, mean age 10.5 years (range 1 to 32 years), were studied a median of 5.8 years following transplantation. The mean (± SD) height Z-score was −0.74 ± 1.26. The mean lumbar spine areal-BMD Z-score was −0.24 ± 1.27. Seven percent of patients had Z-scores less than −2.0. Patients with BMD Z-scores less than −2.0 were more likely to require treatment for rejection, and experienced greater cumulative glucocorticoid exposure in the prior year. The authors did not report whether the height Z-scores were lower in subjects with decreased BMD Z-scores.

The two studies outlined above provide data that liver transplantation has beneficial effects on bone health in children with cirrhosis. These findings contrast sharply with reports of immediate bone loss in adults undergoing liver transplantation, and may be related to the greater potential for bone mineral accrual and modeling in young children.

Hill et al. reported the incidence of fractures in 117 pediatric liver transplant recipients, ages 15 days to 15 years at transplant [23]. Nineteen children sustained a total of 69 fractures, predominantly of the ribs and long bones. Of these 19 children, 13 experienced the fractures prior to transplantation, and 11 of these pretransplant fractures occurred in the absence of identifiable trauma. Among the 6 children fracturing following transplant, 3 were associated with identifiable trauma; one of the children experiencing an atraumatic fracture following transplant had oxalosis. These data do not provide definitive evidence that liver transplant, per se, is associated with increased fracture risk in children.

B. Cardiac Transplantation

Two studies have addressed bone accrual following pediatric cardiac transplantation [107, 108]. The first assessed whole-body, spine, and hip BMD by DXA in 19 adolescents, ages 11 to 20 years [107]. BMD in the hip and spine were significantly decreased compared to the DXA manufacturer's age- and gender-specific controls. However, the study does not report whether the subjects had decreased height for age; therefore, it is not possible to determine whether the DXA results were confounded by short stature.

Subsequently, Daniels et al. evaluated 13 children, ages 9 to 18 years, ranging from 1 to 15 years after cardiac transplant [108]. The height SDS at the time of the DXA scans ranged from −2.3 to 0.20. Two subjects suffered symptomatic vertebral compression fractures. Asymptomatic fractures in the other subjects may have gone undetected. Bone mineral apparent density (BMAD) was calculated from the BMC and area in hip and spine as an estimate of volumetric BMD [94], and was significantly decreased in the spine in cardiac patients compared with age-, gender-, and ethnic-specific reference data. Spine BMD Z-score was not associated with time since transplantation or glucocorticoid exposure in this small, heterogeneous sample.

C. Renal Transplantation

The bone status of pediatric renal transplant recipients has been studied in greater detail [108–119]. One study included bone histomorphometry [114]. In that study, Sanchez et al. evaluated 47 children and adolescents with stable renal function an average of 3.2 years after transplantation. Eleven of 47 children had elevated PTH values. Histomorphometric analysis of the bone biopsies revealed that 31 transplant recipients had normal bone formation rates, 11 had mild hyperparathyroidism, and 5 had adynamic skeletal lesions. Neither the interval since transplantation, serum levels of parathyroid hormone, serum creatinine, nor cumulative prednisone doses differed according to histologic subgroups. Despite normal bone formation rates in many children, all 3 subgroups demonstrated increased eroded bone perimeter, increased osteoid area, and increased osteoid perimeter. Hyperparathyroidism improved or resolved after transplantation in all 14 subjects with high-turnover bone disease prior to transplantation; one patient developed an adynamic lesion following transplantation, however. Bone histology did not change following transplantation among those with normal bone formation prior to transplantation. Bone formation improved in 2 of the 3 children with adynamic bone disease prior to transplantation. In summary, skeletal lesions improved substantially in pediatric patients undergoing successful transplantation, but bone histology did not fully revert to normal in the majority.

DXA studies of bone mineralization in children following transplantation have yielded conflicting results, largely related to the difficulties in interpreting DXA results in children with delayed growth and development, and the limitations of DXA in the setting of renal osteodystrophy [120]. Multiple cross-sectional studies concluded that the decreased BMD in pediatric renal transplant recipients could be largely attributed to height deficits [108, 112–114]. The impact of correction for decreased stature is illustrated in a study by Saland et al. [115]. In 33 renal allograft recipients, lumbar spine BMD Z-scores were calculated relative to height and relative to age. The mean BMD Z-scores were -0.9 ± 1.3 relative to age and $+0.4 \pm 1.4$ relative to height. Simple adjustment for height may yield misleading results, however, since shorter controls will be younger than the renal patients. Skeletal maturity and Tanner stage are key determinants of bone mass, and comparison with less-mature controls is a flawed solution to the influence of bone size. This may account for the increased BMD Z-scores relative to height in such studies.

Two prospective studies concluded that pediatric renal transplant recipients experienced significant bone loss following transplantation. However, both studies are complicated by adjustments for body weight and height in a population with marked and rapid changes in body composition post-transplant. Feber et al. reported DXA results over a 12-month interval in 16 children (ages 5 to 18 years) [109]. Whole-body BMC results were expressed as Z-scores for age, sex, weight, and height [91]. While BMC Z-scores decreased from +0.98 to −0.55 over the first 3 months post-transplantation, body mass index (BMI) Z-scores increased from −0.42 to +0.99 over the same interval. It is therefore unclear whether these patients experienced an absolute reduction in BMC or whether the decreasing BMC Z-scores reflect a decrease in BMC relative to a increase in weight. This may be misleading since the increase in BMC with weight in healthy children is related to lean mass [121], and the increased BMI in such transplant recipients likely represents fat mass.

A randomized trial of methylprednisolone ($n = 14$) versus deflazacort ($n = 13$) in prepubertal transplant recipients demonstrated positive height velocity scores in the deflazacort group and negative height velocity scores in the methylprednisolone group, after 1 year of study. Weight/height ratio increased in the methylprednisolone group and decreased in the deflazacort group over the 12-month interval. The authors reported DXA results divided by body weight and by body surface area. Group differences were significant for changes in lumbar-spine areal-BMD, whole-body areal-BMD, and whole-body BMC, each divided by body weight, but only for whole-body BMC when divided by body surface area. This may be a flawed approach since two patients with comparable weight or body surface area may have markedly different heights. We have shown that DXA BMC relative to height correlated well with bone strength (as measured by pQCT), while DXA BMC relative to weight was not correlated with bone strength [96].

In the two studies just detailed, the interpretation of the results would be aided by presentation of the absolute, unadjusted BMC and BMD at each follow-up interval.

Assessment of radial cortical BMC and forearm muscle cross-sectional area was performed by pQCT in15 renal transplant recipients. These children had decreased height, decreased muscle cross-sectional area, and decreased

BMC for age. Muscle cross-sectional area was normal for height; however, the BMC to muscle cross-sectional area ratio was significantly decreased [118]. The authors concluded that bone strength was not normally adapted to the muscle forces. This study, although small, likely provides the best assessment of BMC relative to bone length in renal transplant recipients.

Two recent studies have assessed fractures following renal transplantation in children [110, 117]. The first was a retrospective cohort study of 11 children undergoing renal transplantation for cystinosis at a single center [117]. DXA results were available in 9 subjects: the spine BMD Z-scores ranged from −1.92 to +0.02 relative to age, and −1.20 to +1.93 relative to height, weight, and pubertal stage. Three subjects experienced 8 long bone fractures. DXA BMD did not correlated with fracture events.

Bartosh recently reported long-term outcomes in 57 adults (mean age 31 years) with a history of pediatric renal transplantation [110]. Overall, 19% of females and 26% of males reported a history of a fracture. The report provides no information on age at fracture, timing relative to transplantation, mechanism of injury, or anatomic site of injury. The authors did not report fracture incidence rates (fracture per patient-year); therefore, it is not possible to determine whether rates were greater in males than females, or whether the rates are greater than those observed in otherwise healthy children and adolescents. For example, in the fracture study by Ma et al. 10% of healthy prepubertal children have a history of fracture [75].

VII. POTENTIAL THERAPIES FOR BONE HEALTH IN TRANSPLANT RECIPIENTS

A. Physical Activity

Physical activity is an important determinant of bone mass accretion during growth; simple loading exercises promote bone accretion in healthy children. Resistance exercise prevents bone loss in adults, as detailed previously. Weight-bearing physical activity should therefore be encouraged in pediatric transplant recipients in an effort to positively affect bone.

B. Vitamins and Minerals

1. Calcium Intake

Multiple prospective randomized double-blind intervention trials have documented that calcium supplementation promotes bone accretion in normal children and adolescents [122–127]. Accordingly, the National Academy of Science's Food and Nutrition Board and the National Institutes of Health Consensus Panel on Calcium Intake increased calcium intake standards for adolescents to 1300 and 1500 mg/day, respectively [128, 129]. These recommendations reflect the need for increasing calcium intake with age to accommodate the calcium needs for the rapidly growing skeleton, especially during the years of the adolescent growth spurt. A national dietary intake survey showed that children's calcium intake declines in all ethnic groups at the ages when calcium requirements increase [130]. Following transplantation, catch-up growth and bone mineral accrual may result in even greater calcium requirements. To our knowledge, no calcium balance studies or calcium supplementation trials have been conducted in children with chronic illness. Calcium intake should therefore be assessed in all pediatric transplant recipients, and should be supplemented to the recommended intakes summarized in Table 6. Caution is raised, however, with excessive calcium intakes, as it has been linked to cardiovascular disease in adult renal transplant patients [131].

2. *Vitamin D Intake*

Vitamin D is essential for the maintenance of adequate calcium levels for bone mineralization, and all pediatric solid-organ transplant recipients are at risk for Vitamin D deficiency, especially during the winter months. Following liver transplantation, serum 25-OH vitamin D levels normalize in most patients and are associated with increased BMD [21]. However, decreased vitamin D levels have been reported in long-term transplantation survivors [106]. Previous studies have defined vitamin D insufficiency at a serum 25-hydroxyvitamin D level that we now recognize as too low, and which affects bone mass [132]. It therefore seems prudent to measure serum 25-hydroxyvitamin D levels when parathyroid hormone levels are elevated [133].

3. *Phosphorus*

Phosphorus is essential for normal bone formation. The renal transplant recipient is at risk for renal phosphate wasting and persistent hyperparathyroidism. Serum phosphorus should be measured at least daily during the first week, weekly during the initial 3 months, and monthly during the 6 months following kidney transplantation. Phosphorus supplementation should be provided to maintain the serum phosphorus within the normal limits for age.

TABLE 6 Recommendations for calcium intake (mg/day)

Food and nutrition board		NIH consensus panel	
Age range (years)	Calcium intake	Age range (years)	Calcium intake
0 to 0.5	210	0 to 0.5	400
0.5 to 1.0	270	0.5 to 1.0	600
1 to 3	500	1 to 5	800
4 to 8	800	6 to 10	800–1200
9 to 13	1300	11 to 18	1200–1500
14 to 18	1300		

C. Recombinant Human Growth Hormone

In addition to its well-established effects on linear growth in childhood and adolescence, growth hormone has both direct and indirect actions on bone mineral accrual [134]. Growth hormone increases lean body mass, muscle strength, and exercise capacity, enabling increased physical activity. *In vitro*, growth hormone stimulates proliferation of osteoblasts and stimulates osteoclast bone resorption [135, 136]. Childhood-onset growth hormone deficiency results in decreased areal-BMD and BMAD, which improves with growth hormone therapy [137, 138]. Until recently, growth hormone therapy in children with growth hormone deficiency was discontinued at completion of linear growth. However, new studies suggest benefit from continued therapy after epiphyseal closure to optimize peak bone mass [134].

The safety and efficacy of growth hormone therapy has been demonstrated in multiple studies in pediatric renal and liver transplant recipients [11]. A single, uncontrolled study conducted in eight liver transplant recipients demonstrated an increase in growth velocity [139]. The largest randomized trial of growth hormone therapy was performed in 90 children at least 12 months after renal transplantation, and revealed increased growth velocity during the first year of therapy [140]. Importantly, there was no evidence of increased allograft rejection or accelerated decline in renal function. Sanchez et al. recently reported the skeletal effects of a randomized trial of growth hormone therapy in 23 stable, prepubertal pediatric kidney recipients, ages 10 $\pm$ 3 years, with a mean interval since transplantation of 3.4 $\pm$ 2.5 years, and with pretherapy histologic findings of either normal bone formation or adynamic bone on transiliac bone biopsies [141]. BMD Z-scores, corrected for height age, decreased in the control group from 0.01 $\pm$ 1.0 to -0.30 ± 1.2 over the 12-month interval. In contrast, the baseline and 12-month values were 1.1 $\pm$ 1.3 and 0.7 $\pm$ 0.8 in the patients treated with growth hormone. Repeat transiliac bone biopsy results for bone formation rates did not increase with growth hormone treatment. This small study suggests that growth hormone protects against bone loss, but may not promote bone formation in prepubertal children with a functioning kidney transplant. Future studies in adolescents are indicated to evaluate effects of bone structure and density. Of note, growth hormone should be used with caution in patients with chronic kidney disease and uncontrolled secondary hyperparathyroidism.

D. Lowest Effect Glucocorticoid Dose

The adverse effects of glucocorticoids on growth in renal allograft recipients are highlighted by reports of improved growth in patients receiving cyclosporine monotherapy [142] or following discontinuation of glucocorticoids [143]. Similarly, studies in liver and heart transplant recipients suggest that the avoidance of glucocorticoid therapy and the withdrawal of glucocorticoids are associated with improved growth [11, 144]. While the impact of glucocorticoid withdrawal on BMD has not been assessed in a controlled trial, it is noteworthy that the liver transplant recipients described by Okajima et al., who were taken off glucocorticoids at six months, manifested dramatic improvements in linear growth and BMD [21]. Prevention of transplant bone disease should therefore include use of the lowest effective glucocorticoid dose, if any are needed.

E. Bisphosphonates

The beneficial effects of bisphosphonates in adults with postmenopausal osteoporosis and glucocorticoid-induced osteoporosis are well recognized. However, concerns regarding the impact on the structure of the modeling skeleton initially tempered enthusiasm for these medications in children. Bisphosphonate therapy results in distinctive radiographic metaphyseal bands in children, but the significance of these bands is uncertain. Pamidronate proved effective in uncontrolled observational studies of children with osteogenesis imperfecta; bone density and size increased and the incidence of fractures decreased [145–147]. The treatment did not alter fracture healing, growth rate, or growth plate appearances. A recent report of osteopetrosis in a child treated with a cumulative pamidronate dose approximately seven times greater than recommended raised concerns regarding the safety of this treatment in growing children [148, 149]. Similar complications have not been observed in children on lower doses [150].

More recently, bisphosphonate therapy has been described in small numbers of children with varied diagnoses, such as connective tissue disorder [151], rheumatic diseases [152], and McCune-Albright syndrome [153]. To our knowledge, only one placebo-controlled clinical trial assessing the safety and efficacy of intravenous pamidronate to treat osteopenia has been performed in children [154]. Henderson et al. treated 6 pairs of children over an 18-month interval. Pamidronate resulted in an 89% increase in BMD of the distal femur, compared with 9% in the control group. Age-normalized Z-scores increased from a mean of −4.0 to −1.8 in the pamidronate group and did not significantly change in the control group (−4.2 to −4.0).

Available data on the long-term effects of bisphosphonates are insufficient to recommend its routine use in pediatric transplant recipients, especially in renal transplant patients at risk for adynamic bone disease. However, future studies may demonstrate an important role for this treatment in patients requiring long-term glucocorticoid therapy.

VIII. SUMMARY

In conclusion, pediatric allograft recipients are at risk for impaired bone mineral accrual, largely due to preexisting bone disease and subsequent glucocorticoid therapy. The impact of transplantation on cortical and trabecular structure, microarchitecture, volumetric density, and turnover are poorly understood, however, largely because of the limitations of DXA technology. Future studies employing QCT and bone histomorphometry are needed to fully appreciate the magnitude of transplant bone disease in children.

The marked increases in height and BMD recently demonstrated in liver transplant recipients provides hope that these children may recover bone deficits and ultimately achieve a normal bone mass. The key to the recovery observed in this population may lie in their young age at transplantation, and the withdrawal of glucocorticoids within six months of transplantation. Alternative therapies may be needed in the adolescent transplant recipient requiring ongoing glucocorticoid therapy. Currently, the prevention of bone disease is best accomplished by providing adequate, but not excessive, calcium and vitamin D stores, and by encouraging physical activity prior to and after transplantation, along with using the minimum effective glucocorticoid dose. Prospective trials of therapeutic agents need to be performed to assess efficacy and safety in the developing skeleton.

REFERENCES

1. Bailey, D.A., McKay, H.A., Mirwald, R.L., Crocker, P.R., and Faulkner, R.A. (1999). A six-year longitudinal study of the relationship of physical activity to bone mineral accrual in growing children: the university of Saskatchewan bone mineral accrual study. *J Bone Miner Res.* 14(10):1672–1679.
2. NIH. (2000). *Osteoporosis prevention, diagnosis, and therapy.* NIH Consensus Statement. 17(1):1–36.
3. University Renal Research and Education Association; United Network for Organ Sharing. 2002 Annual Report of the U.S. Organ Procurement and Transplantation Network and the Scientific Registry of Transplant Recipients: Transplant Data 1992-2001. (2002). from http://www.ustransplant.org/annual.html.
4. Colombani, P.M., Dunn, S. P., Harmon, W.E., Magee, J.C., McDiarmid, S.V., and Spray, T. L. (2003). Pediatric transplantation. *Am J Transplant.* 3 Suppl 4:53–63.
5. Smith, J.M., Ho, P.L., and McDonald, R.A. (2002). Renal transplant outcomes in adolescents: a report of the North American Pediatric Renal Transplant Cooperative Study. *Pediatr Transplant.* 6(6):493–499.
6. Nevins, T. E. (2002). Non-compliance and its management in teenagers. *Pediatr Transplant.* 6(6):475–479.
7. Boucek, M.M., Faro, A., Novick, R.J., Bennett, L.E., Keck, B.M., and Hosenpud, J.D. (2001). The Registry of the International Society for Heart and Lung Transplantation: Fourth Official Pediatric Report—2000. *J Heart Lung Transplant.* 20(1):39–52.
8. North American Pediatric Renal Transplant Cooperative Study Annual Report. (2003). Rockville, MD: Emmes Corporation.
9. Langman, C.B., Mazur, A.T., Baron, R., and Norman, M.E. (1982). 25-hydroxyvitamin D3 (calcifediol) therapy of juvenile renal osteodystrophy: beneficial effect on linear growth velocity. *J Pediatr.* 100(5):815–820.
10. Sanchez, C.P., and Salusky, I.B. (1996). The renal bone diseases in children treated with dialysis. *Adv Ren Replace Ther.* 3(1):14–23.

11. Fine, R.N. (2002). Growth following solid-organ transplantation. *Pediatr Transplant.* 6(1):47–52.
12. Bucuvalas, J.C., Horn, J.A., and Chernausek, S.D. (1997). Resistance to growth hormone in children with chronic liver disease. *Pediatr Transplant.* 1(1):73–79.
13. Bucuvalas, J.C., Horn, J.A., Slusher, J., Alfaro, M.P., and Chernausek, S. D. (1996). Growth hormone insensitivity in children with biliary atresia. *J Pediatr Gastroenterol Nutr.* 23(2):135–140.
14. Collier, J.D., Ninkovic, M., and Compston, J.E. (2002). Guidelines on the management of osteoporosis associated with chronic liver disease. *Gut.* 50 Suppl 1:i1–9.
15. Compston, J.E. (1986). Hepatic osteodystrophy: vitamin D metabolism in patients with liver disease. *Gut.* 27(9):1073–1090.
16. Shiomi, S., Nishiguchi, S., Kubo, S., Tamori, A., Habu, D., Takeda, T., and Ochi, H. (2002). Vitamin K2 (menatetrenone) for bone loss in patients with cirrhosis of the liver. *Am J Gastroenterol.* 97(4):978–981.
17. Argao, E.A., Specker, B.L., and Heubi, J.E. (1993). Bone mineral content in infants and children with chronic cholestatic liver disease. *Pediatrics.* 91(6):1151–1154.
18. Andrews, W.S., Pau, C.M., Chase, H.P., Foley, L.C., and Lilly, J.R. (1981). Fat soluble vitamin deficiency in biliary atresia. *J Pediatr Surg.* 16(3):284–290.
19. Heubi, J.E., Higgins, J.V., Argao, E.A., Sierra, R.I., and Specker, B.L. (1997). The role of magnesium in the pathogenesis of bone disease in childhood cholestatic liver disease: a preliminary report. *J Pediatr Gastroenterol Nutr.* 25(3):301–306.
20. Chongsrisawat, V., Ruttanamongkol, P., Chaiwatanarat, T., Chandrakamol, B., and Poovorawan, Y. (2001). Bone density and 25-hydroxyvitamin D level in extrahepatic biliary atresia. *Pediatr Surg Int.* 17(8):604–608.
21. Okajima, H., Shigeno, C., Inomata, Y., Egawa, H., Uemoto, S., Asonuma, K., Kiuchi, T., Konishi, J., and Tanaka, K. (2003). Long-term effects of liver transplantation on bone mineral density in children with end-stage liver disease: a 2-year prospective study. *Liver Transpl.* 9(4):360–364.
22. Glasgow, J.F., and Thomas, P.S. (1976). The osteodystrophy of prolonged obstructive liver disease in childhood. *Acta Paediatr Scand.* 65(1):57–64.
23. Hill, S.A., Kelly, D.A., and John, P.R. (1995). Bone fractures in children undergoing orthotopic liver transplantation. *Pediatr Radiol.* 25 Suppl 1:S112–117.
24. Kayler, L.K., Rasmussen, C.S., Dykstra, D.M., Punch, J.D., Rudich, S.M., Magee, J.C., Maraschio, M.A., Arenas, J.D., Campbell, D.A., Jr., and Merion, R.M. (2003). Liver transplantation in children with metabolic disorders in the United States. *Am J Transplant.* 3(3):334–339.
25. Ring, E., Wendler, H., Ratschek, M., and Zobel, G. (1989). Bone disease of primary hyperoxaluria in infancy. *Pediatr Radiol.* 20(1-2):131–133.
26. Rego, C., Guerra, A., Guardiano, M., Esteves, P., Pereira, J., Aguiar, A., and Areias, J. C. (2002). Bony density in adolescents after surgical repair of tetralogy of fallot: a comparative study with healthy adolescents. *Cardiol Young.* 12(6):531–536.
27. Marino, B.S. (2002). Outcomes after the Fontan procedure. *Curr Opin Pediatr.* 14(5):620–626.
28. Jenkins, P.C., Flanagan, M.F., Jenkins, K.J., Sargent, J.D., Canter, C.E., Chinnock, R.E., Vincent, R.N., and O'Connor, G.T. (2004). Morbidities in patients with hypoplastic left heart syndrome. *Pediatr Cardiol.* 25(1):3–10.
29. Larson, C.M., and Henderson, R.C. (2000). Bone mineral density and fractures in boys with Duchenne muscular dystrophy. *J Pediatr Orthop.* 20(1):71–74.
30. Nucci, A.M., Reyes, J., Yaworski, J.A., Mazariegos, G., Beserock, N., and Barksdale, E.M., Jr. (2003). Serum growth factors and growth indices pre- and post-pediatric intestinal transplantation. *J Pediatr Surg.* 38(7):1043–1047.
31. Colomb, V., Dabbas, M., Goulet, O., Talbotec, C., Corriol, O., and Ricour, C. (2002). Prepubertal growth in children with long-term parenteral nutrition. *Horm Res.* 58 Suppl 1:2–6.

32. Touloukian, R.J., and Gertner, J.M. (1981). Vitamin D deficiency rickets as a late complication of the short gut syndrome during infancy. *J Pediatr Surg.* 16(3):230–235.
33. Teitelbaum, D.H., and Tracy, T. (2001). Parenteral nutrition-associated cholestasis. *Semin Pediatr Surg.* 10(2):72–80.
34. von Wowern, N., Klausen, B., and Hylander, E. (1996). Bone loss and oral state in patients on home parenteral nutrition. *JPEN J Parenter Enteral Nutr.* 20(2):105–109.
35. Dellert, S.F., Farrell, M.K., Specker, B.L., and Heubi, J.E. (1998). Bone mineral content in children with short bowel syndrome after discontinuation of parental nutrition. *J Pediatr.* 132(3 Pt 1):516–519.
36. Aris, R.M., Renner, J.B., Winders, A.D., Buell, H.E., Riggs, D.B., Lester, G.E., and Ontjes, D. A. (1998). Increased rate of fractures and severe kyphosis: sequelae of living into adulthood with cystic fibrosis. *Ann Intern Med.* 128(3):186–193.
37. Aris, R.M., Neuringer, I.P., Weiner, M.A., Egan, T.M., and Ontjes, D. (1996). Severe osteoporosis before and after lung transplantation. *Chest.* 109(5):1176–1183.
38. Greer, R.M., Buntain, H.M., Potter, J.M., Wainwright, C.E., Wong, J.C., O'Rourke, P.K., Francis, P.W., Bell, S.C., and Batch, J.A. (2003). Abnormalities of the PTH-vitamin D axis and bone turnover markers in children, adolescents and adults with cystic fibrosis: comparison with healthy controls. *Osteoporos Int.* 14(5):404–411.
39. Baroncelli, G.I., De Luca, F., Magazzu, G., Arrigo, T., Sferlazzas, C., Catena, C., Bertelloni, S., and Saggese, G. (1997). Bone demineralization in cystic fibrosis: evidence of imbalance between bone formation and degradation. *Pediatr Res.* 41(3):397–403.
40. Bhudhikanok, G.S., Lim, J., Marcus, R., Harkins, A., Moss, R.B., and Bachrach, L.K. (1996). Correlates of osteopenia in patients with cystic fibrosis. *Pediatrics.* 97(1): 103–111.
41. Bhudhikanok, G. S., Wang, M.C., Marcus, R., Harkins, A., Moss, R.B., and Bachrach, L. K. (1998). Bone acquisition and loss in children and adults with cystic fibrosis: a longitudinal study. *J Pediatr.* 133(1):18–27.
42. Henderson, R.C., and Madsen, C.D. (1996). Bone density in children and adolescents with cystic fibrosis. *J Pediatr.* 128(1):28–34.
43. Gibbens, D.T., Gilsanz, V., Boechat, M.I., Dufer, D., Carlson, M.E., and Wang, C.I. (1988). Osteoporosis in cystic fibrosis. *J Pediatr.* 113(2):295–300.
44. McDiarmid, S.V., Gornbein, J.A., DeSilva, P.J., Goss, J.A., Vargas, J.H., Martin, M.G., Ament, M.E., and Busuttil, R.W. (1999). Factors affecting growth after pediatric liver transplantation. *Transplantation.* 67(3):404–411.
45. Chinnock, R., and Baum, M. (1998). Somatic growth in infant heart transplant recipients. *Pediatr Transplant.* 2(1):30–34.
46. de Broux, E., Huot, C. H., Chartrand, S., Vobecky, S., and Chartrand, C. (2000). Growth and pubertal development following pediatric heart transplantation: a 15-year experience at Ste-Justine Hospital. *J Heart Lung Transplant.* 19(9):825–833.
47. Pradhan, M., Leonard, M.B., Bridges, N.D., and Jabs, K.L. (2002). Decline in renal function following thoracic organ transplantation in children. *Am J Transplant.* 2(7): 652–657.
48. Neau-Cransac, M., Morel, D., Bernard, P.H., Merville, P., Revel, P., Potaux, L., and Saric, J. (2002). Renal failure after liver transplantation: outcome after calcineurin inhibitor withdrawal. *Clin Transplant.* 16(5):368–373.
49. Frost, H.M., and Schonau, E. (2000). The "muscle-bone unit" in children and adolescents: a 2000 overview. *J Pediatr Endocrinol Metab.* 13(6):571–590.
50. Petit, M.A., McKay, H.A., MacKelvie, K.J., Heinonen, A., Khan, K.M., and Beck, T.J. (2002). A randomized school-based jumping intervention confers site and maturity-specific benefits on bone structural properties in girls: a hip structural analysis study. *J Bone Miner Res.* 17(3):363–372.
51. Specker, B., and Binkley, T. (2003). Randomized trial of physical activity and calcium supplementation on bone mineral content in 3- to 5-year-old children. *J Bone Miner Res.* 18(5):885–892.

52. Painter, P.L., Luetkemeier, M.J., Moore, G.E., Dibble, S.L., Green, G.A., Myll, J.O., and Carlson, L. L. (1997). Health-related fitness and quality of life in organ transplant recipients. *Transplantation.* 64(12):1795–1800.
53. Horber, F.F., Hoppeler, H., Herren, D., Claassen, H., Howald, H., Gerber, C., and Frey, F. J. (1986). Altered skeletal muscle ultrastructure in renal transplant patients on prednisone. *Kidney Int.* 30(3):411–416.
54. Braith, R.W., Limacher, M.C., Leggett, S. H., and Pollock, M.L. (1993). Skeletal muscle strength in heart transplant recipients. *J Heart Lung Transplant.* 12(6 Pt 1): 1018–1023.
55. Stephenson, A.L., Yoshida, E.M., Abboud, R.T., Fradet, G., and Levy, R.D. (2001). Impaired exercise performance after successful liver transplantation. *Transplantation.* 72(6):1161–1164.
56. Painter, P.L., Hector, L., Ray, K., Lynes, L., Dibble, S., Paul, S.M., Tomlanovich, S.L., and Ascher, N. L. (2002). A randomized trial of exercise training after renal transplantation. *Transplantation.* 74(1):42–48.
57. Mitchell, M.J., Baz, M.A., Fulton, M.N., Lisor, C.F., and Braith, R.W. (2003). Resistance training prevents vertebral osteoporosis in lung transplant recipients. *Transplantation.* 76(3):557–562.
58. Braith, R.W., Magyari, P.M., Fulton, M.N., Aranda, J., Walker, T., and Hill, J.A. (2003). Resistance exercise training and alendronate reverse glucocorticoid-induced osteoporosis in heart transplant recipients. *J Heart Lung Transplant.* 22(10):1082–1090.
59. Unnithan, V.B., Veehof, S.H., Rosenthal, P., Mudge, C., O'Brien, T.H., and Painter, P. (2001). Fitness testing of pediatric liver transplant recipients. *Liver Transpl.* 7(3):206–212.
60. Pastore, E., Turchetta, A., Attias, L., Calzolari, A., Giordano, U., Squitieri, C., and Parisi, F. (2001). Cardiorespiratory functional assessment after pediatric heart transplantation. *Pediatr Transplant.* 5(6):425–429.
61. Nixon, P.A., Fricker, F.J., Noyes, B.E., Webber, S.A., Orenstein, D.M., and Armitage, J. M. (1995). Exercise testing in pediatric heart, heart-lung, and lung transplant recipients. *Chest.* 107(5):1328–1335.
62. Feber, J., Dupuis, J.M., Chapuis, F., Braillon, P., Jocteur-Monrozier, D., Daudet, G., So, S., Levrey, H., Hadj-Aissa, A., Martin, X., Bellon, G., and Cochat, P. (1997). Body composition and physical performance in children after renal transplantation. *Nephron.* 75(1):13–19.
63. Studies of Pediatric Liver Transplantation: Annual Report. (2003). Rockville, MD: Emmes Corporation.
64. Sarwal, M.M., Vidhun, J.R., Alexander, S.R., Satterwhite, T., Millan, M., and Salvatierra, O., Jr. (2003). Continued superior outcomes with modification and lengthened follow-up of a steroid-avoidance pilot with extended daclizumab induction in pediatric renal transplantation. *Transplantation.* 76(9):1331–1339.
65. Canalis, E., Pereira, R.C., and Delany, A.M. (2002). Effects of glucocorticoids on the skeleton. *J Pediatr Endocrinol Metab.* 15 Suppl 5:1341–1345.
66. Rodino, M.A., and Shane, E. (1998). Osteoporosis after organ transplantation. *Am J Med.* 104(5):459–469.
67. Ortoft, G., Andreassen, T.T., and Oxlund, H. (1999). Growth hormone increases cortical and cancellous bone mass in young growing rats with glucocorticoid-induced osteopenia. *J Bone Miner Res.* 14(5):710–721.
68. WHO. (1994). The WHO Study Group: Assessment of fracture risk and its application to screening for postmenopausal osteoporosis. Geneva, Switzerland.
69. Khosla, S., Melton, L.J., 3rd, Dekutoski, M.B., Achenbach, S.J., Oberg, A.L., and Riggs, B. L. (2003). Incidence of childhood distal forearm fractures over 30 years: a population-based study. *Jama.* 290(11):1479–1485.
70. Chan, G.M., Hess, M., Hollis, J., and Book, L.S. (1984). Bone mineral status in childhood accidental fractures. *Am J Dis Child.* 138(6):569–570.
71. Goulding, A., Cannan, R., Williams, S.M., Gold, E.J., Taylor, R.W., and Lewis-Barned, N. J. (1998). Bone mineral density in girls with forearm fractures. *J Bone Miner Res.* 13(1):143–148.

72. Goulding, A., Jones, I.E., Taylor, R.W., Williams, S.M., and Manning, P.J. (2001). Bone mineral density and body composition in boys with distal forearm fractures: a dual-energy x-ray absorptiometry study. *J Pediatr.* 139(4):509–515.
73. Goulding, A., Jones, I.E., Taylor, R.W., Manning, P.J., and Williams, S.M. (2000). More broken bones: a 4-year double cohort study of young girls with and without distal forearm fractures. *J Bone Miner Res.* 15(10):2011–2018.
74. Ma, D., and Jones, G. (2003). The association between bone mineral density, metacarpal morphometry, and upper limb fractures in children: a population-based case-control study. *J Clin Endocrinol Metab.* 88(4):1486–1491.
75. Ma, D.Q., and Jones, G. (2002). Clinical risk factors but not bone density are associated with prevalent fractures in prepubertal children. *J Paediatr Child Health.* 38(5): 497–500.
76. Cook, S.D., Harding, A.F., Morgan, E.L., Doucet, H.J., Bennett, J.T., O'Brien, M., and Thomas, K.A. (1987). Association of bone mineral density and pediatric fractures. *J Pediatr Orthop.* 7(4):424–427.
77. Skaggs, D.L., Loro, M.L., Pitukcheewanont, P., Tolo, V., and Gilsanz, V. (2001). Increased body weight and decreased radial cross-sectional dimensions in girls with forearm fractures. *J Bone Miner Res.* 16(7):1337–1342.
78. Ma, D., and Jones, G. (2003). Television, computer, and video viewing; physical activity; and upper limb fracture risk in children: a population-based case control study. *J Bone Miner Res.* 18(11):1970–1977.
79. Ellis, K.J., Shypailo, R.J., Hardin, D.S., Perez, M.D., Motil, K.J., Wong, W.W., and Abrams, S. A. (2001). Z score prediction model for assessment of bone mineral content in pediatric diseases. *J Bone Miner Res.* 16(9):1658–1664.
80. Molgaard, C., Thomsen, B.L., Prentice, A., Cole, T.J., and Michaelsen, K.F. (1997). Whole body bone mineral content in healthy children and adolescents. *Arch Dis Child.* 76(1):9–15.
81. Binkley, T.L., Specker, B.L., and Wittig, T.A. (2002). Centile curves for bone densitometry measurements in healthy males and females ages 5-22 yr. *J Clin Densitom.* 5(4):343–353.
82. Hannan, W.J., Tothill, P., Cowen, S.J., and Wrate, R.M. (1998). Whole body bone mineral content in healthy children and adolescents. *Arch Dis Child.* 78(4):396–397.
83. Maynard, L.M., Guo, S.S., Chumlea, W.C., Roche, A.F., Wisemandle, W.A., Zeller, C.M., Towne, B., and Siervogel, R.M. (1998). Total-body and regional bone mineral content and areal bone mineral density in children aged 8-18 y: the Fels Longitudinal Study. *Am J Clin Nutr.* 68(5):1111–1117.
84. van der Sluis, I.M., de Ridder, M.A., Boot, A.M., Krenning, E.P., and de Muinck Keizer-Schrama, S.M. (2002). Reference data for bone density and body composition measured with dual energy x ray absorptiometry in white children and young adults. *Arch Dis Child.* 87(4):341–347.
85. Southard, R.N., Morris, J.D., Mahan, J.D., Hayes, J.R., Torch, M.A., Sommer, A., and Zipf, W.B. (1991). Bone mass in healthy children: measurement with quantitative DXA. *Radiology.* 179(3):735–738.
86. Faulkner, R.A., Bailey, D.A., Drinkwater, D.T., McKay, H.A., Arnold, C., and Wilkinson, A.A. (1996). Bone densitometry in Canadian children 8-17 years of age. *Calcif Tissue Int.* 59(5):344–351.
87. Glastre, C., Braillon, P., David, L., Cochat, P., Meunier, P.J., and Delmas, P.D. (1990). Measurement of bone mineral content of the lumbar spine by dual energy x-ray absorptiometry in normal children: correlations with growth parameters. *J Clin Endocrinol Metab.* 70(5):1330–1333.
88. Bonjour, J.P., Theintz, G., Buchs, B., Slosman, D., and Rizzoli, R. (1991). Critical years and stages of puberty for spinal and femoral bone mass accumulation during adolescence. *J Clin Endocrinol Metab.* 73(3):555–563.

89. del Rio, L., Carrascosa, A., Pons, F., Gusinye, M., Yeste, D., and Domenech, F.M. (1994). Bone mineral density of the lumbar spine in white Mediterranean Spanish children and adolescents: changes related to age, sex, and puberty. *Pediatr Res.* 35(3):362–366.
90. Plotkin, H., Nunez, M., Alvarez Filgueira, M.L., and Zanchetta, J.R. (1996). Lumbar spine bone density in Argentine children. *Calcif Tissue Int.* 58(3):144–149.
91. Braillon, P.M., and Cochat, P. (1998). Analysis of dual energy X-ray absorptiometry whole body results in children, adolescents and young adults. *Appl Radiat Isot.* 49(5-6):623–624.
92. Leonard, M.B., Propert, K.J., Zemel, B.S., Stallings, V.A., and Feldman, H.I. (1999). Discrepancies in pediatric bone mineral density reference data: potential for misdiagnosis of osteopenia. *J Pediatr.* 135(2 Pt 1):182–188.
93. Leonard, M.B., Feldman, H.I., Zemel, B.S., Berlin, J.A., Barden, E.M., and Stallings, V.A. (1998). Evaluation of low density spine software for the assessment of bone mineral density in children. *J Bone Miner Res.* 13(11):1687–1690.
94. Carter, D.R., Bouxsein, M.L., and Marcus, R. (1992). New approaches for interpreting projected bone densitometry data. *J Bone Miner Res.* 7(2):137–145.
95. Kroger, H., Vainio, P., Nieminen, J., and Kotaniemi, A. (1995). Comparison of different models for interpreting bone mineral density measurements using DXA and MRI technology. *Bone.* 17(2):157–159.
96. Leonard, M.B., Shults, J., Elliott, D.M., Stallings, V.A., and Zemel, B.S. (2004). Interpretation of whole body DXA in the assessment of cortical bone health in children: validation with peripheral *QTC Bone.* 34:1044–1052.
97. Parfitt, A.M. (1998). A structural approach to renal bone disease. *J Bone Miner Res.* 13(8):1213–1220.
98. Yamaguchi, T., Kanno, E., Tsubota, J., Shiomi, T., Nakai, M., and Hattori, S. (1996). Retrospective study on the usefulness of radius and lumbar bone density in the separation of hemodialysis patients with fractures from those without fractures. *Bone.* 19(5):549–555.
99. Jamal, S.A., Chase, C., Goh, Y.I., Richardson, R., and Hawker, G.A. (2002). Bone density and heel ultrasound testing do not identify patients with dialysis-dependent renal failure who have had fractures. *Am J Kidney Dis.* 39(4):843–849.
100. Gilsanz, V. (1998). Bone density in children: a review of the available techniques and indications. *Eur J Radiol.* 26(2):177–182.
101. Ferretti, J.L. (1995). Perspectives of pQCT technology associated to biomechanical studies in skeletal research employing rat models. *Bone.* 17(4 Suppl):353S–364S.
102. Leonard, M.B., and Zemel, B.S. (2002). Current concepts in pediatric bone disease. *Pediatr Clin North Am.* 49(1):143–173.
103. Argao, E.A., Balistreri, W.F., Hollis, B.W., Ryckman, F.C., and Heubi, J.E. (1994). Effect of orthotopic liver transplantation on bone mineral content and serum vitamin D metabolites in infants and children with chronic cholestasis. *Hepatology.* 20(3):598–603.
104. Ulivieri, F.M., Lisciandrano, D., Gridelli, B., Lucianetti, A., Roggero, P., Nebbia, G., Cataliotti, E., Prato, P., di Mauro, P., Campanini, F., and Vezzoli, M. (1999). Bone mass and body composition in children with chronic cholestasis before and after liver transplantation. *Transplant Proc.* 31(5):2131–2134.
105. D'Antiga, L., Moniz, C., Buxton-Thomas, M., Cheeseman, P., Gray, B., Abraha, H., Baker, A.J., Heaton, N.D., Rela, M., Mieli-Vergani, G., and Dhawan, A. (2002). Bone mineral density and height gain in children with chronic cholestatic liver disease undergoing transplantation. *Transplantation.* 73(11):1788–1793.
106. Guthery, S.L., Pohl, J.F., Bucuvalas, J.C., Alonso, M.H., Ryckman, F.C., Balistreri, W.F., and Heubi, J.E. (2003). Bone mineral density in long-term survivors following pediatric liver transplantation. *Liver Transpl.* 9(4):365–370.
107. Braith, R.W., Howard, C., Fricker, F.J., Mitchell, M., and Edwards, D.G. (2000). Glucocorticoid-induced osteopenia in adolescent heart transplant recipients. *J Heart Lung Transplant.* 19(9):840–845.

108. Daniels, M.W., Wilson, D.M., Paguntalan, H.G., Hoffman, A.R., and Bachrach, L.K. (2003). Bone mineral density in pediatric transplant recipients. *Transplantation.* 76(4):673–678.
109. Feber, J., Braillon, P., David, L., and Cochat, P. (2001). Body composition in children after renal transplantation. *Am J Kidney Dis.* 38(2):366–370.
110. Bartosh, S.M., Leverson, G., Robillard, D., and Sollinger, H.W. (2003). Long-term outcomes in pediatric renal transplant recipients who survive into adulthood. *Transplantation.* 76(8):1195–1200.
111. Ferraris, J.R., Pasqualini, T., Legal, S., Sorroche, P., Galich, A.M., Pennisi, P., Domene, H., and Jasper, H. (2000). Effect of deflazacort versus methylprednisone on growth, body composition, lipid profile, and bone mass after renal transplantation. The Deflazacort Study Group. *Pediatr Nephrol.* 14(7):682–688.
112. Reusz, G.S., Szabo, A.J., Peter, F., Kenesei, E., Sallay, P., Latta, K., Szabo, A., and Tulassay, T. (2000). Bone metabolism and mineral density following renal transplantation. *Arch Dis Child.* 83(2):146–151.
113. Klaus, G., Paschen, C., Wuster, C., Kovacs, G.T., Barden, J., Mehls, O., and Scharer, K. (1998). Weight-/height-related bone mineral density is not reduced after renal transplantation. *Pediatr Nephrol.* 12(5):343–348.
114. Sanchez, C.P., Salusky, I.B., Kuizon, B.D., Ramirez, J.A., Gales, B., Ettenger, R.B., and Goodman, W.G. (1998). Bone disease in children and adolescents undergoing successful renal transplantation. *Kidney Int.* 53(5):1358–1364.
115. Saland, J.M., Goode, M.L., Haas, D.L., Romano, T.A., and Seikaly, M.G. (2001). The prevalence of osteopenia in pediatric renal allograft recipients varies with the method of analysis. *Am J Transplant.* 1(3):243–250.
116. el-Husseini, A.A., el-Agroudy, A.E., Sobh, M.A., and Ghoneim, M.A. (2003). Bone loss in pediatric renal transplant recipients. *Nefrologia.* 23 Suppl 2:131–134.
117. Zimakas, P.J., Sharma, A.K., and Rodd, C.J. (2003). Osteopenia and fractures in cystinotic children post renal transplantation. *Pediatr Nephrol.* 18(4):384–390.
118. Schoenau, E., Neu, C.M., Beck, B., Manz, F., and Rauch, F. (2002). Bone mineral content per muscle cross-sectional area as an index of the functional muscle-bone unit. *J Bone Miner Res.* 17(6):1095–1101.
119. Ellis, E.N. (2000). Risk factors for bone mineral density loss in pediatric renal transplant patients. *Pediatric Transplantation.* 4(2):146–150.
120. Leonard, M.B., and Bachrach, L.K. (2001). Assessment of bone mineralization following renal transplantation in children: limitations of DXA and the confounding effects of delayed growth and development. *Am J Transplant.* 1(3):193–196.
121. Leonard, M.B., Shults, J., Wilson, B.A., Stallings, V.A., and Zemel, B.S. (2004). Obesity during childhood and adolescence augments bone mass and bone dimensions. *Am J Clin Nutr.* In press.
122. Cadogan, J., Eastell, R., Jones, N., and Barker, M.E. (1997). Milk intake and bone mineral acquisition in adolescent girls: randomised, controlled intervention trial. *Bmj.* 315(7118):1255–1260.
123. Chan, G.M., Hoffman, K., and McMurry, M. (1995). Effects of dairy products on bone and body composition in pubertal girls. *J Pediatr.* 126(4):551–556.
124. Johnston, C.C., Jr., Miller, J.Z., Slemenda, C.W., Reister, T.K., Hui, S., Christian, J.C., and Peacock, M. (1992). Calcium supplementation and increases in bone mineral density in children. *N Engl J Med.* 327(2):82–87.
125. Lee, W.T., Leung, S.S., Wang, S.H., Xu, Y.C., Zeng, W. P., Lau, J., Oppenheimer, S.J., and Cheng, J.C. (1994). Double-blind, controlled calcium supplementation and bone mineral accretion in children accustomed to a low-calcium diet. *Am J Clin Nutr.* 60(5): 744–750.
126. Lloyd, T., Andon, M.B., Rollings, N., Martel, J.K., Landis, J.R., Demers, L.M., Eggli, D.F., Kieselhorst, K., and Kulin, H.E. (1992). Calcium supplementation and bone mineral density in adolescent children. *New England Journal of Medicine.* 327:82–87.

127. Bonjour, J.P., Carrie, A.L., Ferrari, S., Clavien, H., Slosman, D., Theintz, G., and Rizzoli, R. (1997). Calcium-enriched foods and bone mass growth in prepubertal girls: a randomized, double-blind, placebo-controlled trial. *J Clin Invest.* 99(6): 1287–1294.
128. NIH. (1994). NIH Consensus Development Panel on Optimal Calcium Intake. *JAMA*. 272:1942–1948.
129. Food and Nutrition Board, Institute of Medicine. (1997). Dietary reference intakes for calcium, phosphorus, magnesium, vitamin D, and fluoride. Washington, D.C.: National Academy Press.
130. Alaimo, K., McDowell, M. A., Briefel, R.R., Bischof, A.M., Caughman, C.R., Loria, C.M., and Johnson, C.L. (1994). Dietary intake of vitamins, minerals, and fiber of persons ages 2 months and over in the United States: Third National Health and Nutrition Examination Survey, Phase 1, 1988–91. Adv Data(258), 1-28.
131. Chertow, G.M., Raggi, P., McCarthy, J.T., Schulman, G., Silberzweig, J., Kuhlik, A., Goodman, W.G., Boulay, A., Burke, S.K., and Toto, R.D. (2003). The effects of sevelamer and calcium acetate on proxies of atherosclerotic and arteriosclerotic vascular disease in hemodialysis patients. *Am J Nephrol.* 23(5):307–314.
132. Malabanan, A., Veronikis, I.E., and Holick, M.F. (1998). Redefining vitamin D insufficiency. *Lancet.* 351(9105):805–806.
133. Eknoyan, G., Levin, A., and Levin, N.W. (2003). Bone metabolism and disease in chronic kidney disease. *Am J Kidney Dis.* 42(4 Suppl 3):1–201.
134. Mukherjee, A., and Shalet, S.M. (2003). Growth hormone replacement therapy (GHRT) in children and adolescents: skeletal impact. *Med Pediatr Oncol.* 41(3):235–242.
135. Kassem, M., Mosekilde, L., and Eriksen, E.F. (1994). Growth hormone stimulates proliferation of normal human bone marrow stromal osteoblast precursor cells in vitro. *Growth Regul.* 4(3):131–135.
136. Nishiyama, K., Sugimoto, T., Kaji, H., Kanatani, M., Kobayashi, T., and Chihara, K. (1996). Stimulatory effect of growth hormone on bone resorption and osteoclast differentiation. *Endocrinology*. 137(1):35–41.
137. Boot, A.M., Engels, M.A., Boerma, G.J., Krenning, E.P., and De Muinck Keizer-Schrama, S.M. (1997). Changes in bone mineral density, body composition, and lipid metabolism during growth hormone (GH) treatment in children with GH deficiency. *J Clin Endocrinol Metab.* 82(8):2423–2428.
138. Bertelloni, S., Baroncelli, G.I., Ferdeghini, M., Perri, G., and Saggese, G. (1998). Normal volumetric bone mineral density and bone turnover in young men with histories of constitutional delay of puberty. *J Clin Endocrinol Metab.* 83(12):4280–4283.
139. Sarna, S., Sipila, I., Ronnholm, K., Koistinen, R., and Holmberg, C. (1996). Recombinant human growth hormone improves growth in children receiving glucocorticoid treatment after liver transplantation. *J Clin Endocrinol Metab.* 81(4):1476–1482.
140. Guest, G., Berard, E., Crosnier, H., Chevallier, T., Rappaport, R., and Broyer, M. (1998). Effects of growth hormone in short children after renal transplantation. French Society of Pediatric Nephrology. *Pediatr Nephrol.* 12(6):437–446.
141. Sanchez, C.P., Kuizon, B.D., Goodman, W.G., Gales, B., Ettenger, R.B., Boechat, M.I., Wang, Y., Elashoff, R., and Salusky, I.B. (2002). Growth hormone and the skeleton in pediatric renal allograft recipients. *Pediatr Nephrol.* 17(5):322–328.
142. Klare, B., Strom, T.M., Hahn, H., Engelsberger, I., Meusel, E., Illner, W.D., Abendroth, D., and Land, W. (1991). Remarkable long-term prognosis and excellent growth in kidney-transplant children under cyclosporine monotherapy. *Transplant Proc.* 23(1 Pt 2):1013–1017.
143. Soran, A., Shapiro, R., Basar, H., Vivas, C., Scantlebury, V.P., Jordan, M.L., Gritsch, H.A., McCauley, J., Randhawa, P., Hakala, T.R., and Fung, J.J. (1999). Outcome of kidney transplantation under tacrolimus-based immunosuppression in elderly patients. *J Transpl Coord.* 9(2):101–103.

144. Diem, H.V., Sokal, E.M., Janssen, M., Otte, J.B., and Reding, R. (2003). Steroid withdrawal after pediatric liver transplantation: a long-term follow-up study in 109 recipients. *Transplantation*. 75(10):1664–1670.
145. Rauch, F., Plotkin, H., Zeitlin, L., and Glorieux, F. H. (2003). Bone mass, size, and density in children and adolescents with osteogenesis imperfecta: effect of intravenous pamidronate therapy. *J Bone Miner Res*. 18(4):610–614.
146. Glorieux, F.H., Bishop, N.J., Plotkin, H., Chabot, G., Lanoue, G., and Travers, R. (1998). Cyclic administration of pamidronate in children with severe osteogenesis imperfecta. *N Engl J Med*. 339(14):947–952.
147. Glorieux, F.H. (2000). Bisphosphonate therapy for severe osteogenesis imperfecta. *J Pediatr Endocrinol Metab*. 13 Suppl 2:989–992.
148. Marini, J.C. (2003). Do bisphosphonates make children's bones better or brittle? *N Engl J Med*. 349(5):423–426.
149. Whyte, M.P., Wenkert, D., Clements, K.L., McAlister, W.H., and Mumm, S. (2003). Bisphosphonate-induced osteopetrosis. *N Engl J Med*. 349(5):457–463.
150. Glorieux, F.H., Rauch, F., and Shapiro, J.R. (2003). Bisphosphonates in children with bone diseases. *N Engl J Med*. 349(21):2068–2071; author reply 2068-2071.
151. Bianchi, M.L., Cimaz, R., Bardare, M., Zulian, F., Lepore, L., Boncompagni, A., Galbiati, E., Corona, F., Luisetto, G., Giuntini, D., Picco, P., Brandi, M.L., and Falcini, F. (2000). Efficacy and safety of alendronate for the treatment of osteoporosis in diffuse connective tissue diseases in children: a prospective multicenter study. *Arthritis Rheum*. 43(9):1960–1966.
152. Noguera, A., Ros, J.B., Pavia, C., Alcover, E., Valls, C., Villaronga, M., and Gonzalez, E. (2003). Bisphosphonates, a new treatment for glucocorticoid-induced osteoporosis in children. *J Pediatr Endocrinol Metab*. 16(4):529–536.
153. Matarazzo, P., Lala, R., Masi, G., Andreo, M., Altare, F., and de Sanctis, C. (2002). Pamidronate treatment in bone fibrous dysplasia in children and adolescents with McCune-Albright syndrome. *J Pediatr Endocrinol Metab*. 15 Suppl 3:929–937.
154. Henderson, R.C., Lark, R.K., Kecskemethy, H.H., Miller, F., Harcke, H.T., and Bachrach, S. J. (2002). Bisphosphonates to treat osteopenia in children with quadriplegic cerebral palsy: a randomized, placebo-controlled clinical trial. *J Pediatr*. 141(5): 644–651.
155. Roberts, J.P., Brown, R.S., Jr., Edwards, E.B., Farmer, D.G., Freeman, R.B., Jr., Wiesner, R.H., and Merion, R.M. (2003). Liver and intestine transplantation. *Am J Transplant*. 3 Suppl 4:78–90.
156. Pocock, N.A., Noakes, K.A., Majerovic, Y., and Griffiths, M.R. (1997). Magnification error of femoral geometry using fan beam densitometers. *Calcif Tissue Int*. 60(1):8–10.
157. McKay, H.A., Petit, M.A., Bailey, D.A., Wallace, W.M., Schutz, R.W., and Khan, K.M. (2000). Analysis of proximal femur DXA scans in growing children: comparisons of different protocols for cross-sectional 8-month and 7-year longitudinal data. *J Bone Miner Res*. 15(6):1181–1188.

PART IV

Management

CHAPTER 22

Management of Bone Disease in Candidates for Organ Transplant

Susan M. Ott, MD
Division of Metabolism, University of Washington, Seattle, WA

I. INTRODUCTION

Compared to the heart, lungs, kidney, or liver, the skeleton seems to be a stolid organ, which is therefore frequently ignored until it breaks. The bones are actually interesting, complex, and responsive to both mechanical and metabolic changes. In a high proportion of organ transplant recipients, metabolic abnormalities overwhelm the ability of the bone to respond to stress, with resulting structural failure and fractures. In many of these patients, bone disease was present before the transplant, and attention to skeletal risk factors in transplant candidates could reduce the frequency of fractures that occur after the transplant.

The popularity of machines that can measure bone mineral density has shifted the focus of bone health from true strength to radiographic density. When their bone density falls below a committee-defined threshold [1], patients are automatically labelled as having osteoporosis, without consideration of other bone diseases such as osteomalacia, adynamic bone disease, osteitis fibrosis, iron toxicity, or osteogenesis imperfecta. Even more dangerous is the assumption that bone is normal when the bone density is above the threshold, despite diseases that reduce the biomechanical strength of bone, such as fluorosis, osteopetrosis, bisphosphonate-induced osteosclerosis [2], or conditions with poor microarchitecture. Bone can fail in many ways, some of which are associated with low bone density and some of which are not. The bone diseases that result from end-stage hepatic or renal failure are complicated, and the treatments given to women with postmenopausal osteoporosis may not be effective, even when the patients have the same DEXA (dual energy x-ray absorptiometry) score. Furthermore, some of the usual therapeutic recommendations for prevention of osteoporosis do not apply to transplant candidates because they could have more serious side effects.

The relationship between risk factors and bone fractures is not the same in transplant recipients as in the general population. For example, the Study of Osteoporotic Fractures data predict that an 82-year-old woman with a hip DEXA T-score of −3.1 has a spine fracture risk of 18% in the next 5 years [3]. Many transplant patients who are younger and have higher bone density have a higher risk of fracture. This is illustrated by a patient whose risk factors are listed in Table 1, along with the most important risk factors for "ordinary" osteoporosis [4]. This patient did not have the profile usually associated with osteoporosis. His only identified risk factors were prednisone use and limited exercise. Because the bone density was normal, his transplant physicians did not think he was at high risk for any fractures, so preventive therapy was not prescribed. After his transplant, he developed 5 painful vertebral compression fractures within the first 8 months, shown in Figure 1.

Transplant recipients who don't appear to have many risk factors may nevertheless experience fractures, and those who do have "traditional" risk factors have an even greater chance of suffering from a fracture. It is therefore important to check these patients for both major and minor risk factors, and to correct those that are amenable to treatment. Because it is easier to prevent bone loss than it is to restore bone, optimization of factors that relate to bone health should be done as soon as possible.

II. ASSESSMENT OF BONE HEALTH THAT APPLIES TO ALL TRANSPLANT CANDIDATES

Transplant candidates should undergo evaluation of the general risk factors listed below. These apply to all transplant candidates; those with metabolic organ failure may need further specific evaluation.

1. Demographic risk factors
   - age
   - gender
   - race
2. Family history of fractures
3. Lifestyle factors
   - smoking
   - ethanol
   - calcium intake
   - physical activity
4. Medical history
   - any bone fractures
   - height loss
   - weight loss
   - symptoms of hypogonadism
   - history of hyperthyroidism
   - malabsorption

medication history:
- glucocorticoids
- thyroid hormone
- depomedroxyprogesterone
- GNRH agonists
- anticonvulsants
- loop diuretics
- heparin

neurological problems
balance disturbance
history of frequent falls

5. Physical findings
   - height
   - weight
   - kyphosis
   - ability to rise from chair
6. Radiographic studies
   - spine radiographs
   - bone densitometry
7. Laboratory studies
   - routine chemistry panel and blood count
   - calcium
   - phosphate
   - magnesium
   - albumin
   - 25 (OH)vitamin D
   - parathyroid hormone
   - testosterone (in men)
   - thyroid-stimulating hormone
   - 24-hour urine calcium

TABLE 1 Risk factors for osteoporotic fractures

Usual risk factors for osteoporotic fractures	A transplant candidate
Advanced age	44 years
Caucasian or Asian race	African-American
Female gender	Male
Low bone density	T-score at hip +0.2
Family history of osteoporosis	No family history
History of fragility fracture	Never had a fracture
Thin	180 pounds
Excessive use of alcohol	Does not drink alcohol
Cigarette smoking	Stopped smoking 2 years ago
Use of glucocorticoids	Prednisone for 7 years
Diet low in calcium	Drinks 4 glasses milk/day
Inadequate exercise	Exercise limited by breathing

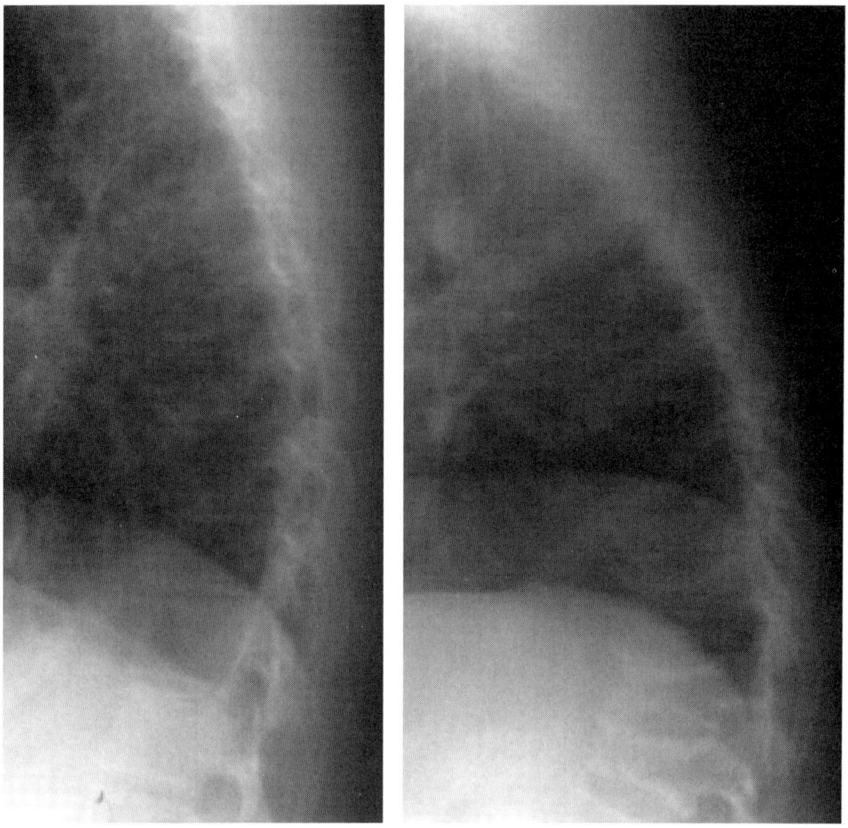

FIGURE 1 Chest x-ray from a patient before and after lung transplantation, showing development of kyphosis from multiple vertebral compression fractures. The bone density was normal before the transplant.

The biochemical indices of bone turnover can help assess bone physiology and response to treatment in some cases. The formation markers include bone specific alkaline phosphatase, osteocalcin, and propeptides of type I collagen. Resorption markers include serum or urine collagen crosslinks (N-telopeptide or C-telopeptide). The markers are altered by renal or hepatic disease, so the biochemical markers are more difficult to interpret in renal or hepatic osteodystrophy. Serum and urine protein electrophoresis should be measured if there is a possibility of myeloma causing fractures.

III. GENERAL MEASURES TO IMPROVE BONE STRENGTH

Many of the recommendations for improving bone health in the general population also apply to transplant candidates. There are, however, important differences for these patients, especially those who are candidates for liver or kidney transplantation. This section discusses general measures and is followed by sections discussing management of candidates for transplant of specific organs.

A. Nutrition

Nutrition is recognized as a vital component in any transplant program. Several individual nutrients are important for bone health, but the patient's overall weight is probably more influential than any of the individual nutrients. Thin people have lower bone density and increased risk of fractures. The ideal body weight for the skeleton is higher than it is for other systems, so there must be a trade-off between what is best for the bones and what is best for the other organs [5]. Clearly, patients who have a body mass index (BMI) lower than 19 are underweight and will benefit from increasing total caloric intake. Weight gain may be difficult in patients who are catabolic due to their underlying disease, or who have frequent infectious complications. Such patients need careful follow-up from nutritional support personnel, because they are also at a higher surgical risk. On the other hand, patients who are obese are usually advised to lose weight to reduce surgical risk, and weight loss is associated with bone loss, even in obese persons. There may be some attenuation of the bone loss associated with weight loss by extra calcium or measures to avoid acidosis [6, 7].

Calcium intake must be adequate for bone health; if intake is too low, bone resorption will increase to supply necessary calcium to the blood. The total calcium intake (diet plus supplements) should be between 1200 and 1500 mg/day [8]. Calcium is a threshold nutrient, and higher intakes do not result in any further benefit. When there is pathologically increased bone resorption, however, calcium intake might exacerbate hypercalcemia or hypercalciuria. These situations are unusual in transplant candidates except for occasional patients with end-stage renal disease and tertiary hyperparathyroidism, or patients with severe sarcoidosis and high levels of $1,25(OH)_2$-vitamin D levels.

The main dietary sources of calcium are usually dairy products, but these must be avoided in patients with renal failure and patients with hepatic failure who are on protein restriction. Supplements should be bioavailable, but studies of dissolution show that many brands (both expensive and inexpensive) do not dissolve sufficiently. OsCal was one brand with good dissolution, and TUMS or other chewable calcium carbonate tablets are bioavailable [9]. Calcium carbonate is better absorbed when taken with food, which also avoids any rebound gastric hyperacidity. Calcium citrate is absorbed as well as calcium carbonate except in fasting persons with achlorhydria. Radioisotope studies show that calcium carbonate and citrate have equivalent intestinal absorption but the urine calcium increases more readily following ingestion of calcium citrate. Calcium citrate is more expensive and thus should be used as a second choice in patients who don't like the other supplements [10]. In renal patients, however, calcium citrate should be avoided because citrate enhances the brain accumulation of aluminum.

Calcium is more effective when given in divided doses, at least twice a day. If patients are also taking iron or thyroid, the calcium should be taken at different times.

Proteins may slightly increase the urine calcium, but this modest negative effect is not as important as the need for adequate protein nutrition. Epidemiological studies have shown that low protein intakes are associated with a higher risk of fractures in elderly people [11]. Although protein restriction should not be recommended for bone health, it may be necessary in liver or renal failure. Thus, the recommended protein will depend on the underlying disease.

Magnesium is discussed and advertised much more often than it is studied. There have been no well-designed clinical trials of magnesium supplementation in postmenopausal osteoporosis. In the large observational study of the Women's Health Initiative, magnesium supplementation was associated with a higher risk of wrist fractures, and no protection from other fractures [12]. Magnesium supplementation therefore should not routinely be given to transplant candidates. After transplantation, antirejection medications may cause renal magnesium losses, and magnesium replacement may be required. It is interesting to notice, however, that the fracture rates in heart transplant recipients were higher in those with higher serum magnesium levels [13].

1. *Vitamin A*

In epidemiological studies, both bone density and fracture rates are increased with either high or low vitamin A intake [14, 15]. Many transplant candidates have vitamin A deficiency and need replacement. Others, however, may be taking more supplements than necessary. Sometimes those with low vitamin D levels are instructed to take 2 multiple vitamins a day, but that may lead to excess vitamin A.

B. Vitamin D

Vitamin D (cholecalciferol) is a steroid hormone that is typically discussed in nutrition sections. In young, healthy persons the major source of vitamin D is production in the skin, after exposure to the same spectrum of radiation that causes sunburn. This steroid is essential for bone health, and has actions on muscles and the immune system as well. Vitamin D levels should be measured on every transplant candidate, because deficiency is common, important, and easily corrected.

Vitamin D metabolism is abnormal in liver and kidney patients, and is discussed further later in this chapter. Patients with malabsorption, granulomatous disease, inherited rickets, or hypophosphatemia also have abnormal vitamin D and require different treatment.

In otherwise healthy persons, the levels of 25-hydroxy-vitamin D (25(OH)D) give a more accurate assessment of the vitamin D status than levels of 1,25-dihydroxy-vitamin D (1,25 $(OH)_2D$). This is partly because 1,25 $(OH)_2D$, the active metabolite, has a short half-life and may transiently be increased when there is moderate vitamin D deficiency [16].

In the last decade, investigators have suggested that the optimal levels of vitamin D are higher than previously recommended. Current target levels of 20 to 40 ng/mL (51 to 102 nmol/L) suppress hyperparathyroidism on a population basis, and allow the intestines to absorb calcium most efficiently [17].

The dose of vitamin D replacement depends on the sunlight exposure, as well as the ability of intestines to absorb fat-soluble vitamins and the catabolic rate of vitamin D. Common doses are 400 to 1000 units a day of cholecalciferol or ergocalciferol. Most multiple vitamins contain between 100 and 400 units of vitamin D. Patients with malabsorption require higher doses. Patients who are vitamin D–deficient (serum 25(OH)D levels below 15 ng/ml) can be replaced initially with 50,000 units daily for 1 or 2 weeks, then start more ordinary doses, with monitoring of the levels. Vitamin D is fat-soluble, and continuous high dosage can lead to toxicity, hypercalcemia, excess bone resorption, and occasionally end-stage renal failure.

Calcitriol may be indicated following transplantation or in patients with malabsorption, renal, or hepatic disease.

C. Exercise

Physical activity is critical to bone health, and exercise is beneficial to many other organ systems as well [18]. This is intellectually easy advice, but in actuality difficult to accomplish. It seems to be human nature to break resolutions about exercise. Reviewing clinical trials of exercise reveals a very high rate of noncompliance; even in the motivated clinical research subjects, only about 50% complete the studies. Exercise that will be incorporated into the patient's lifestyle is therefore the best. Walking is a weight-bearing exercise that can be recommended for most patients. Epidemiological studies of older women show that walkers have lower risk of hip fractures than women who don't walk [4]. Those who prefer workouts in the gym or with equipment should receive reinforcement as well. The subjects of trials who completed exercise studies show modest increases in bone density and more definite improvements in muscle strength.

Transplant candidates present a challenge, because many have limited ability to perform exercise. Patients with end-stage pulmonary disease must often cart around oxygen tanks, and they can become short of breath with minimal exertion. Those with hepatic or renal failure are easily fatigued and have muscle weakness. Cardiac patients may develop angina or arrhythmias. Despite all these difficulties, many patients could do more exercise than they are doing, and rehabilitation programs encouraging exercise can be beneficial to these patients.

D. Other Lifestyle Factors

Ethanol use has a bimodal effect on fracture rates. People with modest intakes have fewer fractures than people who drink no ethanol [19–21]. Higher intakes, however, are associated with lower bone density as well as higher fracture rates. Ethanol inhibits osteoblasts in culture. Patients with hepatic failure should avoid ethanol; other patients should not use it in excess.

Cigarette smoking is harmful to the skeleton, as well as to many other organs [22]. Although it is difficult for patients to stop smoking, it is imperative. Transplant candidates have more motivation to discontinue cigarettes than other patients. Most transplant programs will not list a patient for transplant if he or she continues to smoke cigarettes.

Caffeine slightly increases the loss of calcium in the urine, but this effect is balanced by taking the recommended calcium intake. Up to two caffeinated beverages a day have such minor effects that is not necessary to advise patients to discontinue drinking them [23, 24].

E. Hip Protection

In elderly or frail persons, undergarments with protective pads reduce the risk of hip fracture [25]. Population studies of these hip protectors have sometimes shown no statistical difference in hip fracture rates between those assigned to pads and those not assigned, when using an intention-to-treat analysis, primarily because people did not always comply with wearing the garments. This has led to misunderstanding about the benefits of this simple method. Subjects who actually wore the protectors did have fewer fractures. These hip protectors should be considered in transplant candidates who are thin and have very low bone density, especially if they have a history of falling.

F. Adjustments to Medications

Transplant physicians don't need to be reminded about the deleterious effects of glucocorticoids on the skeleton, but they must be mentioned in any list of medications that cause bone disease [26].

Loop diuretics increase urine calcium loss, and this can have a negative influence on the skeleton. Thiazide diuretics, on the other hand, decrease urine calcium loss [27]. Thiazides also have some beneficial *in vitro* effects on bone cell cultures to inhibit bone resorption. Possibly this is due to weak carbonic anhydrase inhibition. In large observational studies of medication use and fractures, thiazide use is associated with a reduction of 40 to 50% in hip fracture rate. A clinical trial showed a modest but significant beneficial effect on bone density in normal elderly men and women [28]. Some transplant candidates who are receiving low doses of loop diuretics could be changed to thiazide diuretics with a net benefit to the skeleton.

Premenopausal women who use depomedroxyprogesterone acetate for contraception will lose bone density more rapidly than women who use other methods of birth control. This must be taken into consideration in transplant candidates, especially if they have low bone density [29].

Hyperthyroidism increases bone resorption and the risk of osteoporosis. Doses of thyroid hormone should be tailored to keep the thyroid stimulating hormone within the normal range [30].

G. Modification of Other Risk Factors

Malabsorption may be present in transplant candidates, especially those with cirrhosis or cystic fibrosis. These patients will need higher doses of calcium, vitamin D, and other fat-soluble vitamins than usually recommended.

Hypercalciuria is occasionally caused by excess calcium intake; if patients are consuming more than 1500 mg/day of calcium, the urine calcium should be repeated after several weeks of 1000–1200 mg/day. Thiazide diuretics act directly on the kidney to reduce urine calcium losses. Patients with idiopathic hypercalciuria have an increased risk of nephrolithiasis as well as osteoporosis, and they both are improved with thiazides [31].

H. Osteoporosis-Specific Medications

The medications used to treat osteoporosis include estrogen, calcitonin, bisphosphonates, selective estrogen-receptor modulators (SERMS), and intermittent parathyroid hormone (the full 1-84 peptide or the 1-34 amino fragment). These have all been shown to reduce the incidence of osteoporotic fractures in postmenopausal women with osteoporosis [32, 33], and none have been studied in clinical trials with enough power to show significant changes in fracture rates in transplant candidates. Bone density, which is an imperfect surrogate for bone strength, sometimes improves when transplant candidates are treated with osteoporosis medications. The safety profiles of these agents may be altered, depending on the organ which has failed, as summarized in Table 2.

1. Estrogen

In young women who are amenorrheic, estrogen is beneficial to the skeleton, lipid profile, and vasculature. Estrogen should be avoided in patients

TABLE 2 Observations about osteoporosis medications in transplant candidates

	Heart	Lung	Liver	Kidney
Estrogen (women)	greater risk of thrombophlebitis and coronary artery disease	avoid if any history of pulmonary embolism	transdermal doses preferred	less protein binding results in higher blood levels, dose should be cut in half; avoid in polycystic kidney disease
Testosterone (men)	may increase cholesterol	may exacerbate erythrocytosis		
Calcitriol		helpful in cystic fibrosis with malabsorption of vitamin D	useful when there is malabsorption of vitamin D	effective in controlling parathyroid hyperplasia; newer analogs may cause less hypercalcemia; may exacerbate adynamic bone disease
Calcitonin (no known compli-cations)				not studied
Bisphos-phonates		intravenous forms cause severe bone pain in cystic fibrosis	oral forms should be avoided in patients with varices; intra-venous forms have not been adequately investigated	worsens hyperpara-thyroidism; drug is renally excreted; may exacerbate adynamic bone disease
SERM (raloxi-fene)	increases risk of thrombophlebitis			pharmaco-kinetics not well defined
PTH (teriparatide)			no data available	not studied; may worsen hyper-parathyroidism

who are at a high risk of thromboembolism; the relative risk is increased two- to three-fold.

The use of estrogen in postmenopausal women is currently controversial, but there is no debate about the beneficial effect to the skeleton. Estrogen significantly reduces the risk of osteoporotic fractures, including hip fractures, in women regardless of race or bone density [34]. In transplant candidates with low bone density who are within ten years of menopause, estrogen should be considered if they have menopausal symptoms.

The Women's Health Initiative results suggest that addition of progesterone increases the risk of myocardial infarction and breast cancer. Locally applied progesterone might reduce the risk of endometrial hyperplasia without the harmful systemic effects, but this approach has not been studied very carefully. Women who are more than ten years post-menopause usually should avoid initiation of estrogen due to the increased risk of stroke.

Patients with liver or kidney disease have altered estrogen pharmacokinetics, discussed in the following sections.

2. *Selective Estrogen Receptor Modulators*

Raloxifene, a selective estrogen receptor modulator, can be used in postmenopausal women. Raloxifene significantly reduces the risk of vertebral compression fractures, which are the kind of fractures most commonly seen after transplantation [35]. Raloxifene carries the same increased risk of thromboembolism as estrogen. A large clinical trial designed specifically to detect effect of raloxifene on cardiovascular endpoints is still in progress. This drug should be used only in postmenopausal women because it may compete with estrogen in premenopausal women, negating the beneficial skeletal effects of estrogen. In perimenopausal women, raloxifene exacerbates menopausal symptoms of hot flashes, but in women more than a decade beyond menopause the drug is usually well tolerated.

3. *Testosterone*

Testosterone has beneficial musculoskeletal effects in men. In hypogonadal men treated with testosterone, bone density and muscle strength improve, with an acceptable side effect profile. This drug should be avoided in men with a history of prostate cancer, but it has not been shown to increase the risk of developing cancer. Hypogonadal men may have decreased prostate size, which will increase back to normal with hormone replacement. High hematocrit or abnormal cholesterol may limit the use of testosterone. In patients with liver disease, transdermal dosing is preferred.

4. *Calcitonin*

Calcitonin has been shown to reduce the risk of vertebral compression fractures in a randomized clinical trial. Calcitonin is probably the safest osteoporosis drug, with very few side effects (nasal irritation and mild nausea in fewer than 5% of cases). A trial in women with postmenopausal osteoporosis did not show a dose-effect, and the study had a high noncompletion rate, so the benefits are less certain than with the other approved drugs. The bone density does not show much improvement with calcitonin, but there is decreased bone turnover.

5. *Bisphosphonates*

Bisphosphonates are potent antiresorptive medications that reduce incidence of fractures in patients with osteoporosis [36]. The usual recommended doses may be higher than necessary; randomized clinical trials have shown no significant difference in fracture rates between alendronate 5 mg/day and 10 mg/day [37], or between risedronate 2.5 mg/day and 5 mg/day [38]. Once-weekly dosing is effective and usually preferred by patients. Because these medications are poorly absorbed, they must be taken on an empty stomach with water, at least 30 minutes before eating any food. Esophagitis is the most common adverse effect.

Pamidronate is not approved for treatment of postmenopausal osteoporosis and should be reserved for patients who cannot tolerate the oral route. Studies of patients following transplantation have suggested beneficial effects of pamidronate, but data about pre-transplant pamidronate therapy are conflicting. Intravenous forms have the advantage of assured compliance and bioavailabilty, but there are additional side effects of fever, transient leukopenia, hypocalcemia, myalgias, bone pain, and rarely eye inflammation or nephrotic syndrome.

The optimal duration for bisphosphonate therapy has not been defined. These medications deposit in the bone with a half-life greater than ten years, and they cause 60 to 95% reductions in the bone formation rates [39]. Bone density increases because the bone becomes more highly mineralized [40]. Bisphosphonates accumulate within the bone with continuous use, and it is possible that prolonged exposure would limit the ability of the bone to repair microdamage or increase the brittleness of the bone [41]. During the first 5 years of use, controlled trials have demonstrated significant reductions in the incidence of new fractures. A few subjects have taken bisphosphonates for 10 years without obvious harm, but there are no control data on fracture rates [42]. Until more data are available on long-term effects, it is rational to use the bisphophonates mainly in patients who already have osteoporosis.

When patients are referred to my clinic for failure to respond to bisphosphonate therapy, the most frequent causes are vitamin D deficiency or failure to take the drugs correctly. In the clinical trials that have shown benefits of bisphosphonates, the subjects have had adequate calcium and vitamin D intake. Severe hypocalcemia has been reported when bisphosphonates were given to patients with low vitamin D levels or other risk factors for hypocalcemia [43, 44].

6. *Intermittent PTH*

Patients who already have a vertebral compression fracture are at particularly high risk of fracturing more vertebrae after the transplant. They need careful attention to all the other risk factors, and should receive one of the stronger antiresorptive medications (bisphosphonates or raloxifene). In heart or lung transplant candidates who have fractures despite such treatment, another choice is intermittent parathyroid hormone. Teriparatide (recombinant human parathyroid hormone 1-34) has recently been approved for use in postmenopausal women with osteoporosis. It also has been shown to decrease fracture incidence of both vertebral and other clinical fractures [45]. This is the only anabolic agent that is approved in the United States. It has not been studied in transplant candidates, and the role of this agent is still uncertain. It should be considered in patients with compression fractures who have not responded to other medications. Teriparatide caused osteosarcoma in about half the laboratory rats who were exposed to high doses [46], but no cases of osteosarcoma have been reported in humans. Nevertheless, it should not be used in patients with a history of cancer or radiation to the bone. Other side effects include hypercalcemia, nausea, headache, and increased uric acid. The anabolic effect diminishes with time, and the optimal duration of use has not been defined; the clinical trials lasted an average of 18 months. Prior or concomitant use of bisphosphonates attenuates the effect on trabecular bone but increases the effect on cortical bone. The studies of combination use have not been large enough to analyze fracture incidence rates.

I. Glucocorticoid-Treated Patients

Patients who are taking glucocorticoids have more complex bone disease [26]. Bone formation rates are suppressed, bone resorption is increased, gastrointestinal absorption of calcium is decreased, urine calcium losses are increased, and gonadotropic hormones are inhibited. Patients are at greater risk for fracture, and they many fracture more easily than other people with the same bone density. These adverse effects are dose-dependent, and can be seen even with inhaled medication. Treatment is with the same medications just listed [47]. Patients with hypercalciuria will probably benefit from thiazide diuretics before being treated with calcium supplementation. Bisphosphonates have been shown to reduce fracture risk in glucocorticoid-induced osteoporosis. The improvement in bone density is not as great as in patients with idiopathic osteoporosis, probably because the glucocorticoid-treated patients have lower bone formation rates at initiation of therapy.

IV. HEART OR LUNG TRANSPLANT CANDIDATES

A. Fracture Prevalence and Risk Factors

Patients with end-stage cardiac or pulmonary disease frequently have osteoporosis that is usually caused by metabolic abnormalities. A survey of randomly selected hospitalized patients with COPD found an overall prevalence of vertebral fractures of 26%, which was not different from age-matched control inpatients; average age was 71 years. However, the patients with COPD were more likely to have severe compression fractures. Of note, the chest x-ray reports did not mention fracture in 82% of the patients who had vertebral fractures, and osteoporosis therapy was given at discharge to only 18.5% of patients with fractures [48]. In transplant candidates, the reported prevalence of vertebral fractures ranges from 7 to 29% [49–53].

Some of the pathophysiological risk factors leading to decreased bone strength are shown in Figure 2.

Several studies of risk factors seen in transplant candidates have included measurements of bone mineral density, shown in Figure 3 [49–52, 54–60]. The percentage of transplant candidates who already have osteoporosis (BMD lower than 2.5 standard deviations below the mean for young persons) ranges from 21 to 50% at the spine and 19 to 61% at the hip. In longitudinal follow-up, the patients who had fractures after transplantation had lower bone density than those without fractures (Spine T-score −2.8 versus −1.5) [61]. Other risk factors associated with low BMD in the candidates include low body weight, use of glucocorticoids, cigarette smoking, vitamin D insufficiency, hypogonadism, use of loop diuretics [53], and cystic fibrosis [62]. Patients with the lowest FEV1 also had lower BMD [60]. Hypogonadism was untreated in 50% of men and 20% of women, and 15% of patients had hypovitaminosis D [52].

B. Treatment

The general recommendations for patients with osteoporosis or glucocorticoid-induced osteoporosis apply to candidates for heart or lung transplantations. This includes good nutrition, adequate protein and calcium intake, vitamin D sufficient to keep serum 25(OH)D levels in the optimal range (20-40 ng/ml), and exercise. Frail patients should wear hip protectors. Of course they should not smoke cigarettes. If possible, thiazide diuretics should be substituted for loop diuretics. Patients with bone density in the osteoporosis range (T-score below −2.5) should also be treatment with more specific medications as described above.

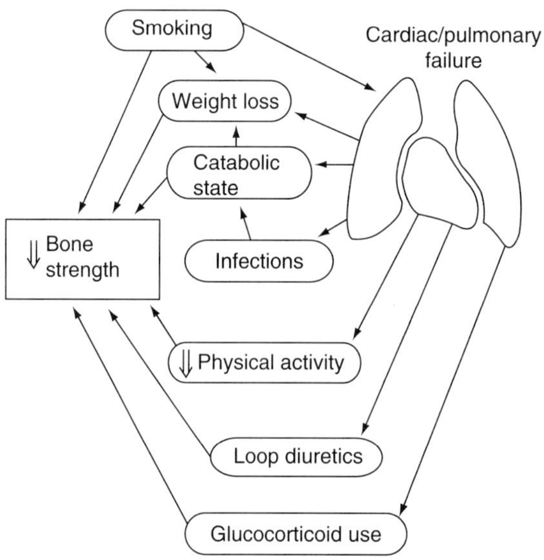

FIGURE 2 Diagram showing pathophysiological risk factors for decreased bone density in candidates for heart or lung transplantation.

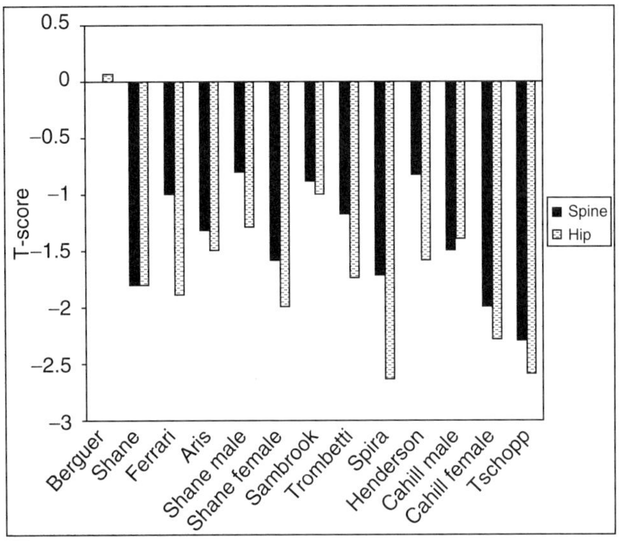

FIGURE 3 Bone density in candidates for heart or lung transplantation. Each bar represents the average result from the studies shown.

Patients with cystic fibrosis also represent a special group. In addition to pulmonary disease, they have malabsorption and an increased risk of osteoporosis and fractures. Vitamin D is especially important, and these patients will require higher doses than other patients [63]. Not only do they fail to absorb dietary vitamin D, but they also have higher metabolic breakdown of vitamin D, perhaps as a result of differences in enterohepatic cycling. Vitamin A is also important, and care must be given in replacement of vitamin A because fracture risk is increased with either high or low levels. The free levels of vitamin A must be determined if patients have low albumin. Patients with cystic fibrosis frequently have pulmonary infections and are catabolic. The catabolic state and weight loss are important risk factors for osteoporosis. Oral bisphosphonates have been shown to increase bone density, but the effect on fracture rates remains uncertain [62]. Intravenous bisphosphonates have been shown to cause such severe bone pain that the investigators terminated their initial study of this medication. They found that pretreatment with glucocorticoids attenuated the bone pain, and resulted in an increase in bone density at the spine, but a decrease at the radius [64]. Thus, the efficacy of bisphosphonates in this group of patients is uncertain.

V. LIVER TRANSPLANT CANDIDATES

A. Fracture Prevalence

Heart or lung transplantation does not improve bone disease, and the skeletal effects are predominantly negative, resulting from antirejection medications or the general catabolic state seen in transplant complications. Liver transplantation, however, can reverse some of the causes of hepatic osteodystrophy. The positive effects of a functional liver partially balance the negative effects of transplantation. After a successful liver transplant, bone density decreases initially, but as antirejection medications are tapered and the patient recovers from surgery, bone density often starts to improve. In transplant candidates, the goal is to strengthen the bones as much as possible, but the bones will never be normal while the liver is failing.

In end-stage liver disease, the prevalence of symptomatic fractures was 15%, and of vertebral fractures 7.5% [65]. Vertebral fracture prevalence in patients at the time of transplant is high, with reported rates that vary from 6.6 to 35%, as seen in Table 3 [65–81].

B. Bone Density

Low bone density is not always seen in patients with cirrhosis, but it is frequent in those who have end-stage disease. In patients with various chronic liver diseases, bone mineral density was significantly lower in patients than in controls at the lumbar spine (Z-score −0.35 versus 0.26 SD) but not at

TABLE 3 Bone density and fracture prevalence in liver transplant candidates

Author	Date	N	BMD	% with osteoporosis	% with fractures
Eastell	91	210	7% lower than control		
Meys	94	16			8%
Abdelhadi	95	25	Not different from control		
Monegal	97	58		33%	29%
Guardiola	99	55	Spine 0.915g/cm2		
Crosbie	99	12	T score= −1.97(spine), −1.8(hip)	42%	
Keogh	99	41	Z score = −0.76 (spine), −0.47 (hip)		
Hussaini	99	56		23%	
Xu	99	38		29%	
Ninkovic	00	37			35%
Trautwein	00	193	Z score = −1 (cholestatic), −0.3 (viral)		
Giannini	01	63			7.5%
Floreani	01	23	Spine = 0.806g/cm2	52%	
Monegal	01	45	Spine =1.06g/cm2, hip= 0.87g/cm2		
Ninkovic	01	243		36%	36%
Ninkovic	02	99	Spine = 0.91g/cm2, hip= 0.75g/cm2	34%	6.6%
Guichelaar	03	33	T score= −2.1(spine)	13%	18%

the femoral neck (Z-score −0.18 versus 0.17 SD) [82]. A recent survey of bone density in 272 patients with primary biliary cirrhosis (PBC) showed bone density that was not different from expected for age in women. The average age was 62 and osteoporosis was present in 35% of the patients. Many of these patients had only mild cirrhosis; only 21 underwent liver transplantation, and in these patients the bone density increased significantly after transplantation [83]. Other studies of PBC, which probably included patients with more-severe disease, have found low bone density [84] and rates of loss twice as fast as controls [66].

Transplant candidates have high rates of osteoporosis, as described in several studies (see Table 3). Osteoporosis was present in 36.6% of 243 candidates for liver transplant, and bone density varied with the liver diagnosis, as shown in Figure 4 [79].

C. Bone Biopsies and Biochemical Markers

As expected from radiological studies of bone density, the bone volume seen on bone biopsies is low in patients with end-stage liver disease. The density, however, does not predict the dynamic properties of the bone, nor the amount of unmineralized osteoid. Biopsies demonstrate that the bone formation rates in hepatic osteodystrophy are distinctly different from postmenopausal osteoporosis; this suggests that therapeutic approaches should also be different.

Osteomalacia was found in 36 to 70% of bone biopsies from patients with cirrhosis in studies done 25 years ago [85–88]. These patients had very low vitamin D levels and malabsorption. More recent studies have not reported osteomalacia [81, 89–99]; of these studies only 2 reported increased bone formation rates [94, 97]. Thus, the preponderance of data suggests that patients with chronic liver disease have low bone formation rates. Osteocalcin, a biochemical marker of bone formation, is also low in these

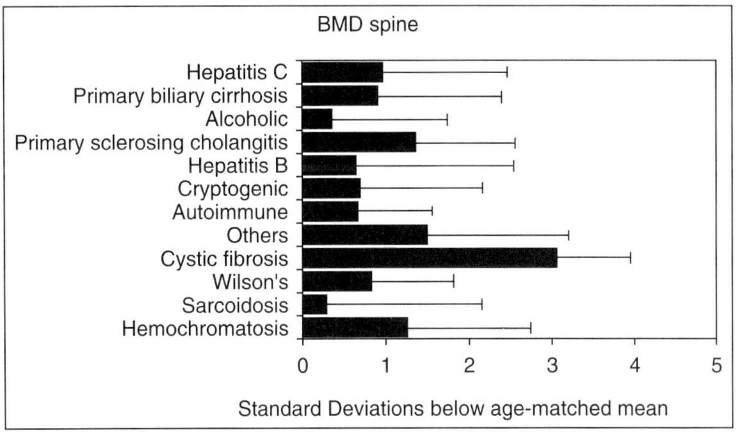

FIGURE 4 Bone density in various kinds of hepatic failure. Data from Ninkovic 2001.

patients [69, 92, 100–103] and it correlates with bone formation rate on bone biopsies [95]. Collagen-based markers of bone formation (carboxy-terminal and amino-terminal propeptides of type I collagen) are increased in liver failure, but these markers correlate with type 3 collagen which reflects hepatic fibrosis [104], and thus are unreliable indices of bone formation.

Bone formation rates in liver transplant patients are low before surgery and show increases after successful transplantation [81, 98, 99]. Osteocalcin also increases after liver transplantation [68, 105-107].

D. Risk Factors

Several factors contribute to the bone disease of patients with cirrhosis, as shown in Figure 5. Malabsorption is frequently seen [85]. Ethanol has a biphasic effect on bone disease; in low amounts it is associated with increased bone density, probably because it activates aromatase, resulting in higher estrogen levels. In higher amounts, however, ethanol is toxic to osteoblasts *in vitro*, and is associated with decreased bone density [19–21]. Patients with alcoholic liver disease are susceptible to abnormalities in vitamin D metabolism [108]. Serum from cirrhotic patients inhibits osteoblasts; the major circulating inhibitor is bilirubin [109]. Iron overload results in increases in iron deposition in the bone [110]. Hemochromatosis is associated with osteoporosis, although the exact mechanisms are not clear [111].

Hypogonadism is seen in patients with cirrhosis; this improves post-transplantation. In men, total testosterone increased from 9.3 nmol/l pretransplant to 15.4 nmol/l after 24 months [112]. Levels of sex hormone binding globulin are increased in liver disease, so free testosterone is even

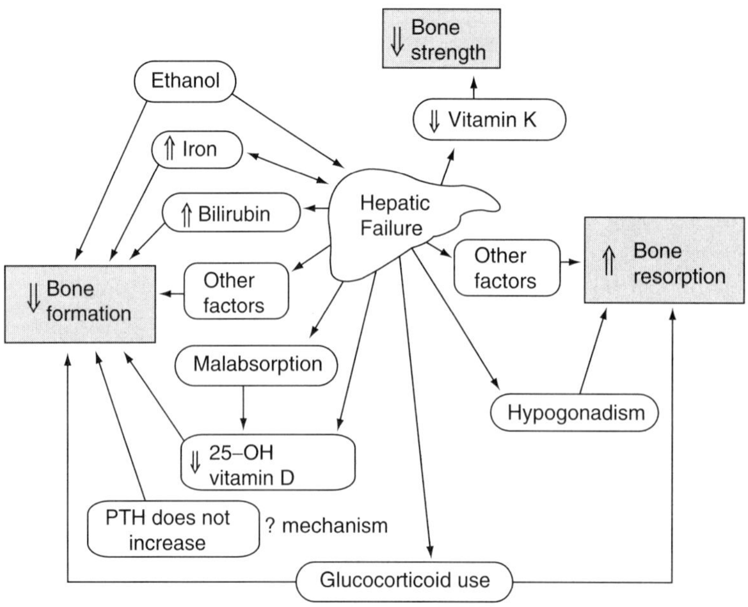

FIGURE 5 Diagram showing pathophysiology of bone disease in hepatic failure.

lower than total testosterone. After liver transplantation the levels increased by 102% at 24 months [77].

Studies of vitamin D receptor gene polymorphisms have shown somewhat conflicting results, analogous to findings in patients without liver disease. In one study of women with PBC, the bb genotype was associated with lower bone density [113]. In another study, bone density did not differ according to genotype at baseline, but those with the bb genotype lost bone less rapidly [70].

In a survey of 72 hospitalized patients with various types of liver disease, the factors significantly associated with low bone density were use of glucocorticoids (odds ratio = 18.9), low body mass index (odds ratio = 14.1), older age, and female sex. Longitudinal measurements showed that the rate of loss was increased at the lumbar spine in patients with more severe hepatic disease [114]. Serum levels of bilirubin correlated independently and positively, and 25(OH)D_3 levels negatively, with bone loss [82]. Another study of 243 consecutive patients undergoing assessment for liver transplant also found that low body weight and older age were associated with low bone density [79].

Several studies have found no independent effect of cholestasis on bone density in transplant candidates [72, 79, 114], but patients with cholestasis were older and therefore had lower bone density. After transplantation, the risk of fracture may be higher in those with cholestatic disease [115].

A prospective study of 130 patients who received liver transplantation showed that fractures after the transplant were six times more likely in patients with a vertebral fracture before the transplant. The mean pretransplant bone density was not different in the patients who fractured post-transplant from those who did not fracture. Those patients with pretransplant BMD T-score less than −2.5, however, did have an increased risk of fractures [115]. Another large study of 153 patients found that fractures after transplantation could not be predicted by several risk factors that are important for post-menopausal osteoporosis, including age, race, menopause, chronic renal insufficiency, family history of osteoporosis, BMD, and T-score [116]. A smaller study of 45 patients did report a higher fracture risk in those with low bone density [112]. Other identified risk factors for fractures following transplantation are older age and lower bone density [112] and higher serum levels of the C-terminal propeptide of collagen [117].

E. Vitamin D and PTH

Vitamin D metabolism is usually normal in mild to moderate liver failure, but in end-stage disease (as is seen in many transplant candidates) the 25-hydroxylation of vitamin D may become impaired. Patients with liver disease frequently have low serum levels of 25(OH)D, but reported levels vary widely, partly because of differences in sunlight exposure and dietary factors, as shown in Table 4 [77, 81, 89, 92, 93, 97, 105, 112, 118–124]. These levels can be low because of reduced exposure to sunlight, malabsorption,

TABLE 4 Vitamin D levels in patients with cirrhosis

Author	Date	Location	N	Patients	Mean serum 25(OH)D ng/mL
Matloff	1982	Boston	10	PBC	19
Hodgson	1985	Minnesota	15	PBC	18
Stellon	1986	England	36	PBC	18
Diamond	1989	Australia	54	Cirrhosis	17
Kirch	1990	Germany	22	Cirrhosis	31
Rabinovitz	1992	Pittsburgh	30	Pre-Transplant	11
Hodgson	1993	Minnesota	24	PBC	16
Compston	1996	England	27	Pre-Transplant	6
Bagur	1998	Argentina	23	PBC	27
Crosbie	1999	Ireland	12	Pre-Transplant	6
Hay	2001	Minnesota	63	Pre-Transplant	15
Monegal	2001	Spain	45	Pre-Transplant	9
Floreani	2001	Italy	23	Pre-Transplant	9
Guanabens	2003	Spain	32	PBC	55
Guichelaar	2003	Minnesota	33	Pre-Transplant	17

increased vitamin D catabolism, higher excretion of polar metabolites, or reduced levels of D-binding protein [125]. D-binding protein and albumin both bind vitamin D, and in chronic liver disease these two proteins are reduced in parallel, so that the free levels of 25(OH)D are higher than suggested by the ordinary serum levels [126]. When serum 25(OH)D is very low, osteomalacia can be seen, but with current medical practice severe vitamin D deficiency is uncommon.

Most studies also show normal or decreased serum PTH levels in liver transplant candidates [77, 89, 95, 105, 112, 119, 123, 124, 127, 128]. The mechanism for this is unclear; with poor calcium absorption and low vitamin D, PTH would be expected to increase. One study found increased PTH levels when using an assay that detected midregion PTH, but normal levels when a different assay which detected the whole sequence was used [119].

After transplantation, the PTH and 25(OH)D levels increase significantly. For example, in one study mean serum PTH level was 26.6 pg/ml at baseline and increased to 61.2 pg/ml in 2 years. Serum 25(OH)D levels were low at baseline and returned to the normal range after 2 years [77].

F. Treatment

1. *Calcium*

A recent guideline for treatment of patients with hepatic disease has been published, which reviews studies of therapy to improve bone density [129]. The same approach is recommended in general for transplant candidates, but the results may not be as favorable because the pretransplant patients have more severe hepatic disease.

The calcium intake in chronic liver disease should probably be the same as for other patients with osteoporosis, at 1200 to 1500 mg/day. This has not been studied very often in this population, but one trial in patients with PBC showed that calcium supplementation had transient beneficial effect [130]. The source of calcium can be either food (predominantly dairy products) or supplements; in patients with encephalopathy, protein restriction may be necessary, in which case supplements are preferred.

2. Vitamin D

Patients with liver disease may need higher doses of vitamin D than those with postmenopausal osteoporosis. A reasonable starting dose is 800 to 1000 units per day, followed by adjustments to achieve and maintain optimal serum levels. 25(OH)D is bound to D-binding-protein and albumin, and in liver failure these both decrease at the same rates. The percentage bound is relatively constant, so it is possible to calculate an "adjusted vitamin D level" in the blood. If albumin is lower than normal, use the following equation, derived from studies by Bikle [126]:

$$\text{"adjusted vitamin D"} = \frac{\text{measured 25(OH)D} \times 4}{\text{Serum albumin (g/dL)}}$$

For example, if measured 25(OH)D is 6 ng/dL and albumin is 2 g/dL, the adjusted 25(OH)D is 12 ng/dL. The optimal range for adjusted serum 25(OH)D is 20 to 30 ng/dL.

In some severe cases of end-stage liver failure, vitamin D is not hydroxylated and levels do not increase even when precursors are given in large amounts. In other cases fat malabsorption results in low levels [131]. These patients then require the active metabolites of vitamin D. Calcitriol in physiological doses (0.25 to 0.5 micrograms/day) will improve calcium absorption. In 34 Japanese women with PBC, calcitriol showed a beneficial effect. The mean annual change in bone mineral density was 0.1% in the treatment group and −3.1% in the control group [132].

Vitamin D therapy alone is not sufficient to reverse bone loss in patients with cirrhosis. Several biopsy studies showed no improvement in bone volume after 25-OH vitamin D [88–90], but in one there was decrease in the bone eroded surface [88].

3. Vitamin K

Vitamin K is low in patients with cirrhosis. Although prothrombin time also depends on vitamin K, it is not a sensitive test for vitamin K levels. Only 1 of 77 subjects with low phylloquinone levels had a prolonged prothrombin time [133]. The role of vitamin K in bone metabolism is not well understood, but vitamin K is necessary for carboxylation of osteocalcin, which allows the osteocalcin to bind to calcium, and for the production of bone morphogenic protein. In elderly women, increased levels of undercarboxylated osteocalcin are associated with osteoporosis [134]. In one study of patients with liver disease, bone density was better with vitamin K treatment than in controls. Serum levels of undercarboxylated osteocalcin decreased [135]. More studies are needed to delineate the benefits of supplementation with vitamin K.

4. *Calcitonin*

In PBC calcitonin was ineffective in halting bone loss [130]. An uncontrolled study showed beneficial effects of calcitriol followed by calcitonin [136]. Calcitonin may have a role in patients who have only mild loss of bone density and side effects from other medications. Calcitonin is not strong enough to prevent bone loss after transplantation [81, 124].

5. *Estrogen and SERMs*

In a retrospective analysis of women with PBC, those who had taken estrogen had better bone density without worsening of their liver disease [137]. In women with PBC, treatment with estrogens for 4 years resulted in a significantly lower rate of bone loss (0.002 versus 0.009 $g/cm^2/yr$). Worsening cholestasis attributable to estrogen replacement therapy did not occur [138]. Another study in women with liver disease showed that hormone replacement caused a statistically significant increase in lumbar spine BMD and total body BMD, whereas control patients showed a significant decrease in lumbar and total body BMD. In contrast to the controls, hormone-treated patients also showed a decrease in truncal fat (−3.8%). Neither of the groups showed any statistically significant changes in the liver function tests [139]. The transdermal route of administration is preferred for estrogen or testosterone.

SERMS (selective estrogen receptor modulators) should theoretically work in these patients because the mechanism of action on the bone is similar to estrogen. Studies in this population have not been published, but a pilot study at the Mayo Clinic showed beneficial effects on bone density [140].

In men who are hypogonadal, transdermal testosterone is a reasonable choice although it has not been studied in this population.

6. *Bisphosphonates*

Bisphosphonates have been studied in patients with liver disease, and they can improve bone density. It is not clear whether they reduce fractures in patients with end-stage liver disease. Oral bisphosphonates should be avoided in patients who have esophageal varices, because the bisphosphonates can cause esophageal erosion or ulceration. Some of the studies of bisphosphonates in liver transplant candidates are summarized in this section.

In a pilot study, 6 patients with PBC were treated with cyclical etidronate, and their bone density was stable after 1 year, whereas 6 control patients lost bone density at the spine. There were no differences at the hip or with bone biochemical markers [141].

Etidronate was also studied in a randomized trial of 67 women who had osteopenia and PBC. After one year, there was no difference between bone density or fracture rates in the placebo and etidronate groups, although the biochemical markers of bone resorption were decreased [142].

Women with PBC were randomly assigned to receive alendronate (10 mg/day) or etidronate (400 mg/day) for 14 days every 3 months. Thirteen patients in each group completed the 2-year trial. Both treatments increased bone mineral density after 2 years, although the increase at the lumbar spine and at the proximal femur was significantly higher in patients receiving alendronate than in patients on etidronate. Gastrointestinal side effects were seen in 6 of 32 patients [120].

Intravenous pamidronate has been studied in patients with cirrhosis [143–145]. In two of the studies, the pamidronate was given before or soon after transplantation, and the effects on post-transplantation bone density and fracture rate were evaluated. These are discussed in the chapter on liver transplantation.

In another study of 12 pretransplant patients, pamidronate was administered randomly to 6. The calcium decreased more than expected from patients without liver disease. After transplantation the PTH was 12 times higher in the group that was pretreated with pamidronate [144].

7. *Summary*

Patients with hepatic osteodystrophy do not always respond to osteoporosis medications. Since most of these patients have low bone formation, the ideal approach would be to give anabolic medications. Intermittent PTH is approved for osteoporosis, but it has not been studied in liver failure. Subjects were excluded from teriparatide studies if they had abnormal liver function. It is possible that osteoblasts in cirrhotic patients would not show the same anabolic response as in patients without cirrhosis, due to inhibition of osteoblasts by serum factors [109]. PTH stimulates bone resorption, and if the anabolic effect is diminished, the net effect could be enhanced bone loss. Therefore, these drugs cannot be recommended without further study. Future drugs, such as SERMs or osteoprotegerin, might be beneficial in these patients.

Physicians should be cautious about using bisphosphonates in patients with gastrointestinal bleeding or esophageal varices. It is unlikely that there will be a large enough study conducted in this population to address effects of potent bisphosphonates on fractures, but more data would be helpful to delineate the effects on serum PTH, serum calcium, and bone formation rate.

Transdermal estrogens can be used in some women, and calcitonin is safe although only modestly effective. Vitamin D is an important therapy in these patients. General measures to improve bone strength (nutrition, physical activity, and reduction of risks) should be encouraged in all transplant candidates.

VI. RENAL OSTEODYSTROPHY

A. Spectrum of Renal Osteodystrophy

Renal osteodystrophy (ROD) is a well-recognized complication of end-stage renal disease. Treatment is difficult because there is a wide spectrum of manifestations of renal osteodystrophy, shown in Figure 6, and because treatments that improve one problem may worsen another. The goal is to preserve bone mass and normal bone formation and resorption rates; maintain steady serum levels of calcium, phosphate, and parathyroid hormone; and avoid accumulation of bone-toxic substances without causing vascular calcification.

It is not possible to provide any simple algorithms for the treatment of renal osteodystrophy. Transplant candidates are managed the same as other patients with end-stage renal disease, with particular attention to controlling hyperparathyroidism. Kidney transplantation will improve many aspects of renal osteodystrophy, but parathyroid hyperplasia may not regress even when normal kidney function returns. Guidelines for management of renal osteodystrophy have recently been proposed [146, 147], and an international group has outlined some of the controversies and new

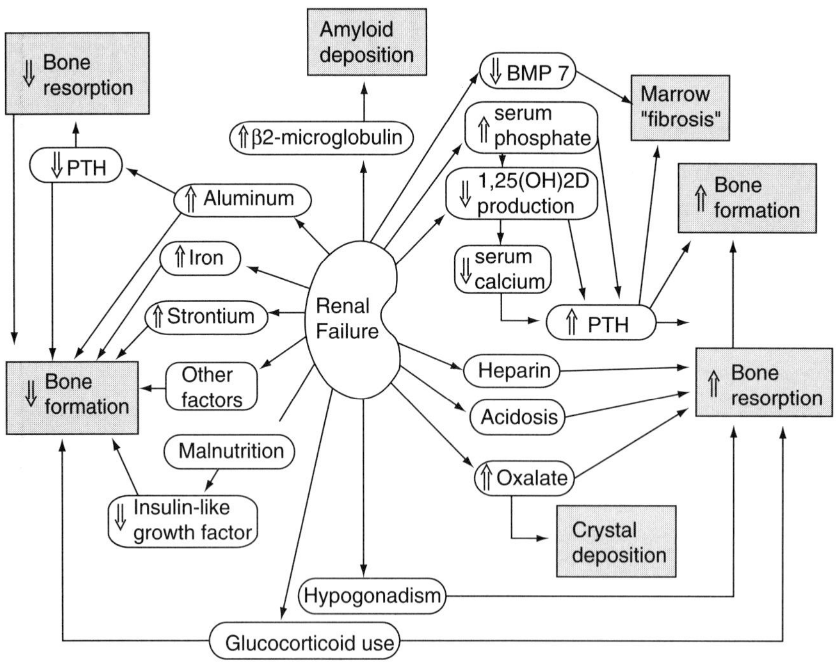

FIGURE 6 Diagram showing pathophysiology of bone disease in renal failure.

therapies [148]. This chapter briefly reviews some of the main aspects of renal osteodystrophy, with emphasis on differences between postmenopausal osteoporosis and renal osteodystrophy.

There are several histologic types of renal osteodystrophy [149]. The most common is high turnover, with increased bone formation and resorption, peritrabecular fibrosis, and often slightly wide, woven osteoid. This is associated with high serum PTH levels, and the "fibrosis" is actually an accumulation of preosteoblasts, which can quickly disappear when parathyroid hormone levels are normalized. The least common type of renal osteodystrophy is osteomalacia, with low bone formation and absence of fibrosis, as seen with excess aluminum, iron, or strontium. Mixed disease combines features of both, with increased resorption and fibrosis as well as increased osteoid. Adynamic bone disease is characterized by low bone formation without evidence of fibrosis. Patients can change from one type to another, but normal bone histology is not usually found [150].

B. Fracture Prevalence

Patients with ROD have an increased risk of fracture. In one center the prevalence of spinal fractures was 52% [151]. Hip fractures occur 4.4 times as often in dialysis patients as in the general population [152]. In dialysis patients who were placed on the renal transplant waiting list in the United States, the rate of hip fractures was 2.9/1000 patients/year, and the relative risk increased by 34% in the first 2 years after transplantation [153].

In postmenopausal osteoporosis, bone density at any location can be used to predict fracture. In renal osteodystrophy, this is not the case. For example, in one study patients with high turnover had more fractures in the appendicular skeleton but fewer in the axial skeleton [154]. Some studies show a higher risk of fractures in patients with low PTH [155, 156], but a large epidemiological survey did not confirm this association [157].

Peripheral vascular disease was independently associated with hip fracture in dialysis patients, with a relative risk of 1.94. Some of the risk factors for fractures are seen in both the general population and in patients with renal osteodystrophy: older age, female gender, Caucasian race, and low weight [157].

After transplantation the fracture rates increase. Pretransplant risk factors for post-transplant fractures include older age and longer duration of renal failure [158]. Bone density does not consistently predict post-transplant fractures [159]. PTH levels also do not consistently predict fracture risk post-transplant [160].

C. Bone Density in Dialysis Patients

Most physicians who treat women with postmenopausal osteoporosis focus on the bone density and do not consider pathophysiology. Nephrologists, on the other hand, have been more concerned about pathological category than bone density. One reason is that the relationships between types of renal osteodystrophy and bone density are not clear. In a group of 62 dialysis patients who had both bone biopsy and measurement of bone density, there were 40 patients with secondary hyperparathyroidism, and the spine bone density Z-score ranged from −3 to +2.5, mean −0.94. Those with mixed osteodystrophy had the lowest mean bone density, Z = −1.71. The 16 patients with low turnover (adynamic bone disease or osteomalacia) had almost the same range as those with secondary hyperparathyroidism (from −2.5 to +1.8, mean −0.32) [161]. Patients commencing hemodialysis also had similar bone densities despite different histological lesions [162].

Other studies comparing biopsy findings to bone density show similar cortical measurements in high or low turnover, but vertebral cancellous bone volume was higher in those with high turnover, probably a result of the increased PTH [154, 163]. In general, bone density in patients with renal osteodystrophy tends to be relatively lower in the forearm and hip (cortical sites) than in the spine (cancellous sites). This pattern is similar to that seen in patients with primary hyperparathyroidism, but not in idiopathic osteoporosis (see Figure 7) [154, 162–197].

Bone density varies widely from study to study (Figure 7), and even among skeletal sites in individual patients. Furthermore, the relationship between bone density and fracture incidence is not consistent. In one center the prevalence of spine fractures was 52% in patients older than 55 years, but this was not associated with low DEXA or heel ultrasound values [151]; in another center the relative risk of vertebral fractures was 2 for each standard deviation decrease in the spine bone density [155]. It is worth emphasizing that bone density does not consistently predict post-transplant fractures [159].

Therefore, a unidimensional approach does not work for renal osteodystrophy. Patients with low bone mass may have either high or low bone formation. Conversely, patients with adynamic bone disease have bone density values ranging from low to high. These findings have led a recent working group on renal bone disease to suggest that terms such as osteopenia and osteoporosis do not apply to patients with end-stage renal disease, and instead patients should be defined according to their type of renal osteodystrophy with modification according to bone density (e.g., "high bone formation with low bone density" or "low bone formation with low bone density") [148].

D. Hyperphosphatemia

Hyperphosphatemia is not encountered in postmenopausal osteoporosis, but it is one of the most important factors in renal osteodystrophy [198]. Patients must ingest a low-phosphate diet, which means they should avoid dairy products. In the past, aluminum was used to bind phosphates, but the

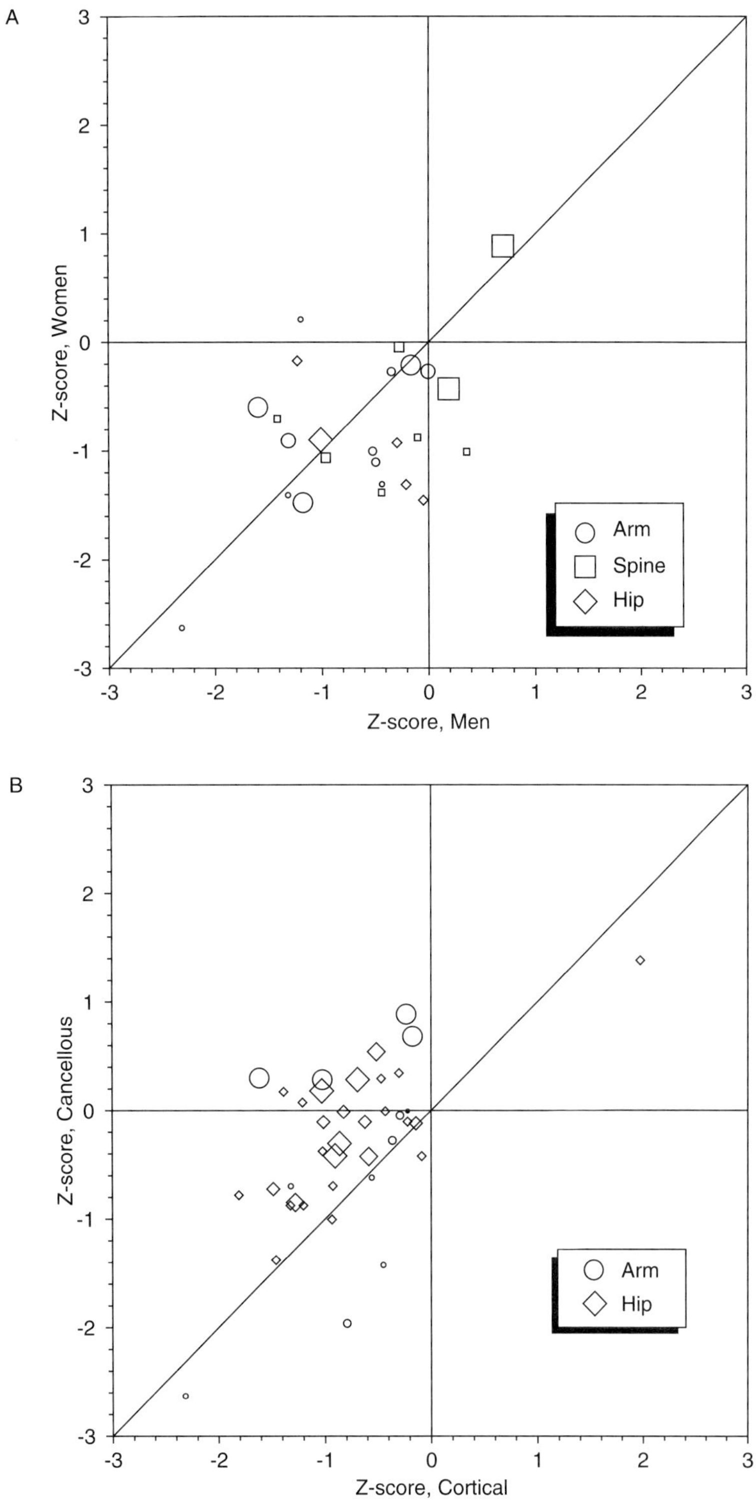

FIGURE 7 **A:** Bone density in patients with end-stage renal failure. Each point represents a study which reported data for both men and women. The size of the points reflects the number of subjects in the study. The points above the 45° line are from studies in which women have higher bone density than men. **B:** Bone density in patients with end-stage renal failure. Each point represents a study which reported data for both spine (cancellous bone) and hip or forearm (cortical bone). The size of the points reflects the number of subjects in the study. The points above the 45° line are from studies in which patients have higher cancellous bone density than cortical bone density. If necessary, data were converted to Z-scores using manufacturers' reference ranges and mean age of subjects.

aluminum can accumulate in the bone and cause osteomalacia. Calcium citrate exacerbates aluminum transfer to the brain, and should be avoided in dialysis patients. High doses of calcium carbonate or acetate have been used to control the phosphate by intestinal binding. This is moderately successful, but the serum calcium increases, which probably worsens vascular calcification. Longer hours of dialysis remove more phosphate, but this is expensive and inconvenient. Newer phosphate binders, such as sevelamer, do not contain calcium and are effective at reducing phosphate [199, 200].

E. Hyperparathyroidism and Vitamin D

Hyperparathyroidism is also a major factor in renal osteodystrophy [201]. The high serum phosphate increases secretion of PTH, and the low $1,25(OH)_2$ vitamin D levels lead to parathyroid hyperplasia. As parathyroid bone disease becomes more severe, bone density decreases. In one study, bone density in patients with mild hyperparathyroid bone disease (as assessed by bone biopsies) was average at the arm and hip and 0.49 standard deviations above age-matched controls at the spine. Bone density was worse in those with moderate hyperparathyroidism, and in patients with severe hyperparathyroid bone disease the Z-score was −0.77 at the spine and −1.94 at the forearm [202]. Parathyroidectomy improves bone density. In one longitudinal study, patients who were losing bone density at the forearm prior to parathyroidectomy started gaining bone postoperatively [203].

In patients with renal disease, fragments of parathyroid hormone are not excreted, and their serum levels rise. The "intact" parathyroid hormone assay actually does not measure the entire molecule (1-84), which largely explains the apparent resistance to PTH in renal patients. Thus, older recommendations suggested that PTH serum levels should be twice the upper limit of normal to prevent bone disease. Newer assays that detect PTH 1-84 ("whole PTH") measure the more physiologic molecule [204]. Advice about the levels of PTH in dialysis patients should be changed in view of these findings, but further studies are needed to define the optimal serum "whole PTH" level. If PTH is too high, the bone density decreases, especially in cortical bone, and fracture rate increases. On the other hand, if PTH is too low, adynamic bone disease develops, which can also lead to fractures. Even if there were a consensus about the optimal PTH level, it would be difficult to achieve this with current therapies, because the parathyroid gland frequently becomes hypertrophied and the PTH secretion cannot be suppressed with medical management. Calcimimetics are new medications that activate the calcium receptor and lower parathyroid levels. The first calcimimetic, cinacalcet, has recently been approved for treatment of secondary hyperparathyroidism [205]. These drugs have great promise for improving the skeletal status of patients with chronic renal failure.

Treatment with calcitriol can lower serum PTH, and if started early in the course of renal failure, it can prevent parathyroid hyperplasia. Calcitriol, however, may cause hypercalcemia (which worsens vascular calcification), and it increases gastroinestinal absorption of phosphate. Calcitriol also may reduce the bone formation rate, although this is probably an indirect effect of suppression of PTH. Newer analogues of vitamin D such as paricalcitol can decrease the parathyroid hormone secretion with less increase in plasma calcium. Active vitamin D analogues are indicated in hypocalcemic patients [206].

The studies of bone loss after transplantation do not show consistent parathyroid effects [170]. Reports show that the bone loss is unrelated to baseline serum PTH [181, 186, 207, 208], that patients with low serum PTH had better post-transplant bone density [209–213], or that low serum PTH predicted unfavorable bone density changes [170].

The potential role of 25(OH)D is currently of interest, as it may have effects on nonskeletal systems. In renal patients who are treated with calcitriol, the optimum levels of 25(OH)D are not established. Previously it was felt that there was no need for the precursors if patients were given the active metabolite, but there is some evidence that 25(OH)D itself plays a role in muscle function. Until more data are available, it seems wise to keep the levels in the same range as recommended for patients without renal failure. Physicians should be aware that some of the multiple vitamins given to renal patients do not contain any vitamin D.

F. Other Factors that Impair Bone Metabolism

In these patients, acidosis may contribute to bone disease, and this can be adjusted with dialysis treatment. Several accumulated toxins affect the bone, including aluminum, iron, strontium, and beta 2 microglobulin (which causes amyloid deposits in bone and joints). Recent studies suggest abnormally low levels of bone morphogenetic protein reduce osteoblast function and retard differentiation of preosteoblasts to mature osteoblasts [214].

G. Treatment of Low Bone Density

Treatment of decreased bone density in patients awaiting kidney transplantation is difficult. Calcitonin is probably safe in renal disease but it has not been examined. Bisphosphonates are widely used in other forms of bone disease, but there are very few data in this population. Some studies suggest that both hyperparathyroidism and adynamic bone disease could worsen with bisphosphonates [215]. In hypercalcemic patients, pamidronate decreased serum calcium and increased bone density but further increased serum PTH. After 3 months, administration of intravenous calcitriol reduced serum PTH in some patients, but effects on vascular calcifications were not measured [211]. Bisphosphonate clearance is entirely renal, so the dosing (if any) should be lower. Intermittent parathyroid hormone 1-34 or 1-84 is anabolic in patients with normal renal function, but it makes little physiological sense to use this in renal patients who already have hyperparathyroidism. Methods to manipulate the serum PTH to achieve periodic peaks could potentially improve osteoblast function, but currently there is no evidence to support this theory.

Estrogen has been shown to improve bone density in a small study of premenopausal women with renal failure [216], but the risks of this hormone in the dialysis population are not known [217]. Women with coronary artery disease who do not have renal disease have a higher risk of myocardial infarction or worsened arterial disease when treated with hormone replacement. Women with chronic renal failure have an increased risk of cardiovascular death, which potentially could worsen with hormone replacement. Pharmacokinetic studies show that the dose of estrogen should be about half that used in women with normal renal function to achieve the same free estradiol levels, because there is reduced protein binding [218]. Estrogen should be avoided in women with polycystic kidney disease because it stimulates hepatic enlargement [219]. Recently, raloxifene has been shown to improve bone density in women on dialysis [220].

Finally, all the usual risk factors that can contribute to postmenopausal osteoporosis can make renal osteodystrophy even worse, and the basic measures outlined for postmenopausal osteoporosis (such as exercise, cessation of smoking, reduction of falls) should be considered in renal transplant candidates.

VII. SUMMARY

Transplant candidates frequently have multiple risk factors for bone fragility. These complex patients present a challenge to their physicians. In addition to risk factors defined by epidemiological studies of the general population, the transplant candidates have risk factors depending on which organ has failed. Therapeutic choices may be limited or ineffective, and side effects may be more pronounced. Definitive studies on the benefits of preventive treatment in transplant candidates are lacking, but these patients have such a high fracture risk that they deserve our best efforts. Attention to all the cumulative risk factors and treatment within the available options will hopefully result in stronger bones with fewer fractures.

REFERENCES

1. Kanis, J.A., Melton, L. Jr, Christiansen, C., et al. (1994). The diagnosis of osteoporosis. *J Bone Miner Res.* 9:1137–1141.

2. Whyte, M.P., Wenkert, D., Clements, K.L., et al. (2003). Bisphosphonate-induced osteopetrosis. *N Engl J Med.* 349:457–463.
3. Cummings, S.R., Karpf, D.B., Harris, F., et al. (2002). Improvement in spine bone density and reduction in risk of vertebral fractures during treatment with antiresorptive drugs. *Am J Med.* 112:281–289.
4. Cummings, S.R., Nevitt, M.C., Browner, W.S., et al. (1995). Risk factors for hip fracture in white women. Study of Osteoporotic Fractures Research Group. *N Engl J Med.* 332:767–773.
5. Ott, S.M. (2004). Diet for the heart or the bone: a biological tradeoff. *Am J Clin Nutr.* 79:4–5.
6. Gougeon-Reyburn, R., Lariviere, F., Marliss, E.B. (1991). Effects of bicarbonate supplementation on urinary mineral excretion during very low energy diets. *Am J Med Sci.* 302:67–74.
7. Grinspoon, S.K., Baum, H.B., Kim, V., et al. (1995). Decreased bone formation and increased mineral dissolution during acute fasting in young women. *J Clin Endocrinol Metab.* 80:3628–3633.
8. Dawson Hughes, B., Harris, S.S., Krall, E.A., et al. (1997). Effect of calcium and vitamin D supplementation on bone density in men and women 65 years of age or older. *N Engl J Med.* 337:670–676.
9. Brennan, M.J., Duncan, W.E., Wartofsky, L., et al. (1991). In vitro dissolution of calcium carbonate preparations. *Calcif Tissue Int.* 49:308–312.
10. Heaney, R.P., Dowell, M.S., Barger-Lux, M.J. (1999). Absorption of calcium as the carbonate and citrate salts, with some observations on method. *Osteoporos Int.* 9:19–23.
11. Munger, R.G., Cerhan, J.R., Chiu, B.C. (1999). Prospective study of dietary protein intake and risk of hip fracture in postmenopausal women. *Am J Clin Nutr.* 69:147–152.
12. Jackson, R., Bassford, T., Cauley, J. ea. (2002). The impact of magnesium intake on fractures: results from the Women's Health Initiative Observational Study. Presented at the American Society for Bone and Mineral Research, held in Minneapolis, MN, September. 2002:1089.
13. Boncimino, K., McMahon, D.J., Addesso, V., et al. (1999). Magnesium deficiency and bone loss after cardiac transplantation. *Journal of Bone and Mineral Research.* 14:295–303.
14. Feskanich, D., Singh, V., Willett, W.C., et al. (2002). Vitamin A intake and hip fractures among postmenopausal women. *Jama.* 287:47–54.
15. Melhus, H., Michaelsson, K., Kindmark, A., et al. (1998). Excessive dietary intake of vitamin A is associated with reduced bone mineral density and increased risk for hip fracture. *Ann Intern Med.* 129:770–778.
16. Hollis, B. (1996). Assessment of Vitamin D nutritional and hormonal status: what to measure and how to do it. *Calcif Tissue Int.* 58:4–5.
17. Heaney, R.P. (2003). Vitamin D, nutritional deficiency, and the medical paradigm. *J Clin Endocrinol Metab.* 88:5107–5108.
18. Wolff, I., van Croonenborg, J.J., Kemper, H.C., et al. (1999). The effect of exercise training programs on bone mass: a meta-analysis of published controlled trials in pre- and postmenopausal women. *Osteoporos Int.* 9:1–12.
19. Baron, J.A., Farahmand, B.Y., Weiderpass, E., et al. (2001). Cigarette smoking, alcohol consumption, and risk of hip fracture in women. *Arch Intern Med.* 161:983–988.
20. Orwoll, E.S., Bevan, L., Phipps, K.R. (2000). Determinants of bone mineral density in older men. *Osteoporos Int.* 11:815–821.
21. Felson, D.T., Zhang, Y., Hannan, M.T. (1995). Alcohol intake and bone mineral density in elderly men and women: the Framingham study. *Am J Epidemiol.* 1995:485–492.
22. Ward, K.D., Klesges, R.C. (2001). A meta-analysis of the effects of cigarette smoking on bone mineral density. *Calcif Tissue Int.* 68:259–270.
23. Cooper, C., Atkinson, E.J., Wahner, H.W., et al. (1992). Is caffeine consumption a risk factor for osteoporosis. *J Bone Miner Res.* 7:465–471.

24. Barrett Connor, E., Chang, J.C., Edelstein, S.L. (1994). Coffee-associated osteoporosis offset by daily milk consumption. The Rancho Bernardo Study. *JAMA*. 271:280–283.
25. Kannus, P., Parkkari, J., Niemi, S., et al. (2000). Prevention of hip fracture in elderly people with use of a hip protector. *N Engl J Med*. 343:1506–1513.
26. Lane, N.E., Lukert, B. (1998). The science and therapy of glucocorticoid-induced bone loss. *Endocrinol Metab Clin North Am*. 27:465–483.
27. Rejnmark, L., Ves which miwtergaard, P., Pedersen, A.R., et al. (2003). Dose-effect relations of loop- and thiazide-diuretics on calcium homeostasis: a randomized, double-blinded Latin-square multiple cross-over study in postmenopausal osteopenic women. *Eur J Clin Invest*. 33:41–50.
28. LaCroix, A.Z., Ott, S.M., Ichikawa, L., et al. (2000). Low-dose hydrochlorothiazide and preservation of bone mineral density in older adults. A randomized, double-blind, placebo-controlled trial. *Ann Intern Med*. 133:516–526.
29. Scholes, D., LaCroix, A.Z., Ichikawa, L.E., et al. (2002). Injectable hormone contraception and bone density: results from a prospective study. *Epidemiology*. 13:581–587.
30. Bauer, D.C., Ettinger, B., Nevitt, M.C., et al. (2001). Risk for fracture in women with low serum levels of thyroid-stimulating hormone. *Ann Intern Med*. 134:561–568.
31. Adams, J.S., Song, C.F., Kantorovich, V. (1999). Rapid recovery of bone mass in hypercalciuric, osteoporotic men treated with hydrochlorothiazide. *Ann Intern Med*. 130:658–660.
32. NIH Consensus Development Panel. (2001). Osteoporosis prevention, diagnosis, and therapy. *Jama*. 285:785–795.
33. Hodgson, S.F., Watts, N.B., Bilezikian, J.P., et al. (2001). American Association of Clinical Endocrinologists 2001 Medical Guidelines for Clinical Practice for the Prevention and Management of Postmenopausal Osteoporosis. *Endocr Pract*. 7:293–312.
34. Rossouw, J.E., Anderson, G.L., Prentice, R.L., et al. (2002). Risks and benefits of estrogen plus progestin in healthy postmenopausal women: principal results from the Women's Health Initiative randomized controlled trial. *Jama*. 288:321–333.
35. Ettinger, B., Black, D.M., Mitlak, B.H. (1999). Reduction of vertebral fracture risk in postmenopausal women with osteoporosis treated with raloxifene. *JAMA*. 282:637–645.
36. Black, D.M., Cummings, S.R., Karpf, D.B., et al. (1996). Randomised trial of effect of alendronate on risk of fracture in women with existing vertebral fractures. Fracture Intervention Trial Research Group [see comments]. *Lancet*. 348:1535–1541.
37. Liberman, U.A., Weiss, S.R., Broll, J., et al. (1995). Effect of oral alendronate on bone mineral density and the incidence of fractures in postmenopausal osteoporosis. The Alendronate Phase III Osteoporosis Treatment Study Group [see comments]. *N Engl J Med*. 333:1437–1443.
38. McClung, M.R., Geusens, P., Miller, P.D., et al. (2001). Effect of risedronate on the risk of hip fracture in elderly women. Hip Intervention Program Study Group. *N Engl J Med*. 344:333–340.
39. Chavassieux, P.M., Arlot, M.E., Reda, C., et al. (1997). Histomorphometric assessment of the long-term effects of alendronate on bone quality and remodeling in patients with osteoporosis. *J Clin Invest*. 100:1475–1480.
40. Boivin, G.Y., Chavassieux, P.M., Santora, A.C., et al. (2000). Alendronate increases bone strength by increasing the mean degree of mineralization of bone tissue in osteoporotic women. *Bone*. 27:687–694.
41. Mashiba, T., Turner, C.H., Hirano, T., et al. (2001). Effects of suppressed bone turnover by bisphosphonates on microdamage accumulation and biomechanical properties in clinically relevant skeletal sites in beagles. *Bone*. 28:524–531.
42. Bone, H.G., Hosking, D., Devogelaer, J.P., et al. (2004). Ten years' experience with alendronate for osteoporosis in postmenopausal women. *N Engl J Med*. 350:1189–1199.

43. Rosen, C.J., Brown, S. (2003). Severe hypocalcemia after intravenous bisphosphonate therapy in occult vitamin D deficiency. *N Engl J Med.* 348:1503–1504.
44. Peter, R., Mishra,V., Fraser,W.D. (2004). Severe hypocalcaemia after being given intravenous bisphosphonate. *Bmj.* 328:335–336.
45. Neer, R.M., Arnaud, C.D., Zanchetta, J.R., et al. (2001). Effect of parathyroid hormone (1-34) on fractures and bone mineral density in postmenopausal women with osteoporosis. *N Engl J Med.* 344:1434–1441.
46. Vahle, J.L., Sato, M., Long, G.G., et al. (2002). Skeletal changes in rats given daily subcutaneous injections of recombinant human parathyroid hormone (1-34) for 2 years and relevance to human safety. *Toxicol Pathol.* 30:312–321.
47. American College of Rheumatology Ad Hoc Committee on Glucocortcoid-Induced Osteoporosis. (2001). Recommendations for the prevention and treatment of glucocorticoid-induced osteoporosis: 2001 update. *Arthritis Rheum.* 44:1496–1503.
48. Papaioannou, A., Parkinson, W., Ferko, N., et al. (2003). Prevalence of vertebral fractures among patients with chronic obstructive pulmonary disease in Canada. *Osteoporos Int.* 14:913–917. Epub 2003 Oct 2009.
49. Shane, E., Silverberg, S.J., Donovan, D., et al. (1996). Osteoporosis in lung transplantation candidates with end-stage pulmonary disease. *American Journal of Medicine.* 101:262–269.
50. Ferrari, S.L., Nicod, L.P., Hamacher, J., et al. (1996). Osteoporosis in patients undergoing lung transplantation. *Eur Respir J.* 9:2378–2382.
51. Trombetti, A., Gerbase, M.W., Spiliopoulos, A., et al. (2000). Bone mineral density in lung-transplant recipients before and after graft: prevention of lumbar spine post-transplantation-accelerated bone loss by pamidronate. *J Heart Lung Transplant.* 19:736–743.
52. Cahill, B.C.,, O.'Rourke, M.K., Parker, S., et al. (2001). Prevention of bone loss and fracture after lung transplantation: a pilot study. *Transplantation.* 72:1251–1255.
53. Lee, A.H., Mull, R.L., Keenan, G.F., et al. (1994). Osteoporosis and bone morbidity in cardiac transplant recipients. *Am J Med.* 96:35–41.
54. Berguer, D.G., Krieg, M.A., Thiebaud, D., et al. (1994). Osteoporosis in heart transplant recipients: a longitudinal study. *Transplant Proc.* 26:2649–2651.
55. Aris, R.M., Neuringer, I.P., Weiner, M.A., et al. (1996). Severe osteoporosis before and after lung transplantation. *Chest.* 109:1176–1183.
56. Shane, E., Rodino, M., ThysJacobs, S., et al. (1997). Comparison of two antiresorptive regimens on rates of bone loss after cardiac transplantation. *Journal of Bone and Mineral Research.* 12:P319–P319.
57. Sambrook, P.N., Kelly, P.J., Keogh, A.M., et al. (1994). Bone loss after heart transplantation: a prospective study. *J Heart Lung Transplant.* 13:116–120; discussion 121.
58. Spira, A., Gutierrez, C., Chaparro, C., et al. (2000). Osteoporosis and lung transplantation: a prospective study. *Chest.* 117:476–481.
59. Henderson, K., Eisman, J., Keogh, A., et al. (2001). Protective effect of short-tem calcitriol or cyclical etidronate on bone loss after cardiac or lung transplantation. *J Bone Miner Res.* 16:565–571.
60. Tschopp, O., Boehler, A., Speich, R., et al. (2002). Osteoporosis before lung transplantation: association with low body mass index, but not with underlying disease. *Am J Transplant.* 2:167–172.
61. Shane, E., Rivas, M., Staron, R.B., et al. (1996). Fracture after cardiac transplantation: a prospective longitudinal study. *J Clin Endocrinol Metab.* 81:1740–1746.
62. Aris, R.M., Lester, G.E., Caminiti, M., et al. (2004). Efficacy of alendronate in adults with cystic fibrosis with low bone density. *Am J Respir Crit Care Med.* 169:77–82. Epub 2003 Oct 2016.
63. Ott, S.M., Aitken, M.L. (1998). Osteoporosis in patients with cystic fibrosis. *Clin Chest Med.* 19:555–567.
64. Haworth, C.S., Selby, P.L., Adams, J.E., et al. (2001). Effect of intravenous pamidronate on bone mineral density in adults with cystic fibrosis. *Thorax.* 56:314–316.

65. Giannini, S., Nobile, M., Dalle Carbonare, L., et al. (2001). Vertebral morphometry by X-ray absorptiometry before and after liver transplant: a cross-sectional study. *Eur J Gastroenterol Hepatol*. 13:1201–1207.
66. Eastell, R., Dickson, E.R., Hodgson, S.F., et al. (1991). Rates of vertebral bone loss before and after liver transplantation in women with primary biliary cirrhosis. *Hepatology*. 14:296–300.
67. Meys, E., Fontanges, E., Fourcade, N., et al. (1994). Bone loss after orthotopic liver transplantation. *Am J Med*. 97:445–450.
68. Abdelhadi, M., Eriksson, S.A., Ljusk Eriksson, S., et al. (1995). Bone mineral status in end-stage liver disease and the effect of liver transplantation. *Scand J Gastroenterol*. 30:1210–1215.
69. Monegal, A., Navasa, M., Guanabens, N., et al. (1997). Osteoporosis and bone mineral metabolism disorders in cirrhotic patients referred for orthotopic liver transplantation. *Calcif Tissue Int*. 60:148–154.
70. Guardiola, J., Xiol, X., Sallie, R., et al. (1999). Influence of the vitamin D receptor gene polymorphism on bone loss in men after liver transplantation. *Ann Intern Med*. 131:752–755.
71. Crosbie, O.M., Freaney, R., McKenna, M.J., et al. (1999). Predicting bone loss following orthotopic liver transplantation. *Gut*. 44:430–434.
72. Keogh, J.B., Tsalamandris, C., Sewell, R.B., et al. (1999). Bone loss at the proximal femur and reduced lean mass following liver transplantation: a longitudinal study. *Nutrition*. 15:661–664.
73. Hussaini, S.H., Oldroyd, B., Stewart, S.P., et al. (1999). Regional bone mineral density after orthotopic liver transplantation. *European Journal of Gastroenterology & Hepatology*. 11:157–163.
74. Xu, H., Eichstaedt, H. (1999). Assessment of serial changes of bone mineral density at lumbar spine and femoral neck before and after liver transplantation. *Chin Med J (Engl)*. 112:379–381.
75. Ninkovic, M., Skingle, S.J., Bearcroft, P.W., et al. (2000). Incidence of vertebral fractures in the first three months after orthotopic liver transplantation. *Eur J Gastroenterol Hepatol*. 12:931–935.
76. Trautwein, C., Possienke, M., Schlitt, H.J., et al. (2000). Bone density and metabolism in patients with viral hepatitis and cholestatic liver diseases before and after liver transplantation. *Am J Gastroenterol*. 95:2343–2351.
77. Floreani, A., Mega, A., Tizian, L., et al. (2001). Bone metabolism and gonad function in male patients undergoing liver transplantation: a two-year longitudinal study. *Osteoporos Int*. 12:749–754.
78. Monegal, A., Navasa, M., Guanabens, N., et al. (2001). Bone mass and mineral metabolism in liver transplant patients treated with FK506 or cyclosporine A. *Calcif Tissue Int*. 68:83–86.
79. Ninkovic, M., Love, S.A., Tom, B., et al. (2001). High prevalence of osteoporosis in patients with chronic liver disease prior to liver transplantation. *Calcif Tissue Int*. 69:321–326.
80. Ninkovic, M., Love, S., Tom, B.D., et al. (2002). Lack of effect of intravenous pamidronate on fracture incidence and bone mineral density after orthotopic liver transplantation. *J Hepatol*. 37:93–100.
81. Guichelaar, M.M.J, Malinchoc, M., Sibonga, J.D., et al. (2003). Bone histomorphometric changes after liver transplantation for chronic cholestatic liver disease. *J Bone Mineral Res*. 18:2190–2199.
82. Ormarsdottir, S., Ljunggren, O., Mallmin, H., et al. (2002). Increased rate of bone loss at the femoral neck in patients with chronic liver disease. *Eur J Gastroenterol Hepatol*. 14:43–48.
83. Newton, J., Francis, R., Prince, M., et al. (2001). Osteoporosis in primary biliary cirrhosis revisited. *Gut*. 49:282–287.

84. Le Gars, L., Grandpierre, C., Chazouilleres, O., et al. (2002). Bone loss in primary biliary cirrhosis: absence of association with severity of liver disease. *Joint Bone Spine.* 69:195–200.
85. Compston, J.E., Thompson, R.P. (1977). Intestinal absorption of 25-hydroxyvitamin D and osteomalacia in primary biliary cirrhosis. *Lancet.* 1:721–724.
86. Reed, J.S., Meredith, S.C., Nemchausky, B.A., et al. (1980). Bone disease in primary biliary cirrhosis: reversal of osteomalacia with oral 25-hydroxyvitamin D. *Gastroenterology.* 78:512–517.
87. Dibble, J.B., Sheridan, P., Hampshire, R., et al. (1981). Evidence for secondary hyperparathyroidism in the osteomalacia associated with chronic liver disease. *Clin Endocrinol (Oxf).* 15:373–383.
88. Davies, M., Mawer, E.B., Klass, H.J., et al. (1983). Vitamin D deficiency, osteomalacia, and primary biliary cirrhosis. Response to orally administered vitamin D3. *Dig Dis Sci.* 28:145–153.
89. Matloff, D.S., Kaplan, M.M., Neer, R.M., et al. (1982). Osteoporosis in primary biliary cirrhosis: effects of 25-hydroxyvitamin D3 treatment. *Gastroenterology.* 83:97–102.
90. Herlong, H.F., Recker, R.R., Maddrey, W.C. (1982). Bone disease in primary biliary cirrhosis: histologic features and response to 25-hydroxyvitamin D. *Gastroenterology.* 83:103–108.
91. Cuthbert, J.A., Pak, C.Y., Zerwekh, J.E., et al. (1984). Bone disease in primary biliary cirrhosis: increased bone resorption and turnover in the absence of osteoporosis or osteomalacia. *Hepatology.* 4:1–8.
92. Hodgson, S.F., Dickson, E.R., Wahner, H.W., et al. (1985). Bone loss and reduced osteoblast function in primary biliary cirrhosis. *Ann Intern Med.* 103:855–860.
93. Stellon, A.J., Webb, A., Compston, J., et al. (1986). Lack of osteomalacia in chronic cholestatic liver disease. *Bone.* 7:181–185.
94. Shih, M.S., Anderson, C. (1987). Does "hepatic osteodystrophy" differ from peri- and postmenopausal osteoporosis? A histomorphometric study. *Calcif Tissue Int.* 41:187–191.
95. Diamond, T.H., Stiel, D., Lunzer, M., et al. (1989). Hepatic osteodystrophy. Static and dynamic bone histomorphometry and serum bone Gla-protein in 80 patients with chronic liver disease. *Gastroenterology.* 96:213–221.
96. Guanabens, N., Pares, A., Marinoso, L., et al. (1990). Factors influencing the development of metabolic bone disease in primary biliary cirrhosis. *Am J Gastroenterol.* 85:1356–1362.
97. Hodgson, S.F., Dickson, E.R., Eastell, R., et al. (1993). Rates of cancellous bone remodeling and turnover in osteopenia associated with primary biliary cirrhosis. *Bone.* 14:819–827.
98. McDonald, J.A., Dunstan, C.R., Dilworth, P., et al. (1991). Bone loss after liver transplantation. *Hepatology.* 14:613–619.
99. Vedi, S., Greer, S., Skingle, S.J., et al. (1999). Mechanism of bone loss after liver transplantation: A histomorphometric analysis. *J Bone Miner Res.* 14:281–287.
100. Fonseca, V., Epstein, O., Gill, D.S., et al. (1987). Hyperparathyroidism and low serum osteocalcin despite vitamin D replacement in primary biliary cirrhosis. *J Clin Endocrinol Metab.* 64:873–877.
101. Pietschmann, P., Resch, H., Muller, C., et al. (1990). Decreased serum osteocalcin levels in patients with liver cirrhosis. *Bone Miner.* 8:103–108.
102. Capra, F., Casaril, M., Gabrielli, G.B., et al. (1991). Plasma osteocalcin levels in liver cirrhosis. *Ital J Gastroenterol.* 23:124–127.
103. Floreani, A., Chiaramonte, M., Giannini, S., et al. (1991). Longitudinal study on osteodystrophy in primary biliary cirrhosis (PBC) and a pilot study on calcitonin treatment. *J Hepatol.* 12:217–223.
104. Guanabens, N., Pares, A., Alvarez, L., et al. (1998). Collagen-related markers of bone turnover reflect the severity of liver fibrosis in patients with primary biliary cirrhosis. *J Bone Miner Res.* 13:731–738.

105. Crosbie, O.M., Freaney, R., McKenna, M.J., et al. (1999). Bone density, vitamin D status, and disordered bone remodeling in end-stage chronic liver disease. *Calcif Tissue Int.* 64:295–300.
106. Floreani, A., Fries, W., Luisetto, G., et al. (1998). Bone metabolism in orthotopic liver transplantation: a prospective study. *Liver Transpl Surg.* 4:311–319.
107. Watson, R.G., Coulton, L., Kanis, J.A., et al. (1990). Circulating osteocalcin in primary biliary cirrhosis following liver transplantation and during treatment with ciclosporin. *J Hepatol.* 11:354–358.
108. Diamond, T., Stiel, D., Lunzer, M., et al. (1989). Ethanol reduces bone formation and may cause osteoporosis. *Am J Med.* 86:282–288.
109. Janes, C.H., Dickson, E.R., Okazaki, R., et al. (1995). Role of hyperbilirubinemia in the impairment of osteoblast proliferation associated with cholestatic jaundice. *J Clin Invest.* 95:2581–2586.
110. Diamond, T., Pojer, R., Stiel, D., et al. (1991). Does iron affect osteoblast function? Studies in vitro and in patients with chronic liver disease. *Calcif Tissue Int.* 48:373–379.
111. Conte, D., Caraceni, M.P., Duriez, J., et al. (1989). Bone involvement in primary hemochromatosis and alcoholic cirrhosis. *Am J Gastroenterol.* 84:1231–1234.
112. Monegal, A., Navasa, M., Guanabens, N., et al. (2001). Bone disease after liver transplantation: a long-term prospective study of bone mass changes, hormonal status and histomorphometric characteristics. *Osteoporos Int.* 12:484–492.
113. Springer, J.E., Cole, D.E., Rubin, L.A., et al. (2000). Vitamin D-receptor genotypes as independent genetic predictors of decreased bone mineral density in primary biliary cirrhosis. *Gastroenterology.* 118:145–151.
114. Ormarsdottir, S., Ljunggren, O., Mallmin, H., et al. (1999). Low body mass index and use of corticosteroids, but not cholestasis, are risk factors for osteoporosis in patients with chronic liver disease. *J Hepatol.* 31:84–90.
115. Leidig-Bruckner, G., Hosch, S., Dodidou, P., et al. (2001). Frequency and predictors of osteoporotic fractures after cardiac or liver transplantation: a follow-up study. *Lancet.* 357:342–347.
116. Hardinger, K.L., Ho, B., Schnitzler, M.A., et al. (2003). Serial measurements of bone density at the lumbar spine do not predict fracture risk after liver transplantation. *Liver Transpl.* 9:857–862.
117. Hockerstedt, K., Isoniemi, H., Risteli, J., et al. (1994). A simple method for predicting bone fractures in PBC patients after liver transplantation. *Transpl Int.* 7 Suppl 1:S121–122.
118. Diamond, T., Stiel, D., Mason, R., et al. (1989). Serum vitamin D metabolites are not responsible for low turnover osteoporosis in chronic liver disease. *J Clin Endocrinol Metab.* 69:1234–1239.
119. Kirch, W., Hofig, M., Ledendecker, T., et al. (1990). Parathyroid hormone and cirrhosis of the liver. *J Clin Endocrinol Metab.* 71:1561–1566.
120. Guanabens, N., Pares, A., Ros, I., et al. (2003). Alendronate is more effective than etidronate for increasing bone mass in osteopenic patients with primary biliary cirrhosis. *Am J Gastroenterol.* 98:2268–2274.
121. Rabinovitz, M., Shapiro, J., Lian, J., et al. (1992). Vitamin D and osteocalcin levels in liver transplant recipients. Is osteocalcin a reliable marker of bone turnover in such cases? *J Hepatol.* 16:50–55.
122. Bagur, A., Mautalen, C., Findor, J., et al. (1998). Risk factors for the development of vertebral and total skeleton osteoporosis in patients with primary biliary cirrhosis. *Calcif Tissue Int.* 63:385–390.
123. Compston, J.E., Greer, S., Skingle, S.J., et al. (1996). Early increase in plasma parathyroid hormone levels following liver transplantation. *J Hepatol.* 25:715–718.
124. Hay, J.E., Malinchoc, M., Dickson, E.R. (2001). A controlled trial of calcitonin therapy for the prevention of post-liver transplantation atraumatic fractures in patients

with primary biliary cirrhosis and primary sclerosing cholangitis. *J Hepatol.* 34:292–298.

125. Mawer, E.B., Klass, H.J., Warnes, T.W., et al. (1985). Metabolism of vitamin D in patients with primary biliary cirrhosis and alcoholic liver disease. *Clin Sci (Lond).* 69:561–570.
126. Bikle, D.D., Halloran, B.P., Gee, E., et al. (1986). Free 25-hydroxyvitamin D levels are normal in subjects with liver disease and reduced total 25-hydroxyvitamin D levels. *J Clin Invest.* 78:748–752.
127. Klein, G.L., Endres, D.B., Colonna, J.D., 2nd, et al. (1989). Absence of hyperparathyroidism in severe liver disease. *Calcif Tissue Int.* 44:330–334.
128. Compston, J.E. (1986). Hepatic osteodystrophy: vitamin D metabolism in patients with liver disease. *Gut.* 27:1073–1090.
129. Collier, J.D., Ninkovic, M., Compston, J.E. (2002). Guidelines on the management of osteoporosis associated with chronic liver disease. *Gut.* 50 Suppl 1:i1–9.
130. Camisasca, M., Crosignani, A., Battezzati, P.M., et al. (1994). Parenteral calcitonin for metabolic bone disease associated with primary biliary cirrhosis. *Hepatology.* 20:633–637.
131. Sitrin, M.D., Bengoa, J.M. (1987). Intestinal absorption of cholecalciferol and 25-hydroxycholecalciferol in chronic cholestatic liver disease. *Am J Clin Nutr.* 46:1011–1015.
132. Shiomi, S., Masaki, K., Habu, D., et al. (1999). Calcitriol for bone loss in patients with primary biliary cirrhosis. *J Gastroenterol.* 34:241–245.
133. Kowdley, K.V., Emond, M.J., Sadowski, J.A., et al. (1997). Plasma vitamin K1 level is decreased in primary biliary cirrhosis. *Am J Gastroenterol.* 92:2059–2061.
134. Hodges, S.J., Pilkington, M.J., Stamp, T.C., et al. (1991). Depressed levels of circulating menaquinones in patients with osteoporotic fractures of the spine and femoral neck. *Bone.* 12:387–389.
135. Shiomi, S., Nishiguchi, S., Kubo, S., et al. (2002). Vitamin K2 (menatetrenone) for bone loss in patients with cirrhosis of the liver. *Am J Gastroenterol.* 97:978–981.
136. Floreani, A., Zappala, F., Fries, W., et al. (1997). A 3-year pilot study with 1,25-dihydroxyvitamin D, calcium, and calcitonin for severe osteodystrophy in primary biliary cirrhosis. *J Clin Gastroenterol.* 24:239–244.
137. Crippin, J.S., Jorgensen, R.A., Dickson, E.R., et al. (1994). Hepatic osteodystrophy in primary biliary cirrhosis: effects of medical treatment. *Am J Gastroenterol.* 89:47–50.
138. Menon, K.V., Angulo, P., Boe, G.M., et al. (2003). Safety and efficacy of estrogen therapy in preventing bone loss in primary biliary cirrhosis. *Am J Gastroenterol.* 98:889–892.
139. Olsson, R., Mattsson, L.A., Obrant, K., et al. (1999). Estrogen-progestogen therapy for low bone mineral density in primary biliary cirrhosis. *Liver.* 19:188–192.
140. Levy, C., Lindor, K.D. (2003). Management of osteoporosis, fat-soluble vitamin deficiencies, and hyperlipidemia in primary biliary cirrhosis. *Clin Liver Dis.* 7:901–910.
141. Wolfhagen, F.H., van Buuren, H.R., den Ouden, J.W., et al. (1997). Cyclical etidronate in the prevention of bone loss in corticosteroid-treated primary biliary cirrhosis. A prospective, controlled pilot study. *J Hepatol.* 26:325–330.
142. Lindor, K.D., Jorgensen, R.A., Tiegs, R.D., et al. (2000). Etidronate for osteoporosis in primary biliary cirrhosis: a randomized trial. *J Hepatol.* 33:878–882.
143. Reeves, H.L., Francis, R.M., Manas, D.M., et al. (1998). Intravenous bisphosphonate prevents symptomatic osteoporotic vertebral collapse in patients after liver transplantation. *Liver Transpl Surg.* 4:404–409.
144. Bishop, N.J., Ninkovic, M., Alexander, G.J., et al. (1999). Changes in calcium homoeostasis in patients undergoing liver transplantation: effects of a single infusion of pamidronate administered pre-operatively. *Clin Sci (Colch).* 97:157–163.
145. Vedi, S., Ninkovic, M., Garrahan, N.J., et al. (2002). Effects of a single infusion of pamidronate prior to liver transplantation: a bone histomorphometric study. *Transpl Int.* 15:290–295.

146. Eknoyan, G., Levin, A., Levin, N.W. (2003). Bone metabolism and disease in chronic kidney disease. *Am J Kidney Dis.* 42:1–201.
147. Elder, G. (2002). Pathophysiology and recent advances in the management of renal osteodystrophy. *J Bone Miner Res.* 17:2094–2105.
148. Cunningham, J., Sprague, S.M., Cannata-Andia, J., et al. (2004). Osteoporosis in chronic kidney disease. *Am J Kidney Dis.* 43:566–571.
149. Martin, K.J., Olgaard, K., Coburn, J.W., et al. (2004). Diagnosis, assessment, and treatment of bone turnover abnormalities in renal osteodystrophy. *Am J Kidney Dis.* 43:558–565.
150. Sherrard, D.J., Hercz, G., Pei, Y., et al. (1993). The spectrum of bone disease in end-stage renal failure—an evolving disorder. *Kidney Int.* 43:436–442.
151. Jamal, S.A., Chase, C., Goh, Y.I., et al. (2002). Bone density and heel ultrasound testing do not identify patients with dialysis-dependent renal failure who have had fractures. *Am J Kidney Dis.* 39:843–849.
152. Alem, A.M., Sherrard, D.J., Gillen, D.L., et al. (2000). Increased risk of hip fracture among patients with end-stage renal disease. *Kidney Int.* 58:396–399.
153. Ball, A.M., Gillen, D.L., Sherrard, D., et al. (2002). Risk of hip fracture among dialysis and renal transplant recipients. *Jama.* 288:3014–3018.
154. Piraino, B., Chen, T., Cooperstein, L., et al. (1988). Fractures and vertebral bone mineral density in patients with renal osteodystrophy. *Clin Nephrol.* 30:57–62.
155. Atsumi, K., Kushida, K., Yamazaki, K., et al. (1999). Risk factors for vertebral fractures in renal osteodystrophy. *Am J Kidney Dis.* 33:287–293.
156. Coco, M., Rush, H. (2000). Increased incidence of hip fractures in dialysis patients with low serum parathyroid hormone. *Am J Kidney Dis.* 36:1115–1121.
157. Stehman-Breen, C.O., Sherrard, D.J., Alem, A.M., et al. (2000). Risk factors for hip fracture among patients with end-stage renal disease. *Kidney Int.* 58:2200–2205.
158. Patel, S., Kwan, J.T., McCloskey, E., et al. (2001). Prevalence and causes of low bone density and fractures in kidney transplant patients. *J Bone Miner Res.* 16:1863–1870.
159. Grotz, W.H., Mundinger, F.A., Gugel, B., et al. (1994). Bone fracture and osteodensitometry with dual energy X-ray absorptiometry in kidney transplant recipients. *Transplantation.* 58:912–915.
160. Monier-Faugere, M.C., Mawad, H., Qi, Q., et al. (2000). High prevalence of low bone turnover and occurrence of osteomalacia after kidney transplantation. *J Am Soc Nephrol.* 11:1093–1099.
161. Gerakis, A., Hadjidakis, D., Kokkinakis, E., et al. (2000). Correlation of bone mineral density with the histological findings of renal osteodystrophy in patients on hemodialysis. *J Nephrol.* 13:437–443.
162. Hutchison, A., Whitehouse, R.W., Boulton, H.F., et al. (1993). Correlation of bone histology with parathyroid hormone, vitamin D3, and radiology in end-stage renal disease. *Kidney Int.* 44:1071–1077.
163. Boling, E., Primavera, C., Friedman, G., et al. (1993). Non-invasive measurements of bone mass in adult renal osteodystrophy. *Bone.* 14:409–413.
164. Aird, E.G.A. Photon absorptiometry in hemodialysis and transplant patients in Newcastle upon Tyne, England, in Proceedings Fourth International Conference on Bone Measurement, Mazess, R., ed. 1980, pp. 217–230. Washington, DC: NIH Publication No. 80-1938.
165. Arici, M., Erturk, H., Altun, B., et al. (2000). Bone mineral density in haemodialysis patients: A comparative study of dual-energy X-ray absorptiometry and quantitative ultrasound. *Nephrol Dial Transplant.* 15:1847–1851.
166. Aroldi, A., Tarantino, A., Montagnino, G., et al. (1997). Effects of three immunosuppressive regimens on vertebral bone density in renal transplant recipients: a prospective study. *Transplantation.* 63:380–386.
167. Asaka, M., Iida, H., Entani, C., et al. (1992). Total and regional bone mineral density by dual photon absorptiometry in patients on maintenance hemodialysis. *Clin Nephrol.* 38:149–153.

168. Barnas, U., Schmidt, A., Seidl, G., et al. (2001). A comparison of quantitative computed tomography and dual X-ray absorptiometry for evaluation of bone mineral density in patients on chronic hemodialysis. *Am J Kidney Dis*. 37:1247–1252.
169. Bianchi, M., Colantonio, G., Montesano, A., et al. (1992). Bone mass status is different degrees of chronic renal failure. *Bone*. 13:225–228.
170. Casez, J.P., Lippuner, K., Horber, F.F., et al. (2002). Changes in bone mineral density over 18 months following kidney transplantation: the respective roles of prednisone and parathyroid hormone. *Nephrol Dial Transplant*. 17:1318–1326.
171. Chan, T., Pun, K.K., Cheng, I.K. (1992). Total and regional bone densities in dialysis patients. *Nephrol Dial Transplant*. 7:835–839.
172. Cohn, S., Ellis, K.J., Caselnova, R.C., et al. (1975). Correlation of radial bone mineral content with total body calcium in chronic renal failure. *J Lab Clin Med*. 86:910–919.
173. De Sevaux, R.G., Hoitsma, A.J., Corstens, F.H., et al. (2002). Treatment with vitamin D and calcium reduces bone loss after renal transplantation: a randomized study. *J Am Soc Nephrol*. 13:1608–1614.
174. Fan, S.L., Almond, M.K., Ball, E., et al. (2000). Pamidronate therapy as prevention of bone loss following renal transplantation1. *Kidney Int*. 57:684–690.
175. Gabay, C., Ruedin, P., Slosman, D., et al. (1993). Bone mineral density in patients with end-stage renal failure. *Am J Nephrol*. 13:115–123.
176. Ghazali, A., Grados, F., Oprisiu, R., et al. (2003). Bone mineral density directly correlates with elevated serum leptin in haemodialysis patients. *Nephrol Dial Transplant*. 18:1882–1890.
177. Grotz, W., Nagel, C., Poeschel, D., et al. (2001). Effect of ibandronate on bone loss and renal function after kidney transplantation. *J Am Soc Nephrol*. 12:1530–1537.
178. Haas, M., Leko-Mohr, Z., Roschger, P., et al. (2003). Zoledronic acid to prevent bone loss in the first 6 months after renal transplantation. *Kidney Int*. 63:1130–1136.
179. Hampson, G., Vaja, S., Evans, C., et al. (2002). Comparison of the humoral markers of bone turnover and bone mineral density in patients on haemodialysis and continuous ambulatory peritoneal dialysis. *Nephron*. 91:94–102.
180. Horber, F.F., Casez, J.P., Steiger, U., et al. (1994). Changes in bone mass early after kidney transplantation. *J Bone Miner Res*. 9:1–9.
181. Julian, B.A., Laskow, D.A., Dubovsky, J., et al. (1991). Rapid loss of vertebral mineral density after renal transplantation. *N Engl J Med*. 325:544–550.
182. Kaji, H., Suzuki, M., Yano, S., et al. (2002). Risk factors for hip fracture in hemodialysis patients. *Am J Nephrol*. 22:325–331.
183. Kaye, M., Rosenthal lL, Hill, R.O., et al. (1993). Long-term outcome following total parathyroidectomy in patients with end-stage renal disease. *Clin Nephrol*. 39:192–197.
184. Lechleitner, P., Krimbacher, E., Genser, N., et al. (1994). Bone mineral densitometry in dialyzed patients: quantitative computed tomography versus dual photon absorptiometry. *Bone*. 15:387–391.
185. Lippuner, K., Casez, J.P., Horber, F.F., et al. (1998). Effects of deflazacort versus prednisone on bone mass, body composition, and lipid profile: a randomized, double blind study in kidney transplant patients. *J Clin Endocrinol Metab*. 83:3795–3802.
186. Mikuls, T.R., Julian, B.A., Bartolucci, A., et al. (2003). Bone mineral density changes within six months of renal transplantation. *Transplantation*. 75:49–54.
187. Mottet, J.J., Horber, F.F., Casez, J.P., et al. (1996). Evidence for preservation of cortical bone mineral density in patients on continuous ambulatory peritoneal dialysis. *J Bone Miner Res*. 11:96–104.
188. Nakashima, A., Yorioka, N., Tanji, C., et al. (2003). Bone mineral density may be related to atherosclerosis in hemodialysis patients. *Osteoporos Int*. 14:369–373. Epub 2003 May 2024.
189. Parfitt, A., Oliver, I., Walczak, N., et al. (1976). The effect of chronic renal failure and maintenance hemodialysis on bone mineral content of the radius. *Am J Roentg*. 126:1292–1293.

190. Rickers, H., Nielsen, A.H., Smith Pederson, R., et al. (1978). Bone mineral loss during maintenance hemodialysis. *Acta Med Scand.* 204:263–267.
191. Russo, C.R., Taccetti, G., Caneva, P., et al. (1998). Volumetric bone density and geometry assessed by peripheral quantitative computed tomography in uremic patients on maintenance hemodialysis. *Osteoporos Int.* 8:443–448.
192. Seeman, E., Miach, P., Cooper, M., et al. (1989). The effect of renal transplantation on bone mass. *Transplant Proc.* 21:2159–2160.
193. Soylemezoglu, O., Derici, U., Arinsoy, T., et al. (2002). Changes in bone mineral density, insulin-like growth factor-1 and insulin-like growth factor binding protein-3 in kidney transplant recipients. A longitudinal study. *Nephron.* 91:468–473.
194. Spindler, A., Paz, S., Berman, A., et al. (1997). Muscular strength and bone mineral density in haemodialysis patients. *Nephrol Dial Transplant.* 12:128–132.
195. Stein, M.S., Packham, D.K., Ebeling, P.R., et al. (1996). Prevalence and risk factors for osteopenia in dialysis patients. *Am J Kidney Dis.* 28:515–522.
196. Taal, M.W., Masud, T., Green, D., et al. (1999). Risk factors for reduced bone density in haemodialysis patients. *Nephrol Dial Transplant.* 14:1922–1928.
197. Yamaguchi, T., Kanno, E., Tsubota, J., et al. (1996). Retrospective study on the usefulness of radius and lumbar bone density in the separation of hemodialysis patients with fractures from those without fractures. *Bone.* 19:549–555.
198. Slatopolsky, E. (2003). New developments in hyperphosphatemia management. *J Am Soc Nephrol.* 14:S297–299.
199. Cozzolino, M., Staniforth, M.E., Liapis, H., et al. (2003). Sevelamer hydrochloride attenuates kidney and cardiovascular calcifications in long-term experimental uremia. *Kidney Int.* 64:1653–1661.
200. Chertow, G.M., Raggi, P., McCarthy, J.T., et al. (2003). The effects of sevelamer and calcium acetate on proxies of atherosclerotic and arteriosclerotic vascular disease in hemodialysis patients. *Am J Nephrol.* 23:307–314. Epub 2003 Aug 2012.
201. Goodman, W.G. (2003). Medical management of secondary hyperparathyroidism in chronic renal failure. *Nephrol Dial Transplant.* 18 Suppl 3:iii2–8.
202. Fletcher, S., Jones, R.G., Rayner, H.C., et al. (1997). Assessment of renal osteodystrophy in dialysis patients: use of bone alkaline phosphatase, bone mineral density and parathyroid ultrasound in comparison with bone histology. *Nephron.* 75:412–419.
203. Copley, J.B., Hui, S.L., Leapman, S., et al. (1993). Longitudinal study of bone mass in end-stage renal disease patients: effects of parathyroidectomy for renal osteodystrophy. *J Bone Miner Res.* 8:415–422.
204. Malluche, H.H., Mawad, H., Trueba, D., et al. (2003). Parathyroid hormone assays—evolution and revolutions in the care of dialysis patients. *Clin Nephrol.* 59:313–318.
205. Quarles, L.D., Sherrard, D.J., Adler, S., et al. (2003). The calcimimetic AMG 073 as a potential treatment for secondary hyperparathyroidism of end-stage renal disease. *J Am Soc Nephrol.* 14:575–583.
206. Slatopolsky E, Finch J, Brown A. (2003). New vitamin D analogs. *Kidney Int Suppl.* 63: S83-87.
207. Isiklar, I., Akin, O., Demirag, A., et al. (1998). Changes in bone mineral density after renal transplantation. *Transplant Proc.* 30:814–815.
208. Kim, H., Chang, K., Lee, T., et al. (1998). Bone mineral density after renal transplantation. *Transplant Proc.* 30:3029–3030.
209. Grotz, W.H., Mundinger, F.A., Rasenack, J., et al. (1995). Bone loss after kidney transplantation: a longitudinal study in 115 graft recipients. *Nephrol Dial Transplant.* 10:2096–2100.
210. Heaf, J., Tvedegaard, E., Kanstrup, I.L., et al. (2003). Hyperparathyroidism and long-term bone loss after renal transplantation. *Clin Transplant.* 17:268–274.
211. Torregrosa JV, Moreno A, Mas M, et al. (2003). Usefulness of pamidronate in severe secondary hyperparathyroidism in patients undergoing hemodialysis. *Kidney Int Suppl.* 63:S88-90.

212. Torres, A., Lorenzo, V., Gonzalez-Posada, J.M. (1986). Comparison of histomorphometry and computerized tomography of the spine in quantitating trabecular bone in renal osteodystrophy. *Nephron*. 44:282–287.
213. Almond, M.K., Kwan, J.T., Evans, K., et al. (1994). Loss of regional bone mineral density in the first 12 months following renal transplantation. *Nephron*. 66:52–57.
214. Lund, R.J., Davies, M.R., Brown, A.J., et al. (2004). Successful treatment of an adynamic bone disorder with bone morphogenetic protein-7 in a renal ablation model. *J Am Soc Nephrol*. 15:359–369.
215. Lu, K.C., Yeung, L.K., Lin, S.H., et al. (2003). Acute effect of pamidronate on PTH secretion in postmenopausal hemodialysis patients with secondary hyperparathyroidism. *Am J Kidney Dis*. 42:1221–1227.
216. Matuszkiewicz-Rowinska, J., Skorzewska, K., Radowicki, S., et al. (1999). The benefits of hormone replacement therapy in pre-menopausal women with oestrogen deficiency on haemodialysis. *Nephrol Dial Transplant*. 14:1238–1243.
217. Mattix, H., Singh, A.K. (2000). Estrogen replacement therapy: implications for postmenopausal women with end-stage renal disease. *Curr Opin Nephrol Hypertens*. 9:207–214.
218. Stehman-Breen, C., Anderson, G., Gibson, D., et al. (2003). Pharmacokinetics of oral micronized beta-estradiol in postmenopausal women receiving maintenance hemodialysis. *Kidney Int*. 64:290–294.
219. Sherstha, R., McKinley, C., Russ, P., et al. (1997). Postmenopausal estrogen therapy selectively stimulates hepatic enlargement in women with autosomal dominant polycystic kidney disease. *Hepatology*. 26:1282–1286.
220. Hernandez, E., Valera, R., Alonzo, E., et al. (2003). Effects of raloxifene on bone metabolism and serum lipids in postmenopausal women on chronic hemodialysis. *Kidney Int*. 63:2269–2274.

CHAPTER 23

Management: Prevention of Bone Loss after Organ Transplantation

Philip Sambrook, MD
Institute of Bone and Joint Research, University of Sydney, Sydney, Australia

I. INTRODUCTION

Large reductions in bone mineral density (BMD) with subsequent increased fracture risk have been reported after most different types of organ transplantation, as discussed in Chapters 11–18.

Although varying reductions in bone density can occur before transplantation depending upon the underlying disease, the most rapid bone loss following transplantation usually occurs in the first 12–18 months, suggesting that interventions to prevent bone loss immediately after transplantation are likely to be most effective in reducing skeletal morbidity. Moreover it is appropriate to consider two different therapeutic situations: (a) primary prevention of rapid bone loss in the early period immediately after transplant and (b) secondary prevention or treatment of "established" transplant-related bone loss in patients at least 12–18 months after transplant, who will almost certainly already have significant reductions in bone mass. Although there is some overlap between this chapter and the next, this chapter focuses on primary prevention of rapid early bone loss after transplantation, whereas Chapter 24 reviews evidence for treatments to reverse "established" bone loss.

As reviewed in Chapter 10, contributing factors for post-transplantation bone loss include (a) immunosuppressive therapy including prednisone and cyclosporine [1], (b) the underlying disease itself, which may be associated with metabolic bone disease prior to transplant so that the degree of loss may vary by type of organ transplanted, and (c) treatment of the underlying disease prior to transplantation. A schematic diagram of possible mechanisms of transplantation bone loss and targets for intervention to

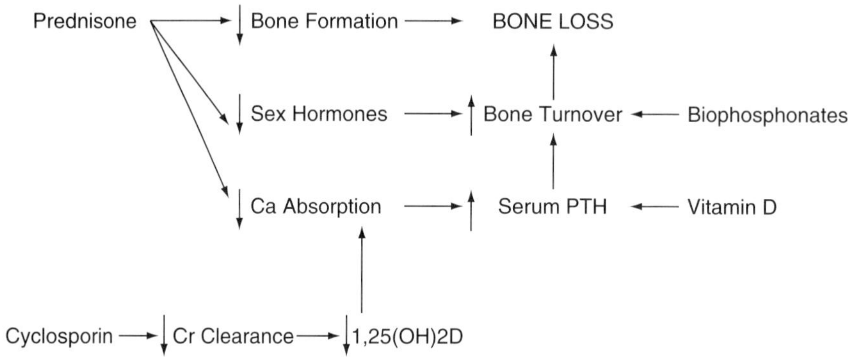

FIGURE 1 Possible mechanisms of transplantation bone loss and targets for therapy.

prevent such loss is shown in Figure 1. Glucocorticoids are an important part of most immunosuppressive regimens after organ transplantation, but they are also known to affect bone metabolism through multiple pathways [2]. Accordingly, many of the studies of agents to prevent bone loss after transplantation have employed similar approaches to those used to prevent glucocorticoid-induced bone loss. The majority of therapeutic trials have focused on the use of vitamin D metabolites and antiresorptive agents, particularly bisphosphonates [3].

II. VITAMIN D

Active vitamin D metabolites such as 1,25 dihydroxy vitamin D (calcitriol) and 1-α hydroxyvitamin D (alfacalcidol) have been shown in some studies to be effective in preventing bone loss in patients starting glucocorticoids [4, 5], suggesting a role for these agents in transplant osteoporosis. Vitamin D metabolites could reduce post-transplantation bone loss by reversing glucocorticoid-induced decreases in intestinal calcium absorption and mitigating secondary hyperparathyroidism [6], which seems a prominent mechanism of bone loss [7] (see Figure 1).

The combination of calcium and simple vitamin D has been used as adjunctive therapy in most transplant clinical trials, but it seems clear that simple vitamin D, in doses of 400–1000 IU/day, cannot prevent significant post-transplantation bone loss [8–10]. Studies of active vitamin D metabolites in the transplant setting have shown better albeit variable results, but their interpretation needs to take account of study quality (many studies were not randomized or used historical controls), small numbers of patients studied, differing doses (remembering 1 mcg of calcitriol is approximately equivalent to 0.5 mcg alfacalcidol), use of concomitant therapy, variable timing after transplant (so that not all studies titled "prevention" are in the early phase of rapid bone loss), and varying immunosuppressive regimens.

For example, Stempfle [11] performed a prospective, randomized, placebo-controlled, double-blind trial of the effect of low-dose calcitriol on bone loss after cardiac transplantation. A total of 132 patients (111 male, 21 female; mean age 51 years) were randomized to calcitriol or placebo. However, the mean dose of calcitriol was low at 0.25 mcg per day, the mean duration before initiating treatment was late at 35 months after transplant (making this a secondary prevention study), and concomitant therapy included sex-hormone therapy in hypogonadal patients (about 20%). BMD increased continuously within the study period in the calcitriol group (over 1 year: 2.2%; over 2 years: 3.9%; over 3 years: 5.7%) but also in the placebo group (over 1 year: 1.8%; over 2 years: 3.7%; over 3 years: 6.1%) with no significant difference between the groups. A greater increase in BMD was seen in hypogonadal patients (most probably because these patients received concomitant hormone replacement) than eugonadal patients, making interpretation of the findings difficult in regard to calcitriol.

Similarly, Neuhaus [12] explored a range of doses of calcitriol, enrolling 509 patients (213 female and 296 male, mean age 47.5 years) in a parallel group but nonrandomized study. Some 283 patients were assigned to 5 treatment groups started just 6 months after liver transplant and followed up for 18 months with 246 patients as controls. The treated patients received either calcitriol 0.25 mcg daily (group 1, 35 patients), calcitriol 0.25 mcg plus calcium 1000 mg daily (group 2, 37 patients), calcitriol 0.5 mcg daily (group 3, 76 patients), or calcitriol 0.5 mcg daily plus calcium 1000 mg daily (group 4, 86 patients). A fifth group received calcitriol 0.5 mcg daily plus 1000 mg of calcium plus sodium fluoride 25 mg daily (49 patients), the latter agent making interpretation of BMD trends in group 5 problematic. Focusing on just the first 4 groups, overall calcitriol led to an improvement of BMD at both the spine and hip in all treatment groups or at least prevented further bone loss. Patients treated with 0.5 mcg of calcitriol (groups 3 and 4) showed a superior response in the spine and hip BMD than patients treated with 0.25 mcg daily. In groups 3 and 4, the mean increment in BMD was surprisingly large at 10% for the spine and 5.6% for the femoral neck. Similarly, patients in group 1 showed quite a large increment of 5.6% for the spine and 4% for the femoral neck. Even better results were obtained in group 2 with an increment of 7.3% for the spine and 3.9% for the femoral neck. However, since after liver transplantation virtually all spinal bone loss occurs in the first 6 months with some recovery evident between 6 and 12 months, this study might be better considered as secondary rather than primary prevention in design. The incidence of atraumatic fractures was significantly lower in the treated patients (2 of 238) in contrast to the control group (7 of 246). Bearing in mind the study was not randomized, these data suggest calcitriol reduced bone loss after liver transplant and that calcitriol 0.5 mcg daily was more effective than 0.25 mcg.

Sambrook [13] also examined the efficacy of treatment with calcitriol in primary prevention in a 2-year, randomized, double-blind study of

65 patients undergoing cardiac or single-lung transplantation. Patients were randomly allocated to receive either placebo or calcitriol (0.5–0.75 mcg/day), the latter for either 12 months or 24 months after transplantation (i.e., there were 3 groups). All groups received calcium 600 mg/day. Bone loss at the proximal femur was significantly reduced or prevented at all 3 sites by treatment with calcitriol for 2 years compared with treatment with calcium alone. Bone loss at 24 months averaged 8.3% for those treated with calcium alone compared to 5.0% for those treated with calcitriol for 2 years. However, treatment with calcitriol for 12 months followed by calcium for 12 months resulted in similar proximal femoral bone loss to that seen in patients treated with calcium alone for 24 months (7.4%), suggesting that prophylaxis with calcitriol needs to be continued beyond 12 months. Although there were no significant differences in lumbar spine BMD between groups, over 2 years 22 new vertebral fractures/deformities occurred in 4 patients treated with calcium alone compared with 1 new vertebral fracture in 1 patient treated with calcitriol. Mild hypercalcemia was common with this dose of calcitriol, as was mild hypercalciuria (59% of patients versus 10% controls), but there were no significant differences between groups in serum creatinine after 2 years. These data suggest calcitriol in doses of 0.5 mcg or greater daily may have a role in reducing bone loss after cardiac or lung transplantation, but treatment needs to be continued beyond 1 year.

The effect of treatment with active vitamin D metabolites on bone loss has also been examined in the first 6 months after renal transplantation [14]. A total of 111 renal transplant recipients (65 men, 46 women; mean age 47 years) were randomized to treatment with either alfacalcidol (0.25 mcg/day) plus calcium (1000 mg/day) or no treatment. In both groups, a significant decrease in lumbar BMD was observed during the first 3 months (alfacalcidol, −3.3 %; $p < 0.0001$; controls −4.1 %; $p < 0.0001$). Between 3 and 6 months, lumbar BMD slightly recovered in the vitamin D group, but it decreased further in the control group (total loss 0 to 6 months: alfacalcidol, −2.6 %; $p < 0.001$; controls, −5.0 %, $p < 0.0001$), and the amount of bone loss at 6 months was significantly different between the groups ($p = 0.02$). Loss of BMD at the various hip sites was also significantly reduced in the alfacalcidol group. Apart from a trend toward more frequent hypercalcemia in the alfacalcidol group (9.2 versus 4.3 %), no clinical or biochemical differences existed between the groups. The authors concluded that treatment with active vitamin D plus calcium partially prevented bone loss at the lumbar spine and proximal femur during the first 6 months after renal transplantation.

Ugur [15] performed a randomized prospective trial in 45 patients after renal transplantation assigned to one of four groups: no treatment, calcium alone, calcium plus calcitriol (0.5mcg/day), or calcium plus calcitriol plus nasal calcitonin (200 IU every second day). However, all patients were more than 12 months after transplant. Patients receiving calcitriol were protected from further bone loss, unlike the calcium and no treatment groups, who lost bone at the spine and hip over the subsequent 12 months. Consistent with studies discussed later in this chapter, addition of calcitonin provided no additional benefit.

In a retrospective cross-sectional analysis, Berczi [16] compared the effect of calcium and alfacalcidol in two historical cohorts comprising 240 patients followed for up to 3 years after renal transplantation. Calcium supplementation appeared superior to alfacalcidol in suppressing hyperparathyroidism and preventing bone loss. Immunosupressive therapy, however, including glucocorticoid doses, was higher in the aflacalcidol group, which may have acted as a confounder and makes interpretation difficult.

Overall, these studies suggest active vitamin D metabolites may have a particular advantage in the transplant setting (compared to glucocorticoid osteoporosis where the data are more conflicting), but are probably not as effective as bisphosphonates, as reviewed in the next section.

III. BISPHOSPHONATES

Bisphosphonates increase BMD and reduce fracture rates in women with postmenopausal osteoporosis and glucocorticoid-induced osteoporosis, and have also been studied in post-transplant osteoporosis.

One of the earliest studies of bisphosphonates was by Van Cleemput [17], who randomized patients to receive either cyclical etidronate (400 mg daily for 14 days every 3 months) or alfacalcidol (starting at 0.25 mcg and going to 1 mcg/day) plus calcium carbonate. In this open-label study in 48 patients after cardiac transplantation, treatment with alfacalcidol reduced bone loss in the spine and femoral neck more than cyclical etidronate, with spinal loss at 6 months averaging 4.6% with alfacalcidol and 7.7% with etidronate. Two vertebral deformities occurred in the alfacalcidol group over 2 years compared with 8 in the etidronate group. There was no control or "untreated" group in this study, however.

To determine whether the rapid phase of bone loss after transplant was a relatively brief phenomenon, Henderson [18] compared the efficacy of 6 months of treatment with 2 cycles of etidronate to calcitriol 0.5 mcg/day immediately after cardiac or lung transplantation in 41 patients. Patients were followed for a further 18 months. There were no significant differences between groups with respect to age or cumulative dose of prednisone or cyclosporine over the 2 years. Bone loss did not differ between groups after 6 months and, despite 6 months prophylaxis with either agent, bone loss was significant in both groups at 6 months and 12 months. However, compared with an untreated historical control group, both therapies offered significant protection at 6 months, and etidronate provided significant protective carryover after therapy had been discontinued. These data suggest short-term prophylaxis with etidronate is partially effective in reducing bone loss after transplantation but probably needs to continue beyond 6 months.

Etidronate is a first-generation bisphosphonate, and subsequent studies have examined more potent agents in this class.

The best studied of these agents has been pamidronate, a second-generation bisphosphonate. Pamidronate is usually administered intravenously every 3 months. The actual doses used and duration of therapy vary considerably between trials, however, and sample sizes have generally been modest. For example, Aris [19] conducted a controlled, randomized, open-label trial of pamidronate (30 mg intravenously every 3 months) plus vitamin D (800 IU/day) and calcium (1 g/day) in 16 patients compared with vitamin D and calcium alone in 18 control subjects after lung transplantation for cystic fibrosis. The treatment groups were similar in age, sex, baseline T scores, renal function, immunosuppressive therapy, and lung function over the study period. The patients treated with pamidronate gained 8.8% and 8.2% in spine and femoral neck BMD, respectively, over 2 years in comparison to control subjects, who gained on average 2.6% and 0.3%, respectively ($p < 0.015$ for both). Seven and 6 fractures occurred in the control and pamidronate groups, respectively ($p > 0.2$). Measures of bone resorption were highest immediately after lung transplant and improved with both pamidronate and time.

Trombetti [20] also studied pamidronate in 42 patients awaiting lung transplantation. Numbers were small, however (14 patients received 30 mg pamidronate IV every 3 months; 5 received hormone replacement therapy, and 10 control patients received only calcium and vitamin D supplementation), and the study was not randomized. Mean age-adjusted lumbar spine and femoral neck BMD was significantly decreased prior to transplantation (Z scores were −0.6 and −1.5 respectively). Pamidronate and hormone replacement therapy decreased the rate of spinal bone loss during the first 6 months and led to a significant increase of BMD at 1 year. One out of 20 patients experienced clinically evident fractures during antiresorptive therapy, as did 3 out of 12 in the calcium plus vitamin D group.

Using a different regimen in another randomized study, Fan [21] assessed prospectively the effect of 12 months treatment with small doses (0.5 mg/kg) of pamidronate IV at the time of renal transplantation and again 1 month later; this treatment was compared to plabeco in 26 male patients. Over the 12-month period, the pamidronate group experienced no significant loss in BMD at the lumbar spine compared to 6.4% loss in the placebo group. BMD at the femoral neck was reduced in the first year by −9.0% in the placebo but did not change in the pamidronate group.

Bianda [22] also conducted a randomized trial in 26 patients after cardiac transplantation with a similar small dose of pamidronate (0.5 mg/kg every 3 months) compared to nasal calcitonin (200 IU/day) plus calcitriol (0.25–0.5 mcg/day). Lumbar spine and hip bone loss in the pamidronate group was 1.9% and 1.4% respectively at 12 months, while in patients randomized to calcitonin plus calcitriol, lumbar spine BMD fell by 7.4% and hip BMD by 6.3%.

In a more recent study, Krieg [23] assessed prospectively the effect of 3 years treatment with 60 mg of pamidronate IV every 3 months combined with 1 g calcium and 1000 IU vitamin D per day. The study was not randomized, however, with therapy given on the basis of baseline BMD. Thus pamidronate was used in 11 heart transplant recipients with T scores below −2.5, whereas calcium and vitamin D was given to 17 heart transplant recipients with T scores above −2.5. Pamidronate was started on average 6 months after heart transplantation, and over the whole treatment period, a continuous increase in BMD at the lumbar spine was noted, reaching 18.3% after 3 years. BMD at the femoral neck was reduced in the first year by 3.4% but recovered totally after 3 years of treatment. Since some of the pamidronate patients were treated up to 14 months after the transplant, however, they may already have passed through the phase of most rapid bone loss. In the control group, a significant decrease in BMD was observed after 6 months following the graft at the lumbar spine (− 6.6%) as well as at the femoral neck (−7.8%). After 2 years, BMD tended to recover at the lumbar spine, whereas the loss persisted after 3 years at the femoral neck.

In another recent trial in which patients were randomized to receive either a single dose of intravenous pamidronate (60 mg) administered 1–3 months prior to liver transplantation or no treatment [24], lumbar BMD did not decline significantly in either the treated or the untreated group during the first post-transplant year, while femoral neck BMD fell comparably in both, and the incidence of new fractures was the same.

Some units have reported experience with pamidronate in "real" clinical practice rather than a formal clinical trial setting. Reeves [25] reported the results of a record review of liver transplant patients treated before or after use of IV pamidronate (given as 60 mg every 3 months before and for 9 months after transplanation). BMD measurements were available in 90 of 136 consecutive first transplants performed from February 1993 to September 1996. Before the use of pamidronate, 7 patients sustained symptomatic vertebral fractures. Their mean spine BMD was lower than in the 38 patients with no clinical evidence of fracture (81.8% versus 94.2%; $p = 0.006$). Following the introduction of pamidronate, no symptomatic vertebral fractures occurred. Of 29 surviving patients with BMD below an arbitrary value of 0.84 g/cm^2 before transplantation, 38% who did not receive treatment with pamidronate suffered spontaneous fracture, whereas 0 of 13 who received treatment suffered such a complication.

Some studies have also used a combination of intravenous and oral bisphosphonates. Shane [26] compared 18 patients who received a single intravenous infusion of pamidronate (60 mg) within 2 weeks of heart transplantation, followed by 4 cycles of oral etidronate and oral calcitriol

0.25 mcg daily, to 52 patients who previously underwent transplantation and did not receive antiresorptive therapy. Both groups received elemental calcium 1000 mg and vitamin D 400 IU daily. At 12 months after transplantation, virtually no lumbar spine bone loss had occurred in the first group, whereas lumbar spine BMD had declined significantly in patients who did not receive antiresorptive therapy (0.2% versus 6.8% , respectively; $p < 0.0001$). Similarly, femoral neck BMD fell by 10.6% in the latter patients and by only 2.7% in the former patients ($p < 0.0001$). Three incident vertebral fractures occurred in 2 bisphosphonate-treated patients, whereas 17 of the other patients sustained 30 incident vertebral fractures, 1 hip fracture, and 3 episodes of rib fractures ($p < 0.02$). Urinary deoxypyridinoline, a marker of bone resorption, fell by 51% in bisphosphonate-treated patients and increased by 65% in the other patients by 3 months after transplantation ($p < 0.0001$).

Another intravenous bisphosphonate, ibandronate, has also been studied in the transplant setting. Grotz [27] performed a randomized controlled 12-month trial in 80 kidney recipients with 40 receiving IV ibandronate (1 mg immediately before transplant and 2 mg at 3, 6, and 9 months) immediately before and at 3, 6, and 9 months after transplantation. Changes in BMD (ibandronate versus controls) were: lumbar spine, −0.9% versus −6.5% ($p < 0.0001$); femoral neck, +0.5% versus −7.7% ($p < 0.0001$); and midfemoral shaft, +2.7 % versus −4.0 % ($p = 0.024$). Fewer spinal deformities developed with ibandronate (7 patients with 7 deformities versus 12 patients with 23 deformities; $p = 0.047$) and loss of body height was 0.5 cm versus 1.1 cm in control subjects ($p = 0.040$). Two bone fractures occurred in each group. Of interest, there were fewer acute rejection episodes with ibandronate (11 versus 22; $p = 0.009$) and graft function after 1 year was comparable. Similarly, a recent randomized trial of ibandronate 2 mg IV every 3 months in 36 liver transplant recipients has also found a significant protective effect on bone mineral density at one year [28].

More recently, the potent oral bisphosphonate alendronate has been studied in a transplant setting. Shane [29] conducted a 1-year, double-blind, randomized trial to compare alendronate 10 mg daily with calcitriol 0.5 mcg daily in 149 patients after cardiac transplantation. Rates of loss were compared to 27 control subjects concurrently transplanted, but not randomized to therapy. Subjects randomized to alendronate and calcitriol did not experience significant bone loss in contrast to the control group. The change in spinal BMD was +0.3% with alendronate, −0.6% with calcitriol, and −3.2% in controls. The change in hip BMD was −1.3% with alendronate, −0.4% with calcitriol, and −6.2% in controls. Urinary N telopeptides fell by 34% with alendronate and 26% with calcitriol but were unchanged with controls. New vertebral fractures occurred in 6.8% of subjects treated with alendronate, 3.6% of subjects treated with calcitriol, and 13.6% of the control subjects. In the second year after discontinuation of both agents, BMD remained stable despite marked increases in bone turnover in the calcitriol group.

Taken together, these studies suggest both parenteral or oral bisphosphonates are effective agents in preventing post transplant bone loss.

IV. COMBINATIONS OF BISPHOSPHONATES AND VITAMIN D

In addition to the study referred to previously [26], a number of studies have examined combinations of bisphosphonates with active vitamin D metabolites. In a small study, Kovac [30] compared 6 renal transplant patients treated with alendronate, calcium carbonate, and low-dose calcitriol to 6 patients treated with calcium carbonate and calcitriol. The daily dose of calcium carbonate was 2 g, calcitriol 0.25 mcg, and alendronate 10 mg. Treatment was introduced 20.3 days (range 11–35 days) after transplantation. One patient from the first group experienced an atraumatic vertebral fracture before dialysis during glucocorticoid treatment, but no patient had any fracture during the dialysis period or in the first 6 months after transplantation. After 6 months of treatment, BMD increased by 6.4% in the alendronate group ($p < 0.05$) and decreased by 9.3% in the non-alendronate group ($p < 0.05$). No patient in either group showed hypercalcemia, and the urinary calcium only temporarily exceeded the upper limit in 4 patients. It was concluded that prevention of bone loss of the lumbar spine after kidney transplantation with combination alendronate, calcium, and low-dose calcitriol in patients with a well-functioning graft was effective and safe in the early post-transplant period, but treatment with calcium and calcitriol alone did not prevent bone loss in the same period.

In another small, secondary prevention study, Giannini [31] enrolled 40 patients (27 men and 13 women, mean age 44.2 years) who had received a renal allograft at least 6 months before, but the mean time since transplant was 61.2 months. At baseline, parathyroid hormone was elevated in 53% of the patients, and bone specific alkaline phosphatase (BSAP) and urinary N telopeptides were elevated ($p < 0.001$). After the first visit, patients were advised to adhere to a diet containing approximately 1000 mg of calcium daily, and BMD was reassessed 1 year later. During this period, BMD decreased at the spine (–2.6%; $p < 0.01$), total femur (–1.4%; $p < 0.05$), and femoral neck (–2.0%; $p < 0.001$). Subsequently, the patients were randomized into two groups: (1) group A received alendronate 10 mg/day, calcitriol 0.50 mcg/day, and calcium carbonate 500 mg/day, and (2) group B received calcitriol 0.50 mcg/day and calcium carbonate 500 mg/day. After a further 12-month treatment period, bone turnover markers showed a nonsignificant fall in group B patients, while both BSAP and N telopeptides decreased significantly in alendronate-treated patients. BMD of the spine (+5.0%), femoral neck (+4.5%), and total femur (+3.9%) increased significantly only in the alendronate-treated patients. However, no trend toward further bone loss was noticed in subjects treated with calcitriol only.

V. OTHER THERAPIES AND APPROACHES

Although calcitonin is able to prevent cyclosporin-induced bone loss in animal models [32], it appears relatively ineffective in preventing bone loss in humans after transplantation, although most studies have been small [33–35]. Valimaki [33] enrolled 69 patients in a randomized trial comparing calcium to nasal calcitonin 400 IU/day after bone marrow transplantation. Only 64% completed 6 months and 52% completed 12 months of follow-up. Neither treatment appeared able to prevent bone loss or influence bone markers. Valero [34] studied the use of calcitonin in patients after liver transplant. Patients with osteoporosis were randomly treated with 40 IU/day of calcitonin by intramuscular injection (n = 17) or cyclical etidronate (n = 23). All patients received calcium supplements. After 12 months of treatment, a significant increment of vertebral mineral density was observed (6.4% and 8.2%, respectively). Hay [35] studied calcitonin in a randomized controlled trial of 63 patients after liver transplant. Patients with osteoporosis were randomly treated with 100 IU/day of salmon calcitonin subcutaneously for 6 months (n = 29) or with no prophylaxis (n = 34). Both groups lost bone at the same rate in the first 4 months (4.7% at the lumbar spine), and after 12 months, BMD loss had stabilized (7.8%), but there was no significant difference between the two groups, suggesting that calcitonin in this dose was ineffective in prevention of transplant-related bone loss.

Two studies have shown encouraging results from exercise training, albeit in small sample sizes. Braith [36] performed a prospective, randomized, controlled study designed to determine the effect of resistance exercise training on bone in heart transplant recipients. Sixteen male heart transplant recipients were randomly assigned to a resistance exercise group for 6 months (mean age 56) or to a control group (mean age 52) that did not perform resistance exercise. The exercise regimen consisted of lumbar extension exercises performed 1 day/week and variable resistance exercises (using a Nautilus machine) performed 2 days/week. Each exercise consisted of 1 set of 10 to 15 repetitions performed to volitional fatigue. BMD of the total body, femoral neck, and lumbar spine were significantly decreased by 2 months after transplantation. Six months of resistance exercise restored BMD of the whole body, femur neck, and lumbar vertebra to within 1%, 1.9%, and 3.6% of pretransplantation levels, respectively. BMD of the control group remained unchanged from the 2-month post-transplantation levels.

In another exercise study, 16 lung transplant candidates were randomly assigned to lumbar extensor exercises or no exercise (control group), with the resistance exercise program initiated 2 months after transplant [37]. Both the exercise and control groups lost BMD at the spine rapidly at 2 months (−14.5%), but between 2 and 8 months the exercise group increased by 9.2%, compared to 5% further loss in the control group.

Apart from the small groups in Trombetti [20] and Stempfle [11], one other study has examined the effect of treatment with hormone replacement therapy on bone mass after transplant. Castelo-Branco [38] evaluated the effect of hormone replacement therapy in patients undergoing autologous bone marrow or bone marrow transplantation with ovarian failure. Thirteen women with previous bone marrow transplantation were treated with a standard dose of conjugated equine estrogen (0.625 mg/day) or with 50 micrograms/day of 17-beta-estradiol in transdermal therapeutic systems plus 5 mg/day of medroxyprogesterone acetate sequentially added to the last 12 days of estrogen therapy. The mean time elapsed between bone marrow transplantation and hormone replacement therapy initiation was 13.0 months (range 3–26 months). Before treatment, 9 patients were osteopenic, and after hormone replacement therapy, bone mass increased in all cases. Following bone marrow transplantation, elevated hepatic enzymes were detected in 3 patients. After 6 and 12 months of treatment, no significant changes were observed in hepatic enzymes. Hormone replacement therapy has also been shown to protect the skeleton in women receiving liver transplants [39]. These data suggest hormone replacement therapy may be useful in the transplant setting, although recent data about increased risk of breast cancer and vascular disease need to be considered. In a recent study evaluating male cardiac transplant recipients treated with intravenous ibandronate, hypogonadal men who received testosterone supplementation showed an improved BMD response at 1 year compared to hypogonadal men who did not receive testosterone [40].

VI. SUMMARY

There is increasing evidence (summarized in Table 1) that a number of agents are effective in prevention of post-transplantation bone loss of various organs. Further clinical trials are necessary to establish the comparative efficacy of different agents, but some form of primary prophylaxis for osteoporosis should be considered in patients undergoing organ transplantation. Data from several clinical trials suggest that bisphosphonates are the most effective agents for the prevention and treatment of post-transplantation osteoporosis. Accordingly, based upon available evidence, prophylaxis should involve a bisphosphonate with active vitamin D metabolites as second line or adjunctive therapy. A potential reduction in immunosuppressive requirements with active vitamin D metabolites is an additional consideration [41], but hypercalcemia and hypercalciuria are also relatively common, and monitoring of urine and serum is required. Testosterone replacement should be reserved for men with true hypogonadism post-transplant. Patients who are receiving anti-osteoporosis therapy prior to transplantation could theoretically experience less bone loss after transplantation, but whether drug therapy for osteoporosis before transplantation reduces bone loss and fracture risk after transplantation is currently unclear.

TABLE 1 Summary of major trials in prevention of transplant bone loss

Reference	Agent	Transplant type	Sample size	Randomized
11	Calcitriol	Cardiac	132	Yes
12	Calcitriol	Liver	509	No
13	Calcitriol	Cardiac	65	Yes
14	Alfacalcidol	Renal	111	Yes
15	Calcitriol	Renal	45	Yes
17	Etidronate/Alfacalcidol	Cardiac	48	Yes
18	Etidronate/Calcitriol	Cardiac	41	Yes
19	Pamidronate	Lung	34	Yes
20	Pamidronate	Lung	42	No
21	Pamidronate	Renal	26	Yes
22	Pamidronate	Cardiac	26	Yes
23	Pamidronate	Cardiac	28	No
24	Pamidronate	Liver	99	Yes
26	Pamidronate/Etidronate	Cardiac	18	Yes
27	Ibandronate	Renal	80	Yes
28	Ibandronate	Liver	36	Yes
29	Alendronate/Calcitriol	Cardiac	149	Yes

REFERENCES

1. Epstein, S., and Shane, E. (1996). Post-transplant bone disease: the role of immuno-suppressive agents on the skeleton. *J Bone Miner Res.* 11:1–7.
2. Sambrook, P., and Lane, N.E. (2001). Corticosteroid osteoporosis, Balliere's Best Practice and Research. *Clinical Rheumatology.* 15(3):401–413.
3. Shane, E., and Cohen, A. (2003). Osteoporosis after solid organ and bone marrow transplantation. *Osteoporosis Int.* 14:617–630.
4. Sambrook, P., Birmingham, J., Kelly, P.J., Kempler, S., Pocock, N.A., and Eisman, J.A. (1993). Prevention of corticosteroid osteoporosis; a comparison of calcium, calcitriol and calcitonin. *New Engl J Med.* 328:1747–1752.
5. Reginster, J.Y., Kuntz, D., Verdickt, W., Wouters, M., Guillevin, L., Menkes, C.J., and Nielsen, K. (1999). Prophylactic use of alfacalcidol in corticosteroid-induced osteoporosis. *Osteop Inter.* 9:75–81.
6. Sambrook P (1999). Alfacalcidol and calcitriol in the prevention of bone loss after organ transplantation. *Calcif Tissue Int.* 65:341–343.
7. Cooper, A.M., Locke, T.J., and Eastell R. (1996). Secondary hyperparathyroidism associated with heart transplantation is reversed by 1 α hydroxyvitamin D. *J Bone Miner Res.* 11:S544.
8. Ferrari, S.L., Nicod, L.P., Hamacher, J. et al. (1996). Osteoporosis in patients undergoing lung transplantation. *Eur Respir J.* 9:2378–2382.
9. Shane, E., Rivas, M., McMahon, D.J et al. (1997). Bone loss and turnover after cardiac transplantation. *J Clin Endocrinol Metab,* 82:1497–1506.
10. Massenkeil, G., Fiene, C., Rosen, O., Michael, R., Reisinger, W., and Arnold, R. (2001). Loss of bone mass and vitamin D deficiency after hematopoietic stem cell transplantation: standard prophylactic measures fail to prevent osteoporosis. *Leukemia.* 15(11):1701–1705.

11. Stempfle, H.U., Werner, C., Echtler, S., Wehr, U., Rambeck, WA., Siebert, U., Uberfuhr P. Angermann, C.E., Theisen, K., and Gartner, R. (1999). Prevention of osteoporosis after cardiac transplantation: a prospective, longitudinal, randomized, double-blind trial with calcitriol. *Transplantation.* 68(4):523–530.
12. Neuhaus, R., Kubo A., Lohmann, R., Rayes, N., Hierholzer, J. and Neuhaus, P. (1999). Calcitriol in prevention and therapy of osteoporosis after liver transplantation. *Transplant Proc.* 31:472–473.
13. Sambrook, P., Henderson, N.K., Keogh, A., MacDonald, P., Glanville, A., Spratt, P., Bergin, P., Ebeling, P., and Eisman, J. (2000). Effect of calcitriol on bone loss after cardiac or lung transplantation. *J Bone Miner Res.* 15(9):1818–1824.
14. De Sevaux, R.G., Hoitsma, A.J., Corstens, F.H., and Wetzels, J.F. (2002). Treatment with vitamin D and calcium reduces bone loss after renal transplantation. A randomized study. *J Amer Soc Nephrol.* 13:1608–1614.
15. Ugur, A., Guvener, N., Isiklar, I., et al. (2000). Efficiency of preventive treatment for osteoporosis after renal transplantation. *Transplant Proc.* 32:556–557.
16. Berczi, C., Asztalos, L., Kincses, Z., Balogh, A., Locsey, L., Balazs, G., and Lukacs, G. (2003). Comparison of calcium and alfacalcidol supplement in the prevention of osteopenia after kidney transplantation. *Osteop Inter.* 14:412–417.
17. Van Cleemput, J., Daenen, W., Geusens, P., Dequeker, J., Van der Werf, F., and Vanhaecke, J. , (1996). Prevention of bone loss in cardiac transplant recipients, a comparison of bisphosphonates and vitamin D. *Transplantation.* 61:1495–1499.
18. Henderson, N.K., Eisman, J.A., Keogh, A., MacDonald, P., Glanville, A., Spratt, P., and Sambrook, P. N. (2001). Protective effect of short term calcitriol or cyclical etidronate on bone loss after cardiac or lung transplantation. *J Bone Miner Res.* 16:565–571.
19. Aris, R.M., Lester, G.E., Renner, J.B., Winders, A., Denene Blackwood, A., Lark, R.K., and Ontjes, D.A. (2000). Efficacy of pamidronate for osteoporosis in patients with cystic fibrosis following lung transplantation. *Amer J Resp Crit Care Med.* 162:941–946.
20. Trombetti, A., Gerbase, M.W., Spiliopoulos, A., Slosman, D.O., Nicod, L.P., and Rizzoli, R. (2000). Bone mineral density in lung-transplant recipients before and after graft: prevention of lumbar spine post-transplantation-accelerated bone loss by pamidronate. *J Heart Lung Transpl.* 19(8):736–743.
21. Fan, S., Almond, M.K., Ball, E. et al. (2000). Pamidronate therapy as prevention of bone loss following renal transplantation. *Kidney Int.* 57:684–690.
22. Bianda, T., Linka, A., Junga, G. et al. (2000). Prevention of osteoporosis in heart transplant recipients: a comparison of calcitriol with calcitonin and pamidronate. *Calcif Tissue Int.* 67:116–121.
23. Krieg, M.A., Seydoux, C., Sandini, L., Goy, J.J., Berguer, D.G., Thiebaud, D., and Burckhardt, P. (2001). Intravenous pamidronate as treatment for osteoporosis after heart transplantation. A prospective study. *Osteoporosis Inter.* 12(2):112–116.
24. Ninkovic, M., Love, S., Tom, B.D. et al. (2002). Lack of effect of intravenous pamidronate on fracture incidence and bone mineral density after orthotopic liver transplantation. *J Hepatol.* 37:93–100.
25. Reeves, H.L., Francis, R.M., Manas, D.M., Hudson, M., and Day, C.P. (1998). Intravenous bisphosphonate prevents symptomatic osteoporotic vertebral collapse in patients after liver transplantation. *Liver Transpl Surg.* 4(5):404–409.
26. Shane, E., Rodino, M.A., McMahon, D.J., Addesso, V., Staron, R.B., Seibel, M.J., Mancini, D., Michler, R. E., and Lo, S. H. (1998). Prevention of bone loss after heart transplantation with antiresorptive therapy: a pilot study. *J Heart Lung Transpl.* 17(11):1089–1096.
27. Grotz, W., Nagel, C., Poeschel, D., Cybulla, M., Petersen, K.G., Uhl, M., Strey, C., Kirste, G., Olschewski, M., Reichelt, A., and Rump, L. C. (2001). Effect of ibandronate on bone loss and renal function after kidney transplantation. *J Amer Soc Nephrol.* 12:1530–1537.
28. Hommann, M., Abendroth, K., Lehmann, G. et al. (2002). Effect of transplantation on bone: osteoporosis after liver and multivisceral transplantation. *Transplant Proc.* 34: 2296–2298.

29. Shane, E., Addesso, V., Namerow, P.B., McMahon, D. J., Lo, S. H., Staron, R.B., Zucker, M., Pardi, S., Maybaum, S., and Mancini, D. (2004). Alendronate or calcitriol and prevention of bone loss after cardiac transplantation. *New Engl J Med.* 350:767–776.
30. Kovac, D., Lindic, J., Kandus, A., and Bren, A.F. (2000). Prevention of bone loss with alendronate in kidney transplant recipients. *Transplantation.* 70(10):1542–1543.
31. Giannini, S., Dangel, A., Carraro, G., Nobile, M., Rigotti, P., Bonfante L., Marchini, F., Zaninotto, M., Dalle Carbonare, L., Sartori L., and Crepaldi, G. (2001). Alendronate prevents further bone loss in renal transplant recipients. *J Bone Miner Res.* 16(11): 2111–2117.
32. Stein, B., Takizawa, M., Katz, I. et al. (1991). Salmon calcitonin prevents cyclosporin A induced high turnover bone loss. *Endocrinology.* 129:92–98.
33. Valimaki, M., Kinnunen, K., Volin, L. et al. (1999). A prospective study of bone loss and turnover after allogeneic bone marrow transplantation: effect of calcium supplementation with or without calcitonin. *Bone Marrow Transplant.* 23:355–361.
34. Valero, M.A., Loinaz, C., Larrodera, L., Leon, M., Moreno, E., and Hawkins, F. (1995). Calcitonin and bisphosphonates treatment in bone loss after liver transplantation. *Calcif Tissue Internat.* 57(1):15–19.
35. Hay, J.E., Malinchoc, M., and Dickson, E. R. (2001). A controlled trial of calcitonin therapy for the prevention of post-liver transplantation atraumatic fractures in patients with primary biliary cirrhosis and primary sclerosing cholangitis. *J Hepatol.* 34:292–298.
36. Braith, R.W., Mills, R.M., Welsch, M.A., Keller, J.W., and Pollock, M.L. (1996). Resistance exercise training restores bone mineral density in heart transplant recipients. *J Amer Coll Cardiol.* 28(6):1471–1477.
37. Mitchell, M.J., Baz, M.A., Fulton, M.N., Lisor, C.F., and Braith, R.W. (2003). Resistance training prevents vertebral osteoporosis in lung transplant recipients. *Transplantation.* 76:557–562.
38. Castelo-Branco, C., Rovira, M., Pons, F., Duran, M., Sierra, J., Vives A., Balasch, J., Fortuny, A., and Vanrell, J. (1996). The effect of hormone replacement therapy on bone mass in patients with ovarian failure due to bone marrow transplantation. *Maturitas.* 23(3):307–312.
39. Isoniemi, H., Appelberg, J., Nilsson, C.G. et al. (2001). Transdermal oestrogen therapy protects postmenopausal liver transplant women from osteoporosis. A 2-year follow-up study. *J Hepatol.* 34:299–305.
40. Fahrleitner, A., Prenner, G., Tscheliessnigg, K.H. et al. (2002). Testosterone supplementation has additional benefits on bone metabolism in cardiac transplant recipients receiving intravenous bisphosphonate treatment: a prospective study. *J Bone Miner Res.* 17:S388.
41. Henderson-Briffa, K., Keogh, K., Sambrook, P.N., and Eisman, J.A., (2003). Reduction by calcitriol of immunosuppressive therapy requirements in heart transplantation. *Transplantation.* 75:2133–2134.

CHAPTER 24

Management: Established Osteoporosis in Organ Transplant Recipients

Ian R. Reid, MD
Dept. of Medicine, University of Auckland, Auckland, New Zealand

I. INTRODUCTION

It is now widely recognized that osteoporosis is potentially a major problem in patients who have undergone organ transplantation. As outlined in the preceding chapters, this has led to efforts to optimize bone density before transplantation, and to put in place specific measures to prevent bone loss in the postoperative period. In spite of this, a substantial number of patients with transplants are osteoporotic, whether defined in terms of bone density or the occurrence of fractures after minor trauma. The reasons for this are manifold. Many chronic illnesses, particularly those associated with inflammation, weight loss, or hypoxia, are associated with bone loss (see Table 1). The immobility often associated with chronic illness contributes to the loss of both bone and muscle, the latter increasing the risk of falls and thus compounding the risk of fractures. Immobility is also likely to be associated with reduced sunlight exposure leading to vitamin D deficiency, which impacts adversely on both bone and muscle. Chronic illness is often associated with hypogonadism, and sex hormones are among the most important regulators of bone metabolism. The conditions that lead to organ failure sometimes require treatment with drugs that cause bone loss. Glucocorticoids are the most common offender in this regard, but other immunosuppressive agents and loop diuretics may also contribute. Following transplantation, the combination of glucocorticoids and other immunosuppressive drugs provides a potent cause of bone loss.

In addition to the disease-specific and pharmacological causes of bone loss, the same factors that contribute to the development of osteoporosis in the general population are operative in recipients of transplants. These

TABLE 1 Conditions and drugs associated with osteoporosis

Inflammatory Disorders	**Disorders Associated with Immobilisation**
Rheumatoid arthritis	Parkinson's disease
Inflammatory bowel disease	Poliomyelitis
Cystic fibrosis	Cerebral palsy
Bone Marrow Disorders	Paraplegia
Multiple myeloma	**Defective Synthesis of Connective Tissue**
Mastocytosis	Osteogenesis imperfecta
Leukaemia	Marfan's syndrome
Disorders Associated with Hypogonadism	Homocystinuria
Athletic amenorrhoea	**Endocrinological Disorders**
Haemochromatosis	Thyrotoxicosis
Turner's syndrome	Hyperparathyroidism
Klinefelter's syndrome	**Miscellaneous**
Post-chemotherapy	Pregnancy/lactation
Hypopituitarism	Ankylosing spondylitis
Disorders Associated with Low Body Weight	Hypercalciuric nephrolithiasis
Anorexia nervosa	**Drugs**
Type 1 diabetes mellitus	Glucocorticoids
Disorders Associated with Malabsorption	Alcohol
Coeliac disease	Caffeine
Post-gastrectomy	Medroxyprogesterone acetate
Liver disease	Anti-convulsants
Total parenteral nutrition	Methotrexate
	Heparin
	Agents used post-transplantation

factors contribute to one-half of women and one-third of men suffering fractures after the age of 50, in a typical white population. In women, menopause is a key contributor to the increase in fracture risk, and the more gradual development of hypogonadism in men may also be significant. Genetic contributions to bone density and bone architecture are likely to be important contributors to fracture risk, since a family history of fractures significantly increases an individual's risk. Smoking and, in men, alcohol intake are important lifestyle risk factors for osteoporosis, and are sometimes involved in the pathogenesis of the condition that has led to the patient having a transplantation in the first place. Globally, the single most important contributor to osteoporotic fractures is age, and many patients requiring transplantation are in older age groups. Osteoporotic fractures can occur at the other end of life, however, particularly when chronic illness has interfered with normal growth and the timing of puberty.

These considerations are important because the clinical trials literature relating to the management of established osteoporosis in subjects with organ transplants is very limited. Few studies have been published, and of those that are available, a high proportion are not randomized, are short term, have small numbers, or do not provide adequate data to assess antifracture efficacy. The clinicians advising post-transplant patients with osteoporosis must therefore look elsewhere for the evidence base they need. To some extent, they can draw upon the larger database addressing the prevention of bone loss in the immediate post-transplant period, reviewed in the previous chapter. Since glucocorticoids are a major contributor to post-transplant osteoporosis, the literature on the management of glucocorticoid-induced osteoporosis is also important. Finally, because osteoporosis after transplantation almost always has a multifaceted pathogenesis, the broader literature on the management of osteoporosis in older men and women is also a very important guide. Before the evidence relating to each of the available treatment interventions is considered, it is important to consider how fracture risk is assessed and at what levels of risk intervention is appropriate.

II. FRACTURE RISK ASSESSMENT

The need for therapeutic interventions is judged from an individual's fracture risk rather than any arbitrary level of bone density. Since both bone density and fracture risk are continuously distributed, there is no single diagnostic threshold that determines when treatment should be advised, but rather the key issue is to assess fracture risk, then determine which interventions are cost-effective for a given level of risk. Fracture risk can be assessed from the combination of clinical risk factors and bone density measurements.

A. Clinical Risk Factors for Fracture

In a patient with an organ transplant, history of disease and drug use, particularly the cumulative dose of glucocorticoids, contributes to fracture risk. Table 1 provides a list of conditions and drugs associated with bone loss, many of which are common in transplanted patients. These factors operate on top of the large number of risk factors that are independent of transplantation, the most important of which are listed in Table 2. Possibly the most powerful predictor of future fractures is past history of fracture. The presence of a deformed vertebra on a lateral spine or chest x-ray increases future fracture risk as much as five-fold, and a similar effect is seen with a past history of fractures at other sites also [1]. Therefore, treatment is

TABLE 2 Important clinical risk factors for fracture

European or Asian race
Female sex
Age*
Previous history of fracture*
Bone density
Weight <60 kg*
Smoking*
Family history of fracture*
Systemic use of glucocorticoid drugs*

*These risk factors are, in part, independent of bone density

Based in part on data in Eddy et al, Osteoporosis: Review of the evidence for prevention, diagnosis, and treatment and cost-effectiveness analysis. *Osteoporos. Int.* 8 (suppl 4), 1-88.

sometimes indicated following fracture even if the bone density is not particularly low.

B. Bone Densitometry

There is a continuous, inverse relationship between fracture risk and bone density. A difference in bone density of one population standard deviation (about 10%) is associated with a two-fold difference in fracture risk. Most sites of bone density measurement give comparable prediction of global fracture risk. However, fracture at a given site is best predicted by bone density measurement at that site, e.g., hip bone density predicts hip fracture risk better than measurements elsewhere. The most commonly assessed sites are the hip and spine. The fact that hip fracture is the single most important osteoporotic fracture argues in favor of using the hip as the preferred measurement site. The precision of measurement is greater in the spine, however, and spine bone density is more responsive to changes, such as those that occur after transplantation. Similarly, treatment effects are more readily observed at the spine. With advancing age, the value of spine scans diminishes because of artifacts associated with degenerative joint and disc disease. Because of these conflicting issues, it is common practice to measure bone density in both the lumbar spine and proximal femur. In the femur, the "total hip" region is now often preferred to the femoral neck, because it is larger and contains more trabecular bone, and so has precision and responsiveness characteristics closer to those of the spine. In the past, the forearm was a common site of measurement because that was all that was technically feasible. Modern densitometers can also measure bone density in the forearm, but there is no reason to prefer it to the spine and hip, when these are available.

Absolute values of bone mineral density are not comparable between different sites, measurement techniques, and manufacturers. This problem has been addressed by reporting bone densities with reference to the young normal population range for that particular device, using standard deviation units (T-scores). The WHO has adopted this approach in its definitions of osteopenia (T-score < −1) and osteoporosis (T-score < −2.5, i.e., a bone density that is more than 2.5 standard deviations below the mean value in the young normal population). This "definition" of osteoporosis is sometimes used as a threshold for intervention, but this does not take into account the fact that the clinical risk factors listed in Tables 1 and 2 are multiplicative with the risk estimated from bone density measurement. For example, a T-score of −2.5 in an 80-year-old woman with a history of vertebral fracture is associated with a considerably higher risk of fracture over the next 5 years than is the same density in a 50-year-old woman with no fracture history. There is a move to combine these factors to produce estimates of absolute fracture risk. While the algorithms that make this possible are undergoing refinement, it is possible to incorporate this approach into clinical practice now, by using different bone density thresholds for treatment according to coexistent risk factors (see Table 3). This particular analysis was conducted in the context of postmenopausal osteoporosis. However, glucocorticoid use appears to confer a risk additional to that assessed from bone density, which is comparable to that associated with a prevalent fracture [2], so the intervention threshold in transplanted patients would usually be a T-score of −1.5 to −2.0.

TABLE 3 Thresholds of cost-effectiveness for treatment of postmenopausal osteoporosis with alendronate

Risk factors	T-Score
None	−3.0 to −2.2
Previous non-vertebral fracture	−2.5 to −1.8
Previous vertebral fracture	−2.5 to −1.7
Previous vertebral fracture plus 1 other risk factor*	−1.9 to −1.1
Previous vertebral fracture plus >1 other risk factor*	−1.8 to −1.1

Data are bone densities at the femoral neck (given as standard deviations below the mean value in the young normal population, i.e. T-scores). In general, the lower densities within the indicated range apply to younger postmenopausal women, and the upper end of the given ranges to women of about 80 years of age.

*Possible risk factors are: low weight, smoking, family history. Steroid use was not noted as a risk factor in this analysis, but it is probably as important as prevalent fracture [2]. Based on data in Eddy et al, Osteoporosis: Review of the evidence for prevention, diagnosis, and treatment and cost-effectiveness analysis. *Osteoporos. Int.* 8 (suppl 4), 1-88.

C. Biochemical Markers

In the last decade a number of biochemical tests have been developed that assess the activity of either osteoblasts or osteoclasts. These are collectively referred to as biochemical markers of bone turnover. There are now several studies that suggest that high bone turnover is an independent risk for fracture in normal older women. There is some inconsistency between the published studies, and it is not clear whether the available markers are equivalent for predicting fracture risk. There is also considerable biological and assay variability in these measurements. For these reasons, they are not routinely used in fracture risk assessment in nontransplanted subjects at present, and it is unwise to extrapolate these results to the transplantation population, since glucocorticoids and illness can directly impact bone turnover.

III. NONPHARMACOLOGICAL INTERVENTIONS

Some of the measures that might reduce fracture risk or increase bone density can be inferred from the risk factors set out in Table 2. Cessation of smoking, maintenance of normal body weight (e.g., > 60 kg in women of average height), avoidance of high alcohol intakes, and minimization of glucocorticoid doses are all to be recommended. Discontinuation or reduction of dose of glucocorticoids produces substantial benefits to bone mass [3]. In addition, substantial literature documents the small but consistent gains in bone density that are associated with weight-bearing and muscle-strengthening exercise [4]; such programs typically increasing bone mineral density by 1–2% in nontransplanted subjects [5]. Exercise may have its greatest benefits through reducing the risk of falls. In frail subjects [6] falls may also be reduced in frequency through training related to balance and gait, reduction in home hazards (e.g., power cords, loose carpets), discontinuation of psychotropic medication, and improvement in vision [7, 8]. When falls can't be prevented, there may be some benefit resulting from force attenuation devices, such as hip protectors [9], though this is not a universal finding [10].

IV. PHARMACOLOGICAL INTERVENTIONS

The management of post-transplant osteoporosis draws on the same potential therapies as postmenopausal or glucocorticoid-induced osteoporosis. The evidence for the use of each of these treatments in these broader contexts will be briefly reviewed, together with a consideration of what data are available specifically relating to osteoporosis in patients after transplantation.

A. Calcium

Calcium is the principal mineral constituent of bone. Its concentration in the extracellular fluid is tightly regulated, and when obligatory losses of calcium in the urine and feces are not met by dietary intake, secretion of parathyroid hormone increases and the calcium necessary to maintain normal circulating concentrations is mobilized from the skeleton. For these reasons, it has been postulated that the provision of additional calcium may reduce bone loss in subjects at risk of osteoporosis.

This question has been addressed through a large number of observational studies of normal subjects, which have produced conflicting results [11]. However, the data from more than 20 randomized controlled trials (RCTs) [12] are much more consistent, demonstrating an increase in bone density of 0.5–1% over periods of 2–4 years. This beneficial effect is seen throughout the skeleton, and may be more marked in late postmenopausal women, in subjects with a lower baseline calcium intake, and with the use of more bioavailable calcium preparations.

There are reasonable observational data on the effect of calcium supplementation on glucocorticoid-induced bone loss, in that the "control" groups in trials of most other agents have been given calcium [13, 14]. These data indicate that considerable bone loss still occurs despite calcium supplementation. However, calcium does reduce biochemical indices of bone resorption in glucocorticoid-treated patients [15], and hydroxyapatite tablets have been shown to slow forearm bone loss in one study [16]. No authoritative data addresses the effects of calcium alone in the management of post-transplant osteoporosis.

Several small studies now suggest a beneficial effect of calcium monotherapy on fracture incidence in nontransplanted, non-glucocorticoid-treated subjects, despite the between-groups differences in bone density observed as being less than 2%. These findings should be interpreted with caution, however, since meta-analysis of these and similar data does not show a convincing effect, though a trend to benefit is discernible [17]. Fracture data from calcium studies in subjects receiving glucocorticoids or with organ transplants are not available.

Calcium is generally well tolerated, and reports of significant side effects are rare. Some individuals complain of constipation when taking supplements. There has been concern that high calcium intakes will lead to urinary calculi in susceptible subjects. Observational data suggest that dietary calcium intake is inversely related to the risk of stone formation, whereas the use of calcium supplements may increase stone risk by 20% [18]. This apparent inconsistency may arise from a reduction in intestinal oxalate absorption when calcium is taken with a meal. It has been suggested that high calcium intakes (e.g., highest quintile versus lowest, or supplements of about 1 g) are associated with a reduced risk of colorectal cancer, reduced blood pressure, and reduced serum lipid concentrations, but these possibilities require further investigation.

Most authorities recommend that individuals with osteoporosis maintain a calcium intake of 1000–1500 mg/day, equivalent to 4 to 6 servings of dairy products. In those who would prefer to take their calcium in the form of a supplement, daily doses of 500–1000 mg are usually given to achieve a total calcium intake within or slightly above the target range. Present evidence suggests that food sources of calcium are of comparable benefit to calcium preparations. Of the principal food sources of calcium, dairy products have higher calcium availability than vegetables, and cheese may be superior to milk. When choosing a calcium supplement, the balance of current evidence suggests more soluble salts (e.g., lactate, gluconate, or citrate) to be more effective.

B. Vitamin D

Vitamin D, or calciferol, is produced in the skin as a result of the action of ultraviolet light on 7-dehydrocholesterol. The efficiency of this conversion is reduced with age and with skin pigmentation. In the absence of the fortification of foods, the diet is relatively unimportant in determining vitamin D status. In recent years, there has been an increasing recognition that vitamin D deficiency is common in chronic illness and old age, particularly in those who are no longer fully independent and are therefore less exposed to sunlight. The problem is greater at higher latitudes, though in some very hot climates individuals avoid sunlight and are also at risk. It is also common in transplant populations, recently being reported in two-thirds of subjects undergoing liver transplantation [19], in whom it was associated with lower bone density. Vitamin D deficiency leads to secondary hyperparathyroidism and a resulting increase in bone loss [20].

In normal elderly populations, physiological supplements of calciferol (e.g., 400–800 IU/day) reduce parathyroid hormone concentrations, and lead to increases in bone density, particularly at the femoral neck [21]. Similar changes in biochemical end-points can be achieved with regular sunlight exposure for 15–30 minutes daily [22]. Two large studies have assessed the effect on fracture rates of calciferol supplementation alone. Lips et al. [23] showed no change in fracture incidence in 2578 men and women over the age of 70 years randomized to oral calciferol 400 IU/day or placebo, whereas Heikinheimo et al. [24] showed that 150,000 IU annually of parenteral vitamin D reduced symptomatic fracture rates by 25% in a cohort of 800 elderly subjects in Finland. Two further major studies have been reported in which calcium was coadministered with calciferol to elderly subjects. Chapuy et al. [25] demonstrated a reduction of more than 25% in nonvertebral and hip fracture rates in a cohort of 3000 elderly women studied over a period of 3 years. Dawson-Hughes et al. [26] demonstrated a reduction of nonvertebral fracture rates by more than 50% in 400 older men and women randomized to calcium 500 mg/day plus 700

IU vitamin D, or to placebo. It is not possible to determine whether the calcium, the vitamin D, or the combination was the essential component to the success of these two studies, but they do point to the possibility of a major reduction in morbidity in D-deficient patients as a result of a safe and inexpensive intervention.

In the context of glucocorticoid-induced osteoporosis, there have been two major studies of calcium and vitamin D combinations. Buckley et al. studied patients with rheumatoid arthritis receiving low-dose prednisone who were randomized to receive placebo or calcium 500 mg/day plus vitamin D 500 IU/day over a 2-year period [27]. Those receiving calcium and vitamin D showed 5% more positive changes in bone density than those receiving placebo. The vitamin D status of the study subjects was not assessed. In contrast, Adachi et al. [28] failed to show any benefit on lumbar spine density from the use of calciferol 50,000 u/week plus calcium 1000 mg/day in a RCT over 3 years.

In transplanted subjects, most studies have been of prevention starting soon after transplantation; they are reviewed in the previous chapter. In general, these studies provide confirmation of the results from nontransplanted subjects, in that calcium and vitamin D increase BMD in D-deficient subjects following transplantation [29], and in one study, 25-hydroxyvitamin D had progressive positive effects on BMD over an 18-month period, which were greater than those associated with the use of calcitonin or etidronate [30]. Both these studies used 25-hydroxyvitamin D, which is produced directly from vitamin D itself, with little regulation. It is therefore usually regarded as being therapeutically equivalent to dosing with the parent compound, and the use of either compound in replacement doses can regarded as treating a deficiency of the substrate necessary for normal vitamin D metabolism.

When supplementing vitamin D in deficient subjects, it is important to consider the optimal target to be achieved. This has been addressed by Malabanan et al. [31] in a study of the effect of vitamin D supplementation on circulating levels of parathyroid hormone. They demonstrated that vitamin D supplementation suppressed parathyroid hormone levels only in subjects whose baseline serum 25-hydroxyvitamin D was less than 50 nmol/L (20 ng/dL). This suggests that when optimizing vitamin D status, 50 nmol/L is an appropriate target concentration for serum 25-hydroxyvitamin D. Vitamin D supplementation seems to produce no benefit in early postmenopausal women who are already vitamin D replete. The use of pharmacological doses of calciferol, which raises serum 25-hydroxyvitamin D concentrations well above the normal range, has not been demonstrated to confer any beneficial effects on bone density.

While there is no compelling evidence for vitamin D having a specific role in the treatment of post-transplantation osteoporosis, there is increasing evidence of deleterious effects of vitamin D deficiency on the skeleton. Since some transplanted patients are less frequently outdoors, assessment of vitamin D status (by a measurement of serum 25-hydroxyvitamin D) and, where necessary, supplementation with vitamin D itself (e.g., calciferol 500–1000 u/day or 20,000–50,000 u/month) is appropriate.

C. Vitamin D Metabolites

The use of physiological doses of calciferol or 25-hydroxyvitamin D is quite distinct from the use of the 1α-hydroxylated metabolites (calcitriol and alfacalcidol), which are much more potent stimulators of both intestinal calcium absorption and osteoclastic bone resorption. The production of the physiologically-produced compound, calcitriol, is tightly regulated in the kidney, but its therapeutic use bypasses the homeostatic controls of vitamin D metabolism and carries a risk of increasing bone resorption, hypercalcemia, and hypercalcuria. The potential benefit of these agents is that they increase intestinal calcium absorption, which is clearly reduced by the use of glucocorticoids. Thus, the balance of these opposing effects will determine whether there is a therapeutic benefit from their use in either transplanted or nontransplanted subjects.

The vitamin D metabolites are used in some countries for treating postmenopausal osteoporosis. Both increased and decreased fracture rates have been demonstrated in trials using calcitriol, and even in the positive studies, its effects on bone density are less than those of the bisphosphonates. There is now some evidence that calcitriol, when combined with estrogen/progestogen therapy or a bisphosphonate, has an additive effect on bone density, but combination therapy is expensive and its antifracture efficacy unknown.

In glucocorticoid-treated subjects calcitriol has been assessed in several RCTs. Dykman et al. [32] found no difference between calcitriol 0.4 μg/day and placebo in their effects on forearm bone density. Sambrook [13] reported a 1-year study in which patients beginning glucocorticoid therapy were randomly assigned to receive calcium, calcium plus calcitriol (mean dose 0.6 μg/day), or these two agents combined with calcitonin. Bone losses from the lumbar spine were 4.3%, 1.3%, and 0.2% in the respective groups. There was a similar, nonsignificant trend in distal radial bone loss but no evidence of reduced bone loss in the proximal femur (3% in all groups). A trial comparing the use of calcitriol 0.5 μg/day with hormone replacement therapy in hypogonadal young women with systemic lupus erythematosus, showed progressive bone loss in those taking the vitamin analogue in comparison with increases in density observed in those receiving hormones (between-groups difference at the spine of 3.7% at 2 years) [33]. There was also a significant difference between groups at the distal radius.

As reviewed in the previous chapter, calcitriol immediately after organ transplantation has produced mixed results. Sambrook et al., in a small

RCT, showed that calcitriol prevented bone loss in the femur following heart or lung transplantation, but had no benefit in the spine. Despite this, there appeared to be fewer vertebral fractures in the calcitriol group [34]. The same group has subsequently reported that neither calcitriol nor etidronate are able to completely prevent bone loss in a similar group of patients, though there was no randomly allocated placebo group in this study [35]. Stempfle [36] showed increases in bone density in patients randomized to either calcitriol or placebo, though these were only significant in the calcitriol group, where spine bone density at 24 months was 14% above baseline. This is a very substantial increase, and it is probably contributed to by other interventions, such as hormone replacement therapy, which were introduced not long before the initiation of the study.

Some studies with calcitriol do address the treatment of post-transplantation osteoporosis. Neuhaus [37] reported a large, nonrandomized, open-label study of 509 subjects who had undergone liver transplantation 6 months before entry to the study. Approximately half received no specific intervention during the 18-month study period, while others took calcitriol in doses of 0.25 or 0.5 μg with or without a 1 g calcium supplement. There were increases in spinal bone density of 5–10% in the various calcitriol groups, but it is not clear from the paper what the rate of change during the same observation period was in the control subjects, or what the results of the formal statistical comparison between these groups is. Thus, the study is suggestive of a benefit but certainly not conclusive.

Stempfle [38] randomized 132 adults to therapy with calcitriol 0.25 μg/day or placebo. The study started an average of 35 months following cardiac transplantation. Bone density increased by about 6% in both groups over the 3 years of the study, with no significant difference between groups. The population had normal levels of 25-hydroxyvitamin D at baseline (mean value 120 nmol/L).

Cueto-Manzano carried out a small RCT of 30 subjects who had received a renal transplant at least 2 years before. The provision of calcitriol 0.25 μg/day plus calcium carbonate made no difference to the rate of change of bone density in the forearm, spine, or femur over a 12-month period of follow-up [39].

The other 1α-hydroxylated metabolite, alfacalcidol, has been shown to slow femoral neck and lumbar spine bone loss immediately following cardiac transplantation, more effectively than etidronate, though the loss in both groups was substantial [40]. A similar attenuation of lumbar spine bone loss has been reported in a predominantly nontransplant population with the use of alfacalcidol 1 μg/day, though femoral bone density was not measured in this study [41]. In a population of patients with established steroid osteoporosis, Ringe has shown a beneficial effect of alfacalcidol 1 μg/day in comparison with calciferol plus calcium supplements (2.5% between-groups at the lumbar spine at 3 years) [42]. There was no significant effect in the proximal femur.

The variability of outcomes with these agents makes it difficult to assess their value following transplantation. In general, their effects are less than those of the bisphosphonates. Their best use may be as adjunctive therapy to bisphosphonates in patients with severe glucocorticoid-induced osteoporosis, or as a second-line therapy in patients for whom other agents are not acceptable.

D. Sex Hormone Replacement

The pivotal role played by reduced concentrations of estrogen in the genesis of postmenopausal bone loss suggested that estrogen replacement was likely to have a beneficial effect on bone in older women. This was first explored in detail by Lindsay et al. [43] in a study of women undergoing oophorectomy, who were randomized to treatment with estrogen or placebo and followed up for 15 years. Bone loss at the metacarpal was completely prevented by estrogen replacement, whereas nearly one-third of baseline bone mineral was lost in the placebo group. Over the first 9 years of the study, patients receiving placebo gained 3.2 kg in weight, lost 0.9 cm in height, and had an average of 1.6 vertebral deformities, whereas there was no significant change in any of these indices in the individuals receiving estrogen.

The beneficial effects of estrogen on bone mineral density in nontransplanted women have now been confirmed in a number of studies ranging from the early perimenopausal period through to women in their seventies. By far the largest of these studies is the Women's Health Initiative, which was carried out in nonosteoporotic women aged 50–79 years at the beginning of the study [44]. Over 5 years of follow-up, this showed a one-third reduction in the risk of hip and spine fractures, and reduction in total fracture events by 25%. At the same time as definitively establishing the skeletal efficacy of oral estrogen/progestogen replacement, the Women's Health Initiative highlighted the potential risks of this therapy. It showed increases in the risk of breast cancer, coronary heart disease, strokes, and thromboembolic disease with hormone use. The increase in the number of these adverse outcomes was greater than the number of hip fractures prevented, but less than the reduction in total fracture numbers.

In the context of ongoing glucocorticoid treatment, estrogen/progestogen therapy clearly has a beneficial effect on bone mass in the spine and femur, comparable to that seen in non-steroid-treated subjects [45, 46]. The limited data available suggest that the same is true following transplantation. Isoniemi [47] described a cohort of 33 postmenopausal women who had undergone liver transplantation. Treatment with transdermal estradiol for 2 years was associated with increases in bone density at the spine of 6.5% and at the hip of 4.5%. Castelo-Branco [48] reported a similar series of 13 women who had previously undergone bone marrow transplantation for malignant hematopoietic disorders. Treatment with either oral conjugated estrogen or transdermal estradiol plus medroxyprogesterone acetate resulted in increases in bone density in all subjects. Despite these positive data, the recent evidence regarding vascular adverse effects of estrogen/progestogen therapy suggest that the risks of this intervention will exceed the benefits in most individuals, so other agents (such as bisphosphonates) are preferred in most women.

In glucocorticoid-treated men, circulating testosterone levels are reduced by almost one half, a factor likely to contribute to the development of osteopenia. We have shown that testosterone replacement (250 mg testosterone esters per month) produces a 5% increase in lumbar spine bone mineral density after 12 months, as well as reversing the accumulation of body fat and loss of lean tissue that accompany glucocorticoid therapy [49]. In this study, mean serum testosterone concentrations had returned to baseline at the end of the one-month interdose interval, suggesting that greater benefits may be possible with a more sustained normalization of circulating sex-hormone levels. This might be achieved by administration of these depot preparations at 2–3 week intervals, or by the use of transdermal delivery systems. In some glucocorticoid-treated men, testosterone replacement is associated with a significant increase in well-being.

E. Selective Estrogen Receptor Modulators (SERMs)

SERMs are a new and expanding class of pharmaceuticals that have mixed estrogen agonist/antagonist activities, which vary from tissue to tissue. Thus, the prototypic SERM, raloxifene, acts as an estrogen agonist in bone, but as an antagonist in the breast and endometrium. Raloxifene reduces bone resorption and increases bone density, but is less potent than both estradiol and bisphosphonates in this regard. It decreases the incidence of vertebral fractures but does not have any effect on nonvertebral fractures, despite having been used in a study of almost 8000 women [50]. It has the other exciting property of reducing the incidence of breast cancer by 75%, and studies are ongoing to assess its effects on vascular disease. Its efficacy in women following transplantation has not been assessed, but it is likely to have the beneficial effects on BMD seen in other postmenopausal women.

F. Bisphosphonates

The pharmacological management of osteoporosis has come to be dominated by the bisphosphonates. These are relatively simple phosphate salts that have a very high affinity for the surface of bone but are very poorly absorbed from the gastrointestinal tract. Thus, only 1–2% of an oral dose is absorbed, about half of this is rapidly deposited on the bone surface, and the balance is excreted unchanged in the urine. When osteoclasts resorb bone, they ingest the bisphosphonate and are effectively poisoned by it. This results in a reduction of bone resorption, and a consequent redressing of the imbalance between bone formation and resorption. Bisphosphonate on the bone surface remains there for many years and is gradually incorporated into the structure of bone, so that it can inhibit remodeling cycles that occur years after the time of dosing. The long duration of bisphosphonate action makes intermittent administration a possibility.

The low oral bioavailability of bisphosphonates is a critical issue in their use. They must be taken fasting, with water alone, if they are to be absorbed at all. Amino-bisphosphonates, such as alendronate, can cause upper gastrointestinal irritation, so patients must not lie down for 30–60 minutes after oral dosing. Failure to observe this caution may permit reflux of the tablet into the esophagus, resulting in local inflammation and possibly ulceration. This does not appear to be such a problem for the less potent, non-amino-bisphosphonate etidronate.

1. Pamidronate

Post-transplantation osteoporosis is one of the areas in which the use of intravenous bisphosphonates has been pioneered. In most cases, this has been using intravenous pamidronate, in both preventative and treatment roles. Reeves et al. [51] described a cohort of patients undergoing liver transplantation whose baseline bone density was towards the lower end of the age-appropriate normal range. These individuals were given 4 infusions of pamidronate at 3-month intervals and had no symptomatic vertebral fractures, in contrast to a historical control group in which the fracture rate was 38%.

Aris [52] conducted an RCT giving 30 mg of pamidronate every 3 months over a 2-year period and comparing this with calciferol and calcium supplementation in patients undergoing lung transplantation for cystic fibrosis. Treatment was initiated within 1–12 months after transplantation, but the average T-score at baseline was in the region of −2.5, indicating that this was a predominantly osteoporotic population. The patients treated with pamidronate showed increases in spine and femur densities of 8.8 and 8.2% respectively, in comparison with gains of 2.6 and 0.3% in control subjects. Both these differences were statistically significant. Similar results were found in an RCT for prevention of bone loss from the time of heart transplantation, again using infusions of pamidronate every 3 months [53]. This study demonstrated the superiority of this regimen to combined therapy with calcitriol and calcitonin. Fan et al. [54] demonstrated a similar prevention of post-transplant bone loss in both spine and femur in patients receiving renal grafts, and Thrombetti produced similar results for lung transplant recipients [55]. In the latter study, many subjects had osteoporotic bone densities at baseline. Krieg [56] described a cohort of heart transplant recipients who were allocated to treatment with pamidronate 60 mg every 3 months, because their bone densities at 6 months post-transplantation were in the osteoporotic range. Over 3 years of follow-up, lumbar spine BMD increased by 18% in those receiving pamidronate, but there was no net change in density in the femoral neck.

One recent paper [57] contrasts with the other pamidronate studies. This is a prevention study in patients undergoing liver transplantation who were given a single infusion of pamidronate 60 mg at the time of transplantation or up to 12 weeks beforehand. Over the following 12 months there was no significant spinal bone density loss in either the treatment or control groups. In the femur, bone loss did take place but was not different between groups. The marked contrast between results of this study and the others just cited implies that more frequent treatment with pamidronate or the use of larger doses is necessary for an optimal skeletal result.

2. *Etidronate*

It has been more traditional to give bisphosphonates orally rather than intravenously in the management of postmenopausal osteoporosis. The longest experience is with cyclical etidronate, which is typically given in 2-week courses of 400 mg/day, repeated at 3-month intervals. A number of groups have used etidronate alone or in combination with other agents in the prevention of post-transplant bone loss, with mixed results. Riemens [58] showed that bone loss still occurs after liver transplantation despite the combined use of etidronate and alfacalcidol. As mentioned previously, Van Cleemput [40] found that alfacalcidol was superior to etidronate, and Garcia-Delgado [59] showed that 25-hydroxyvitamin D was superior to etidronate. Henderson et al. [35] found that calcitriol and etidronate were equivalent in the first 6 months after heart or lung transplantation, but both permitted significant bone loss during this period.

Arlen et al. [60] have provided data on the treatment of osteoporosis following renal transplantation. In a nonrandomized study, they compared bone loss in 25 individuals treated with etidronate and 24 control subjects. They were, on average, 1 year post-transplantation at the time of initiation of the study. With 12 months of etidronate treatment, lumbar spine BMD increased 4.3%, in comparison with 0.6% increase in the control subjects. In the femoral trochanter the difference between groups was even greater (10.3% compared to 2.2%). Both these comparisons were statistically significant. Valero et al. have reported similar data in patients with low bone density 17 months after liver transplantation [61]. Cyclical etidronate in these subjects increased BMD in the spine by 8.2%, though there was no placebo-treated comparator group. Thus, etidronate may not be adequate to prevent the rapid bone loss that occurs immediately after transplantation, but it does appear to have significant beneficial effects on bone density once a more stable baseline has developed subsequently.

3. *Alendronate*

Alendronate is the most widely used agent in many forms of osteoporosis, and it has now been studied in the management of osteoporosis post-transplantation. Giannini et al. [62] randomized 40 patients, who had had kidney transplants an average of 6 years previously, to treatment with alendronate 10 mg/day, calcitriol 0.5 μg/day, and calcium 500 mg/day, or to calcitriol and calcium. Alendronate produced changes in the density of the lumbar spine and hip that were about 5% greater than those seen with calcitriol alone (see Figure 1). More recently, Torregrosa et al. [63] have reported a series of 12 patients with BMD T scores < −2.5 one to two years after renal transplantation. They found similar benefits in bone density over a 12-month treatment period to those described by Giannini.

4. *Other Bisphosphonates*

In general, the various members of the bisphosphonate class are comparably effective if used in appropriate dosages. Therefore, it is to be expected that other bisphosphonates would have similar effects to those outlined previously. Risedronate is widely used for the management of postmenopausal osteoporosis, and is also effective in glucocorticoid-induced osteoporosis [64]. It would therefore be expected to be a satisfactory management for osteoporosis in patients following transplantation, though this does not appear to have been specifically examined to date. Ibandronate has been reported to prevent bone loss, reduce the number of fractures, and reduce the number of rejection episodes when given every 3 months from the time of renal transplantation in an RCT in 80 subjects [65].

G. Other Therapies

Calcitonin has been used to treat post-transplantation osteoporosis, just as it has been used in postmenopausal [66] and glucocorticoid-induced osteo-

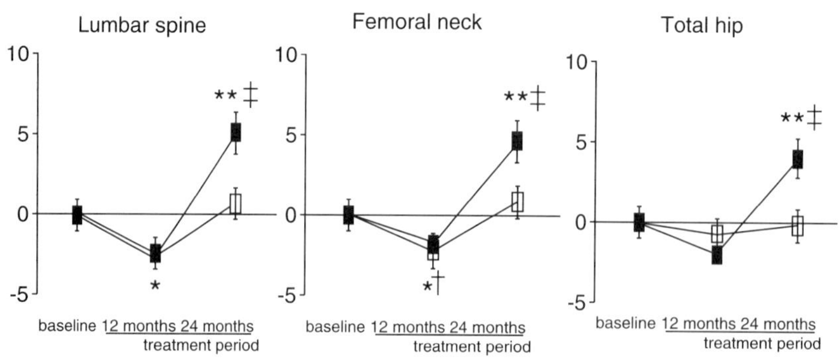

FIGURE 1 BMD in renal allograft recipients who were observed for 12 months, then randomized to alendronate (closed symbols) or placebo (open symbols). There were significant between-groups effects at the end of the study at all sites ($P < 0.05$). From Giannini et al. (2001). Alendronate prevents further bone loss in renal transplant recipients. *J Bone Miner Res.* 16:2111–2117; reproduced with permission from the American Society for Bone and Mineral Research.

porosis [67]. In the latter conditions, its efficacy appears to be less than that of the bisphosphonates, and this is probably true in transplantation disease as well. Valero [61] found intramuscular calcitonin to be almost as effective as etidronate in treating subjects with established bone loss, but intramuscular administration has a low patient acceptability and is little used these days. The available studies with intranasal calcitonin have not shown significant beneficial effects [53, 59, 68].

Fluoride has been used to treat established osteoporosis in patients with transplants [69] as it has been in other forms of bone loss. Beneficial effects on bone density are seen, but the failure of these improvements to translate into reduced fracture rates in other forms of osteoporosis [70] has led to a lack of enthusiasm for the use of this compound in osteoporosis in general.

Parathyroid hormone, given by daily injection, has recently shown spectacular effects on bone density and fractures in postmenopausal osteoporosis [71] and has also shown impressive effects on bone density in glucocorticoid-treated patients [72]. As yet, there are no data specifically in the transplant situation, but there is no reason to believe that this anabolic agent would not be effective in this context. One possible exception to this would be in patients with persisting renal impairment and secondary hyperparathyroidism, in whom the addition of yet more parathyroid hormone may be counterproductive.

H. Treatment Decisions

Figure 2 sets out an approach to both the evaluation of a patient following organ transplantation and to the making of therapeutic decisions. Optimization of dietary and lifestyle variables is applicable to all such

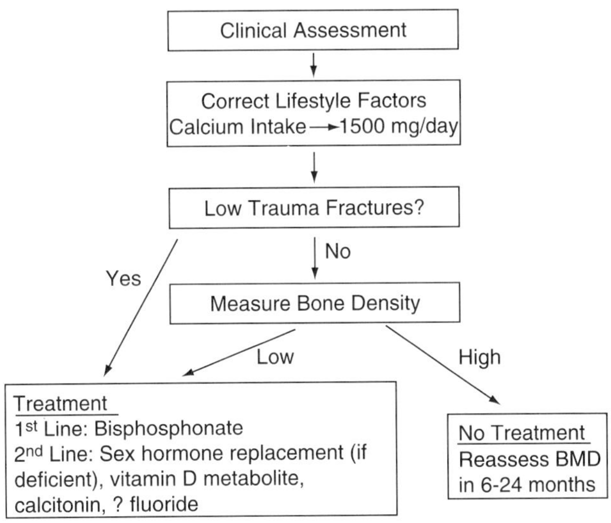

FIGURE 2 Flowchart for the evaluation and treatment of osteoporosis in patients following organ transplantation. Copyright © I.R. Reid; reproduced with permission.

individuals. In those with a history of minimal trauma fracture, treatment will usually be offered, but bone densitometry is still useful since it further defines the fracture risk and provides a baseline against which to assess subsequent change. In individuals whose bone density is at the lower end of the young normal range (i.e., T-score < -1.5), intervention with a single agent, usually a bisphosphonate, is appropriate, though sex-hormone replacement is an option in those with demonstrable deficiency. In a patient with marked bone loss, these agents can be combined with each other, and/or with other interventions such as alfacalcidol, though the antifracture efficacy of such combination regimens is unknown.

The availability of effective interventions for this condition places a responsibility of any physician caring for patients following organ transplantation to assess fracture risk in these patients and to provide prophylaxis against bone loss. The widespread adoption of this strategy will result in many fewer patients having to accept the morbidity of multiple fractures in addition to that of their other medical conditions.

REFERENCES

1. Klotzbuecher, C.M., Ross, P.D., Landsman, P.B., Abbott, T.A,. and Berger, M. (2000). Patients with prior fractures have an increased risk of future fractures: A summary of the literature and statistical synthesis. *J Bone Mineral Res.* 15:721–739.
2. Van Staa, T.P., Laan, R.F., Barton, I.P., Cohen, S., Reid, D.A. and Cooper, C. (2003). Bone density threshold and other predictors of vertebral fracture in patients receiving oral glucocorticoid therapy. *Arthritis Rheum.* 48:3224–3229.
3. Laan, R.F.J.M., Vanriel, P.L.C.M., Vandeputte, L.B.A., Vanerning, L.J.T.O., Vanthof, M.A. and Lemmens, J.A.M. (1993). Low-dose prednisone induces rapid reversible axial bone loss in patients with rheumatoid arthritis—a randomized, controlled study. *Ann Intern Med.* 119:963–968.
4. Marcus, R. (2001). Role of exercise in preventing and treating osteoporosis. *Rheum Dis Clin N Amer.* 27:131–141.
5. Kohrt, W. M., Ehsani, A. A. and Birge, S. J. (1997). Effects of exercise involving predominantly either joint-reaction or ground-reaction forces on bone mineral density in older women. *J Bone Mineral Res.* 12:1253–1261.
6. Campbell, A.J., Robertson, M.C., Gardner, M.M., Norton, R.N., Tilyard, M.W. and Buchner, D. M. (1997). Randomised controlled trial of a general practice programme of home based exercise to prevent falls in elderly women. *BMJ.* 315:1065–1069.
7. Close, J., Ellis, M., Hooper, R., Glucksman, E., Jackson, S. and Swift, C. (1999). Prevention of falls in the elderly: a randomised controlled trial. *Lancet.* 353:93–97.
8. Tinetti, M. E. (2003). Clinical practice. Preventing falls in elderly persons. *N Engl J Med.* 348:42–49.
9. Kannus, P., Parkkari, J., Niemi, S., Pasanen, M., Palvanen, M., Jarvinen, M. and Vuori, I. (2000). Prevention of hip fracture in elderly people with use of a hip protector. *N Engl J Med.* 343:1506–1513.
10. van Schoor, N.M., Smit, J.H., Twisk, J.W.R., Bouter, L.M. and Lips, P. (2003). Prevention of hip fractures by external hip protectors—A randomized controlled trial. *JAMA.* 289:1957–1962.
11. Reid, I.R. (1998). The roles of calcium and vitamin D in the prevention of osteoporosis. *Endocrinol Metabol Clin Nth Amer.* 27:389ff.

12. Nordin, B.E.C. (1997). Calcium and osteoporosis. *Nutrition*. 13:664–686.
13. Sambrook, P., Birmingham, J., Kelly, P., Kempler, S., Nguyen, T., Pocock, N. and Eisman, J. (1993). Prevention of corticosteroid osteoporosis—a comparison of calcium, calcitriol, and calcitonin. *N Engl J Med*. 328:1747–1752.
14. Reid, I.R., King, A.R., Alexander, C.J. and Ibbertson, H.K. (1988). Prevention of steroid-induced osteoporosis with (3-amino-1-hydroxypropylidene)-1,1-bisphosphonate (APD). *Lancet* i:143–146.
15. Reid, I.R. and Ibbertson, H.K. (1986). Calcium supplements in the prevention of steroid-induced osteoporosis. *Am J Clin Nutr*. 44:287–290.
16. Nilsen, K.H., Jayson, M.I.V. and Dixon, A.S. (1978). Microcrystalline calcium hydroxyapatite compound in corticosteroid-treated rheumatoid patients: A controlled study. *BMJ*. ii:1124.
17. Shea, B., Wells, G., Cranney, A., Zytaruk, N., Robinson, V., Griffith, L., Ortiz, Z., Peterson, J., Adachi, J., Tugwell, P. and Guyatt, G. (2002). Meta-analysis of calcium supplementation for the prevention of postmenopausal osteoporosis. *Endocrine Rev*. 23:552–559.
18. Curhan, G.C., Willett, W.C., Speizer, F.E., Spiegelman, D. and Stampfer, M.J. (1997). Comparison of dietary calcium with supplemental calcium and other nutrients as factors affecting the risk for kidney stones in women. *Ann Intern Med*. 126:497ff.
19. Segal, E., Baruch, Y., Kramsky, R., Raz, B., Tamir, A. and Ish-Shalom, S. (2003). Predominant factors associated with bone loss in liver transplant patients—after prolonged post-transplantation period. *Clin Transplant*. 17:13–19.
20. Isaia, G., Giorgino, R., Rini, G.B., Bevilacqua, M., Maugeri, D. and Adami, S. (2003). Prevalence of hypovitaminosis D in elderly women in Italy: clinical consequences and risk factors. *Osteoporos Int*. 14:577–582.
21. Ooms, M.E., Roos, J.C., Bezemer, P.D., Vandervijgh, W.J.F., Bouter, L.M. and Lips, P. (1995). Prevention of bone loss by vitamin D supplementation in elderly women: A randomized double-blind trial. *J Clin Endocrinol Metab*. 80:1052–1058.
22. Reid, I.R., Gallagher, D.J.A. and Bosworth, J. (1986). Prophylaxis against vitamin D deficiency in the elderly by regular sunlight exposure. *Age Ageing*. 15:35–40.
23. Lips, P., Graafmans, W.C., Ooms, M.E., Bezemer, P.D. and Bouter, L.M. (1996). Vitamin D supplementation and fracture incidence in elderly persons—a randomized, placebo-controlled clinical trial. *Ann Intern Med*. 124:400–406.
24. Heikinheimo, R.J., Inkovaara, J.A., Harju, E.J., Haavisto, M.V., Kaarela, R.H., Kataja, J. M., Kokko, A. M., Kolho, L. A. and Rajala, S. A. (1992). Annual injection of vitamin D and fractures of aged bones. *Calcif Tissue Int*. 51:105–110.
25. Chapuy, M.C., Arlot, M.E., Duboeuf, F., Brun, J., Crouzet, B., Arnaud, S., Delmas, P.D. and Meunier, P. J. (1992). Vitamin-D3 and calcium to prevent hip fractures in elderly women. *N Engl J Med*. 327:1637–1642.
26. Dawson-Hughes, B., Harris, S.S., Krall, E.A. and Dallal, G.E. (1997). Effect of calcium and vitamin D supplementation on bone, density in men and women 65 years of age or older. *N Engl J Med*. 337:670–676.
27. Buckley, L.M., Leib, E.S., Cartularo, K.S., Vacek, P.M. and Cooper, S.M. (1996). Calcium and vitamin D-3 supplementation prevents bone loss in the spine secondary to low-dose corticosteroids in patients with rheumatoid arthritis—a randomized, double-blind, placebo-controlled trial. *Ann Intern Med*. 125:961–968.
28. Adachi, J.D., Bensen, W.G., Bianchi, F., Cividino, A., Pillersdorf, S., Sebaldt, R.J., Tugwell, P., Gordon, M., Steele, M., Webber, C. and Goldsmith, C.H. (1996). Vitamin D and calcium in the prevention of corticosteroid induced osteoporosis—a 3 year followup. *J Rheumatol*. 23:995–1000.
29. Talalaj, M., Gradowska, L., Marcinowskasuchowierska, E., Durlik, M., Gaciong, Z. and Lao, M. (1996). Efficiency of preventive treatment of glucocorticoid-induced osteoporosis with 25-hydroxyvitamin D3 and calcium in kidney transplant patients. *Transplant Proc*. 28:3485–3487.

30. Garciadelgado, I., Prieto, S., Gilfraguas, L., Robles, E., Rufilanchas, J.J. and Hawkins, F. (1997). Calcitonin, etidronate, and calcidiol treatment in bone loss after cardiac transplantation. *Calcif Tissue Int.* 60:155–159.
31. Malabanan, A., Veronikis, I. E. and Holick, M. F. (1998). Redefining vitamin D insufficiency. *Lancet.* 351:805–806.
32. Dykman, T.R., Haralson, K.M., Gluck, O.S., Murphy, W.A., Teitelbaum, S.L., Hahn, T.J. and Hahn, B.H. (1984). Effect of oral 1,25-dihydroxy-vitamin D and calcium on glucocorticoid-induced osteopenia in patients with rheumatic diseases. *Arthritis Rheum.* 27:1336–1343.
33. Kung, A.W.C., Chan, T.M., Lau, C.S., Wong, R.W.S. and Yeung, S.S.C. (1999). Osteopenia in young hypogonadal women with systemic lupus erythematosus receiving chronic steroid therapy: a randomized controlled trial comparing calcitriol and hormonal replacement therapy. *Rheumatology.* 38:1239–1244.
34. Sambrook, P., Henderson, N.K., Keogh, A., Macdonald, P., Glanville, A., Spratt, P., Bergin, P., Ebeling, P. and Eisman, J. (2000). Effect of calcitriol on bone loss after cardiac or lung transplantation. *J Bone Miner Res.* 15:1818–1824.
35. Henderson, K., Eisman, J., Keogh, A., MacDonald, P., Glanville, A., Spratt, P. and Sambrook, P. (2001). Protective effect of short-term calcitriol or cyclical etidronate on bone loss after cardiac or lung transplantation. *J Bone Miner Res.* 16:565–571.
36. Stempfle, H.U., Werner, C., Siebert, U., Assum, T., Wehr, U., Rambeck, W.A., Meiser, B., Theisen, K. and Gartner, R. (2002). The role of tacrolimus (FK506)-based immunosuppression on bone mineral density and bone turnover after cardiac transplantation: a prospective, longitudinal, randomized, double-blind trial with calcitriol. *Transplantation.* 73:547–552.
37. Neuhaus, R., Kubo, A., Lohmann, R., Rayes, N., Hierholzer, J. and Neuhaus, P. (1999). Calcitriol in prevention and therapy of osteoporosis after liver transplantation. *Transplant Proc.* 31:472–473.
38. Stempfle, H.U., Werner, C., Echtler, S., Wehr, U., Rambeck, W.A., Siebert, U., Uberfuhr, P., Angermann, C.E., Theisen, K. and Gartner, R. (1999). Prevention of osteoporosis after cardiac transplantation—A prospective, longitudinal, randomized, double-blind trial with calcitriol. *Transplantation.* 68:523–530.
39. Cueto-Manzano, A.M., Konel, S., Freemont, A.J., Adams, J.E., Mawer, B., Gokal, R. and Hutchison, A. J. (2000). Effect of 1,25-dihydroxyvitamin D-3 and calcium carbonate on bone loss associated with long-term renal transplantation. *Amer J Kidney Dis.* 35: 227–236.
40. Van Cleemput, J., Daenen, W., Geusens, P., Dequeker, J., Van de Werf, F. and Vanhaecke, J. (1996). Prevention of bone loss in cardiac transplant recipients—a comparison of biphosphonates and vitamin D. *Transplantation.* 61:1495–1499.
41. Reginster, J.Y., Kuntz, D., Verdickt, W., Wouters, M., Guillevin, L., Menkes, C.J. and Nielsen, K. (1999). Prophylactic use of alfacalcidol in corticosteroid-induced osteoporosis. *Osteoporos Int.* 9:75–81.
42. Ringe, J.D., Coster, A., Meng, T., Schacht, E. and Umbach, R. (1999). Treatment of glucocorticoid-induced osteoporosis with alfacalcidol/calcium versus vitamin D/calcium. *Calcif Tissue Int.* 65:337–340.
43. Lindsay, R., Hart, D.M., Forrest, C. and Baird, C. (1980). Prevention of spinal osteoporosis in oophorectomised women. *Lancet.* ii:1151–1153.
44. Writing Group for the Women's Health Initiative Investigators. (2002). Risks and benefits of estrogen plus progestin in healthy postmenopausal women. *JAMA.* 288: 321–333.
45. Hall, G.M., Daniels, M., Doyle, D.V. and Spector, T.D. (1994). Effect of hormone replacement therapy on bone mass in rheumatoid arthritis patients treated with and without steroids. *Arthritis Rheum.* 37:1499–1505.
46. Grey, A.B., Cundy, T.F. and Reid, I.R. (1994). Continuous combined oestrogen/progestin therapy is well tolerated and increases bone density at the hip and spine in postmenopausal osteoporosis. *Clin Endocrinol.* 40:671–677.

47. Isoniemi, H., Appelberg, J., Nilsson, C.G., Makela, P., Risteli, J. and Hockerstedt, K. (2001). Transdermal oestrogen therapy protects postmenopausal liver transplant women from osteoporosis. A 2-year follow-up study. *J Hepatol.* 34:299–305.
48. Castelo-Branco, C., Rovira, M., Pons, F., Duran, M., Sierra, J., Vives, A., Balasch, J., Fortuny, A. and Vanrell, J. (1996). The effect of hormone replacement therapy on bone mass in patients with ovarian failure due to bone marrow transplantation. *Maturitas.* 23:307–312.
49. Reid, I.R., Wattie, D.J., Evans, M.C. and Stapleton, J.P. (1996). Testosterone therapy in glucocorticoid-treated men. *Arch Int Med.* 156:1173–1177.
50. Ettinger, B., Black, D.M., Mitlak, B.H., Knickerbocker, R.K., Nickelsen, T., Genant, H. K., Christiansen, C., Delmas, P.D., Zanchetta, J.R., Stakkestad, J., Gluer, C.C., Krueger, K., Cohen, F.J., Eckert, S., Ensrud, K.E., Avioli, L.V., Lips, P. and Cummings, S.R. (1999). Reduction of vertebral fracture risk in postmenopausal women with osteoporosis treated with raloxifene—Results from a 3-year randomized clinical trial. *JAMA.* 282:637–645.
51. Reeves, H.L., Francis, R.M., Manas, D.M., Hudson, M. and Day, C.P. (1998). Intravenous bisphosphonate prevents symptomatic osteoporotic vertebral collapse in patients after liver transplantation. *Liver Transplant Surg.* 4:404–409.
52. Aris, R.M., Lester, G.E., Renner, J.B., Winders, A., Blackwood, A.D., Lark, R.K. and Ontjes, D. A. (2000). Efficacy of pamidronate for osteoporosis in patients with cystic fibrosis following lung transplantation. *Amer J Respir Crit Care Med.* 162:941–946.
53. Bianda, T., Linka, A., Junga, G., Brunner, H., Steinert, H., Kiowski, W. and Schmid, C. (2000). Prevention of osteoporosis in heart transplant recipients: A comparison of calcitriol with calcitonin and pamidronate. *Calcif Tissue Int.* 67:116–121.
54. Fan, S.L.S., Almond, M.K., Ball, E., Evans, K. and Cunningham, J. (2000). Pamidronate therapy as prevention of bone loss following renal transplantation. *Kidney Int.* 57:684–690.
55. Trombetti, A., Gerbase, M.W., Spiliopoulos, A., Slosman, D.O., Nicod, L.P. and Rizzoli, R. (2000). Bone mineral density in lung-transplant recipients before and after graft: Prevention of lumbar spine post-transplantation-accelerated bone loss by pamidronate. *J Heart Lung Transplant.* 19:736–743.
56. Krieg, M.A., Seydoux, C., Sandini, L., Goy, J.J., Berguer, D.G., Thiebaud, D. and Burckhardt, P. (2001). Intravenous pamidronate as treatment for osteoporosis after heart transplantation: A prospective study. *Osteoporos Int.* 12:112–116.
57. Ninkovic, M., Love, S., Tom, B.D.M., Bearcroft, P.W.P., Alexander, G.J.M. and Compston, J. E. (2002). Lack of effect of intravenous pamidronate on fracture incidence and bone mineral density after orthotopic liver transplantation. *J Hepatol.* 37:93–100.
58. Riemens, S.C., Oostdijk, A., Vandoormaal, J.J., Thijn, C.J.P., Drent, G., Piers, D.A., Groen, E.W.J., Meerman, L., Slooff, M.J.H. and Haagsma, E.B. (1996). Bone loss after liver transplantation is not prevented by cyclical etidronate, calcium and alphacalcidol. *Osteoporos Int.* 6:213–218.
59. Garcia-Delgado, I., Prieto, S., Gilfraguas, L., Robles, E., Rufilanchas, J.J. and Hawkins, F. (1997). Calcitonin, etidronate, and calcidiol treatment in bone loss after cardiac transplantation. *Calcif Tissue Int.* 60:155–159.
60. Arlen, D.J., Lambert, K., Ioannidis, G. and Adachi, J.D. (2001). Treatment of established bone loss after renal transplantation with etidronate. *Transplantation.* 71:669–673.
61. Valero, M.A., Loinaz, C., Larrodera, L., Leon, M., Moreno, E. and Hawkins, F. (1995). Calcitonin and bisphosphonates treatment in bone loss after liver transplantation. *Calcif Tissue Int.* 57:15–19.
62. Giannini, S., Dangel, A., Carraro, G., Nobile, M., Rigotti, P., Bonfante, L., Marchini, F., Zaninotto, M., Dalle Carbonare, L., Sartori, L. and Crepaldi, G. (2001). Alendronate prevents further bone loss in renal transplant recipients. *J Bone Mineral Res.* 16:2111–2117.
63. Torregrosa, J.V., Moreno, A., Gutierrez, A., Vidal, S. and Oppenheimer, F. (2003). Alendronate for treatment of renal transplant patients with osteoporosis. *Transplant Proc.* 35:1393–1395.
64. Wallach, S., Cohen, S., Reid, D.M., Hughes, R.A., Hosking, D.J., Laan, R.F., Doherty, S.M., Maricic, M., Rosen, C., Brown, J., Barton, I. and Chines, A.A. (2000). Effects of

risedronate treatment on bone density and vertebral fracture in patients on corticosteroid therapy. *Calcif Tissue Int.* 67:277–285.
65. Grotz, W., Nagel, C., Poeschel, D., Cybulla, M., Petersen, K.G., Uhl, M., Strey, C., Kirste, G., Olschewski, M., Reichelt, A. and Rump, L. C. (2001). Effect of ibandronate on bone loss and renal function after kidney transplantation. *J Amer Soc Nephrol.* 12:1530–1537.
66. Chestnut, C.H., Silverman, S., Adriano, K., Genant, H.K., Gimona, A., Harris, S., Kiel, D., LeBoff, M., Maricic, M., Miller, P., Moniz, C., Peacock, M., Richardson, P., Watts, N. and Baylink, D. (2000). A randomized trial of nasal spray salmon calcitonin in postmenopausal women with established osteoporosis: the prevent recurrence of osteoporotic fractures study. *Am J Med.* 109:267–276.
67. Wu, F. and Reid, I.R. (2000). Calcitonin in the prevention and treatment of glucocorticoid-induced osteoporosis. *Clin Exp Rheumatol.* 18:S53-S56.
68. Hay, J.E., Malinchoc, M. and Dickson, E. R. (2001). A controlled trial of calcitonin therapy for the prevention of post-liver transplantation atraumatic fractures in patients with primary biliary cirrhosis and primary sclerosing cholangitis. *J Hepatol.* 34:292–298.
69. Meys, E., Terreaux-Duvert, F., Beaume-Six, T., Dureau, G. and Meunier, P.J. (1993). Bone loss after cardiac transplantation: effects of calcium, calcidiol and monofluorophosphate. *Osteoporos Int.* 3:322–329.
70. Riggs, B.L., Hodgson, S.F., O'Fallon, W.M. and al., e. (1990). Effect of fluoride treatment on the fracture rate in postmenopausal women with osteoporosis. *N Engl J Med.* 322:802–809.
71. Neer, R.M., Arnaud, C.D., Zanchetta, J.R., Prince, R., Gaich, G.A., Reginster, J.Y., Hodsman, A.B., Eriksen, E.F., Ish-Shalom, S., Genant, H.K., Wang, O.H. and Mitlak, B. H. (2001). Effect of parathyroid hormone (1-34) on fractures and bone mineral density in postmenopausal women with osteoporosis. *N Engl J Med.* 344:1434–1441.
72. Lane, N.E., Sanchez, S., Modlin, G.W., Genant, H.K., Pierini, E. and Arnaud, C.D. (1998). Parathyroid hormone treatment can reverse corticosteroid-induced osteoporosis—results of a randomized controlled clinical trial. *J Clin Invest.* 102:1627–1633.

Index